Gonzalo Bearman • Silvia Munoz-Price
Daniel J. Morgan • Rekha K. Murthy
Editors

Infection Prevention

New Perspectives and Controversies

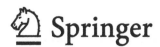 Springer

Editors
Gonzalo Bearman
VCUHS Epidemiology and Infection Control
North Hospital
Richmond, VA, USA

Daniel J. Morgan
University of Maryland
Baltimore, MD, USA

Silvia Munoz-Price
Medical College of Wisconsin
Milwaukee, WI, USA

Rekha K. Murthy
Department of Medical Affairs and Division
  of Infectious Diseases
Cedars-Sinai Health System
Los Angeles, CA, USA

ISBN 978-3-319-86975-9   ISBN 978-3-319-60980-5   (eBook)
DOI 10.1007/978-3-319-60980-5

Printed on acid-free paper

This Springer imprint is published by Springer Nature
The registered company is Springer International Publishing AG
The registered company address is: Gewerbestrasse 11, 6330 Cham, Switzerland

Dedicated to all of the mentors and patients who have inspired us.

Contents

Contributors

Salma Muhammad Abbas Department of Internal Medicine, Infectious Diseases, Virginia Commonwealth University, Richmond, VA, USA

David Banach Infectious Diseases, University of Connecticut School of Medicine, Farmington, CT, USA

Tinzar Basein Division of Geographic Medicine and Infectious Diseases, Tufts Medical Center, Boston, MA, USA

Gonzalo Bearman VCUHS Epidemiology and Infection Control, North Hospital, Richmond, VA, USA

Ana Berbel Caban Department of Internal Medicine, University of Miami Hospital/Jackson Memorial Hospital, Miami, FL, USA

Natalia Blanco Epidemiology and Public Health, University of Maryland School of Medicine, Baltimore, MD, USA

Kristina A. Bryant University of Louisville, Healthcare Epidemiologist, Norton Children's Hospital, Louisville, KY, USA

Megan Buller OhioHealth Physician Group-Infectious Diseases, Columbus, OH, USA

Jose Cadena Medicine/Infectious Diseases, University of Texas Health Science at San Antonio and South Texas Veterans Healthcare System, San Antonio, TX, USA

Philip C. Carling Department of Infectious Diseases, Boston University School of Medicine and Carney Hospital, Boston, MA, USA

Teena Chopra Division of Infectious Diseases, Harper University Hospital, Detroit Medical Center/Wayne State University, Detroit, MI, USA

Theodore J. Cieslak Biocontainment Unit, Nebraska Medicine, Omaha, NE, USA

College of Public Health, Department of Epidemiology, University of Nebraska Medical Center, Omaha, NE, USA

Cornelius J. Clancy Infectious Diseases Section, VA Pittsburgh Healthcare System, University Drive C, Medicine IIIE-U, Pittsburgh, PA, USA

Lindsay Croft Division of Epidemiology, Department of Internal Medicine, University of Utah School of Medicine, Salt Lake City, UT, USA

Brooke K. Decker Infectious Diseases Section, VA Pittsburgh Healthcare System, University Drive C, Medicine IIIE-U, Pittsburgh, PA, USA

E. Patchen Dellinger Department of Surgery, University of Washington Medical Center, Seattle, WA, USA

Michelle Doll Department of Internal Medicine-Division of Infectious Diseases, VCU Medical Center, Richmond, VA, USA

Infectious Diseases/Epidemiology, Virginia Commonwealth University Health System, Richmond, VA, USA

Shira Doron Division of Geographic Medicine and Infectious Diseases, Tufts Medical Center, Boston, MA, USA

Briana Ehnes Department of Human Ecology, University of Alberta, Edmonton, AB, Canada

Allison Gibble Department of Pharmacy, Froedtert & The Medical College of Wisconsin, Milwaukee, WI, USA

Bryan D. Harris Department of Medicine, Vanderbilt University Medical Center, Nashville, TN, USA

Oryan Henig Department of Infectious Diseases, Assaf Harofeh Medical Center, Zerifin, Israel

Angela Hewlett Division of Infectious Diseases, Internal Medicine, Infectious Diseases, University of Nebraska Medical Center, Omaha, NE, USA

Biocontainment Unit, Nebraska Medicine, Omaha, NE, USA

Angela M. Huang Department of Pharmacy, Froedtert & The Medical College of Wisconsin, Milwaukee, WI, USA

Claudia Denisse Jarrin Tejada Berkley, MI, USA

David E. Katz Department of Infectious Diseases, Assaf Harofeh Medical Center, Zerifin, Israel

Amar Krishna Division of Infectious Diseases, Harper University Hospital, Detroit Medical Center/Wayne State University, Detroit, MI, USA

Surbhi Leekha Epidemiology and Public Health, University of Maryland School of Medicine, Baltimore, MD, USA

John J. Lowe Biocontainment Unit, Nebraska Medicine, Omaha, NE, USA

Environmental, Agricultural, and Occupational Health, University of Nebraska Medicine, Omaha, NE, USA

Andrew D. Ludwig Department of Surgery, University of Washington Medical Center, Seattle, WA, USA

Derya Mahmutoglu Department of Medicine-Division of Infectious Diseases, Froedtert & the Medical College of Wisconsin, Froedtert Hospital, Milwaukee, WI, USA

Dror Marchaim Department of Infectious Diseases, Assaf Harofeh Medical Center, Zerifin, Israel

John Daniel Markley Department of Internal Medicine, Division of Infectious Diseases, Virginia Commonwealth University Medical Center, Richmond, VA, USA

Elise Martin Medical Affairs, Cedars-Sinai Health System, Los Angeles, CA, USA

Eriko Masuda Internal Medicine, LAC+USC Medical Center, Los Angeles, CA, USA

Rachel H. McQueen Department of Human Ecology, University of Alberta, Edmonton, AB, Canada

Daniel J. Morgan Departments of Epidemiology, Public Health and Medicine, University of Maryland School of Medicine and Baltimore VA Medical Center, Baltimore, MD, USA

Luisa Silvia Munoz-Price Department of Medicine-Division of Infectious Disease, Froedtert & the Medical College of Wisconsin, Froedtert Hospital, Milwaukee, WI, USA

Rekha K. Murthy Cedars-Sinai Health System, Virginia Commonwealth University School of Medicine, University of North Carolina, Chapel Hill, NC, USA

Medical Affairs, Cedars-Sinai Health System, Los Angeles, CA, USA

Tara N. Palmore Hospital Epidemiology Service, National Institutes of Health Clinical Center, Bethesda, MD, USA

Vivek Pandrangi Virginia Commonwealth University School of Medicine, Richmond, VA, USA

Whitney Perry Division of Internal Medicine, Tufts Medical Center, Boston, MA, USA

Kyle J. Popovich Internal Medicine, Infectious Disease, Rush University Medical Center and Stroger Hospital of Cook County, Chicago, IL, USA

Sara Revolinski Department of Pharmacy, Froedtert & The Medical College of Wisconsin, Milwaukee, WI, USA

Medical College of Wisconsin School of Pharmacy, Milwaukee, WI, USA

Zachary Rubin Medical Affairs, Cedars-Sinai Health System, Los Angeles, CA, USA

Shelly Schwedhelm Biocontainment Unit, Nebraska Medicine, Omaha, NE, USA

Infection Prevention & Emergency Preparedness, Nebraska Medicine, Omaha, NE, USA

Edward J. Septimus Infection Prevention and Epidemiology, Clinical Services Group, HCA, Nashville, TN, USA

Internal Medicine, Texas A&M Health Science Center College of Medicine, Houston, TX, USA

Maroun Sfeir Department of Medicine, Division of Infectious Disease, New York Presbyterian Hospital/Weill Cornell Medical Center, New York, NY, USA

Luis A. Shimose Critical Care Medicine, Cleveland Clinic, Cleveland, OH, USA

Matthew S. Simon Department of Medicine, Division of Infectious Disease, New York Presbyterian Hospital/Weill Cornell Medical Center, New York, NY, USA

Geetika Sood Department of Medicine, Division of Infectious Diseases, Johns Hopkins University, Baltimore, MD, USA

Pranavi V. Sreeramoju Internal Medicine-Infectious Diseases, UT Southwestern Medical Center, Dallas, TX, USA

Michael P. Stevens Department of Internal Medicine, Division of Infectious Diseases, Virginia Commonwealth University Medical Center, Richmond, VA, USA

Infectious Diseases/Epidemiology, Virginia Commonwealth University Health System, Richmond, VA, USA

Thomas R. Talbot Department of Medicine, Vanderbilt University Medical Center, Nashville, TN, USA

David Thomas Infectious Diseases, University of Connecticut School of Medicine, Farmington, CT, USA

Angela M. Vasa Biocontainment Unit, Nebraska Medicine, Omaha, NE, USA

David Jay Weber Division of Infectious Diseases, University of North Carolina at Chapel Hill School of Medicine, Chapel Hill, NC, USA

Jenna Wick Division of Geographic Medicine and Infectious Diseases, Tufts Medical Center, Boston, MA, USA

Deborah S. Yokoe Department of Medicine, Brigham and Women's Hospital and Harvard Medical School, Boston, MA, USA

HAI Controversies: Contact Precautions

Elise Martin, Zachary Rubin, and Rekha K. Murthy

Introduction

Despite the widespread use of contact precautions in acute care hospitals, even after decades of experience, the use of contact precautions (CPs) remains controversial [1]. This paper aims to review the current controversies related to CP in acute care hospital settings, identifies potential areas for future study, and provides updated information where available.

Current Guideline Recommendations for Contact Precautions in Acute Care Facilities

Current national guidelines from the Healthcare Infection Control Practices Advisory Committee (HICPAC) and Centers for Disease Control and Prevention (CDC) broadly recommend that contact precautions (CPs) be implemented routinely in "all patients infected with target MDROs and for patients that have been previously identified as being colonized with target MDROs" without identifying explicitly which MDROs are to be included [2]. In addition, multiple guidelines address strategies for preventing cross-transmission of methicillin-resistant *Staphylococcus aureus* (MRSA) and vancomycin-resistant *Enterococcus* (VRE) in acute care settings that reference the use of CP. The Society for Healthcare Epidemiology of America (SHEA) and the Infectious Diseases Society of America (IDSA) jointly recommend that CP be used for MRSA-infected and MRSA-colonized patients in acute care settings for the control of MRSA in both endemic and outbreak settings [3]. A SHEA/

E. Martin • Z. Rubin • R.K. Murthy (✉)
Medical Affairs, Cedars-Sinai Health System,
8700 Beverly Boulevard, Suite 2211, Los Angeles,
CA 90048, USA
e-mail: EMartin@mednet.ucla.edu; zacharyarubin@gmail.com;
Rekha.Murthy@cshs.org

IDSA joint guidance document also recommends that CP be used for patients with *C. difficile* infection for the duration of illness, and notes that some authors recommend CP for up to 48 h after resolution of diarrhea [4].

Despite these recommendations, recent publications have identified variations in policies among acute care facilities [1]. An increasing number of acute care hospitals surveyed do not apply CP for endemic MRSA and, in some cases, for endemic VRE, in the setting of high compliance with hand hygiene, environmental cleaning, or other horizontal infection control strategies [1].

In this chapter, we review the controversies associated with the use of CP for MRSA, VRE, multidrug-resistant gram-negative organisms (MDR-GNR), and *Clostridium difficile* in endemic or non-outbreak settings.

History of Isolation Precautions

In 1970, the CDC first sought to standardize the application of what are now called "transmission-based precautions" with the publication of the first edition of *Isolation Techniques for Use in Hospitals* [5]. The goal of this document was to prevent the spread of infectious pathogens within the hospital milieu and, at the same time, tried to minimize what they saw as the costs of isolation: added expense, inconvenience, decreased visits by providers, and psychological duress. In order to balance these sometimes competing goals, the CDC developed a graded isolation scheme based upon the mode of pathogen transmission. The categories were to be placed on colored cards on room doors and provide directions for incoming providers and visitors. The categories included the following terms, which would later be classified into standard precautions and contact precautions: strict isolation; enteric precautions; wound and skin precautions; discharge precautions, which included excretion precautions; secretion precautions; and blood precautions [6]. Clinical staff determined which category patients best fit into based upon a combination of clinical syndromes and the isolation of specific pathogens. The second edition of *Isolation Techniques*

© Springer International Publishing AG 2018
G. Bearman et al. (eds.), *Infection Prevention*, DOI 10.1007/978-3-319-60980-5_1

for Use in Hospitals published in 1975 did not significantly alter the scheme [7].

In 1983, CDC significantly revised isolation precaution schemes in the CDC Guideline for Isolation Precautions in Hospitals [8]. This document still included both category- and disease-specific isolation systems and required end-users to determine the best category. Soon after the 1983 document was published, however, the HIV epidemic led to the adoption of "universal precautions" for all blood and body fluids, other than sweat in the mid-1980s [9, 10].

Ultimately, the 1996 guidelines refined and simplified isolation precautions further and into its current form [6]. Instead of the complex and often subjective categories of previous guidelines, the categories of isolation practices were simplified into three transmission-based categories: contact, airborne, and droplet precautions. Additionally, "universal precautions" and body substance isolation were combined into the "standard precautions" in use today. The most recently published guideline from 2007 essentially upheld this general simplified scheme intact with some minor updates [11].

Vertical Versus Horizontal Infection Control Strategies

Acute care hospitals employ a number of strategies to decrease healthcare-associated infections (HAIs) and the spread of resistant organisms between patients. In general, these infection prevention strategies can be grouped into two types of programs, vertical and horizontal strategies [12, 13]. Vertical approaches focus on specific pathogens and utilize targeted programs, such as active surveillance testing (AST) to identify patients with specific organisms, followed by interventions to specifically prevent the spread of those organisms [12]. Horizontal programs are more broadly focused and aim to decrease the spread of any pathogen that could lead to an HAI through programs, such as hand hygiene and standard precautions, that are applied to all patients in the health system, not only those with resistant pathogens [12]. There are pros and cons to both strategies, and many hospitals use a combination of these interventions [14].

Vertical infection prevention programs are aimed at decreasing HAIs by focusing on high-risk pathogens that may be transmitted from patient to patient [12, 13, 15]. These programs are based on first identifying patients with a particular pathogen and then decreasing spread. Vertical programs have been used for a variety of high-risk pathogens, including methicillin-resistant *Staphylococcus aureus* (MRSA), vancomycin-resistant *Enterococcus* (VRE), *Clostridium difficile*, multidrug-resistant gram-negative pathogens, and others [12]. Most of these programs are centered on the use of AST, in addition to identifying infected patients, to detect patients who are MDRO carriers as well. Infection prevention strategies are then employed to prevent spread of these particular pathogens through interventions such as CP, isolation, and cohorting of patients. Decolonization strategies may also be applied for patients for a specific pathogen, such as MRSA, through the use of chlorhexidine gluconate (CHG) bathing or mupirocin [12]. While these strategies may decrease the spread of each of these specific organisms, each strategy only targets one specific pathogen, and not all important organisms, such as MRDO gram negatives and VRE, have options for decolonization.

Horizontal infection preventions strategies have a much broader focus. Instead of targeting a single high-risk pathogen, they focus on initiatives that reduce HAIs from any pathogen. One of the most well-known strategies is standard precautions, which include effective hand hygiene and use of personal protective equipment when encountering body fluids [12]. Hospitals can also develop antimicrobial stewardship programs to decrease development of resistant organisms, remove unnecessary medical devices to decrease the risk of device-associated infections, and improve environmental cleaning to decrease the risk of infection to subsequent patients [12]. Some of the interventions used for a specific organism, such as gloving, use of other personal protective equipment, and decolonization with CHG, can be applied universally to all patients, not just those with a specific pathogen. These programs decrease the risk of infections from multiple organisms, including pathogens that have not yet been identified in the patient.

Groups have attempted to determine which of these is the optimal strategy to reduce HAIs [12, 13, 15]. Given MRSA-focused interventions have become increasingly common, Wenzel RP et. al. developed a model to assess the impact on mortality with a hospital intervention to reduce MRSA blood stream infections (BSI) versus all causes of BSI [15]. Based on their calculations, even a 50% decrease in the rate of MRSA BSI would not impact mortality as much as can be achieved with just a 25% decrease in overall BSI [15] The authors of this study argue that focusing on a single pathogen may be insufficient to reduce HAIs and, instead, hospitals should employ a variety of evidence-based interventions to optimally reduce the risk of HAIs to patients.

While there are two main categories of infection preventions strategies, they are not mutually exclusive and are often used in combination to decrease the spread of resistant organism and HAIs [12] (Table 1.1).

MRSA and the Impact of Contact Precautions

The Center for Disease Control (CDC) and the Society for Healthcare Epidemiology of America (SHEA) still

Table 1.1 Examples of vertical and horizontal infection prevention strategies

Vertical infection preventions strategies
Focus: specific pathogens (examples: MRSA, VRE, CRE)
Active surveillance testing to identify patients with specific pathogens
Contact precautions for specific pathogens
Spore precautions for specific pathogens
Targeted decolonization for specific pathogens
Horizontal infection prevention strategies
Focus: all pathogens, universal
Standard precautions (hand hygiene, barrier precautions when encountering fluids)
Universal gowning and gloving
Universal decolonization of all patients
Environmental cleaning and disinfection
Antimicrobial stewardship
Minimizing unnecessary medical devices

Modified from Refs. [12, 13]
MRSA methicillin-resistant *Staphylococcus aureus*, *VRE* vancomycin-resistant *Enterococcus*, *CRE* carbapenem-resistant *Enterobacteriaceae*

recommend the use of CP to decrease the transmission of methicillin-resistant *Staphylococcus aureus* (MRSA) in acute care hospitals, but the practice has become increasingly controversial [1, 3, 16]. Concerns include both the lack of evidence clearly showing benefit and data suggesting potential patient harm associated with CP. Despite the controversy, recent surveys have demonstrated that more than 90% of US acute care hospitals still use CP for MRSA [1, 14].

Although MRSA rates have been declining, MRSA remains a serious threat according to the CDC's 2013 Antimicrobial Resistance Threat report [17]. The CDC estimates that there are 80,461 invasive MRSA infections and 11,285 deaths related to MRSA every year in the USA and the majority of the severe infections occur during or shortly after inpatient care [17]. For this reason, efforts have been made to decrease the spread of MRSA in healthcare settings through various initiatives, including CP. According to published reports, up to 18% of patients are isolated for MRSA in acute care hospitals [18, 19].

Multiple studies have attempted to examine the benefit of CP for MRSA. The Veterans Affairs hospitals developed an "MRSA bundle," composed of universal surveillance, CP, improved hand hygiene, and an institutional culture change, that was associated with a decrease in transmissions of and infections with MRSA. The study showed that MRSA infections in ICUs decreased by 62% after the implementation of the bundle, from 1.64 to 0.62 infections per 1000 patient-days (PD) ($p < 0.001$). MRSA infections also decreased in non-ICUs by 45% from 0.47 per to 0.26 per 1000 PD ($p < 0.001$). Another study by Huang SS et al., in 2006, utilized an interrupted time series to look at multiple interven-

tions over a 9 year period and found that routine surveillance cultures and subsequent contact precautions lead to a 67% hospital-wide reduction in MRSA bacteremia ($p = 0.002$) [20]. A study from a French hospital found that MRSA acquisition decreased in their facility from 7.0 to 2.8% after instituting weekly MRSA surveillance screening followed by CP [21]. A study evaluating universal gowning and gloving also decreased MRSA acquisition in ICU patients by 2.98 acquisitions per 1000 person-days ($p = 0.046$), although the primary outcome of MRSA/VRE acquisition was not met [22]. A large study from three hospitals found a reduction in MRSA disease during admission and 30 days after discharge with the introduction of universal surveillance and isolation for MRSA [23]. While these studies do show benefit with the use of CP, because these studies all used a combination of strategies, it is difficult to tease out whether it was the gowns and gloves specifically or if other factors drove the improvement. In addition, several of these studies were based in the ICU, and it is unknown if the results are generalizable to non-ICU settings.

Several other studies looking at the impact of CP for MRSA have not shown a benefit. A group from a Swiss teaching hospital performed a prospective, interventional cohort study with crossover on a surgical ward and found that MRSA nosocomial infection was not reduced with CP, AST, and targeted decolonization [24]. Another group performed a cluster-randomized trial in 18 ICUs to evaluate the impact of enhanced surveillance for MRSA colonization and expanded use of CP and found no reduction in the transmission of MRSA, although the use of CP by providers was less than expected [25].

Given the conflicting data about the benefit of CP, multiple institutions have evaluated the impact of discontinuing CP for endemic MRSA [1]. One health system eliminated routine CP for MRSA in both their hospitals and started universal CHG bathing [26]. They found no increase in MRSA infections or colonization. The study also demonstrated a $643,776 cost savings in 1 year and significant savings in healthcare worker time. Another study looked at the impact of discontinuing CP on device-associated infections and found no increase in these infections after they removed routine CP in both the ICUs and the wards [27]. A study from a surgical ICU compared the use of universal gloving to standard CP and found that universal gloving in their unit was associated with improved hand hygiene compliance and skin health and was not associated with a significant change in the rates of device-associated infection, *Clostridium difficile* infection, or multidrug-resistant organism acquisition [28].

A number of studies have evaluated the possible negative impacts of CP and the potential harms to those placed in isolation. Several studies have shown decreased contact with healthcare providers, including fewer bedside visits from healthcare providers, shorter contact time during those visits, fewer physical examinations by attending physicians, and fewer progress notes documenting their visits when compared to patients not on CP [29–34]. Patients on CP can also experience delays in transitions of care, including from the emergency room and discharge to skilled nursing facilities [34–37]. There is also evidence that patients on CP have higher rates of anxiety and depression during their hospitalization and lower satisfaction with their care [34, 38, 39]. The data on other adverse events have been conflicting. While some have found an association with increased preventable adverse events, such as pressure ulcers, falls, and medication administration errors, others have found a decrease in adverse events in patients on CP [34, 40, 41].

Although the data on the efficacy of routine CP for endemic MRSA is controversial, it remains common practice [1, 14]. Currently, at least 30 US hospitals have discontinued routine CP for MRSA and are instead using other horizontal infection prevention strategies, such as improved hand hygiene, HAI bundles, decolonization, and syndromic indications for precautions (i.e., draining wounds) [1]. While the early data on discontinuing CP is encouraging, future research with larger trials is needed to conclusively determine whether or not CPs are necessary for endemic MRSA. Further data are also needed on whether select populations may benefit from MRSA CP and the optimal strategies for continuing CP.

Vancomycin-Resistant *Enterococcus* (VRE)

In a recent survey of US-based physicians conducted by the Emerging Infections Network (EIN), 92% of 364 respondents reported routinely use CP for vancomycin-resistant *Enterococcus* [14]. As with MRSA, CPs are commonly used for VRE, and although multiple publications have reported the benefits of CP in terminating VRE outbreaks, few published studies have actually examined the use of CP alone as an intervention to reduce VRE acquisition, particularly in non-outbreak settings [1].

Bearman et al. conducted two quasi-experimental studies where CP for patients with VRE was compared with universal glove use [28, 42]. The authors found no difference in VRE acquisition and found higher healthcare-associated infection rates with universal glove use in one of the studies. In a systematic review and meta-analysis of measures taken to control VRE in ICU settings, De Angelis et al. reported results from three studies in which application of CP was the only intervention. In these studies, CP did not significantly reduce the VRE acquisition rate (pooled relative risk, 1.08 [95% CI, 0.63–1.83]) [43]. Three other studies that examined the impact of CP on VRE acquisition in ICUs were cluster-randomized trials [22, 25, 44]. Huskins et al. compared CP in the intervention group after active screening cul-

tures (ASC) to standard precautions and found that the incidence of colonization or infection with VRE did not differ between the two groups ($P = 0.53$) [25]. In a cluster-randomized trial among ICUs, Harris et al. evaluated intervention ICUs where HCP wore gowns and gloves for all patient contacts and room entries in comparison with control ICUs where CP was used only for patients with known antibiotic-resistant bacteria. No difference in VRE outcomes was found by investigators [22]. Similarly, a study in the setting of universal chlorhexidine body washes and hand hygiene improvement identified no benefit to ASC for addressing VRE or other MDROs [44].

Although the majority of US hospitals use CP for endemic VRE, Morgan et al. identified at least 30 hospitals that reported not using CP for VRE and instead employ horizontal infection control methods, with CP reserved only for syndromes correlated with greater contamination (e.g., diarrhea, wounds) [1, 14]. Several of these institutions focus on general horizontal approaches to limiting transmission VRE, such as hand hygiene, bathing patients with chlorhexidine, or environmental cleaning and disinfection. However, these hospitals continue to apply CP for *Clostridium difficile* and multidrug-resistant gram-negative rods. Martin et al. assessed laboratory identified culture rates of VRE before and after discontinuing CP for endemic MRSA and VRE and expansion of chlorhexidine bathing to all hospital units. The study found no significant change in the average rate of positive cultures for VRE before and after the intervention which were 0.48 and 0.40 cultures/100 admissions for VRE ($P = 0.14$), respectively [26]. Furthermore, discontinuing routine CP for endemic VRE did not result in increased rates of VRE after 1 year. The authors concluded that, with cost savings on materials, decreased healthcare worker time, and no concomitant increase in possible infections, elimination of routine CP may add substantial value to inpatient care delivery.

In conclusion, although CPs are widely used for VRE based on current national guidelines, no clear evidence has been identified to substantiate a benefit to CP over standard precautions in acute care settings for controlling the transmission of VRE in non-outbreak settings. Unfortunately, no study has compared CP with standard precautions alone, and other studies are limited by likely positive publication bias and generally low study quality. Alternative approaches using horizontal infection control strategies have been employed at some acute care facilities without adverse impact on VRE acquisition rates, although confidence in the achievement and sustainment of successful horizontal infection control strategies has been a common factor among these institutions [26, 45, 46]. Given the lack of robust clinical data to establish clear evidence-based guidelines, the experience from hospitals using these alternate approaches suggests that individual institutions should assess local factors, needs, and resources (e.g., availability of single rooms, VRE acquisition and infection data, potential susceptibility of patient populations such as immunocompromised patients, etc.) to determine the risks and benefits of modifying current policies on the use CP for VRE. Finally, higher-quality research on the risks and benefits of CP in endemic VRE in acute care hospitals is needed to determine more definitive recommendations.

Contact Precautions for Gram-Negative Rods and *Clostridium difficile*

While we have previously discussed that a lack of evidence for the benefits of CP for endemic MSRA and VRE has led some institutions to abandon CP for these indications, many of these same institutions have continued CP for gram-negative rods (GNRs) and *Clostridium difficile* infection (CDI) [1].

Any discussion of CP for GNRs is hampered by the great diversity of these organisms and the different approaches taken by various institutions to each. For example, Ronald Reagan UCLA Medical Center does not isolate extended-spectrum beta-lactamase (ESBL) organisms but has isolated carbapenem-resistant GNRs, while Cedars-Sinai Medical Center, just a few miles away, applies CP to both. We see the same complexity in reviewing the literature on CP. It is unclear whether CP and other interventions against GNRs can and should be generalized across different species and resistance phenotypes. Interestingly, the HICPAC's 2007 Guideline for Isolation Precautions and the 2006 Management of Multidrug-Resistant (MDR) Organisms in Healthcare Settings recommend CP for drug-resistant GNRs in general [11, 47]. Neither guideline explicitly differentiates between different classes of GNR organisms. The authors of the latter HICPAC document posit a general, though largely untested, rationale for the general use of CP for all GNRs. Because MDR-GNRs and *C. difficile* are thought to be correlated with environmental contamination—the reasoning goes in the 2007 document—CP should decrease the risk of indirect transmission of infectious agents. Though the strongest rationale supporting CP is not entirely borne out by medical research, hospitals persist in their use of CP for MDR-GNRs and CDI for a host of assumptions:

1. There is a greater perceived institutional threat from the rising incidence of these emerging pathogens compared to MRSA and VRE [48, 49].
2. MDR-GNRs and CDI are thought to be more highly correlated to indirect contact transmission than MRSA and VRE because of a higher environmental burden.
3. MDR-GNRs require extra control measures because they may be higher pathogenicity organisms than MRSA and VRE.
4. Because there is a lower incidence of MDR-GNRs currently compared to more widespread MRSA and VRE in the community, these organisms are more amenable to successful control with CP.
5. MDR-GNRs and CDI are likely controlled less effectively by horizontal infection prevention strategies than MRSA and VRE.

There are many difficulties in reviewing the literature regarding CP for MDR-GNRs not only owing to the lack of prospective, controlled data but also to the inherent diversity and complexity of the organisms themselves. As stated above, the definition of "MDR" may vary between institutions and public health entities, leading to significant variations in practice. Second, GNRs include a broad and diverse category of organisms, including organisms like *Pseudomonas aeruginosa*, *Acinetobacter*, *Enterobacteriaceae*, etc., that may have very different colonization and transmission characteristics. They also differ in regard to susceptibilities to environmental cleaners. Not only does this diversity make it hard to extrapolate a study of a single organism to others, it also leads to confusion when trying to use data-driven practice in individual hospitals.

Adding to the confusion, as institutions and public health departments increasingly employ molecular testing methodologies, we are learning that the previously established correlation between phenotypic and genotypic resistance that has been used clinically to define MDR status can be tenuous and can change rapidly. Certain types of resistance, such as plasmid encoded genes, are transferred between organisms more readily, while chromosomal genes are not – even though the organisms may look similar phenotypically. Organisms can add or drop plasmids quickly, even in a single patient over time, so that the same *Klebsiella* phenotype can look different from one culture to the next and can cause considerable confusion among clinical staff trying to monitor these organisms. Additionally, as MDR-GNRs increase in frequency in previously hospitalized patients, it is becoming clear that CP applied only to those who have positive clinical isolates of MDR-GNR will exclude many asymptomatic carriers. As a result, the CDC and other organizations have recommended active surveillance cultures, at least in the case of carbapenem-resistant *Enterobacteriaceae* (CRE), for some populations [50]. As with MRSA and VRE, it is doubtful that CPs are as effective without active surveillance.

There is ample, though not entirely supportive, evidence that CP is successful when applied to outbreak situations due to MDR-*Enterobacteriaceae*. As with all papers describing control of outbreaks, it is difficult to separate out any single intervention, given that CP was used in addition to other control measures. Additional measures used to control outbreaks include monitored hand hygiene programs, active surveillance testing, and cohorting. There is also lower-level evidence of a similar effect with regard to *Pseudomonas* outbreaks [51, 52]. However, robust evidence is lacking to support CP for endemic MDR-GNRs. Most work has been done with ESBLs, but these studies usually include only a single institution, often lack comparison groups, and do not offer detailed information about their CP practices. The most recent example, an interrupted time series analysis that monitored ESBL rates after discontinuation of CP, demonstrated a transmission rate of 2.6 % without CP, compared to 1.5% with CP in place at the same hospital [53, 54]. This difference was deemed not clinically significant by the investigators. A study in Germany which performed ESBL surveillance after initiation of CP found a low overall transmission risk, but as there was no comparison group, it is difficult to make any conclusions [55]. Another study showed no changes in the incidence of nosocomial ESBL *E. coli* and *Klebsiella* organisms after active screening of urine isolates and CP for all positive cases [56]. One study of active surveillance and CP of ESBL *Klebsiella* in a neonatal ICU in Israel showed a significant decrease in carriage, from 24 to 11%, though the high baseline rate of transmission suggests an outbreak and not a normal, endemic carriage pattern [57]. Aside from significant methodologic concerns as discussed above, a significant confounder for all of these studies is that most were performed in hospitals with rooms that housed two to four patients. There is evidence from a number of studies that placing patients in private rooms decreases transmission of MDR-GNR organisms and furthermore reduces the overall infection rate, though many of these studies do not include control wards [58]. While ESBL presents a confusing problem because of the lack of controlled data, the case for carbapenem-resistant *Enterobacteriaceae* (CRE) is even less clear. The majority of studies or CRE are in outbreak settings and used a bundle of interventions, making it difficult to extrapolate to endemic settings [59, 60].

Preventing CDI transmission in hospitals, like all the other organisms we have discussed in this chapter, is likely best done with a bundle of interventions. As in the other cases discussed, there are few studies that study only CP in isolation from other interventions for the control of CDI. Though hospitals across the country generally follow CP for CDI, according to the most recent population-based data in the USA, CDI has proved more difficult to control and causes over 100,000 annual hospital acquired cases [61]. Indeed, in recent data from the state of California, CDI rates have actually increased despite falls for other HAI types [62]. The transmission characteristics of CDI, like GNRs, are not well worked understood. Because hospitals do not have the techniques to characterize CDI genotypes easily, we

rely on relatively few studies that have looked at CDI at individual institutions. What these studies continue to demonstrate is that there are often multiple distinct CDI organisms causing disease in hospitals at any given time, suggesting that community acquisition is common and that many patients may enter hospitals already colonized with the organisms that will ultimately cause their infections [63–66]. One Australian study found a strong correlation between hospital and community strains of both symptomatic CDI and asymptomatic carriage, suggesting that transmission may be common outside the healthcare setting [67]. In this model, patients' immune status and bowel flora disruption with antibiotics, and not direct transmission, may be the most common contributing factors to development of CDI in the hospitals. In this model, CP may have only a limited role in decreasing hospital transmission.

We believe it is important to note that the lack of evidentiary support for CP for management of endemic MDR-GNRs and CDI should not be taken to prove that CPs are ineffective. Because most hospitals currently use CP to control CDI and MDR-GNRs, and most epidemiologic studies have been unable to simultaneously compare transmission without CP, it is difficult to make a strong argument either way. It is very possible that CDI and MDR-GNR transmission within hospitals and the community would be more common without CP. Nevertheless, because CP has financial impact to hospitals and may have negative clinical impacts to patient care, it is clear that more prospective, controlled research in this area should be performed. In the meantime, while we await the final verdict on CP, it is important that hospitals not ignore the importance of basic elements of infection control which have been shown to be effective for over a century: hand hygiene, environmental disinfection, and the judicious use of antibiotics [68].

References

1. Morgan DJ, Murthy R, Munoz-Price LS, et al. Reconsidering contact precautions for endemic methicillin-resistant *Staphylococcus aureus* and vancomycin-resistant enterococcus. Infect Control Hosp Epidemiol. 2015;36:1163–72.
2. CDC/HICPAC. Prevention of transmission of multidrug resistant organisms 2009. (2009). http://www.cdc.gov/hicpac/mdro/mdro_5.html. Accessed Nov 2016.
3. Calfee DP, Salgado CD, Milstone AM, et al. Strategies to prevent methicillin-resistant *Staphylococcus aureus* transmission and infection in acute care hospitals: 2014 update. Infect Control Hosp Epidemiol. 2014;35:772–96.
4. Dubberke ER, Carling P, Carrico R, et al. Strategies to prevent Clostridium difficile infections in acute care hospitals: 2014 update. Infect Control Hosp Epidemiol. 2014;35:628–45.
5. Center NCD. Isolation techniques for use in Hospitals. 1st ed. Washington, DC: US Government Printing Office; PHS publication no 2054; 1970. https://books.google.com/books?id=3mmDVeUjUsYC&pg=PR8&lpg=PR8&dq=control+of+infectious+diseases+in+

general+hospitals+1967+american+public+health&source=bl&ots =dU8T6AeRoZ&sig=rwL8zwmqsPpYzEQ13KLYfcO1DuM&hl= en&sa=X&ved=0ahUKEwjs3KKj94XQAhVJrVQKHUopAAkQ6 AEIKDAE-v=onepage&q&f=false. Accessed 31 Oct 2016

6. Garner JS. Guideline for isolation precautions in hospitals. The Hospital Infection Control Practices Advisory Committee. Infect Control Hosp Epidemiol. 1996;17:53–80.

7. Center NCD. Isolation techniques for use in Hospitals. 2nd ed. Washington, DC: US Government Printing Office; PHS Publication No; 1975.

8. Garner JS, Simmons B. CDC guideline for isolation precautions in hospitals. US Department of Health and Human Services, Public Health Service, Centers for Disease Control. Infect Control. 1983;4:245–325.

9. Centers for Disease Control. Update: universal precautions for prevention of transmission of human immunodeficiency virus, hepatitis B virus, and other bloodborne pathogens in health-care settings. MMWR Morb Mortal Wkly Rep. 1988;37:377–82. 387–378

10. Centers for Disease Control. Recommendations for preventing transmission of infection with human T-lymphotropic virus type III/lymphadenopathy-associated virus in the workplace. MMWR Morb Mortal Wkly Rep. 1985;34:681–6. 691–685

11. Siegel JD, Rhinehart E, Jackson M. 2007 Guideline for isolation precautions: preventing transmission of infectious agents in health-care settings. The Hospital Infection Control Practices Advisory Committee 2007.

12. Septimus E, Weinstein RA, Perl TM, Goldmann DA, Yokoe DS. Approaches for preventing healthcare-associated infections: go long or go wide? Infect Control Hosp Epidemiol. 2014;35(Suppl 2):S10–4.

13. Wenzel RP, Edmond MB. Infection control: the case for horizontal rather than vertical interventional programs. Int J Infect Dis. 2010;14(Suppl 4):S3–5.

14. Russell D, Beekmann SE, Polgreen PM, Rubin Z, Uslan DZ. Routine use of contact precautions for methicillin-resistant Staphylococcus aureus and vancomycin-resistant enterococcus: which way is the pendulum swinging? Infect Control Hosp Epidemiol. 2016;37:36–40.

15. Wenzel RP, Bearman G, Edmond MB. Screening for MRSA: a flawed hospital infection control intervention. Infect Control Hosp Epidemiol. 2008;29:1012–8.

16. Muto CA, Jernigan JA, Ostrowsky BE, et al. SHEA guideline for preventing nosocomial transmission of multidrug-resistant strains of Staphylococcus aureus and enterococcus. Infect Control Hosp Epidemiol. 2003;24:362–86.

17. Antibiotic Resistance Threats in the United States 2013. 2013. http://www.cdc.gov/drugresistance/pdf/ar-threats-2013-508.pdf.

18. Jain R, Kralovic SM, Evans ME, et al. Veterans Affairs initiative to prevent methicillin-resistant Staphylococcus aureus infections. N Engl J Med. 2011;364:1419–30.

19. Day HR, Perencevich EN, Harris AD, et al. Do contact precautions cause depression? A two-year study at a tertiary care medical centre. J Hosp Infect. 2011;79:103–7.

20. Huang SS, Yokoe DS, Hinrichsen VL, et al. Impact of routine intensive care unit surveillance cultures and resultant barrier precautions on hospital-wide methicillin-resistant Staphylococcus aureus bacteremia. Clin Infect Dis. 2006;43:971–8.

21. Lucet JC, Paoletti X, Lolom I, et al. Successful long-term program for controlling methicillin-resistant Staphylococcus aureus in intensive care units. Intensive Care Med. 2005;31:1051–7.

22. Harris AD, Pineles L, Belton B, et al. Universal glove and gown use and acquisition of antibiotic-resistant bacteria in the ICU: a randomized trial. JAMA. 2013;310:1571–80.

23. Robicsek A, Beaumont JL, Paule SM, et al. Universal surveillance for methicillin-resistant Staphylococcus aureus in 3 affiliated hospitals. Ann Intern Med. 2008;148:409–18.

24. Harbarth S, Fankhauser C, Schrenzel J, et al. Universal screening for methicillin-resistant Staphylococcus aureus at hospital admission and nosocomial infection in surgical patients. JAMA. 2008;299:1149–57.

25. Huskins WC, Huckabee CM, O'Grady NP, et al. Intervention to reduce transmission of resistant bacteria in intensive care. N Engl J Med. 2011;364:1407–18.

26. Martin EM, Russell D, Rubin Z, et al. Elimination of routine contact precautions for endemic methicillin-resistant Staphylococcus aureus and vancomycin-resistant enterococcus: a retrospective quasi-experimental study. Infect Control Hosp Epidemiol. 2016;37:1323–30.

27. Edmond MB, Masroor N, Stevens MP, Ober J, Bearman G. The impact of discontinuing contact precautions for VRE and MRSA on device-associated infections. Infect Control Hosp Epidemiol. 2015;36:978–80.

28. Bearman G, Rosato AE, Duane TM, et al. Trial of universal gloving with emollient-impregnated gloves to promote skin health and prevent the transmission of multidrug-resistant organisms in a surgical intensive care unit. Infect Control Hosp Epidemiol. 2010;31:491–7.

29. Dashiell-Earp CN, Bell DS, Ang AO, Uslan DZ. Do physicians spend less time with patients in contact isolation?: a time-motion study of internal medicine interns. JAMA Intern Med. 2014;174:814–5.

30. Evans HL, Shaffer MM, Hughes MG, et al. Contact isolation in surgical patients: a barrier to care? Surgery. 2003;134:180–8.

31. Masse V, Valiquette L, Boukhoudmi S, et al. Impact of methicillin resistant Staphylococcus aureus contact isolation units on medical care. PLoS ONE. 2013;8:e57057.

32. Morgan DJ, Pineles L, Shardell M, et al. The effect of contact precautions on healthcare worker activity in acute care hospitals. Infect Control Hosp Epidemiol. 2013;34:69–73.

33. Saint S, Higgins LA, Nallamothu BK, Chenoweth C. Do physicians examine patients in contact isolation less frequently? A brief report. Am J Infect Control. 2003;31:354–6.

34. Stelfox HT, Bates DW, Redelmeier DA. Safety of patients isolated for infection control. JAMA. 2003;290:1899–905.

35. Gilligan P, Quirke M, Winder S, Humphreys H. Impact of admission screening for methicillin-resistant Staphylococcus aureus on the length of stay in an emergency department. J Hosp Infect. 2010;75:99–102.

36. McLemore A, Bearman G, Edmond MB. Effect of contact precautions on wait time from emergency room disposition to inpatient admission. Infect Control Hosp Epidemiol. 2011;32:298–9.

37. Goldszer RC, Tamplin E, Yokoe DS, Shadick N, Bardon CG, Johnson PA, Hogan J, Kahlert T, Whittermore A. A program to remove patients from unnecessary contact precautions. J Clin Outcomes Manag. 2002;9:553–6.

38. Catalano G, Houston SH, Catalano MC, et al. Anxiety and depression in hospitalized patients in resistant organism isolation. South Med J. 2003;96:141–5.

39. Day HR, Morgan DJ, Himelhoch S, Young A, Perencevich EN. Association between depression and contact precautions in veterans at hospital admission. Am J Infect Control. 2011;39:163–5.

40. Karki S, Leder K, Cheng AC. Patients under contact precautions have an increased risk of injuries and medication errors: a retrospective cohort study. Infect Control Hosp Epidemiol. 2013;34:1118–20.

41. Croft LD, Liquori M, Ladd J, et al. The effect of contact precautions on frequency of hospital adverse events. Infect Control Hosp Epidemiol. 2015;36:1268–74.

42. Bearman GM, Marra AR, Sessler CN, et al. A controlled trial of universal gloving versus contact precautions for preventing the transmission of multidrug-resistant organisms. Am J Infect Control. 2007;35:650–5.

43. De Angelis G, Cataldo MA, De Waure C, et al. Infection control and prevention measures to reduce the spread of vancomycin-resis-

tant enterococci in hospitalized patients: a systematic review and meta-analysis. J Antimicrob Chemother. 2014;69:1185–92.

44. Derde LP, Cooper BS, Goossens H, et al. Interventions to reduce colonisation and transmission of antimicrobial-resistant bacteria in intensive care units: an interrupted time series study and cluster randomised trial. Lancet Infect Dis. 2014;14:31–9.

45. Edmond M. Panel on clinical controversies in ID. Abstract 18. Paper presented at: IDWeek 2014; Philadelphia; (2014).

46. Gandra S, Barysauskas CM, Mack DA, Barton B, Finberg R, Ellison RT 3rd. Impact of contact precautions on falls, pressure ulcers and transmission of MRSA and VRE in hospitalized patients. J Hosp Infect. 2014;88:170–6.

47. Siegel JD, Rhinehart E, Jackson M, et al. Management of Multidrug-resistant organisms in healthcare settings, 2006. Am J Infect Control. 2007;35(10 Suppl 2):S165–93.

48. CDC. Antibiotic resistance threats I the United States. http://www.cdc.gov/drugresistance/pdf/ar-threats-2013-508.pdf. (2013). Accessed 29 Nov 2016.

49. Smith, AM, Wuerth BA, Wiemken TL, Arnold FW. Prevalence of Clostridium difficile infection presenting to US EDs. Am J Emerg Med. 2015;33:238–43. Lessa FC, Mu Y, Bamberg WM, et al. Burden of Clostridium difficile infection in the United States. NEJM. 2015;372:825–34.

50. CDC. Facility guidance for control of carbapenem-resistant Enterobacteriaceae: November 2015 Update- CRE Toolkit. http://www.cdc.gov/hai/pdfs/cre/cre-guidance-508.pdf. Accessed 1 Dec (2016).

51. Tacconelli E, Cataldo MA, Dancer SJ, et al. ESCMID guideline for the management of infection control measures to reduce transmission of multidrug-resistant Gram-negative bacteria in hospitalized patients. Clin Microbiol Infect. 2014;20:1–55.

52. Wilson AP, Livermore DM, Otter JA, et al. Prevention and control of multi-drug-resistant Gram-negative bacteria: recommendations from a joint working party. J Hosp Infect. 2016;92:S1–44.

53. Tschudin-Sutter S, Frei R, Schwahn F, et al. Prospective validation of cessation of contact precautions for extended spectrum B-lactamase-producing E. coli. Emerg Infect Dis. 2016;22:1094–7.

54. Tschudin-Sutter S, Frei R, Dangel M, et al. Rate of transmission of extended-spectrum beta-lactamase-producing enterobacteriaceae without contact isolation. Clin Infect Dis. 2012;55:1505–11.

55. Kola A, Holst M, Chaberny IF, et al. Surveillance of ESBL-producing bacteria and routine use of contact isolation: experience from a three-year study. J Hosp Infect. 2007;66:46–51.

56. Han JH, Bilker WB, Nachamkin I, et al. The effect of a hospital-wide urine culture screening intervention on the incidence of ESBL-producing E. coli and Klebsiella species. Infect Control Hosp Epidemiol. 2013;34:1160–6.

57. Benenson S, Levin PD, Block C, et al. Continuous surveillance to reduce ESBL Klebsiella pneumonia colonization in the neonatal ICU. Neonatology. 2013;103:155–60.

58. Teltsch DY, Hanley J, Loo V, et al. Infection acquisition following intensive care unit room privatization. Arch Intern Med. 2011;171:32–8.

59. Munoz-Price LS, Quinn JP. Deconstructing the infection control bundles for the containment of carbapenem-resistant Enterobacteriaceae. Curr Opin Infect Dis. 2013;26:378–87.

60. Sypsa V, Psichogiou M, Bouzala GA, et al. Transmission dynamics of carbapenemase-producing Klebsiella pneumonia and anticipated impact of infection control strategies in a surgical unit. PLoS ONE. 2012;7:e41068.

61. Lessa FC, Mu Y, Bamberg WM, et al. Burden of Clostridium difficile infections in the United States. NEJM. 2015;372:825–34.

62. California Department of Public Health. Healthcare-associated infections in California hospitals annual report for January to December (2015). https://www.cdph.ca.gov/programs/hai/Documents/2015-HAI-in-CA-Hospitals-Annual-Report-2015.pdf

63. Jin D, Luo Y, Huang C, et al. Molecular epidemiology of Clostridium Difficile infection in hospitalized patients in Eastern China. J Clin Microbiol. doi:10.1128/JCM.01898-16.

64. Tian TT, Zhao JH, Yang J, et al. Molecular characterization of Clostridium difficile isolates from human subjects and the environment. PLoS ONE. 2016;11:e0151964.

65. Freeman J, Vernon J, Morris K, et al. Pan-European longitudinal surveillance of antibiotic resistance among Clostridium difficile ribotypes. Clin Microbiol Infect. 2015;21:e9–248.

66. Foster NF, Collins DA, Ditchburn SL, et al. Epidemiology of Clostridium difficile infection in two tertiary-care hospitals in Perth, Western Australia: a cross-sectional study (n.d.).

67. Furuya-Kanamori L, Riley TV, Paterson DL, et al. A comparison of Clostridium difficile ribotypes circulating in Australian hospitals and communities. J Clin Microbiol. 2016;JCM.01779–16.

68. Weber DJ, Rutala WA, Miller MB, et al. Role of hospital surfaces in the transmission of emerging health care-associated pathogens: norovirus, Clostridium difficile and Acinetobacter species. Am J Infect Control. 2010;38:S25–33.

Hand Hygiene Monitoring Technologies: Implementation and Outcomes

Claudia Denisse Jarrin Tejada

Introduction

Although hand hygiene (HH) is the most important measure for preventing of healthcare-associated infections, its compliance among healthcare workers (HCW) is extremely low with an average of 40% [1] even after simplifying the procedure by replacing soap and water with alcohol-based hand rubs (ABHR) – except in the case of confirmed or suspected *Clostridium difficile* infection [2].

The First Global Patient Safety Challenge, "Clean Care is Safer Care," was a campaign initiated by the WHO in 2005 to promote system change, training and education, observation, and feedback, in order to improve HH compliance. The WHO describes five moments recommended for HH: before patient contact, before performing an aseptic procedure, after exposure to body fluids, after patient contact, and after contact with patient's surroundings [1].

Monitoring Hand Hygiene Compliance

Monitoring HH compliance plays a crucial role in decreasing hospital-acquired infections. The gold standard method for monitoring HH is direct observation [3]. With the advances in technology, different modalities such as video monitoring and electronic surveillance have emerged. Importantly, these modalities also allow real-time feedback which can provide important and durable increases in HH compliance rates.

The majority of studies evaluating technologies for monitoring HH are quasi-experimental. To date, there is no consensus on which technology has better outcomes in terms of monitoring and achieving sustainable levels of HH compliance.

Srigley et al. performed a systematic review that included experimental and quasi-experimental studies of HH monitoring technologies [4]. The study contained only seven peer-reviewed articles. Interestingly, no study measured direct observation. In this review, the authors divided the studies into three categories: studies using hand hygiene monitoring technologies (HHMT) that provided real-time reminders without feedback, studies using HHMT that provided feedback without reminders, and studies using HHMT that provided both feedback and real-time reminders. The second group included three studies but only two with interpretable results. The studies in this group showed an important and prolonged increase in hand hygiene with an increase in HH from 6.5 to 81% [5] and from 30 to 82% [6], respectively. In addition, in both studies, the compliance percentage remained around 80% for 75% and 48 weeks, respectively.

Another systematic review found that in four studies, there was no difference in the HH compliance rates achieved with direct observation versus any other newer technology [7].

Methods for Monitoring HH Compliance

Direct Observation

This is the current gold standard for HH monitoring and allows evaluation of proper HH technique. Its main disadvantage is the possibility of Hawthorne effect [8] which can be prevented by the use of covert observers as it was demonstrated at a Taiwanese hospital where covered observers found a 44% HH compliance rate versus 74% and 94% rates recorded by non-covert observers (i.e., infection control nurses and HH ambassadors) [9]. Furthermore, direct observation is subject to observer interpretation, lack of experience, and fatigue. The latter issue becomes very important as many observers may not be able to adequately capture all events for long periods of time. Recently, there has been a development of a number of electronic apps such as iScrub [10] that replace the role of pencil and pen allowing a more convenient and standardized recording. Some propose that, given the popularity use of smartphones and devices, this modality of recording could provide more accurate rates and decrease the Hawthorne effect.

C.D. Jarrin Tejada (✉)
2057 Wiltshire Road, Berkley, MI 48072, USA
e-mail: claudiajarrin@gmail.com

© Springer International Publishing AG 2018
G. Bearman et al. (eds.), *Infection Prevention*, DOI 10.1007/978-3-319-60980-5_2

Measuring Product Consumption

The measurement of HH product consumption indirectly assesses HH compliance by measuring weight or volume of product used or the amounts purchased [11] and should be used in conjunction with other modalities. There are several studies using electronic counters placed in alcohol rub dispensers, but usually data from these counters does not correlate with data from direct observation [8]. For instance, a study comparing rates of HH via disinfectant usage versus direct observation in two units found a twofold difference between these two methods. Compliance measured by disinfectant usage was around 21% and 24% versus 43% and 47% measured by direct observation [12].

Moreover, when compared to direct observation or video surveillance techniques, measuring product consumption does not identify the individual performing HH nor does it provide information on the HH technique [3, 8], missing opportunity for feedback. This method, however, is particularly useful when comparing pre- and post-intervention results [13, 14].

The cost of installing these monitoring devices in one patient unit ranges from $30,000 to 40,000 [13]. In addition, battery monitoring for both electronic dispenser counters and automated monitoring devices is also critical in order to prevent gaps or inaccurate measurements. A study performed at a hospital in Brazil measured HH compliance at two hospital entrances using video surveillance and electronic counters in alcohol dispensers via radio-frequency identification. The cost for each device was of $1500. In this study there is also an important discrepancy between the rates measured by the electronic devices (16 and 8%) and those measured by the human observer (1.25 and 0.82%). It is important to note that this study involved anyone who entered the hospital, not just healthcare workers [15].

In summary, given its many potential pitfalls such as poor correlation between HH by direct observation and product consumption and inability to determine the individual and technique for performing HH, this method should be used in conjunction with others and can be very useful in measuring post-intervention results.

Video Surveillance and Feedback

The two major quasi-experimental studies on video-monitored direct observation, by Armellino et al. [5] and Davis et al. [16], show very different rates in increased compliance: an approximate 70% increase in the study by the former author and 40% increase in the study by the latter. Of note, only the second study used covert cameras.

In the first study, independent auditors reviewed clips that recorded HH at room entry and exit. Importantly, during the study real-time feedback was provided. The authors divided the study in three periods: a 16-week pre-feedback period, a 16-week post-feedback period, and a 75-week maintenance period. Hand hygiene compliance rates in each period were 6.5%, 81.5%, and 88%, respectively. These results show the importance of real-time feedback not only in achieving important increases in HH compliance but also in providing long-term benefits. The installation of video cameras in one unit costs about $50,000 dollars. As a side note, the pre-study internal hospital-based HH rates collected by direct observation were 60% (vs. <10% recorded in the pre-feedback period) [5].

The study by Davis et al. had two periods: a 6-month pre-intervention and a 6-month post-intervention period. Covert cameras were implemented in a surgical ICU, and the intervention consisted on the placement of red tape on the floor which directed individuals to use the hand rub dispenser. A hand hygiene compliance rate of 24% was recorded in the first period which went up to 62% during the intervention [16].

As described above, this technology has certainly showed increases in HH compliance, especially with the addition of real-time feedback. An important downside of this technology is the lack of patient privacy due to the installed cameras, which, concomitantly, may contribute to the Hawthorne effect.

Electronic Surveillance and Alerts

Technology has allowed the development of motion sensors capable of detecting room entry and exit, as well as sensors attached to badges worn by the HCW and to sinks or alcohol dispensers which can capture when HH is performed via Wi-Fi, radio-frequency identification (RFID), ANT, and ZigBee [17] and transmitted to a central server. Some authors recommend the use of two wireless systems to capture HH in order to assure the most accurate results.

These devices can also provide real-time feedback in the form of visual or auditory alerts which have been proven to increase HH compliance rates with promising results [17–20]. For instance, the use of alcohol-sensing badge has been implemented with a 26% increase in compliance among HCW [18]. During this study, HCW had to hold his or her hands after HH. If alcohol was sensed by the badges, a green light would appear, if not, a red light and a beep would appear. The type of alert (i.e., vibration vs. sound) is also important as it may interfere with patient care. Venkatesh et al. implemented real-time feedback via automatic beeps or voice alerts at a hematology unit and noted and increase in HH compliance rates from 38 to 62%. Importantly, there was a temporary, nonstatistically significant, reduction in the rate of VRE transmission during the intervention period [19].

Two studies, however, have shown significant differences in measurements by these automated systems when compared to direct observation. In Swoboda's study, phase 1 monitoring devices measured a compliance of approximately 20% vs. 44% obtained by direct observation [21]. Similarly, the network system used by Cheng et al. showed a higher compliance measured by direct observation (95%) than by technology (88%) [22].

Other limitations of wireless HH surveillance technologies include the need for a specific infrastructure; high cost (RFID); the need for batteries (all but RFID), computers, and onboard storage; and sensing a false event by proximity.

Electronic surveillance is a promising technology as it provides real-time assessment of compliance allowing for feedback opportunities, and it has been proven to capture 95–100% of HH events. Importantly, it does not capture WHO moments 2 and 3 for HH. Its biggest limitation is the cost which varies among the different systems used.

Summary

Hand hygiene is critical in preventing the transmission of infections. It is of utmost importance in this era of multidrug resistance. Unfortunately, rates among HCW remain less than 50% in the majority of studies. Direct observation remains the gold standard method for monitoring, and new technologies include video surveillance and electronic monitors. With these recent developments, feedback, especially, real-time, has become extremely useful in increasing the rates. Some studies have even shown a sustained increase over time when real-time feedback is implemented. The main limitations of the newer methods include cost and the need for special infrastructure which prevent their implementation in limited resource settings. Therefore, it is important to keep in mind that while monitoring and feedback are important, HH education at early stages, such as during early years of medical and/or nursing school, plays a very important role in achieving good rates of HH compliance and therefore, preventing nosocomial infections.

References

1. World Health Organization. WHO guidelines on hand hygiene in health care: first global patient safety challenge clean care is safer care. Geneva: World Health Organization; 2009. p. 16. Hand hygiene practices among health-care workers and adherence to recommendations. Available from: http://www-ncbi-nlm-nih-gov.proxy.library.vcu.edu/books/NBK144026/. Accessed 16 Mar 2014.
2. Jabbar U, Leischner J, Kasper D, et al. Effectiveness of alcohol-based hand rubs for removal of *Clostridium difficile* spores from hands. Infect Control Hosp Epidemiol. 2010;31:565–70.
3. The Joint Commission. Measuring hand hygiene adherence: overcoming the challenges. In: Developing a strategy for measuring hand hygiene. The Joint Commission. (2009). http://www.jointcommission.org/assets/1/18/hh_monograph.pdf. Accessed 16 Mar 2014.
4. Srigley JA, Gardam M, Fernie G, et al. Hand hygiene monitoring technology: a systematic review of efficacy. J Hosp Infect. 2015;89:51–60.
5. Armellino D, Hussain E, Schilling ME. Using high-technology to enforce low-technology safety measures: the use of third-party remote video auditing and real-time feedback in healthcare. Clin Infect Dis. 2012;54:1–7.
6. Armellino D, Trivedi M, Law I, et al. Replicating changes in hand hygiene in a surgical intensive care unit with remote video auditing and feedback. Am J Infect Control. 2013;41:925–7.
7. Ward MA, Schweizer ML, Polgreen PM, et al. Automated and electronically assisted hand hygiene monitoring systems: a systematic review. Am J Infect Control. 2014;42:472–8.
8. Boyce JM. Measuring healthcare worker hand hygiene activity: current practices and emerging technologies. Infect Control Hosp Epidemiol. 2011;32:1016–28.
9. Pan SC, Tien KL, Hung IC, et al. Compliance of health care workers with hand hygiene practices: independent advantages of overt and covert observers. PLoS ONE. 2013;8:e53746. doi:10.1371/journal.pone.0053746.
10. Marra AR, Camargo TZ, Cardoso VJ, et al. Hand hygiene compliance in the critical care setting: a comparative study of 2 different alcohol handrub formulations. Am J Infect Control. 2013;41:136–9.
11. Jarrin Tejada C, Bearman G. Hand hygiene compliance monitoring: the state of the art. Curr Infect Dis Rep. 2015;17:16.
12. Scheithauer S, Oberröhrmann A, Haefner H. Compliance with hand hygiene in patients with methicillin-resistant *Staphylococcus aureus* and extended-spectrum β-lactamase-producing enterobacteria. J Hosp Infect. 2010;76:320–3.
13. Morgan DJ, Pineles L, Shardell M, et al. Automated hand hygiene count devices may better measure compliance than human observation. Am J Infect Control. 2012;40:955–9.
14. Marra AR, Moura DF Jr, Paes AT, et al. Measuring rates of hand hygiene adherence in the intensive care setting: a comparative study of direct observation, product usage and electronic counting devices. Infect Control Hosp Epidemiol. 2010;31:796–801.
15. Vaidotas M, Yokota PK, Marra AR, et al. Measuring hand hygiene compliance rates at hospital entrances. Am J Infect Control. 2015;43:694–6.
16. Davis CR. Infection-free surgery: how to improve hand-hygiene compliance and eradicate methicillin-resistant *Staphylococcus aureus* from surgical wards. Ann R Coll Surg Engl. 2010;92:316–9.
17. Polgreen PM, Hlady CS, Severson MA, et al. Method for automated monitoring of hand hygiene adherence with our radio-frequency identification. Infect Control Hosp Epidemiol. 2010;31:1294–7.
18. Edmond MD, Goodell A, Zuelzer W, et al. Successful use of alcohol sensor technology to monitor and report hand hygiene compliance. J Hosp Infect. 2010;76:364–5.
19. Venkatesh AK, Lankford MG, Rooney DM, et al. Use of electronic alerts to enhance hand hygiene compliance and decrease transmission of vancomycin-resistant *Enterococcus* in a hematology unit. Am J Infect Control. 2008;36:199–205.
20. Pineles LL, Morgan DJ, Limper HM, et al. Accuracy of a radio-frequency identification (RFID) badge system to monitor hand hygiene behavior during routine clinical activities. Am J Infect Control. 2014;42:144–7.
21. Swoboda SM, Earsing K, Strauss K, et al. Electronic monitoring and voice prompts improve hand hygiene and decrease nosocomial infections in an intermediate care unit. Crit Care Med. 2004;32:358–63.
22. Cheng VC, Tai JW, Ho SK, et al. Introduction of an electronic monitoring system for monitoring compliance with moments 1 and 4 of the WHO "My 5 moments for hand hygiene" methodology. BMC Infect Dis. 2011;11:151.

Universal Glove and Gown Use for the Prevention of Methicillin-Resistant *Staphylococcus aureus* (MRSA) or Vancomycin-Resistant *Enterococcus* (VRE)

3

Lindsay Croft and Daniel J. Morgan

Background

Over 100,000 healthcare-associated infections (HAIs) occur in the USA annually [1]. Many are caused by multidrug-resistant organisms (MDROs) like methicillin-resistant *Staphylococcus aureus* (MRSA) and vancomycin-resistant *Enterococcus* (VRE) [1, 2]. MRSA and VRE are associated with worse outcomes than antibiotic-sensitive counterparts [3, 4], and the estimated cost of antibiotic resistance in the USA is more than $4 billion per year [5].

Transmission of MRSA and VRE in healthcare settings is believed to occur from patient to patient through contamination of healthcare workers (HCWs) and the environment [6]. Patients who are colonized with MRSA or VRE commonly contaminate the room environment, and HCWs leaving the rooms of these patients are contaminated 10–25% of the time [7–10].

The use of gloves and gowns as a barrier to contamination is a commonly employed method for preventing transmission of MRSA, VRE, and other pathogens [11]. Theoretically, this barrier will become contaminated during care but will be removed at room exit, reducing burden of HCW contamination. By reducing HCW contamination, gloves and gowns should decrease the likelihood of contaminating subsequent patients. Gloves and gowns are recommended as a part of standard precautions for any patient with uncontrolled secretions and as a part of contact precautions for MDROs of importance, such as MRSA or VRE [11]. Evidence for effectiveness of contact precautions is limited, leading to various interpretations of CDC guidance [12, 13]. Gloves and gowns can also be used in a universal fashion in which all HCWs use gloves and gowns for every patient contact or room entry regardless of colonization or infection with an MDRO. Universal glove and gown (UGG) use has been employed in relatively limited fashion in response to outbreaks or in specific hospital units with high risk of spread for MDROs [14–18]. A recent randomized cluster trial found universal glove and gown use in intensive care units had no impact on the primary outcome of MRSA or VRE acquisition but appeared to decrease MRSA in secondary analysis [14].

Policies

Universal glove and gown use is not part of CDC recommendations [11]. SHEA recommendations for MRSA prevention include UGG as an option for "special approaches" where endemic MRSA rates are not effectively controlled despite compliance with basic practices [19]. "Special approaches include recommendations where the intervention is likely to reduce HAI risk but where there is concern about the risks for undesirable outcomes, where the quality of evidence is low, or where evidence supports the impact of the intervention in select settings." The evidence for using UGG for all patient contact and the patient care environment was rated moderate.

Controversies (Table 3.1)

Effectiveness of Universal Glove and Gown Use

Beyond the Benefits of Universal Glove and Gown (BUGG) cluster trial finding a decrease in MRSA as a secondary outcome, follow-up of five sites compared UGG intervention-phase HCW clothing contamination to post-intervention usual

L. Croft
Division of Epidemiology, Department of Internal Medicine,
University of Utah School of Medicine, Salt Lake City, UT, USA
e-mail: lindsay.croft@hsc.utah.edu

D.J. Morgan (✉)
Departments of Epidemiology, Public Health and Medicine,
University of Maryland School of Medicine and Baltimore
VA Medical Center, 10 S. Pine Street, MSTF 334, Baltimore,
MD 21201, USA
e-mail: dmorgan@som.umaryland.edu

© Springer International Publishing AG 2018
G. Bearman et al. (eds.), *Infection Prevention*, DOI 10.1007/978-3-319-60980-5_3

Table 3.1 Controversies related to universal glove and gown use

Controversial subject	Argument for	Argument against
Prevents endemic MRSA or VRE	Gloves and gown are theoretically effective as a barrier to MRSA and VRE, which frequently contaminate HCWs. MRSA acquisition decreased in the BUGG randomized controlled trial (RCT)	The primary outcome of BUGG study was no effect on MRSA or VRE acquisition. Practice is laborious and expensive
Causes adverse events and other harm	UGG is similar to contact precautions which may cause adverse events	A cluster RCT found a trend toward fewer adverse events with UGG. Many nonrandomized studies showing an increase in events have uncontrolled confounding from severity of illness
Improves hand hygiene	In BUGG RCT as well as observational studies of contact precautions, better hand hygiene compliance noted	HCWs will believe hands are clean due to glove use and will not perform hand hygiene

care and found a 70% relative reduction in HCW clothing contamination with UGG (7.1% of HCW clothing contaminated during UGG; 23% during usual care) [20]. Another single-center outbreak study which employed UGG for an outbreak of *A. baumannii* found UGG reduced VRE and MRSA acquisition over a 6-month period [18]. Likewise, a small individual-level patient trial from the 1980s found that children requiring mechanical ventilation and at least 3-day intensive care unit (ICU) stay randomized to either standard care or empiric gloving and gowning had a significant delay in median time to nosocomial colonization when gloving and gowning was used [17]. Likewise, in a burn unit, an MRSA outbreak was rapidly terminated after implementing UGG with all patients (rate ratio [R_tR] post-outbreak endemic rate vs. baseline, 0.48; 95% confidence interval [CI], 0.14–1.53; $p = 0.10$) [16]. A similar intervention of universal glove use during respiratory syncytial virus (RSV) season versus standard care during non-RSV time periods was evaluated in a retrospective cohort of all patients in a tertiary care hospital's pediatric units from 2002 to 2010 [15]. They found that overall risk of HAI was 25% lower during universal gloving versus non-glove time periods (relative risk [RR], 0.75; 95% CI, 0.69–0.93; $p = 0.01$). Universal gloving was also evaluated during a before-after study in a single ICU. This study found no difference in rate of MDRO acquisition when emollient-impregnated universal gloving was used rather than contact precautions [21].

In nursing homes, patients at high risk of infection were assigned to UGG regardless of colonization status with MRSA or VRE in a bundled intervention [22]. Investigators found a decrease in both prevalence density of MDROs (R_tR 0.77; 95% CI 0.62–0.94) and MRSA acquisition in the intervention compared to control nursing homes (RtR 0.78; 95% CI, 0.64–0.96).

However, many studies have raised questions over the effectiveness of UGG. In the only cluster trial of UGG, no decrease was noted for the primary outcome of composite VRE or MRSA (1.71 fewer acquisitions per 1000 person-days with UGG but $p = 0.57$). There was also no decrease in the secondary outcome of VRE acquisition (0.89 fewer acquisitions per 1000 person-days with UGG compared to usual care, $p = 0.70$) and only a possible decrease in the secondary outcome of MRSA acquisition (2.98 fewer acquisitions per 1000 person-days with UGG, $p = 0.046$; reduction in acquisition from baseline to end of intervention period of 40.2% in UGG and 15% in control) [14]. Other studies have found a lack of effect with universal glove and gown or universal gloving. In a single ICU cohort study, no difference was noted among eight beds assigned to UGG (93 patients) and eight beds assigned to universal gloving (88 patients) [23]. Twenty-four patients (25.8%) in UGG acquired VRE, while 21 patients (23.9%) in glove-only acquired VRE ($p > 0.05$). In a medical intensive care unit study comparing 3 months of CDC guideline contact precautions to 3 months of universal gloving, there was no difference in VRE acquisition (14% universal glove vs. 18% standard contact precautions; $p = 0.19$) or MRSA acquisition (5.0% universal glove vs. 5.7% standard contact precautions; $p = 0.92$) [24]. In addition, the rate of bloodstream infections was actually higher in the universal glove phase (14.1 vs. 6.2 per 1,000 device days; $p < 0.001$). One difficulty in interpreting results of these studies is that the comparison of UGG to universal gloving would require gowns to add meaningful extra benefit beyond the contribution of glove use in order to show an effect.

The STAR*ICU trial was a cluster randomized trial which investigated an intervention of placing all patients on universal gloving until discharge or admission surveillance cultures were reported negative. The study found no difference in MRSA or VRE colonization or infection rate [25].

A 2015 Cochrane systematic review of contact precautions (not UGG) found great variation in studies and comparison groups, potential sources of bias, low intervention effectiveness, etc. and concluded no recommendation for or against CP effectiveness could be made [26].

Cost-Effectiveness of Universal Glove and Gown

The cost-effectiveness of UGG has been debated with some results suggesting it could be more cost-effective than other interventions. One systematic review of MRSA infection control interventions looked at cost-benefit analyses [27].

Contact precautions were implemented preemptively (until test results were known) in 12 studies, although all of the studies employed bundled interventions, making it difficult to assess how much of the effect (and cost) was due to UGG versus other aspects. In the review, the cost-benefit ratio varied wildly from 1.7 times higher cost than savings to 13.5 times savings with intervention employing preemptive gown and glove use. In contrast, Gidengil et al. used a hypothetical 10,000-person cohort to model the cost-effectiveness of various infection control approaches for MRSA and concluded that UGG was not cost-effective [28]. While UGG averted 387 cases of MRSA colonization and 107 infections, UGG as a lone intervention cost an estimated $8.15 million, while MRSA disease cost was $6.58 million.

Possible Unintended Consequences/Adverse Events from UGG

Only one study of adults has examined possible harms related to UGG. In the BUGG trial, fewer HCW visits per hour were noted among UGG units (4.28 visits vs. 5.24 visits per hour; $p = 0.02$) [14]. This study also found no statistical difference in adverse events and a trend toward fewer adverse events with UGG (58.7 adverse events per 1000 patient-days among UGG vs. 74.4 per 1000 patient-days with usual care; $p = 0.24$). Most studies of adverse events are with contact precautions. However, association between gloving and gowning and adverse events has not been identified for UGG. In the study of pediatric empiric gloving and gowning versus standard care, Klein et al. found that children in each group were touched and handled with the same frequency [17].

Studies of contact precautions have found more potential negative effects of gloves and gowns (although also had more bias toward being applied to sicker patients) [29]. Forty-six (59%) physicians surveyed in one study reported they were less likely to examine isolated patients [30]. Likewise, greater depression, anxiety, and adverse events have been reported in some studies. In a retrospective cohort study, Stelfox et al. reported a doubling in rate of adverse events and an almost sevenfold increase in preventable adverse events among patients placed on contact precautions compared to non-isolated [31]. Day et al. observed higher depression scores in veterans on contact precautions [32] as well as among patients placed on contact precautions at an academic medical center [33]. In addition, lower patient satisfaction has been noted with contact precautions, with isolated patients being twice as likely to report concerns with care [34]. Some have also argued that the use of contact precautions may interfere with a homelike environment in long-term care facilities (LTCFs) [35].

Hand hygiene has been generally noted to increase with universal glove and gown use, especially upon room exit [14, 36]. Some studies report increases in HH compliance with UGG as compared to traditional contact precautions or with usual care [14, 21]. Others report no change. While one quasi-experimental study of universal gloving compared to traditional contact precautions found a significant decrease in hand hygiene with universal gloving [24], a cluster trial found hand hygiene compliance was higher with UGG (78.3% UGG vs. 62.9% control; $p = 0.02$) [14].

A possible effect of UGG relates to compliance. Requiring gloves and gowns for contact with all patients might result in lower compliance. The STAR*ICU trial noted lower compliance with universal gloving than with contact precautions; the median compliance for contact precautions in intervention ICUs was 82% for gloves, 77% for gowns, and 69% for hand hygiene. However, for universal gloving in intervention ICUs, compliance was 72% for gloves and 62% for hand hygiene [25]. Issues with compliance may especially be the case outside of clinical studies with increased attention to compliance.

The simplicity of universal glove and gown has been proposed as a benefit. Instead of relying on active surveillance, which can be laborious and expensive, UGG could be implemented. Furthermore, this overcomes the weakness of active surveillance that colonized patients will not be isolated rapidly [37]. Active surveillance followed by usual contact precautions is not cost-effective. Modeling suggests universal MRSA screening followed by contact precautions for positives would be a net loss to a hospital of approximately $104,000 per 10,000 admissions (95% CI, $83,000–126,000) [38].

Practical Resolutions

Universal glove and gown use is one of the most rigorously tested interventions for infection control. Results of the BUGG study did not find strong evidence that it prevents MRSA and VRE, but UGG likely has some benefit on MRSA acquisition. MRSA acquisition under endemic settings is relatively rare, and only a portion of those patients develop actual infection with MRSA. The intervention of UGG is labor and resource intense and not easily implemented.

Institution-specific decisions relating to UGG should be based on endemic MRSA rates after compliance with standard precautions and/or traditional contact precautions has been maximized or considered for use in higher risk populations. UGG may have a favorable effort to effect ratio in situations such as outbreaks [16, 18] or for high-risk patient groups such as those with recent skin abscesses [39] or high-risk LTCF residents [22].

Future Research

Given the strength of the BUGG RCT, it is unlikely there will be further trials for UGG. Observational or quasi-experimental studies could be helpful for examining the effect on specific pathogens or settings where UGG would be most useful. A randomized cluster trial of the related, and controversial, intervention of contact precautions versus standard precautions for endemic MRSA or VRE would advance the field of infection control approaches [19].

Conclusions

Despite obvious theoretical benefits to UGG as a barrier to transmission, real-world effects on preventing infections are likely modest and limited to MRSA. Given staff effort and resources, UGG is unlikely to be adopted in hospitals beyond outbreaks or in patients with high risk of infection.

References

1. Magill SS, Edwards JR, Bamberg W, Beldavs ZG, Dumyati G, Kainer MA, Lynfield R, Maloney M, McAllister-Hollod L, Nadle J, Ray SM, Thompson DL, Wilson LE, Fridkin SK, Emerging Infections Program Healthcare-Associated Infections and Antimicrobial Use Prevalence Survey Team. Multistate point-prevalence survey of health care-associated infections. N Engl J Med. 2014;370:1198–208.
2. Dantes R, Mu Y, Belflower R, et al. National burden of invasive methicillin-resistant Staphylococcus aureus infections, United States, 2011. JAMA Intern Med. 2013;173:1970–8.
3. Cosgrove SE, Sakoulas G, Perencevich EN, Schwaber MJ, Karchmer AW, Carmeli Y. Comparison of mortality associated with methicillin-resistant and methicillin-susceptible Staphylococcus aureus bacteremia: a meta-analysis. Clin Infect Dis. 2003;36:53–9.
4. DiazGranados CA, Jernigan JA. Impact of vancomycin resistance on mortality among patients with neutropenia and enterococcal bloodstream infection. J Infect Dis. 2005;191:588–95.
5. Talbot GH, Bradley J, Edwards JE Jr, et al. Bad bugs need drugs: an update on the development pipeline from the antimicrobial availability task force of the Infectious Diseases Society of America. Clin Infect Dis. 2006;42:657–68.
6. Siegel JD, Rhinehart E, Jackson M, Chiarello L, Healthcare Infection Control Practices Advisory Committee. Management of multidrug-resistant organisms in health care settings, 2006. Am J Infect Control. 2007;35:S165–93.
7. Morgan DJ, Rogawski E, Thom KA, et al. Transfer of multidrug-resistant bacteria to healthcare workers' gloves and gowns after patient contact increases with environmental contamination. Crit Care Med. 2012;40:1045–51.
8. Morgan DJ, Liang SY, Smith CL, et al. Frequent multidrug-resistant Acinetobacter baumannii contamination of gloves, gowns, and hands of healthcare workers. Infect Control Hosp Epidemiol. 2010;31:716–21.
9. Hayden MK, Blom DW, Lyle EA, Moore CG, Weinstein RA. Risk of hand or glove contamination after contact with patients colonized with vancomycin-resistant Enterococcus or the colonized patients' environment. Infect Control Hosp Epidemiol. 2008;29:149–54.
10. Snyder GM, Thom KA, Furuno JP, et al. Detection of methicillin-resistant Staphylococcus aureus and vancomycin-resistant enterococci on the gowns and gloves of healthcare workers. Infect Control Hosp Epidemiol. 2008;29:583–9.
11. Siegel J, Rhinehart E, Jackson M, Chiarello L. 2007 guideline for isolation precautions: preventing transmission of infectious agents in health care settings. Am J Infect Control. 2007;35:S65–164.
12. Morgan DJ, Murthy R, Munoz-Price LS, et al. Reconsidering contact precautions for endemic methicillin-resistant Staphylococcus aureus and vancomycin-resistant Enterococcus. Infect Control Hosp Epidemiol. 2015;36:1163–72.
13. Morgan DJ, Kaye KS, Diekema DJ. Reconsidering isolation precautions for endemic methicillin-resistant I and vancomycin-resistant Enterococcus. JAMA. 2014;312:1395–6.
14. Harris AD, Pineles L, Belton B, et al. Universal glove and gown use and acquisition of antibiotic-resistant bacteria in the ICU: a randomized trial. JAMA. 2013;310:1571–80.
15. Yin J, Schweizer M, Herwaldt L, Pottinger J, Perencevich E. Benefits of universal gloving on hospital-acquired infections in acute care pediatric units. Pediatrics. 2013;131:e1515–20.
16. Safdar N, Marx J, Meyer N, Maki D. Effectiveness of preemptive barrier precautions in controlling nosocomial colonization and infection by methicillin-resistant Staphylococcus aureus in a burn unit. Am J Infect Control. 2006;34:476–83.
17. Klein BS, Perloff WH, Maki DG. Reduction of nosocomial infection during pediatric intensive care by protective isolation. N Engl J Med. 1989;320:1714–21.
18. Wright M, Hebden JN, Harris AD, et al. Aggressive control measures for resistant Acinetobacter baumannii and the impact on acquisition of methicillin-resistant Staphylococcus aureus and vancomycin-resistant Enterococcus in a medical intensive care unit. Infect Control Hosp Epidemiol. 2004;25:167–8.
19. Calfee DP, Salgado CD, Milstone AM, et al. Strategies to prevent methicillin-resistant Staphylococcus aureus transmission and infection in acute care hospitals: 2014 update. Infect Control Hosp Epidemiol. 2014;35:S108–32.
20. Williams C, McGraw P, Schneck EE, et al. Impact of universal gowning and gloving on health care worker clothing contamination. Infect Control Hosp Epidemiol. 2015;36:431–7.
21. Bearman G, Rosato AE, Duane TM, et al. Trial of universal gloving with emollient-impregnated gloves to promote skin health and prevent the transmission of multidrug-resistant organisms in a surgical intensive care unit. Infect Control Hosp Epidemiol. 2010;31:491–7.
22. Mody L, Krein SL, Saint SK, et al. A targeted infection prevention intervention in nursing home residents with indwelling devices: a randomized clinical trial. JAMA Intern Med. 2015;175:714–23.
23. Slaughter S, Hayden MK, Nathan C, et al. A comparison of the effect of universal use of gloves and gowns with that of glove use alone on acquisition of vancomycin-resistant enterococci in a medical intensive care unit. Ann Intern Med. 1996;125:448–56.
24. Bearman GM, Marra AR, Sessler CN, et al. A controlled trial of universal gloving versus contact precautions for preventing the transmission of multidrug-resistant organisms. Am J Infect Control. 2007;35:650–5.
25. Huskins WC, Huckabee CM, O'Grady NP, et al. Intervention to reduce transmission of resistant bacteria in intensive care. N Engl J Med. 2011;364:1407–18.
26. Cohen C, Cohen B, Shang J. Effectiveness of contact precautions against multidrug-resistant organism transmission in acute care: a systematic review of the literature. J Hosp Infect. 2015;90:275–84.
27. Farbman L, Avni T, Rubinovitch B, Leibovici L, Paul M. Cost–benefit of infection control interventions targeting methicillin-resistant Staphylococcus aureus in hospitals: systematic review. Clin Microbiol Infect. 2013;19:E582–93.
28. Gidengil CA, Gay C, Huang SS, Platt R, Yokoe D, Lee GM. Cost-effectiveness of strategies to prevent methicillin-resistant Staphylococcus aureus transmission and infection in an intensive care unit. Infect Control Hosp Epidemiol. 2015;36:17–27.
29. Morgan DJ, Diekema DJ, Sepkowitz K, Perencevich EN. Adverse outcomes associated with contact precautions: a review of the literature. Am J Infect Control. 2009;37:85–93.

30. Khan FA, Khakoo RA, Hobbs GR. Impact of contact isolation on health care workers at a tertiary care center. Am J Infect Control. 2006;34:408–13.
31. Stelfox H, Bates D, Redelmeier D. Safety of patients isolated for infection control. JAMA. 2003;290:1899–905.
32. Day H, Morgan D, Himelhoch S, Young A, Perencevich E. Association between depression and contact precautions in veterans at hospital admission. Am J Infect Control. 2011;39:163–5.
33. Day HR, Perencevich EN, Harris AD, et al. Do contact precautions cause depression? A two-year study at a tertiary care medical centre. J Hosp Infect. 2011;79:103–7.
34. Mehrotra P, Croft L, Day H, Perencevich E, Pineles L, Harris A, Weingart S, Morgan D. Effects of contact precautions on patient perception of care and satisfaction: a prospective cohort study. Infect Control Hosp Epidemiol. 2013;34:1087–93.
35. Stone ND. Revisiting standard precautions to reduce antimicrobial resistance in nursing homes. JAMA Intern Med. 2015;175:723–4.
36. Morgan D, Pineles L, Shardell M, et al. The effect of contact precautions on healthcare worker activity in acute care hospitals. Infect Control Hosp Epidemiol. 2013;34:69–73.
37. Kypraios T, D O'Neill P, Huang SS, Rifas-Shiman SL, Cooper BS. Assessing the role of undetected colonization and isolation precautions in reducing methicillin-resistant Staphylococcus aureus transmission in intensive care units. BMC Infect Dis. 2010;10:1.
38. McKinnell JA, Bartsch SM, Lee BY, Huang SS, Miller LG. Cost-benefit analysis from the hospital perspective of universal active screening followed by contact precautions for methicillin-resistant Staphylococcus aureus carriers. Infect Control Hosp Epidemiol. 2015;36:2–13.
39. Talbot TR, Nania JJ, Wright PW, Jones I, Aronsky D. Evaluation of the microbiology of soft-tissue abscesses in the era of community-associated strains of methicillin-resistant Staphylococcus aureus: an argument for empirical contact precautions. Infect Control Hosp Epidemiol. 2007;28:730–2.

Isolation Precautions for Visitors to Healthcare Settings

Maroun Sfeir, Matthew S. Simon, and David Banach

Introduction

Transmission of infectious organisms within healthcare settings is an increasingly recognized threat to the safety of patients and healthcare personnel. There has been much attention on healthcare providers as potential vectors of infection transmission and many infection-prevention strategies focus on this population. However, visitation to healthcare facilities by individuals other than healthcare personnel is common. Additionally, hospital visitors spend significant time with patients within the healthcare setting, often for longer periods than healthcare personnel [1]. Data on the topic remains sparse, though the Society of Healthcare Epidemiology of America (SHEA) has recently issued guidance on the topic to assist healthcare institutions in addressing specific infection control questions pertinent to visitors [2]. The goal of this chapter is to review the potential role of visitors in the transmission of organisms in the healthcare setting and address specific situations in which infection prevention strategies may be appropriate in order to protect both patients and visitors.

Visitors and Transmission/Outbreaks

Visitors to healthcare facilities have been linked to hospital-acquired infections and rarely healthcare-associated infection outbreaks. Such events have been infrequently reported in the medical literature, but underreporting and the inherent difficulty in proving transmission from hospital visitors to patients and/or healthcare personnel likely underestimate the frequency of such occurrences. More commonly, it is suspected that visitors play a role in the initiation or propagation of a healthcare-associated infection outbreak. For this reason, visitor restriction is one commonly employed strategy as part of an outbreak response plan.

Nosocomial transmission of *Mycobacterium tuberculosis* has been clearly linked to hospital visitors. Since adults are more likely than children to be infectious with active tuberculosis, recognition of symptomatic disease in visitors accompanying suspected pediatric tuberculosis patients is crucial for infection prevention and control efforts. At a pediatric hospital, 24 pediatric patients developed active tuberculosis after exposure to a patient's mother with cavitary pulmonary disease [3]. Another report documented the development of latent tuberculosis infection in two hospital contacts of a visitor with active pulmonary disease on a pediatric ward [4]. Data suggests the parents or other primary caregivers are commonly the source of infection in pediatric patients with active tuberculosis [5]. Over a 6-year period, investigators at a children's hospital in Texas prospectively screened adults accompanying children with suspected tuberculosis to determine the frequency of undiagnosed disease in visitors. Of 105 adults screened, 16 (15%) had previously undetected pulmonary tuberculosis. These adults were associated with 14 (24%) of the 59 children admitted to the hospital with suspected tuberculosis during the study period. Consequently, the US Centers for Disease Control and Prevention (CDC) recommends screening the caregivers of pediatric tuberculosis patients for active disease [6]. Infection control practitioners should be aware of the strong association between pediatric tuberculosis and active disease in family members, recognize the risk of transmission from these visitors to other patients and staff, develop protocols for the screening of visitors when tuberculosis is suspected in a pediatric patient, and facilitate prompt evaluation and/or reporting to local public health departments when indicated.

Influenza and other respiratory viruses are likely the most common infections transmitted from visitors to

M. Sfeir (✉) • M.S. Simon
Department of Medicine, Division of Infectious Disease,
New York Presbyterian Hospital/Weill Cornell Medical Center,
New York, NY, USA
e-mail: mas9469@nyp.org; mss9008@med.cornell.edu

D. Banach
Infectious Diseases, University of Connecticut School of
Medicine, Farmington, CT, USA
e-mail: DBanach@uchc.edu

© Springer International Publishing AG 2018
G. Bearman et al. (eds.), *Infection Prevention*, DOI 10.1007/978-3-319-60980-5_4

patients due to their high seasonal prevalence, the potential for asymptomatic viral shedding, and the potential for indirect transmission from the environment. Following an outbreak of H3N2 influenza on a geriatric ward, genetic sequence analysis identified three distinct influenza clusters [7]. Two out of three were linked to healthcare personnel, while the third was assumed to be introduced by a visitor to the facility. Similarly, studies on the molecular and genetic diversity of nosocomial respiratory syncytial virus outbreaks suggest multiple strains tend to circulate during a hospital outbreak [8]. These data support the potential role visitors can play as a source of healthcare-associated transmission of respiratory viruses particularly when community prevalence is high. In one example during the 2009 H1N1 influenza pandemic, a hospital visitor was reported to be the source of an outbreak of six cases on a pediatric hematology-oncology ward [9]. Control measures included oseltamivir prophylaxis, isolation of cases, strict adherence to personal protective equipment, and visitor restriction. Visitor restriction has also been a key component in controlling respiratory syncytial virus, metapneumovirus, and parainfluenza outbreaks especially among immunocompromised patient populations [10]. Because visitor restriction typically occurs simultaneously with other control interventions, the incremental effectiveness of this measure on reducing transmission is difficult to ascertain.

A hospital outbreak of *Bordetella pertussis* was linked to a hospital visitor in at least one instance, and nosocomial transmission from visitors has been suspected in other outbreaks [11–13]. The hospital outbreak occurred following delayed diagnosis in the mother of a confirmed pertussis neonatal patient who was hospitalized in the pediatric intensive care unit. The patient's mother, who was later confirmed to have pertussis infection, was the likely source of infection for two other pediatric intensive care unit patients and five healthcare personnel.

Visitor restriction has been frequently employed to control healthcare-associated outbreaks of norovirus. Norovirus is capable of spreading rapidly through healthcare settings because of its low infectious dose and its ability to persist in the environment. As support for the effectiveness of visitor restrictions in decreasing the risk of norovirus transmission in healthcare settings, a prospective analysis of 49 nursing homes in the Netherlands found that restricting symptomatic visitors was the only control measure to significantly reduce the odds of norovirus acquisition in multivariate analysis [14]. In a large US hospital outbreak affecting over 500 patients and staff, all hospital visitations were temporarily restricted after transmission continued to occur following symptom screening of visitors [15]. The CDC's guidelines for norovirus prevention in healthcare settings include a category 1B recommendation to "Restrict nonessential visitors from affected areas of the facility during outbreaks of norovirus gastroenteritis [16]." If this is not practical or not deemed to be necessary, CDC recommends symptom screening and exclusion of visitor with symptoms consist with norovirus and ensuring visitor compliance with hand hygiene and contact precautions.

The outbreak of severe acute respiratory syndrome (SARS) virus is perhaps the most dramatic example that highlights the important role hospital visitors may play in the transmission and propagation of an infectious disease outbreak. Several reports documented visitors to healthcare settings acquiring SARS and becoming sources of transmission to patients, healthcare personnel, family members, and other community members [17, 18]. For instance, in Singapore, at least 21 SARS cases were reported resulting from transmission by hospital visitors to family and other community contacts [18]. Following recognition of the significance of visitors in SARS transmission dynamics, more stringent restrictions were placed on visitation. Visitors were tracked using logs and exposed visitors were quarantined. Visitors initially were allowed to visit SARS wards with full personal protective equipment, but due to continued transmission, all visitation at some affected hospitals was prohibited [18]. In Toronto, hospitals implemented a visitor and healthcare personnel screening with a questionnaire and temperature assessment prior to hospital entrance [19]. Visitors with concerning symptoms were referred to the emergency room. In Taiwan, infrared thermography was used to screen 72,327 outpatients and visitors over a 2-month period with identification of three probable SARS cases [20]. The lessons learned from SARS regarding the pivotal role visitors may play in the transmission of a communicable disease have informed public health guidance about more recent emerging infectious diseases such as Ebola and Middle East respiratory syndrome coronavirus (MERS-CoV).

Improved understanding of the role visitors play in healthcare-associated transmission of pathogens is an important area for further investigation, particularly as diagnostics are enhanced with routine use of rapid multiplex polymerase chain reaction assays in the clinical microbiology lab. Infection control practitioners play a vital role in engaging and educating healthcare personnel on the importance of screening visitors for communicable diseases and implementing and enforcing visitor restriction policies when necessary. The intensity of visitor symptom screening should be tailored based on individual hospital need and patient population. For instance, screening can be augmented for visitors to hospital locations with vulnerable patient populations such as neonates, the elderly, or immunocompromised particularly when community prevalence of respiratory viruses is high or when healthcare-associated transmission is recognized. Hospital administrators should support infection control programs to scale up enforcement of visitor-related infection control policies in such instances.

Visitors and Standard Precautions

In 2007, the CDC published a two-tiered strategy to prevent transmission of organisms throughout the healthcare setting focusing on standard precautions and transmission-based precautions [21]. Standard precautions are a group of infection prevention practices that apply to any individual who may have direct patient contact or contact with patient body fluids which may contain transmissible organisms. These include hand hygiene; respiratory cough etiquette; the use of barrier protection such as gloves, gowns, masks, or face shields depending on anticipated exposures; and safe injection practices. Although healthcare visitors do not usually have contact with blood, body fluids, or secretions and do not administer injections to patients, the practice of hand hygiene is an important infection prevention practice applicable to all hospital visitors. Respiratory etiquette among visitors will be discussed later in this chapter.

Hand Hygiene

Standard precautions remain the basic level of infection control in healthcare settings, and hand hygiene is an essential component of any infection prevention strategy [21]. The World Health Organization [22] and the CDC [23] have published evidence-based guidelines outlining essential components to hand hygiene in healthcare settings. These guidelines are focused on healthcare personnel though many of the principles can be applied to visitors to healthcare settings with contact with patients and the healthcare environment. These include the performance of hand hygiene before and after contact with patients, after any contact with patient body fluids, and after contact with the patient surrounding environment. Generally, use of either an alcohol-based hand hygiene product or soap and water is acceptable means of performing hand hygiene in most healthcare settings. Soap and water, when available, are preferred following contact with a patient with suspected or proven infection with a spore-forming organism such as *Clostridium difficile*.

Published data has shown that the hands of visitors are often colonized with multiple organisms including organisms of clinical significance and multidrug-resistant organisms and that hand hygiene can reduce the microbial burden on the hands of visitors [24]. There is limited data evaluating hand hygiene among visitors to healthcare settings, and most studies have been observational with significant heterogeneity in study design and setting. Generally, hand hygiene varied markedly between studies, usually lower than healthcare providers [25, 26], though a study in Japan showed high rates of adherence [27]. Increased hand hygiene rates have been identified among visitors to patients receiving care on contact precautions. Additionally, some interventional studies have shown that interventions can improve visitor adherence to hand hygiene practices [25, 26]. These include improving access to sinks and alcohol-based hand hygiene stations and the use of reminders to encourage visitors to perform hand hygiene before entering and after exiting patient rooms. The optimal strategy to encourage hand hygiene among visitors is unclear, but visual reminders through signs posted throughout the healthcare setting, verbal education, and reminders from healthcare personnel may improve hand hygiene rates among visitors.

Visitors and Contact Precautions

Contact precautions are measures used to prevent transmission of epidemiologically important organisms within the healthcare setting [21]. These precautions focus on organisms, usually antibiotic-resistant organisms, which are spread through direct contact between individuals or indirect contact with the organism through the patient environment. Care for patients in contact precautions is typically provided in a single room by healthcare personnel wearing barrier protection, including gloves and a protective gown when interacting with these patients or their environment.

The use of barrier precautions among visitors to healthcare settings remains a controversial topic, with very limited scientific literature to guide practices. Institutional decisions regarding the use of barrier precautions among visitors should take into account the organism of concern, the endemicity of the organism to a specific healthcare setting, as well as the likelihood of transmission to the visitor and other patients within the facility [2]. Organisms of high virulence with limited therapeutic options, including carbapenem-resistant *Enterobacteriaceae* (CRE), may warrant increased efforts to reduce spread including the use of barrier precautions among visitors. Gastrointestinal pathogens, including norovirus and *Clostridium difficile*, may infect and cause significant disease in normal hosts at a relatively high rate. Visitors to patients infected with these organisms may directly benefit from the use of barrier precautions in addition to standard precautions to prevent infecting themselves. Conversely, the benefit of barrier precautions use among visitors to patients with colonization or infection caused by methicillin-resistant *Staphylococcus aureus* (MRSA) or vancomycin-resistant enterococci (VRE), both endemic in many healthcare settings, may be limited. Many household contacts of these patients may likely be colonized themselves [28, 29]. However, in settings of suspected high rates of transmission of these organism within a healthcare setting (outbreak or epidemic), the use of barrier precautions among visitors may be appropriate in order to maximize attempts to reduce transmission.

Scabies and head lice are parasites that were described in hospital outbreaks where patients and visitors played a role in spreading the infection [30–32]. In order to prevent the spread of these ectoparasitic infections in the healthcare facility, contact precautions should be implemented for all visitors of patients with these infections until patients are treated because household members might not yet be infected or in the incubation period themselves. Symptomatic visitors should have visitation restricted until appropriate treatment has been initiated [21].

Additionally, in circumstances when visitors may be visiting multiple patients, such as clergy, adherence to contact precautions may be appropriate. These visitors have the potential to spread organisms, including multidrug-resistant organisms (MDRO), between patients within a healthcare facility and may be viewed in a manner similar to healthcare personnel. Institutions should attempt to identify these visitors and extend extra effort in educating them on infection prevention strategies.

Survey data suggests that visitors have an understanding of contact precautions and their role in preventing organism transmission [33]. Ensuring visitor adherence to contact precautions remains a consistent challenge in the healthcare setting. To date, most institutions do not routinely monitor visitor adherence to barrier precautions in the healthcare setting [2]. Additionally, published data on this topic is limited to observational studies in heterogeneous settings. Based on the available data, adherence to all components within contact precautions among visitors is low, particularly glove use and hand hygiene [34–36]. One study demonstrated higher rates of adherence to gown and glove use among visitors to patients in the intensive care unit compared to those on the medical wards [35]. Some studies included the use of gowns and gloves by visitors in the control of multidrug-resistant organisms but did not perform a separate analysis to determine whether their use by visitors had a measurable impact [37–39].

The overall risk of transmission associated of multidrug-resistant organisms through visitors as vectors as well as the optimal use of barrier precautions among healthcare visitors remain important areas of future study.

Visitors and Droplet Precautions

Droplet precautions are used when entering a room with a person with a respiratory infection by wearing a surgical mask [21]. Examples of infectious agents that are transmitted via the droplet route include *Bordetella pertussis* [40], influenza virus [41], adenovirus [40], rhinovirus [42], *Mycoplasma pneumoniae* [43], SARS-associated coronavirus (SARS-CoV) [44], group A streptococcus [45], and *Neisseria meningitides* [46]. Although respiratory syncytial virus may be transmitted by the droplet route, direct contact with infected respiratory secretions is the most important determinant of transmission, and consistent adherence to standard plus contact precautions is recommended to prevent transmission in healthcare settings [8]. SHEA suggests using surgical masks for visitors to rooms of patients on droplet precautions. Visitors of pediatric patients could be considered an exception because of the interference with bonding and the potential adverse psychological impact. Additionally, visitors who have had extensive exposure to the patient prior to hospitalization could also be considered an exception because they might either be immune to the infectious organism or already exposed [2]. Both the CDC and SHEA guidance recommends restricting visitation by any ill individual or family member with active respiratory symptoms (Table 4.1) [2, 21]. However, during periods of increased prevalence of respiratory infections in the community, surgical masks should be offered to coughing patients and other symptomatic persons who accompany ill patients upon entry into the facility [47], and these individuals should be encouraged to maintain a distance of at least 3 ft from others in common waiting areas [40, 41].

Visitors have been identified as the source of transmission of respiratory viral infections in the healthcare facilities [8, 48–50]. Consequently, patients, family members, healthcare personnel, infection control practitioners, and visitors should be partners in preventing transmission of infections in healthcare settings [11, 51, 52].

Influenza

The CDC recommends limiting visitors of patients in isolation for suspected or confirmed influenza to persons who are necessary for the patient's emotional well-being and care [21]. The CDC also recommends that visitors to patients in isolation for influenza should be screened for symptoms of acute respiratory illness before entering the hospital, instructed on hand hygiene before entering patients' rooms, limiting surfaces touched and their movement within the facility, and use of personal protective equipment (PPE) according to current facility policy while in the patient's room [21, 53, 54]. Visitors should not be present during aerosol-generating procedures [3]. They also should be encouraged to receive influenza vaccination [21, 55]. Visitors who have been in contact with the patient before and during hospitalization are a possible source of influenza for other patients, visitors, and staff [7, 9, 56–61]. Tan et al. [62] surveyed the attitudes of ten visitors toward influenza A (H1N1) response measures instituted within a tertiary hospital in Singapore with a high level of perceived inconvenience among respondents. Restriction of visitors who

Table 4.1 Summary of recommendations for visitors based on some common contagious organisms and the possible subsequent related challenges to consider [2, 21]

Organism	General recommendations for visitors	Comments or challenges
Measles virus	Airborne precautions	Difficulty in assessing immune status against measles. Fit testing for N95 respirators may be impractical. Visitor restriction should be considered.
Varicella zoster virus	Airborne and contact precautions recommended for non-immune persons in primary infection or disseminated disease.	Difficulty to assess immunity status against varicella due to inability to obtain serology to document immunity.
		Visitor restriction should be considered for non-immune visitors.
Mycobacterium tuberculosis	Airborne precautions	Fit testing for N95 respirators may be impractical. Difficult to impose to the patient to wear a surgical mask during the presence of visitors. isitors who are close contacts may have already been infected.
Influenza virus and other respiratory viruses	Droplet precautions	Recommend against visitation in case of outbreaks or if visitors are symptomatic (eg. cough, fever…)
Bordetella pertussis	Droplet precautions	Difficulty assessing vaccine history among visitors.
Highly virulent or novel organisms (Ebola virus, MERS-coV, SARS, etc.)	Visitor restriction/limitation	Videoconferencing could be considered
	Guidance from local and national public health authorities should be sought.	Consider exceptions based on end-of-life situations or when a visitor is essential for the patient's well-being and care.
MRSA and VRE	Standard precautions may be acceptable. Contact precautions could be considered in outbreak situations, among immunocompromised visitors, visitors visiting multiple patients or those unable to perform hand hygiene.	Contact precautions might be of limited value for visitors.
		General high prevalence of these organisms in the community and family members may likely be colonized.
Enteric pathogens (*Clostridium difficile*, norovirus)	Contact precautions with visitor education promoting handwashing with soap and water.	General low prevalence of these organisms in the community.
		Visitors are susceptible to infections caused by these organisms which are associated with significant morbidity and mortality.
CRE	Contact precautions should be considered	General low prevalence of these organisms in the community.
		Visitors are susceptible to infections caused by these organisms which are associated with limited therapeutic options.
Scabies and head lice	Contact precautions	Individualized considerations should be undertaken for visitors spending extended time with their hospitalized child.

MERS-CoV Middle East Respiratory Syndrome Coronavirus, *SARS* Severe Acute Respiratory Syndrome

were symptomatic or who had contact with contagious patients has been an essential strategy in influenza A outbreaks control [9, 61, 63–67].

Bordetella pertussis

Bordetella pertussis, the bacterial cause of whooping cough, is another example of infectious agent that is transmitted by droplet route [21, 40]. It is classically recognized as a disease of infants and children [40]. Reported incidence in adolescents and adults has increased globally at a significant rate over the past decade [68]. Similarly, nosocomial transmis-

sion of pertussis has increased [69, 70] due to unsuspected (asymptomatic/subclinical) pertussis patients who serve as vectors of infection to other susceptible contacts, including patients, healthcare personnel, and even their own children at home, resulting in substantial costs to the healthcare system [69]. Christie et al. [13] described the measures and procedures for visitors that were followed in order to contain a pertussis outbreak in a pediatric facility in Cincinnati. Those measures included wearing surgical masks; limiting visitation to neonatal unit to parents, grandparents, and guardians only; and creating a temporary child care service [13].

Visitors and Airborne Precautions

Airborne transmission occurs by dissemination of either airborne droplet nuclei or small particles in the respirable size range containing infectious agents that remain infective over time and distance (e.g., *Mycobacterium tuberculosis* [71], rubeola virus (measles) [72], and varicella-zoster virus (chickenpox) [73]. In addition to a negative pressure isolation room, CDC currently recommends N95 or higher level respirators to prevent acquisition of airborne infectious agents [21]. SHEA recommends N95 respirator as the gold standard for visitors to patients on airborne precautions, best used with training and fit testing [2]. Less optimal options include the use of surgical masks by the visitors which has been recommended by the SHEA guidelines for visitors' isolation precautions [2] or the use of surgical mask by the patient [74], particularly in situations where visitor fit testing is not feasible. Visitors may be exempted from wearing a mask if they have significant documented exposure to the symptomatic patient and are not ill themselves [2]. Hospital infection control programs should be involved in making these decisions regarding personal protective equipment use in these settings.

Measles

Measles is a highly contagious rash illness that is transmitted by respiratory droplets and airborne spread [21, 72]. Approximately nine out of ten susceptible persons with close contact to a measles patient will develop measles [75]. The majority of people who were infected with measles were unvaccinated or did not have a history of natural immunity against measles [75]. Individuals are considered communicable from 4 days before rash onset to 4 days after rash onset [21]. According to the CDC guidelines, all staff entering the room of a patient with suspected measles should use respiratory protection consistent with airborne precautions regardless of presumptive immunity status [21, 76]. SHEA guidelines for visitors' isolation have no recommendation for type of mask to be worn by visitors based on their immunity [2]. Visitors who were born before 1957 have been most likely exposed to measles and subsequently immune [77].

Immunocompromised Visitors

Immunocompromised individuals may be at risk for opportunistic infections and severe infections from organisms that may cause mild disease in immunocompetent hosts. These groups may include patients receiving immunosuppressing medications in the setting of organ transplantation or treatment of cancer or acquired or hereditary immunodeficien-

cies. The risk to hospital visitors with immunocompromising conditions likely varies by organism, mode of transmission, and other patient and environmental factors impacting infectivity. No professional societies or public health authorities have issued specific guidelines for this special population of hospital visitors. The American Society of Transplantation has published a guideline for safe living strategies among transplant recipients [78]. Although they do not specifically address hospital visitation, general principles outlined may be applicable to hospital visitation. Among immunocompromised visitors, hand hygiene is a particularly important infection prevention strategy. Generally, avoiding close contact with individuals with respiratory illness is recommended, and the use of a surgical mask should be considered for the immunocompromised visitor if contact cannot be avoided. The use of barrier precautions, particularly gown and glove use, may be useful among these visitors. It may be reasonable for immunocompromised individuals to avoid visiting patients with suspicion or proven infection with airborne pathogens (disseminated varicella, tuberculosis) or other virulent pathogens, particularly if they have not been fitted for an appropriate respirator [71].

Emerging Infections and Visitors to Healthcare Settings

Globalization and the ease of international travel pose new challenges for infection prevention and control of emerging infectious diseases. Outbreaks of communicable diseases in seemingly remote areas of the world have necessitated preparedness efforts for US healthcare facilities in the event of an imported case. The recent outbreak of Ebola in West Africa and the emergence of MERS-CoV in the Middle East are two such examples. The largest outbreak of MERS-CoV outside of the Middle East occurred in South Korea due to an imported case resulting in 186 secondary cases and 36 deaths. During this outbreak, hospital visitors were implicated in amplifying transmission in a similar fashion as was observed during the SARS outbreak [79–81]. Although imported cases of Ebola and MERS-CoV in the USA have been extremely rare, the high consequences of such events have led to greater recognition of the importance of hospital preparedness for emerging infectious diseases. To this end, CDC has issued explicit guidelines for managing visitors to healthcare facilities with hospitalized patients with MERS-CoV [82]. Recommendations include the following:

1. Establish procedures for monitoring, managing, and training visitors.
2. Screen visitors for respiratory illness prior to entering the hospital.

3. Restrict visitors from entering the room of patients with MERS-CoV with consideration of exceptions for end-of-life situations when the visitor is otherwise essential for patient's well-being and care.
4. Maintain a log of all visitors to patient rooms.
5. Educate visitors on respiratory hygiene, cough etiquette, hand hygiene, personal protective equipment, and limiting contact with environmental surfaces in the room.
6. Instruct visitor to limit their movement within the facility.
7. Visitors to MERS-CoV patients should be scheduled and controlled to allow for the above.

CDC has issued similar guidance for managing visitors of patients with suspected or confirmed Ebola [83]. Guidance from SHEA includes a recommendation to explore alternative methods of communication between visitors and patients (e.g., videoconferencing) following recognition of a novel or virulent organism. Videoconferencing was provided for family members to communicate with the first imported case of Ebola virus infection in Dallas, Texas [84]. In circumstances where a novel or highly contagious pathogen is identified, implementation of the above recommendations for screening, monitoring, and educating visitors necessitates close collaboration between hospital infection control practitioners, local government, public health authorities, hospital leadership, and healthcare personnel.

Ethical Considerations in Isolation Precautions for Visitors to Healthcare Facilities

Visitor restriction policies raise important bioethical questions that merit consideration. In the context of an infectious disease outbreak, restriction of visitation can conflict with the individual freedoms of patients and caregivers and the philosophy of patient-/family-centered care. Infection control practitioners must be cognizant of the powerful psychosocial impact denying visitation rights may have on patients and families. Such restrictions can be justified to protect public health on the basis of the epidemiological evidence demonstrating the role visitors can play in transmission of high-consequence infections such as SARS [85]. Accounting for the disease-specific consequences of infection and transmission can inform the public health justifications for visitor restrictions. For instance, in the case of MERS-CoV, the public health rationale for such stringent visitor precautions includes the lack of a safe and effective vaccine and chemoprophylaxis, the high rate of morbidity and mortality among infected patients, and incompletely defined modes of transmission [82]. Survey data from a Canadian hospital affected by the SARS outbreak demonstrated that the majority of healthcare personnel (90%), patients (80%), and family members (76%) supported visitor restrictions [86]. Communication to patients and families explaining visitation restriction policies should be clear and sensitive. Moreover, in some exceptional circumstances, the adverse psychosocial impact of visitor restriction and the patient's and family's emotional needs may necessitate flexibility in restricting visitation, particularly at the end of life. Understanding the short- and long-term psychosocial implications of visitor restriction, and the impact of transmission-based precautions on visitation and relationships between patients and visitors, in settings of both endemic and epidemic disease, warrants further investigation.

Isolation precautions and visitor restriction in pediatric populations pose unique ethical issues as such precautions may have additional adverse consequences such as interference with bonding, breastfeeding, and negative psychosocial impact for both children and parents. Parents and guardians may have extended stays in a patient's room, including overnight visitation, and likely have had substantial exposure to the infection prior to the child's admission. SHEA guidance questions the practicality and effectiveness of using gowns and gloves and masks for such visitors and emphasizes the importance of standard precautions, good hand hygiene practices, and individualized considerations [2].

References

1. Cohen B, et al. Frequency of patient contact with health care personnel and visitors: implications for infection prevention. Jt Comm J Qual Patient Saf. 2012;38(12):560–5.
2. Munoz-Price LS, et al. Isolation precautions for visitors. Infect Control Hosp Epidemiol. 2015;36(7):747–58.
3. Weinstein JW, et al. Nosocomial transmission of tuberculosis from a hospital visitor on a pediatrics ward. Pediatr Infect Dis J. 1995;14(3):232–4.
4. George RH, et al. An outbreak of tuberculosis in a children's hospital. J Hosp Infect. 1986;8(2):129–42.
5. Munoz FM, et al. Tuberculosis among adult visitors of children with suspected tuberculosis and employees at a children's hospital. Infect Control Hosp Epidemiol. 2002;23(10):568–72.
6. Jensen PA, et al. Guidelines for preventing the transmission of Mycobacterium tuberculosis in health-care settings, 2005. MMWR Recomm Rep. 2005;54(Rr-17):1–141.
7. Eibach D, et al. Routes of transmission during a nosocomial influenza A (H3N2) outbreak among geriatric patients and healthcare workers. J Hosp Infect. 2014;86(3):188–93.
8. Hall CB. Nosocomial respiratory syncytial virus infections: the "Cold War" has not ended. Clin Infect Dis. 2000;31(2):590–6.
9. Buchbinder N, et al. Pandemic a/H1N1/2009 influenza in a paediatric haematology and oncology unit: successful management of a sudden outbreak. J Hosp Infect. 2011;79(2):155–60.
10. Dykewicz CA. Guidelines for preventing opportunistic infections among hematopoietic stem cell transplant recipients: focus on community respiratory virus infections. Biol Blood Marrow Transplant. 2001;7 Suppl:19s–22s.
11. Valenti WM, Pincus PH, Messner MK. Nosocomial pertussis: possible spread by a hospital visitor. Am J Dis Child. 1980;134(5):520–1.

12. Vranken P, et al. Outbreak of pertussis in a neonatal intensive care unit – Louisiana, 2004. Am J Infect Control. 2006;34(9):550–4.

13. Christie CD, et al. Containment of pertussis in the regional pediatric hospital during the greater Cincinnati epidemic of 1993. Infect Control Hosp Epidemiol. 1995;16(10):556–63.

14. Friesema IH, et al. Norovirus outbreaks in nursing homes: the evaluation of infection control measures. Epidemiol Infect. 2009;137(12):1722–33.

15. Johnston CP, et al. Outbreak management and implications of a nosocomial norovirus outbreak. Clin Infect Dis. 2007;45(5):534–40.

16. Updated norovirus outbreak management and disease prevention guidelines. MMWR Recomm Rep. 2011;60(Rr-3): 1–18.

17. Mukhopadhyay A, et al. SARS in a hospital visitor and her intensivist. J Hosp Infect. 2004;56(3):249–50.

18. Gopalakrishna G, et al. SARS transmission and hospital containment. Emerg Infect Dis. 2004;10(3):395–400.

19. Dwosh HA, et al. Identification and containment of an outbreak of SARS in a community hospital. CMAJ. 2003;168(11):1415–20.

20. Chiu WT, et al. Infrared thermography to mass-screen suspected SARS patients with fever. Asia Pac J Public Health. 2005;17(1):26–8.

21. Siegel JD, et al. 2007 guideline for isolation precautions: preventing transmission of infectious agents in health care settings. Am J Infect Control. 2007;35(10 Suppl 2):S65–164.

22. Pittet D, The World Health Organization, et al. Guidelines on hand hygiene in health care and their consensus recommendations. Infect Control Hosp Epidemiol. 2009;30(7):611–22.

23. Boyce JM, et al. Guideline for hand hygiene in health-care settings. Recommendations of the healthcare infection control practices Advisory committee and the HICPAC/SHEA/APIC/IDSA hand hygiene task force. Society for Healthcare Epidemiology of America/Association for Professionals in Infection Control/ Infectious Diseases Society of America. MMWR Recomm Rep. 2002;51(RR-16):1–45. quiz CE1–4

24. Birnbach DJ, et al. An evaluation of hand hygiene in an intensive care unit: are visitors a potential vector for pathogens? J Infect Public Health. 2015;8(6):570–4.

25. Birnbach DJ, et al. Do hospital visitors wash their hands? Assessing the use of alcohol-based hand sanitizer in a hospital lobby. Am J Infect Control. 2012;40(4):340–3.

26. Fakhry M, et al. Effectiveness of an audible reminder on hand hygiene adherence. Am J Infect Control. 2012;40(4):320–3.

27. Nishimura S, et al. Handwashing before entering the intensive care unit: what we learned from continuous video-camera surveillance. Am J Infect Control. 1999;27(4):367–9.

28. Fritz SA, et al. *Staphylococcus aureus* colonization in children with community-associated *Staphylococcus aureus* skin infections and their household contacts. Arch Pediatr Adolesc Med. 2012;166(6):551–7.

29. Rafee Y, et al. Increased prevalence of methicillin-resistant *Staphylococcus aureus* nasal colonization in household contacts of children with community acquired disease. BMC Infect Dis. 2012;12:45.

30. Belvisi V, et al. Large nosocomial outbreak associated with a Norwegian scabies index case undergoing TNF-alpha inhibitor treatment: management and control. Infect Control Hosp Epidemiol. 2015;36(11):1358–60.

31. Sfeir M, Munoz-Price LS. Scabies and bedbugs in hospital outbreaks. Curr Infect Dis Rep. 2014;16(8):412.

32. Sharma D, Kaliaperumal C, Choudhari KA. An overview of head lice infestation in neurosurgical patients. Br J Nurs. 2007;16(16):982–6.

33. Roidad N, Khakoo R. Knowledge and attitudes of visitors to patients in contact isolation. Am J Infect Control. 2014;42(2):198–9.

34. Afif W, et al. Compliance with methicillin-resistant *Staphylococcus aureus* precautions in a teaching hospital. Am J Infect Control. 2002;30(7):430–3.

35. Manian FA, Ponzillo JJ. Compliance with routine use of gowns by healthcare workers (HCWs) and non-HCW visitors on entry into the rooms of patients under contact precautions. Infect Control Hosp Epidemiol. 2007;28(3):337–40.

36. Weber DJ, et al. Compliance with isolation precautions at a university hospital. Infect Control Hosp Epidemiol. 2007;28(3):358–61.

37. Simor AE, et al. An outbreak due to multiresistant Acinetobacter baumannii in a burn unit: risk factors for acquisition and management. Infect Control Hosp Epidemiol. 2002;23(5):261–7.

38. Puzniak LA, et al. To gown or not to gown: the effect on acquisition of vancomycin-resistant enterococci. Clin Infect Dis. 2002;35(1):18–25.

39. Hanna H, et al. Management of an outbreak of vancomycin-resistant enterococci in the medical intensive care unit of a cancer center. Infect Control Hosp Epidemiol. 2001;22(4):217–9.

40. Musher DM. How contagious are common respiratory tract infections? N Engl J Med. 2003;348(13):1256–66.

41. Bridges CB, Kuehnert MJ, Hall CB. Transmission of influenza: implications for control in health care settings. Clin Infect Dis. 2003;37(8):1094–101.

42. Dick EC, et al. Aerosol transmission of rhinovirus colds. J Infect Dis. 1987;156(3):442–8.

43. Steinberg P, et al. Ecology of Mycoplasma pneumoniae infections in marine recruits at Parris Island, South Carolina. Am J Epidemiol. 1969;89(1):62–73.

44. Seto WH, et al. Effectiveness of precautions against droplets and contact in prevention of nosocomial transmission of severe acute respiratory syndrome (SARS). Lancet. 2003;361(9368):1519–20.

45. Hamburger M Jr, Robertson OH. Expulsion of group A hemolytic streptococci in droplets and droplet nuclei by sneezing, coughing and talking. Am J Med. 1948;4(5):690–701.

46. Gehanno JF, et al. Nosocomial meningococcemia in a physician. Infect Control Hosp Epidemiol. 1999;20(8):564–5.

47. Beck M, et al. Wearing masks in a pediatric hospital: developing practical guidelines. Can J Public Health. 2004;95(4):256–7.

48. Garcia R, et al. Nosocomial respiratory syncytial virus infections: prevention and control in bone marrow transplant patients. Infect Control Hosp Epidemiol. 1997;18(6):412–6.

49. Whimbey E, et al. Community respiratory virus infections among hospitalized adult bone marrow transplant recipients. Clin Infect Dis. 1996;22(5):778–82.

50. Maltezou HC, Drancourt M. Nosocomial influenza in children. J Hosp Infect. 2003;55(2):83–91.

51. Srinivasan A, et al. Foundations of the severe acute respiratory syndrome preparedness and response plan for healthcare facilities. Infect Control Hosp Epidemiol. 2004;25(12):1020–5.

52. McGuckin M, et al. Evaluation of a patient education model for increasing hand hygiene compliance in an inpatient rehabilitation unit. Am J Infect Control. 2004;32(4):235–8.

53. Roberts L, et al. Effect of infection control measures on the frequency of upper respiratory infection in child care: a randomized, controlled trial. Pediatrics. 2000;105(4 Pt 1):738–42.

54. White C, et al. The effect of hand hygiene on illness rate among students in university residence halls. Am J Infect Control. 2003;31(6):364–70.

55. Martinello RA, Jones L, Topal JE. Correlation between healthcare workers' knowledge of influenza vaccine and vaccine receipt. Infect Control Hosp Epidemiol. 2003;24(11):845–7.

56. Aschan J, et al. Influenza B in transplant patients. Scand J Infect Dis. 1989;21(3):349–50.

57. Meibalane R, et al. Outbreak of influenza in a neonatal intensive care unit. J Pediatr. 1977;91(6):974–6.

58. Weingarten S, et al. Influenza surveillance in an acute-care hospital. Arch Intern Med. 1988;148(1):113–6.

59. Pachucki CT, et al. Influenza A among hospital personnel and patients. Implications for recognition, prevention, and control. Arch Intern Med. 1989;149(1):77–80.

60. Sagrera X, et al. Outbreaks of influenza A virus infection in neonatal intensive care units. Pediatr Infect Dis J. 2002;21(3):196–200.
61. Chen LF, et al. Cluster of oseltamivir-resistant 2009 pandemic influenza A (H1N1) virus infections on a hospital ward among immunocompromised patients – North Carolina, 2009. J Infect Dis. 2011;203(6):838–46.
62. Tan WM, Chlebicka NL, Tan BH. Attitudes of patients, visitors and healthcare workers at a tertiary hospital towards influenza A (H1N1) response measures. Ann Acad Med Singap. 2010;39(4):303–4.
63. Carnicer-Pont D, et al. Influenza A outbreak in a community hospital in south east Wales, February 2005. Euro Surveill. 2005;10(2):E050217 2.
64. Fanella ST, et al. Pandemic (H1N1) 2009 influenza in hospitalized children in Manitoba: nosocomial transmission and lessons learned from the first wave. Infect Control Hosp Epidemiol. 2011;32(5):435–43.
65. Munoz FM, et al. Influenza A virus outbreak in a neonatal intensive care unit. Pediatr Infect Dis J. 1999;18(9):811–5.
66. Kashiwagi S, et al. An outbreak of influenza A (H3N2) in a hospital for the elderly with emphasis on pulmonary complications. Jpn J Med. 1988;27(2):177–82.
67. Cunney RJ, et al. An outbreak of influenza A in a neonatal intensive care unit. Infect Control Hosp Epidemiol. 2000;21(7):449–54.
68. Edwards KM, Talbot TR. The challenges of pertussis outbreaks in healthcare facilities: is there a light at the end of the tunnel? Infect Control Hosp Epidemiol. 2006;27(6):537–40.
69. Wright SW, Decker MD, Edwards KM. Incidence of pertussis infection in healthcare workers. Infect Control Hosp Epidemiol. 1999;20(2):120–3.
70. De Serres G, et al. Morbidity of pertussis in adolescents and adults. J Infect Dis. 2000;182(1):174–9.
71. Riley RL. Aerial dissemination of pulmonary tuberculosis. Am Rev Tuberc. 1957;76(6):931–41.
72. Bloch AB, et al. Measles outbreak in a pediatric practice: airborne transmission in an office setting. Pediatrics. 1985;75(4):676–83.
73. Leclair JM, et al. Airborne transmission of chickenpox in a hospital. N Engl J Med. 1980;302(8):450–3.
74. Dooley SW Jr, et al. Guidelines for preventing the transmission of tuberculosis in health-care settings, with special focus on HIV-related issues. MMWR Recomm Rep. 1990;39(RR-17):1–29.
75. McLean HQ, et al. Prevention of measles, rubella, congenital rubella syndrome, and mumps, 2013: summary recommendations of the Advisory Committee on Immunization Practices (ACIP). MMWR Recomm Rep. 2013;62(RR-04):1–34.
76. Bolyard EA, et al. Guideline for infection control in healthcare personnel, 1998. Hospital Infection Control Practices Advisory Committee. Infect Control Hosp Epidemiol. 1998;19(6):407–63.
77. Kim DK, et al. Advisory committee on immunization practices recommended immunization schedule for adults aged 19 years or older – United States, 2015. MMWR Morb Mortal Wkly Rep. 2015;64(4):91–2.
78. Avery RK, Michaels MG, A.S.T.I.D.C.o. Practice. Strategies for safe living after solid organ transplantation. Am J Transplant. 2013;13(Suppl 4):304–10.
79. Chowell G, et al. Transmission characteristics of MERS and SARS in the healthcare setting: a comparative study. BMC Med. 2015;13:210.
80. Lee SS, Wong NS. Probable transmission chains of Middle East respiratory syndrome coronavirus and the multiple generations of secondary infection in South Korea. Int J Infect Dis. 38:65–7.
81. Yang JS, et al. Middle East respiratory syndrome in 3 persons, South Korea, 2015. Emerg Infect Dis. 2015;21(11):2084–7.
82. Centers for Disease Control and Prevention. Interim infection prevention and control recommendations for hospitalized patients with middle east respiratory syndrome coronavirus (MERS-CoV). Available from: http://www.cdc.gov/coronavirus/mers/infection-prevention-control.html. 31 Jan 2016.
83. Centers for Disease Control and Prevention. Infection prevention and control recommendations for hospitalized patients under investigation (PUIs) for Ebola Virus Disease (EVD) in U.S. Hospitals. Available from: http://www.cdc.gov/vhf/ebola/healthcare-us/hospitals/infection-control.html. 31 Jan 2016.
84. NBC News. Dallas Ebola patient's family too upset to watch video link. Available from: http://www.nbcnews.com/storyline/ebola-virus-outbreak/dallas-ebola-patients-family-too-upset-watch-video-link-n2208312014. 31 Jan 2016.
85. Rogers S. Why can't I visit? The ethics of visitation restrictions – lessons learned from SARS. Crit Care. 2004;8(5):300–2.
86. Quinlan B, et al. Restrictive visitor policies: feedback from healthcare workers, patients and families. Hosp Q. 2003;7(1):33–7.

Bacterial Contamination of the Anesthesia Work Area: Hands, Patients, and Things

Derya Mahmutoglu and Luisa Silvia Munoz-Price

One of the most prominent contemporary figures in infection control, Dr. Robert Weinstein, previously stated that proving the role of the hospital environment on the transmission of multidrug-resistant organisms is easier asked than answered [1]. As nicely summarized in a 2012 Editorial, the healthcare environment was a major concern in the 1950s [1]. Later on in the 1960s, collective interest in the healthcare environment decreased, including interest in cleaning and disinfection. During the last couple of decades, we have experienced another shift with resurgence of interest in the healthcare environment. Several publications have described the relevance of the environment as a reservoir for various organisms, such as methicillin-resistant *Staphylococcus aureus* (MRSA), vancomycin-resistant enterococcus (*VRE*), *Clostridium difficile*, *Enterobacteriaceae* (e.g., *Klebsiella pneumoniae, Escherichia coli*), and other non-lactose fermenters such as *Acinetobacter baumannii*. Most of these organisms are carried in the stool and then contaminate the healthcare environment, particularly patient's rooms. This environmental contamination was named by Weinstein as *fecal patina* [1] which stands for the invisible veneer of stool organisms that contaminate environmental surfaces in a concentric fashion with the highest level of contamination next to the anus and with decreasing bacterial loads that further away from this anatomical site. In many cases, hands of medical providers act as transient carriers (vectors) of pathogens between the environment and patients, forming a triad of transmission between hands, environment, and patient's body surfaces.

Even though the above concepts have been explored, analyzed, and described outside the operating rooms, their relevance in the operating room is not as well stablished. This is especially interesting given that patients are placed for many hours in an environment that has been used by others equally sick, transiently immunocompromised (i.e., surgery, hypothermic), and exposed to multiple hand contacts by nursing and anesthesia providers. The role of anesthesia providers and their interactions with the anesthesia work area are particularly interesting. During a surgical procedure, anesthesia providers have the potential of undertaking hundreds of contacts with surfaces, not only environment but also patient's body surfaces, at a high pace (e.g., induction) and while wearing gloves. The flow and pace of these interactions makes hand hygiene very challenging which has the potential to further increase the contamination of their environment. In addition, the anesthesia area (e.g., anesthesia machine) is frequently not cleaned between patients or terminally at the end of the day. What does this mean for our patients? What are the roles of the environment and healthcare workers' hands in this transmission?

This chapter will start with a brief summary of data published on the horizontal transmission of pathogens outside the operating room. We will focus on MRSA, *VRE*, and *A. baumannii*. Then we will discuss the majority of evidence dealing with environmental contamination, hand providers' contamination, and contamination of patients' body surfaces in the operating room environment. Additionally, we will argue about the long-term clinical implications of intraoperative exposures during anesthesia.

MRSA and *VRE*

MRSA and *VRE* are considered preeminent healthcare pathogens [2], and as described in this section, both organisms are known to contaminate the hospital environment. Even though these organisms can survive in the environment for up to 2–3 months, routine cleaning and disinfection can easily eradicate them.

A study performed at the University of Maryland analyzed environmental cultures from 360 rooms. Samples were obtained in rooms that underwent routine cleaning ($n = 242$) and terminal cleaning ($n = 118$) [3]. The authors found that

D. Mahmutoglu • L.S. Munoz-Price (✉)
Department of Medicine-Division of Infectious Diseases, Froedtert & the Medical College of Wisconsin, Froedtert Hospital, 9200 W Wisconsin Ave, Milwaukee, WI 53226, USA
e-mail: dmahmutoglu@mcw.edu; smunozprice@mcw.edu

© Springer International Publishing AG 2018
G. Bearman et al. (eds.), *Infection Prevention*, DOI 10.1007/978-3-319-60980-5_5

the overall loads of MRSA in routine and terminal cleaning rooms were 79 and 0.12 CFU/100 cm², respectively. Similarly, VRE loads were 42 and 1 CFU/100 cm² in the routine and terminal cleaning rooms, respectively. Environmental sites were cultured using three sponges. Composite 1 included bed rails, remote control, call button, and phone. Composite 2 included overbed table, intravenous pole, and inside room handle. Composite 3 included portable commode, bedpan, or bathroom. Cultures of routinely cleaned rooms showed composite 1 with the highest number of CFUs/cm² (mean 3800), followed by composite 3 (mean 2900), and lastly composite 3 (mean 1570). Terminally cleaned rooms had 444, 244, and 436 CFU/cm² for composites 1, 2, and 3, respectively.

In a 2014 multicenter trial, 1023 environmental cultures were obtained among 45 rooms occupied by patients infected or colonized with MRSA or VRE [4]. Twenty-four rooms (53%) with colonized patients had at least one positive environmental culture. Interestingly, the number of CFUs in rooms occupied by colonized patients was higher than the CFUs found in rooms occupied by infected patients. This contamination of the environment by VRE-positive patients has been shown by others. Bala and colleagues showed in 2009 that 21% of environmental surfaces belonging to rooms occupied by VRE-positive patients were detected as VRE positive prior to cleaning [5].

It has been shown that VRE causes environmental contamination as a target-like pattern such as concentric circles with greatest effect of contamination, which happens around patient's rectum. Beezhold et al. screened 14 patients with VRE bacteremia and found that rectal colonization of VRE in all infected patients [6]. In the same study, colonization of the inguinal area and/or the antecubital fossa was found as 86%. A more recent paper published by Ford and colleagues showed that VRE was present on room surfaces of 10% of terminally cleaned room [7]. Curtains are room items that are logistically challenging to change or clean between discharges. Ohl and colleagues cultured 43 curtains in two ICUs, finding 42% of them positive for VRE [8]. Interestingly, eight of these curtains yielded VRE in a recurrent basis. Thus, future studies should look into the significance of contamination of curtains on the horizontal transmission of pathogens. Contamination of the environment occurs also in the outpatient setting although its significance is unclear. Smith et al. cultured the environment before and after the outpatient visits of 11 cancer patients colonized with VRE, and 29% of encounters resulted in VRE contamination [9].

The impact of environmental contamination on future room occupants was nicely shown in a paper by Huang SS and colleagues [10]. The authors performed admission and weekly screening for MRSA and VRE in eight ICUs. During 20 months, 3.9% of patients admitted to rooms with a previous MRSA-positive occupant acquired MRSA compared to 2.9% of patients admitted to a room previously not occupied

by a MRSA-positive patient (adjusted odds ratio=1.4; $p = 0.02$). For VRE this difference was 4.5% vs. 2.8%, respectively (adjusted odds ratio=1.4; $p = .02$). A similar experience was published by Drees et al. (CID 2008) in which two ICUs underwent weekly environmental cultures and twice-weekly patient surveillance cultures. The study found that having a VRE-colonized prior room occupant increased the risk for VRE acquisition almost three times (hazard ratio 3.1; 95% CI. 1.6–5.8). This increased risk remained even if the VRE-colonized patient was discharged from the room within the previous 2 weeks (HR = 2.7; 95% CI: 1.4–5.3). A similar risk was seen if the room had previous positive environmental cultures (HR = 3.4; CI: 1.2–9.6). This association remained present even after adjusting for colonization pressure.

A landmark study showing the relevance of VRE environmental contamination was published by Hayden et al. [11]. The authors cultured the hands of providers going in and out of rooms occupied by VRE-colonized patients, while concomitantly observing the activities of providers inside the rooms. Providers that touched both the patient and the room contaminated their hands in 70% of instances. More significantly for the purposes of this chapter, providers that touched only the environment contaminated their hands in 52% of instances. Wearing gloves decreased the likelihood of hand contamination from 37 to 5%. Although, this finding might have different implications within the operating room setting as we will discuss later in the chapter.

In 1995, a group from Chicago inoculated VRE on the fingertips and gloved fingertips of healthy volunteers and environmental surfaces [12]. Enterococcal strains survived for 60 min on ungloved and gloved fingertips and up to 7 days on dry surfaces.

Drees and colleagues also looked at the room contamination of 142 VRE-colonized patients, finding that 25% of this cohort had VRE+ environmental cultures (Drees ICHE 2008). During adjusted analyses, only higher mean colonization pressure in the ICU was associated with higher risk of room contamination (aHR = 1.44; CI:1.04–2.04), and no antibiotic usage was associated with lower risk of room contamination (aHR = 0.21; CI: 0.05–0.89). Another study by Bonten and colleagues [13] evaluated the presence of VRE colonization, acquisition, and concomitant environmental contamination in 97 MICU admissions. They found that out of 13 patients exposed to VRE contaminated environment (ascertained by VRE environmental cultures), three (23%) acquired VRE during hospitalization.

Gram-Negative Organisms

Among Gram-negative rods, *Acinetobacter* is probably one of the organisms with the highest level of environmental contamination, which seems to be the case due to Acinetobacter's ability to resist desiccation and to survive for months on dry surfaces [14].

Morgan et al. cultured 585 healthcare worker/patient interactions and found that the organism most frequently transferred to gowns/gloves was *A. baumannii* [15]. The strongest independent risk factor for transfer of *Acinetobacter* was the presence of environmental contamination with the same organism. More importantly, pulse field gel electrophoresis determined the relatedness between strains isolated in the environment, hands, and patient's body surface. Nutman and colleagues evaluated the degree of environmental contamination in rooms occupied by carbapenem-resistant Acinetobacter (CRAB) patients [16]. Among the 34 patients included, environmental surfaces were found to be contaminated on all patients. Rosa and colleagues published environmental culture results of 586 rooms, out of which 134 were occupied by CRAB-positive patients [17]. Among the patients colonized in the rectum, the odds of having bed rails contaminated with CRAB was 2.55 times the odds among patients colonized in the respiratory tract. The opposite was observed for intravenous pumps, in which case patients colonized in the respiratory tract had 2.72 times the odds of having the pumps contaminated compared to the patients colonized in the rectum.

A subsequent study evaluated the risk of acquiring CRAB after inadvertent exposure to a CRAB-positive room environment [18]. The authors found that the risk of acquiring CRAB if exposed to a contaminated environment was 2.77 times the risk if not exposed to a known contaminated environment.

The air has also been found to be positive in rooms occupied by CRAB-positive patients [19]. Shimose et al. cultured the air of 25 patients: 17 colonized by CRAB in the respiratory tract and 8 colonized in the rectum. Air cultures were obtained using open plates left next to the ceiling tiles for 24 h periods. Among patients rectally colonized, 38% of air samples were positive for *A. baumannii* and 13% of air samples were *Acinetobacter* positive among patients with respiratory colonization. However, these findings have not been replicated in newer publications [20]. These contradictory findings warrant further investigations in hospital settings with various humidity levels and geographic locations [21].

Intraoperative Anesthesia Work Area

Environmental Contamination

Loftus and collaborators cultured 61 randomly selected patients undergoing anesthesia in the operating room, their anesthesia machines (adjustable pressure limiting valve), and the intravenous stopcocks [22]. Cultures of the anesthesia machine showed that the number of colony-forming units (CFUs) increased by a mean of 115 by the end of surgery

($p < 0.001$). Similarly, 32% of stopcocks were found contaminated by the end of the case. It is important to notice that most of the bacteria isolated were skin organisms; however, MRSA, *VRE*, and *Enterobacter cloacae* were identified.

In order to examine the relative contribution of environment, hands, and patients to stopcock contamination, the same group from Dartmouth evaluated 578 surgical cases [23]. They included the first and second cases within the same day (pairs). In addition to culturing the providers' hands, stopcocks, and anesthesia machine before and after cases, patients were cultured from their nasopharynx and their axillae. All similar strains within a same pair were typed using pulsed field gel electrophoresis. The authors found contamination of the stopcock in 23% of instances (126 out of 548). There were 14 pairs in which the stopcock from the second case got contaminated with organisms found in the first case. These organisms were fundamentally skin flora, such as *Staphylococcus epidermidis*. Ten of the 14 cases originated from the environment (including one *Pseudomonas* and one *Serratia*), two originated from the attending staffing the first case, and two from the patients' axillae (*S. epidermidis* and *S. aureus*).

Three subsequent studies from the same group used the above framework to describe the transmission of *S. aureus* [24], enterococcus [25], and Gram-negative rods [26]. Please note that the main caveat of all these three studies is that they only cultured two body surfaces (the axillae and the nasopharynx). In particular for enterococcus and Gram-negative rods, this restriction of body surfaces could have incurred in several false-negative results under-reporting patients already colonized [27].

Even though frequently overlooked, contamination of the floor of the operating room should be evaluated in future studies. Our personal observations showed that intravenous tubing, EKG cables, drapes, patient's fasteners to operating room bed, etc. are commonly in contact with the floor and placed back on the patients' body surfaces [28]. However, at this time the relevance of the operating room's floor on cross transmission is unclear.

Hand Hygiene

Several independent observations have described low rates of hand hygiene in the anesthesia area during surgical procedures. A Dutch study evaluated the frequency of hand hygiene during 28 operations totaling 60 h of observations [29]. The frequency of hand hygiene was below once an hour (mean, 0.14 events per hour). However, these observations included other staff members in the operating room, such as surgeons, surgical nurses, and medical students. The authors also determined compliance with hand hygiene upon entry and exit of the operating rooms, finding 2% (7/363) and 8% (28/333) compliance, respectively. A different study documented 8 h of hand hygiene frequency and contacts of anesthesia providers in the operating room area [30]. A total of 1132 contacts were observed, and the most frequently touched objects were the anesthesia machines and keyboards. Only 13 hand disinfections were witnessed throughout the 8 h of observation. Stopcocks were accessed 66 times, and disinfection was witnessed only in 10 of these manipulations. All procedures, such as bronchoscopies, line insertions, and blood exposures, were not followed by hand hygiene.

In another study, Koff et al. evaluated the impact of a portable hand sanitizer dispenser on hand hygiene frequency during 111 surgical procedures [31]. In addition to dispensing hand sanitizer, the dispenser also tallied the hand hygiene events and their timing. Attending providers had a baseline hand hygiene of 0.15 events per hour, and this frequency increased to 7.1 events per hour with the device ($p = 0.008$). Similarly, other providers had a baseline hand hygiene frequency of 0.38 events per hour which later increased to 8.7 events per hour with the device. Concomitant contamination of the stopcocks was evaluated which showed that at baseline (without the device) stopcock contamination was 32.8% compared to 7.5% with the device. Similarly, contamination of the anesthesia machine also decreased by a mean of 77 CFUs per site ($p = 0.01$).

The relevance of hand contamination was evaluated in a study by Loftus in 2011 [32]. The first and second operative procedures in 92 randomly selected ORs were evaluated for hand and environmental contamination before and after each of the cases. Interestingly, 66% of provider's hands were contaminated at the beginning of the first case with noteworthy findings of 18% of culture positivity showing *S. aureus* and 49% positive for Gram-negative rods. Bacterial transmission from hands to environment occurred in 17 out of 146 cases (12%) and from hands to the stopcocks in 19 out of 164 cases (11.5%). Four stopcocks belonging to the second case of the day were contaminated with the same organism (by pulsed field electrophoresis) found in the hands of anesthesia providers at the beginning of the first case.

The World Health Organization's five moments for hand hygiene might not be suitable for the anesthesia work area, especially during induction when there is a high frequency of activities. The high frequency during induction was shown in a study by Munoz-Price and colleagues in which induction was compared against maintenance [33]. The frequency of contacts during induction was compared to maintenance xx. At the same time, hand hygiene events were observed at a frequency of 154.8 ± 7.7 (mean ± standard error) during induction and 60 ± 3.1 during maintenance. Nevertheless, a study by Biddle evaluated the WHO opportunities for hand hygiene among anesthesia providers [34]. They found 34–41 opportunities per hour with peaks up to 54 opportunities per hour. Compliance with hand hygiene based on these criteria was in average 18%. The opportunities with lowest hand

hygiene compliance included moving between patients, placing preoperative nerve blocks, keyboard use with soiled hands, during placement of intravenous lines, preparing drugs and equipment for the case with soiled hands, soiled gloves left after airway manipulation such as endotracheal intubation, suctioning of airways, intubation, etc.

A couple of additional studies looked at interventions for increasing hand hygiene among anesthesia providers. Rodriguez-Aldrete et al. evaluated electronic visual reminders geared to anesthesia providers which said "Please Sanitize Your Hands" which was shown for 60 s every 15 min [35]. Each of the 20 anesthesia providers was exposed to this reminder four times over 1 h per observation. Providers were observed during anesthesia procedures with and without the reminders. Frequency of hand hygiene without the reminders was 0.2 events per hour and with the reminders 2.1 events per hour were observed ($p = 0.006$).

Based on feedback by anesthesia providers on hand hygiene barriers in the operating room, a hand sanitizer holder was evaluated to increase hand hygiene compliance [36]. This study randomized anesthesia providers to either the intervention (hand sanitizer holder on the anesthesia machine) versus control (no holder; hand sanitizer dispenser was on the operating room wall). After the initial intervention, the anesthesia providers were evaluated in the opposite group. The use of the dispenser on the anesthesia machine increased the frequency of hand hygiene from 0.5 to 0.8 hand hygiene events per hour. Even though the difference was significant ($p = 0.01$), the clinical impact of this difference might be limited, especially when compared to the impact of portable hand sanitizer devices evaluated by Koff [31]. The impact of the hands of anesthesia providers during anesthesia care was also evaluated by Mermel and colleagues [37]. The authors cultured the manifolds of newly placed intravenous peripheral catheters. Out of 70 stopcocks cultured, 12 (17%) had growth which suggests intraoperative contamination.

An innovative intervention to bypass the need of hand hygiene immediately after intubation was published by Birnbach and colleagues [38]. The intervention consisted of wearing double gloves during intubation on the degree of environmental contamination (measured by the spread of fluorescent gel placed on a mannequin). The number of sites that were found contaminated with the fluorescent marker decreased from 20.3 ± 1.4 (mean ± standard error) to 5.0 ± 0.7 with single versus double gloves, respectively.

Increased Surgical Site Infections and Mortality

In a 2008 paper by Loftus [22], patients with contaminated stopcock sets were found to have no difference in nosocomial infection rates (odds ratio=3.08; 95% CI: 0.56–17.5), but higher mortality was observed (0 out of 40 in the non-contaminated group vs. 2 of 20 in the contaminated group). However, these determinations were done solely by chart review, and it is unknown if the review was blinded to the contamination status of the stopcocks.

In a 2009 paper by Koff [31], patients that underwent surgery with the use of a hand hygiene dispenser device had a decrease incidence of nosocomial infections (17.2% vs. 3.8%, $p = 0.02$). In regard to mortality, none of the patients in the device group expired compared to 2 out of 58 in the control. In this paper, the chart reviewers were blinded to the use of the hand hygiene dispenser, and none of the patients were lost to follow-up at 6 weeks.

A study designed to evaluate the intraoperative transmission of organisms was also used to determine the impact of stopcock contamination on mortality [23]. Unfortunately the authors only published the associations without the distribution of mortality in the two groups. The adjusted odds ratio was determined to be 58.5 ($p = 0.014$).

Compliance with Cleaning and Disinfection

Outside the operating room, we have known for approximately a decade that hospital surfaces are not regularly disinfected. Phil Carling came up with a novel technology for evaluating cleaning over 48 h using fluorescent markers and ultraviolet lamps [39]. Various subsequent studies have shown that less than 50% of objects in patient rooms are wiped at least once within a 48 h period. Carling and colleagues also evaluated the degree of environmental cleaning in the operating room [40]. The authors tested ten standardized objects including main and second overbed table lights, main and second operating room doors, Bovie control panel and radiology equipment, anesthesia machine and anesthesia cart, main operating room light switch, and storage cabinet handle. Markers were placed after terminal cleaning was performed and inspected with an ultraviolet lamp after the room had been terminally cleaned two or three times. Seventy-one operating rooms were evaluated across six hospitals with a total of 946 objects observed. The mean overall thoroughness of cleaning was 25% (95% CI: 9.4–50%). The anesthesia cart had a mean cleaning rate of 20.65 (range 0–73) and the anesthesia machine's mean was 28% (range 10–50%).

In a separate study, fluorescent markers were used to evaluate cleaning rates in the anesthesia area and the impact of feedback and education of the environmental services cleaning staff. At baseline, we found only 47% of objects were cleaned over a 24 h period and 10.7% of these surfaces were contaminated with Gram-negative rods. After feedback and education, cleaning rates increased to 82% ($p < 0.0001$) and Gram-negative rod contamination decreased to 2.3% ($p = 0.015$).

Conclusions and Controversies

Similarly to what occurs outside the operating room, the anesthesia work area seems to follow a cycle of transmission of pathogens involving the environment, the patients, and the hands of healthcare workers. Controversies in this area of hospital epidemiology include the following topics that should be considered for future research:

1. The long-term clinical significance of exposure to pathogens in the anesthesia work area.
2. The optimal ways to clean and disinfect the operating room are uncertain at this time.
3. Approaches to improve compliance with hand hygiene among anesthesia providers during an anesthesia procedure.
4. Given the high frequency of contacts with the environment and patient's body surfaces, especially during anesthesia induction and emergence, the practical/realistic timing for hand hygiene during anesthesia care in the operating room is still uncertain.

References

1. Weinstein RA. Intensive care unit environments and the fecal patina: a simple problem? Crit Care Med. 2012;40(4):1333–4.
2. Centers for Disease Control. Antibiotic resistance threats. Available at: https://www.cdc.gov/drugresistance/pdf/ar-threats-2013-508.pdf
3. Shams AM, Rose LJ, Edwards JR, et al. Assessment of the overall and multidrug-resistant organism bioburden on environmental surfaces in healthcare facilities. Infect Control Hosp Epidemiol. 2016;37(12):1426–32.
4. Knelson LP, Williams DA, Gergen MF, et al. A comparison of environmental contamination by patients infected or colonized with methicillin-resistant *Staphylococcus aureus* or vancomycin-resistant enterococci: a multicenter study. Infect Control Hosp Epidemiol. 2014;35(7):872–5.
5. Hota B, Blom DW, Lyle EA, Weinstein RA, Hayden MK. Interventional evaluation of environmental contamination by vancomycin-resistant enterococci: failure of personnel, product, or procedure? J Hosp Infect. 2009;71(2):123–31.
6. Beezhold DW, Slaughter S, Hayden MK, et al. Skin colonization with vancomycin-resistant enterococci among hospitalized patients with bacteremia. Clin Infect Dis. 1997;24(4):704–6.
7. Ford CD, Lopansri BK, Gazdik MA, et al. Room contamination, patient colonization pressure, and the risk of vancomycin-resistant Enterococcus colonization on a unit dedicated to the treatment of hematologic malignancies and hematopoietic stem cell transplantation. Am J Infect Control. 2016;44(10):1110–5.
8. Ohl M, Schweizer M, Graham M, Heilmann K, Boyken L, Diekema D. Hospital privacy curtains are frequently and rapidly contaminated with potentially pathogenic bacteria. Am J Infect Control. 2012;40(10):904–6.
9. Smith TL, Iwen PC, Olson SB, Rupp ME. Environmental contamination with vancomycin-resistant enterococci in an outpatient setting. Infect Control Hosp Epidemiol. 1998;19(7):515–8.

10. Huang SS, Datta R, Platt R. Risk of acquiring antibiotic-resistant bacteria from prior room occupants. Arch Intern Med. 2006;166(18):1945–51.
11. Hayden MK, Blom DW, Lyle EA, Moore CG, Weinstein RA. Risk of hand or glove contamination after contact with patients colonized with vancomycin-resistant enterococcus or the colonized patients' environment. Infect Control Hosp Epidemiol. 2008;29(2):149–54.
12. Noskin GA, Stosor V, Cooper I, Peterson LR. Recovery of vancomycin-resistant enterococci on fingertips and environmental surfaces. Infect Control Hosp Epidemiol. 1995;16(10):577–81.
13. Bonten MJ, Hayden MK, Nathan C, et al. Epidemiology of colonisation of patients and environment with vancomycin-resistant enterococci. Lancet. 1996;348(9042):1615–9.
14. Munoz-Price LS, Weinstein RA. Acinetobacter infection. N Engl J Med. 2008;358(12):1271–81.
15. Morgan DJ, Rogawski E, Thom KA, et al. Transfer of multidrug-resistant bacteria to healthcare workers' gloves and gowns after patient contact increases with environmental contamination. Crit Care Med. 2012;40(4):1045–51.
16. Nutman A, Lerner A, Schwartz D, Carmeli Y. Evaluation of carriage and environmental contamination by carbapenem-resistant Acinetobacter baumannii. Clin Microbiol Infect. 2016;22(11):949. e5–7.
17. Rosa R, Depascale D, Cleary T, Fajardo-Aquino Y, Kett DH, Munoz-Price LS. Differential environmental contamination with Acinetobacter baumannii based on the anatomic source of colonization. Am J Infect Control. 2014;42(7):755–7.
18. Rosa R, Arheart KL, Depascale D, et al. Environmental exposure to carbapenem-resistant Acinetobacter baumannii as a risk factor for patient acquisition of A. baumannii. Infect Control Hosp Epidemiol. 2014;35(4):430–3.
19. Shimose LA, Masuda E, Sfeir M, et al. Carbapenem-resistant Acinetobacter baumannii: concomitant contamination of air and environmental surfaces. Infect Control Hosp Epidemiol. 2016;37(7):777–81.
20. Rock C, Harris AD, Johnson JK, Bischoff WE, Thom KA. Infrequent air contamination with Acinetobacter baumannii of air surrounding known colonized or infected patients. Infect Control Hosp Epidemiol. 2015;36(7):830–2.
21. Munoz-Price LS. Acinetobacter in the air: did Maryland get it wrong? Infect Control Hosp Epidemiol. 2015;36(7):833–4.
22. Loftus RW, Koff MD, Burchman CC, et al. Transmission of pathogenic bacterial organisms in the anesthesia work area. Anesthesiology. 2008;109(3):399–407.
23. Loftus RW, Brown JR, Koff MD, et al. Multiple reservoirs contribute to intraoperative bacterial transmission. Anesth Analg. 2012;114(6):1236–48.
24. Loftus RW, Koff MD, Brown JR, et al. The epidemiology of Staphylococcus aureus transmission in the anesthesia work area. Anesth Analg. 2015;120(4):807–18.
25. Loftus RW, Koff MD, Brown JR, et al. The dynamics of enterococcus transmission from bacterial reservoirs commonly encountered by anesthesia providers. Anesth Analg. 2015;120(4):827–36.
26. Loftus RW, Brown JR, Patel HM, et al. Transmission dynamics of Gram-negative bacterial pathogens in the anesthesia work area. Anesth Analg. 2015;120(4):819–26.
27. Munoz-Price LS, Weinstein RA. Fecal patina in the anesthesia work area. Anesth Analg. 2015;120(4):703–5.
28. Munoz-Price LS, Birnbach DJ, Lubarsky DA, et al. Decreasing operating room environmental pathogen contamination through improved cleaning practice. Infect Control Hosp Epidemiol. 2012;33(9):897–904.
29. Krediet AC, Kalkman CJ, Bonten MJ, Gigengack ACM, Barach P. Hand-hygiene practices in the operating theatre: an observational study. Br J Anaesth. 2011;107(4):553–8.
30. Munoz-Price LS, Lubarsky DA, Arheart KL, et al. Interactions between anesthesiologists and the environment while providing anesthesia care in the operating room. Am J Infect Control. 2013;41(10):922–4.
31. Koff MD, Loftus RW, Burchman CC, et al. Reduction in intraoperative bacterial contamination of peripheral intravenous tubing through the use of a novel device. Anesthesiology. 2009;110(5):978–85.
32. Loftus RW, Muffly MK, Brown JR, et al. Hand contamination of anesthesia providers is an important risk factor for intraoperative bacterial transmission. Anesth Analg. 2011;112(1):98–105.
33. Munoz-Price LS, Riley B, Banks S, et al. Frequency of interactions and hand disinfections among anesthesiologists while providing anesthesia care in the operating room: induction versus maintenance. Infect Control Hosp Epidemiol. 2014;35(8):1056–9.
34. Biddle C, Shah J. Quantification of anesthesia providers' hand hygiene in a busy metropolitan operating room: what would Semmelweis think? Am J Infect Control. 2012;40(8):756–9.
35. Rodriguez-Aldrete D, Sivanesan E, Banks S, et al. Recurrent visual electronic hand hygiene reminders in the anesthesia work area. Infect Control Hosp Epidemiol. 2016;37(7):872–4.
36. Munoz-Price LS, Patel Z, Banks S, et al. Randomized crossover study evaluating the effect of a hand sanitizer dispenser on the frequency of hand hygiene among anesthesiology staff in the operating room. Infect Control Hosp Epidemiol. 2014;35(6):717–20.
37. Mermel LA, Bert A, Chapin KC, LeBlanc L. Intraoperative stopcock and manifold colonization of newly inserted peripheral intravenous catheters. Infect Control Hosp Epidemiol. 2014;35(9):1187–9.
38. Birnbach DJ, Rosen LF, Fitzpatrick M, Carling P, Arheart KL, Munoz-Price LS. Double gloves: a randomized trial to evaluate a simple strategy to reduce contamination in the operating room. Anesth Analg. 2015;120(4):848–52.
39. Carling PC, Parry MF, Von Beheren SM. Healthcare environmental hygiene study group. Identifying opportunities to enhance environmental cleaning in 23 acute care hospitals. Infect Control Hosp Epidemiol. 2008;29(1):1–7.
40. Jefferson J, Whelan R, Dick B, Carling P. A novel technique for identifying opportunities to improve environmental hygiene in the operating room. AORN J. 2011;93(3):358–64.

Infection Control in the Outpatient Setting

John Daniel Markley and Michael P. Stevens

Introduction

As healthcare continues to evolve, economic forces and technological advancements have facilitated the transition of healthcare delivery from acute care hospitals to a myriad of different outpatient care settings such as ambulatory surgery centers, physician offices, dialysis centers, home care, and other specialized settings [1]. The number of outpatient visits and procedures continues to rise, with 929 million physician office visits occurring in the United States in 2012, or 301 visits per 100 persons [2]. Surgical procedures occurring in ambulatory surgical centers rose threefold between 1999 and 2005 and now represent 75% of all surgical procedures performed [3]. Outpatient oncologic care is also significant, with an estimated 1.1 million cancer patients per year receiving outpatient chemotherapy or radiation [4]. Approximately 500,000 patients per year receive infusion therapy for maintenance hemodialysis, nutritional support, home intravenous antimicrobial therapy, or cancer chemotherapy in the outpatient setting [5]. While healthcare in the outpatient setting is on the rise, the overall number of inpatient hospital admissions is decreasing (35,522,000 in 2008 to 34,217,000 in 2012) [6]. These pivotal trends provide a major impetus to develop sound infection control processes and practices in the outpatient setting.

J.D. Markley (✉)
Department of Internal Medicine, Division of Infectious Diseases, Virginia Commonwealth University Medical Center, VMI Building, 2nd Floor, Suite 205, 1000 E. Marshall Street, PO Box 980049, Richmond, VA 23298, USA
e-mail: john.markley@vcuhealth.org

M.P. Stevens
Department of Internal Medicine, Division of Infectious Diseases, Virginia Commonwealth University Medical Center, Richmond, VA, USA

Infectious Diseases/Epidemiology, Virginia Commonwealth University Health System, Richmond, VA, USA
e-mail: michael.stevens@vcuhealth.org

It is estimated that healthcare-associated infections (HAIs) occur in nearly two million patients per year in the United States, culminating in a total of 99,000 deaths and a cost of approximately $33 billion each year [7]. These estimates are primarily derived from infection surveillance in acute care settings including central line-associated bloodstream infections (CLABSI), ventilator-associated pneumonia (VAP), catheter-associated urinary tract infection (CAUTI), and surgical site infections (SSI). Indeed, since the Institute of Medicine (IOM) released the siren call, "To Err is Human: Building a Safer Health System," in 1999, hospital-based infection control and patient safety research has experienced a period of intense growth [8, 9]. Spurred by the IOM report, mandatory reporting and other requirements from the Joint Commission on Accreditation of Hospitals and Healthcare Organizations (JCAHO), the Department of Health and Human Services (DHHS), and the Centers for Medicare and Medicaid Services (CMS) have led to the development of refined approaches to surveillance, isolation, outbreak investigation, environmental cleaning, and antimicrobial stewardship in the hospital setting. These efforts have been highly fruitful, as evidenced by the most recent Centers for Disease Control and Prevention (CDC) HAI Prevalence Survey which found a 46% decrease in CLABSI between 2008 and 2013, a 19% decrease in select SSIs, an 8% decrease in hospital-onset MRSA bacteremia between 2011 and 2013, and a 10% decrease in hospital-onset *C. difficile* infections between 2011 and 2013 [10].

Unfortunately, infection control in the outpatient setting has not experienced a parallel evolutionary trend and, when compared to hospital-based infection control, is largely in its nascency. Regulatory emphasis has primarily focused on acute care settings, though in the coming years this emphasis will be shifting to the outpatient setting as outlined in "Phase Two" of the DHHS *National Action Plan to Prevent Health Care-Associated Infections: Road Map to Elimination* [11]. Historically, infection control in the outpatient setting has been managed by affiliated hospital programs. Private offices and unaffiliated, freestanding ambulatory care centers have

G. Bearman et al. (eds.), *Infection Prevention*, DOI 10.1007/978-3-319-60980-5_6

very little written infection-control policies and lacked formal training procedures for their personnel [12]. The problem has been amplified by a lack of resources to support infection control and prevention in the outpatient setting.

To date, there is a paucity of data describing the rates and risks for HAIs in the outpatient setting. However, numerous outbreaks of *Staphylococcus aureus*, hepatitis B and C, non-tuberculous mycobacteria, *Clostridium difficile*, and multi-drug-resistant organisms (MDROs) have been described and have increased public awareness of the dire need for improvement in outpatient infection control and prevention practices. Outbreaks in ambulatory surgery centers have stemmed from lapses in basic infection control processes such as reusing syringes, mishandling of injectable medications from single-dose vials (SDVs) or multi-dose vials (MDVs), breaches in sterilization protocols of endoscopy equipment, and the breakdown in use of personal protective equipment (PPE), to name a few [13]. In 2012, one of the largest outbreaks in US history took place due to steroid injections with infected lots of methylprednisolone acetate from the New England Compounding Center (NECC). Out of the nearly 14,000 patients at risk, a total of 753 cases of fungal infections spanning 20 states culminated in 64 deaths and untold morbidity [14]. A congressional hearing concluded that greater oversight and standards for nontraditional compounding be implemented, and The Drug Quality and Security Act was passed by the Senate on November 27, 2013.

Several regulatory and expert bodies have begun outlining recommendations to guide infection control and prevention programs in the outpatient setting. In 2015, the CDC released a summary guide of infection prevention recommendations for outpatient (ambulatory care) settings that includes evidence-based guidelines produced by the CDC and the Healthcare Infection Control Practices Advisory Committee (HICPAC). The guide focuses on the basic elements of standard precautions and proclaims itself to be "the minimum infection prevention expectations for safe care in ambulatory care settings" [15]. This document serves as a major step forward to assist infection control and prevention professionals to develop more robust outpatient programs.

As healthcare delivery shifts to the outpatient setting, regulatory measures are implemented, and more outpatient HAIs are recognized, infection control and prevention programs will be called upon to translate hospital-based approaches to the outpatient setting. More and more complex patient populations including immunocompromised hosts are receiving a myriad of diagnostic and treatment modalities in ambulatory settings, with heightened potential risk for infection acquisition. Basic infection control practices including surveillance of infection rates, isolation, environmental cleaning, sterilization of devices/tools, outbreak investigation, antimicrobial stewardship, personnel training, and mandatory reporting and monitoring should be applied to the outpatient setting.

Definitions

For the purposes of consistency, this chapter will employ the following definitions as outlined by the recent recommendations from the CDC's "Guide to Infection Prevention for Outpatient Settings: Minimum Expectations for Safe Care" [15].

Outpatient care: care provided in facilities where patients do not remain overnight (e.g., hospital-based outpatient clinics, non-hospital-based clinics and physician offices, urgent care centers, ambulatory surgical centers, public health clinics, imaging centers, oncology clinics, behavioral health clinics and physical therapy and rehabilitation centers) [15].

Healthcare personnel (HCP): all persons, paid and unpaid, working in outpatient settings who have the potential for exposure to patients and/or to infectious materials, including body substances, contaminated medical supplies and devices, contaminated environmental surfaces, or contaminated air. This includes persons not directly involved in patient care (e.g., clerical, housekeeping, and volunteers) but potentially exposed to infectious agents that can be transmitted to and from HCP and patients [15].

In this chapter, we aim to outline the basic principles of infection control and prevention in the outpatient setting, as well as emphasize common scenarios that represent the highest infectious risk to patients and HCP. It is beyond the scope of this chapter to discuss every particular outpatient setting currently in use; however, we will review major concepts that can be applied to all outpatient settings and highlight a few particularly high-risk scenarios. For an exhaustive review of practices and protocols, we refer you to our references. We will not discuss home healthcare and dental offices; for guidance on these topics, the reader is referred to recent reviews [16–18].

Applying the Principles of Hospital Infection Control to Outpatient Infection Control

Across the vast spectrum of outpatient care settings, there are many unique patient care environments, some of which are wholly dissimilar from hospital settings. However, the principles of infection control and prevention remain constant regardless of the patient care location. Generally speaking, there are two basic epidemiologic approaches to infection control and prevention: (1) broad programs which attempt to reduce the rates of all infections due to all pathogens, so-called horizontal process measures, and (2) narrow programs focusing on a single pathogen or single anatomic site, so-called vertical process measures [19]. When conceptualizing the approach to outpatient infection control, it is helpful to evoke this concept. Horizontal process measures span both the inpatient and outpatient settings. While there will always be exceptional infection control situations, one need not think of outpatient infection control as a field within a field. But rather, it is the application of core principles of infection control across the entire continuum of care. With that said, the outpatient setting does pose distinct challenges when compared to inpatient settings that should not be overlooked. Herein we aim to expound on the key principles of outpatient infection control and how they compare to inpatient practices.

Infrastructure

Infection control programs are tasked with coordinating and directing a large number of activities that are vital to patient safety and quality care. Implementing the most current and credible scientific evidence and guidelines, detecting and investigating outbreaks, surveillance of HAIs, educating healthcare personnel (HCP), intervening to prevent infections, and antimicrobial stewardship are but a few functions of any robust program. A program must be outfitted with sufficient equipment, supplies, and trained personnel to carry out these tasks. In the hospital setting, mandatory compliance with state and federal regulations has led to significant resources being funneled to infection control programs; however, the same cannot be said of outpatient setting.

Unfortunately, as the CDC indicated in its summary document, Guide to Infection Prevention for Outpatient Settings: Minimum Expectation for Safe Care, compared to inpatient acute care settings, outpatient settings have traditionally lacked infrastructure and resources to support infection prevention and surveillance activities [15]. Because many outpatient care settings are not certified by CMS or licensed by states, they do not invest appropriate funding to develop robust infection control programs. However, as the number of patients undergoing increasingly complex medical treatment in the ambulatory setting continues to grow, a parallel increase in risk of iatrogenic infection can be anticipated [12]. One must conclude that outpatients deserve care that is as effective and safe as that received by inpatients.

Standard Precautions

Standard precautions include a bundle of practices that apply to all patients and HCWs across the entire spectrum of healthcare (see Table 6.1). As outlined in the HICPAC 2007 Guideline for Isolation Precautions, the "implementation of Standard Precautions constitutes the primary strategy for the

Table 6.1 Essential standard precautions

Standard precautions	Hand hygiene
	Use of personal protective equipment (e.g., gloves, gowns, masks)
	Safe injection practices
	Safe handling of potentially contaminated equipment or surfaces in the patient environment
	Respiratory hygiene/cough etiquette

Adapted from: Guide to infection prevention in outpatient settings: minimum expectations for safe care [15]

prevention of healthcare-associated transmission of infectious agents among patients and healthcare personnel" [20]. These practices should be employed wherever healthcare is delivered, including outpatient settings, regardless of whether or not the patient is suspected of having an infection. True rates of compliance with standard precautions across the spectrum of outpatient settings are currently unknown but are likely below expectations owing to the relative absence of surveillance when compared to the inpatient setting.

The individual components of standard precautions as they pertain to outpatient settings will be expanded upon below. We refer the reader to the CDC website and current guidelines for a detailed review of standard precautions in the outpatient setting [20, 21].

Hand Hygiene

In terms of overall impact on infection rates, it is difficult to overstate the vital importance of proper hand hygiene. The hands of HCWs are the most common vectors by which microorganisms are transmitted to patients [22]. Beginning with the establishment of germ theory by Ignaz Semmelweis in the 1840s, the association between hand hygiene and reduction of HAIs has been demonstrated in various settings, and hand hygiene is now widely regarded as one of the most important of all infection control practices [23, 24]. It serves as the backbone of any effective infection control program. Despite a strong consensus of its effectiveness among infection control professionals and the widespread dissemination of convenient access to alcohol-based hand sanitizers, hand hygiene compliance rates remain far below expectations, perhaps as low as 40% in inpatient settings [23, 25]. The reasons for this are many, including an overestimation of self-compliance, inconvenient location of sinks, understaffing or busy work setting, skin irritation, poor attention to guidelines, and more [23, 25]. To date, there is no comprehensive analysis of surveillance data for hand hygiene compliance across the wide spectrum of outpatient care settings; however, individual settings have been studied and rates of compliance seem to be extremely poor (as low as 18% among HCWs) [26, 27].

Why Is Hand Hygiene Compliance So Poor in the Outpatient Setting?

In contrast to inpatient settings, the physical layout of outpatient settings is more variable. Often times, there is no alcohol-based hand rub (ABHR) outside of examination rooms. Sinks and/or ABHR is often inside the examination room. The examination room door is closed when an HCW is seeing a patient, essentially eliminating the ability to covertly observe the process [28]. Furthermore, hand hygiene compliance monitoring is performed less often than in the inpatient setting due to the absence of infection control staff, dedicated resources, and regulations mandating that monitoring be performed. These factors and likely many more effect compliance rates, but due to the paucity of research in this area, much of this is speculation.

Recommendations

In the outpatient setting, the CDC and WHO recommend ABHR due to its broad antimicrobial activity, superior compliance rates, expediency, and convenience when compared to soap and water [15, 29]. When hands are visibly soiled or after caring for patients with infectious diarrhea (e.g., *Clostridium difficile*, norovirus, etc.), soap and water is preferred [15, 30] (see Table 6.2).

For comprehensive guidance on how and when hand hygiene should be performed, we refer you to the *Guideline for Hand Hygiene in Health-Care Settings Recommendations of the Healthcare Infection Control Practices Advisory*

Table 6.2 Key recommendations for hand hygiene in ambulatory care settings

Key situations where hand hygiene should be performed	Before touching a patient, even if gloves will be worn
	Before exiting the patient's care area after touching the patient or the patient's immediate environment
	After contact with blood, body fluids or excretions, or wound dressings
	Prior to performing an aseptic task (e.g., placing an IV, preparing an injection)
	If hands will be moving from a contaminated-body site to a clean-body site during patient care
	After glove removal

Adapted from: Guide to infection prevention in outpatient settings: minimum expectations for safe care [15]

Committee and the HICPAC/SHEA/APIC/IDSA Hand Hygiene Task Force [30].

Injection Practices

Safe injection practices are considered to be part of standard precautions. The CDC defines injection safety as "practices intended to prevent transmission of infectious diseases between one patient and another, or between a patient and healthcare provider during preparation and administration of parenteral medications" [15]. Injections are invasive procedures, and, as with any invasive procedure, they pose a risk of infection to the patient and the HCW. Consequently, the Occupational Safety and Health Administration (OSHA) has developed the "Bloodborne Pathogens Standard" which can be found in the Code of Federal Regulations. The standard OSHA has set forth outlines what employers must do to protect workers who are occupationally exposed to blood or other potentially infectious materials (OPIM), as defined in the standard. However, despite having clear guidelines to maximize injection safety, major safety breeches continue to plague the outpatient care setting. There have been many significant outbreaks linked to ambulatory care procedures reported in the last 20 years. Outbreaks have been tied to common source exposures such as single- and multi-dose medication vials, intravenous solutions, vaccine administration, insulin needles, and, more recently, a multistate fungal meningitis outbreak linked to glucocorticoid injections originating from compounding pharmacies [31–35].

Much progress is needed in ensuring safe injections practices in the United States. Traditionally, problems with injection practices were thought to be a problem of low- and middle-income countries. In the year 2000, the estimated global incidence of infections related to unsafe injection practices included a total of >20 million hepatitis B virus infections, > two million hepatitis C virus infection, and >250,000 HIV infections [36]. However, the Unites States is not exempted from this alarming trend. A comprehensive review of patient notification of blood-borne pathogen exposure occurring between 2001 and 2011 identified 35 patient notification events related to unsafe injection practices in at least 17 states, resulting in an estimated total of 130,198 patients notified. Eighty-three percent involved outpatient care settings and 74% occurred since 2007. The most common breach identified (≥16 events; 44%) was syringe reuse to access shared medications (e.g., single-dose or multi-dose vials). Most notification events were linked to viral hepatitis transmission (22 events; 63%), and 13 (37%) notification events were prompted by the discovery of unsafe injection practices [35]. Another review evaluating outpatient viral hepatitis outbreaks in the United States between 1998 and 2008 identified a total of 33 outbreaks that occurred in non-hospital settings (outpatient clinics ($N = 12$), dialysis centers ($N = 6$), and long-term care facilities ($N = 15$)), resulting in 448 cases of HBV or HCV infection [37].

Breeches in safe injection practices have led to catastrophic consequences. In 2008, an endoscopy clinic in Las Vegas was linked to the largest hepatitis C outbreak in US history. Investigation of the outbreak uncovered that transmission of hepatitis C stemmed from the routine reuse of single-dose vials of propofol from one patient to another. Ultimately, 114 cases of hepatitis C acquisition were linked to the clinic and over 40,000 patients required notification of potential exposure to blood-borne diseases [38]. In 2002, unsafe practices at an outpatient pain clinic in Oklahoma led to 71 patients acquiring hepatitis C and 31 patients acquiring hepatitis B. A total of 908 people required notification of potential exposure [39]. Investigation of the outbreak determined that the Certified Registered Nurse Anesthetist (CRNA) responsible routinely prepared three needles and syringes per day (one for each medication) and reused them on multiple patients during each clinic session.

Misconceptions about injection safety are common. A survey among nurse anesthetists in the Unites States revealed that nearly 4% have administered medications from the same syringe to multiple patients, 18% had reused a needle on the same patient, and 82% had refilled used syringes [40]. Furthermore, the study found that 22% had reused a syringe or needle to withdraw medication from a multi-dose vial, and nearly 50% had reentered a single-use medication vial to prepare doses for multiple patients [40]. After analyzing four major outbreaks of hepatitis B and C in four unique outpatient settings (a pain clinic, private medical practice, endoscopy clinic, and hematology-oncology clinic), HICPAC concluded that the primary breaches in infection control practices were the following:

1. Reinsertion of used needles into a multiple-dose vial or solution container (e.g., saline bag)
2. Use of a single needle/syringe to administer intravenous medication to multiple patients [20]

Other common lapses include the preparation of medications in close proximity to contaminated supplies or equipment and the failure to wear a facemask (e.g., surgical mask) when placing a catheter or injecting material into the epidural or subdural space [15]. There are many more examples of injection safety breeches, though the reported events are likely only the tip of the iceberg. The true prevalence of unsafe injection practices is unknown.

Injection safety is a complex public health problem requiring coordination on multiple levels within healthcare organizations as well as enforcement and oversight on the state and federal level. Safe injection practices are a key element of standard precautions. Definitive guidance on safe

injection practices can be accessed via the 2007 Guideline for Isolation Precautions [20]. The numerous outbreaks stemming from breeches in injection safety should serve as a beacon to encourage heightened infection control attention in this area. Recently, the CDC has partnered with the Safe Injection Practices Coalition (SIPC) to develop a public health campaign called the "One & Only Campaign," to raise awareness among patients and healthcare providers about safe injection practices and to promote said practices. The CDC website on injection safety also provides numerous resources including an injection safety toolkit for infection control programs (see Table 6.3) [15, 41].

Table 6.3 Safe injection practices

Key recommendations for safe injection practices in outpatient settings	Use aseptic technique when preparing and administering medications
	Cleanse the access diaphragms of medication vials with alcohol before inserting a device into the vial
	Never administer medications from the same syringe to multiple patients, even if the needle is changed or the injection is administered through an intervening length of intravenous tubing
	Do not reuse a syringe to enter a medication vial or solution
	Do not administer medications from single-dose or single-use vials, ampoules, or bags or bottles of intravenous solution to more than one patient
	Do not use fluid infusion or administration sets (e.g., intravenous tubing) for more than one patient
	Dedicate multi-dose vials to a single patient whenever possible. If multi-dose vials will be used for more than one patient, they should be restricted to a centralized medication area and should not enter the immediate patient treatment area (e.g., operating room, patient room/cubicle)
	Dispose of used sharps at the point of use in a sharps container that is closable, puncture resistant, and leak-proof
	Wear a facemask (e.g., surgical mask) when placing a catheter or injecting material into the epidural or subdural space (e.g., during myelogram, epidural, or spinal anesthesia)

Adapted from: Guide to infection prevention in outpatient settings: minimum expectations for safe care [15]

Surveillance

Surveillance is defined as the ongoing, systematic collection, analysis, interpretation, and dissemination of data regarding a health-related event for use in public health action to reduce morbidity and mortality and to improve health [15]. Conducting outcomes-based infection surveillance in the outpatient setting is inherently challenging. In contrast to the hospital setting where a patient is under close observation, outpatient encounters are sporadic and short lived. Patients that develop outpatient HAIs do not become symptomatic until returning home and subsequently might not report to the same facility where the HAI developed. Therefore, surveillance in the outpatient setting typically requires retrospective reviews of medical records or prospective audits. Cross talk and data extraction between electronic medical record (EMR) systems is lacking or nonexistent, further complicating the process of data procurement. Novel methods to track infections across the continuum of care are needed in order to capture the true rates of outpatient HAIs. Research in this area is underway, for example, researchers at Duke developed an automated system for prospective surveillance for post-ERCP bacteremia in order to establish an institutional baseline rate of post-ERCP bloodstream infections [42]. Further developments in technology are needed so that outpatient HAIs can be promptly identified.

Generally speaking, surveillance data in outpatient care facilities is largely absent [43]. For example, a mere 20 ASCs reported data to the National Healthcare Safety Network (NHSN) between 2006 and 2008, compared with data reported by 1,545 hospitals [44]. The majority of data related to HAIs comes primarily from hospitals, which, in contrast to outpatient settings, have established infrastructure with dedicated infection control personnel to carry out HAI surveillance. Furthermore, regulations requiring surveillance and reporting of HAIs in the outpatient setting are far less robust than their inpatient counterparts are [11]. However, due to several unprecedented outbreaks in the outpatient setting, public awareness has been significantly heightened in the past decade and more oversight is forthcoming.

Currently, the CDC recommends that at a minimum outpatient care settings adhere to local, state, and federal regulations regarding reportable diseases, as well as performing regular audits and competency evaluations of HCW adherence to infection prevention practices (see Table 6.4 below) [15]. As opposed to outcomes data (e.g., rates of CLABSI at hemodialysis centers), performing surveillance on process measures such as HCW compliance with existing infection prevention guidelines would potentially be less complicated and may serve as a good start in the process of enhancing surveillance in the outpatient setting.

Table 6.4 Recommendations

Key recommendations for HAI surveillance and reporting in outpatient settings	Educate patients who have undergone procedures at the facility regarding signs and symptoms of infection that may be associated with the procedure and instruct them to notify the facility if such signs and symptoms occur
	Adhere to local, state, and federal requirements regarding HAI surveillance, reportable diseases, and outbreak reporting
	Perform regular audits of HCP adherence to infection prevention practices

Adapted from: Guide to infection prevention in outpatient settings: minimum expectations for safe care [15]

More stringent federal regulations regarding surveillance in the outpatient setting are forthcoming as outlined in Phase Two of the DHHS *National Action Plan to Prevent Health Care-Associated Infections: Road Map to Elimination.* Based on previous trends, without government-mandated surveillance and reporting, the likelihood of outpatient care settings investing in infection control programs to carry out high-quality surveillance is low (see section below for further discussion of this topic) (see Table 6.4).

Regulations, Mandatory Reporting, and Monitoring

Unlike acute care settings which are highly regulated and where accreditation is the standard, outpatient care settings are not held to the same regulatory standard and are operating more under the auspices of trust. For example, despite ambulatory care centers (ASCs) being subject to the same regulatory requirements for Medicare participation as inpatient facilities for similar services provided, the majority of monitoring of regulatory compliance has been left to individual states, and direct observation has not been required [3]. Only a minority, 20–25% of ASCs, are accredited by one of the official accreditation organizations deemed by CMS (see Table 6.5) [11].

Generally speaking, surveillance data for these facilities is largely absent. For example, only 20 ASCs reported data to the National Healthcare Safety Network (NHSN) between 2006 and compared with data reported by 1545 hospitals [44]. However, due to several high-profile cases of HAIs in ASCs revealing significant lapses in infection control practices, the outpatient setting has come under heightened scrutiny. One such example involved approximately 40,000 patients in Nevada that were potentially exposed to hepatitis C, HIV, and other blood-borne pathogens over a 4-year period [38]. Cases such as this prompted an investigation of

Table 6.5 Accrediting organization deemed by CMS

Accrediting organization deemed by CMS	The Joint Commission (TJC)
	Accreditation Association for Ambulatory Health Care (AAAHC)
	Accreditation Association for Ambulatory Health Care (AAAHC)
	American Association for Accreditation of Ambulatory Surgery Facilities (AAAASF)
	American Osteopathic Association (AOA)

Table 6.6 Identifying potentially infectious patients in the outpatient setting

Identifying potentially infectious patients in the outpatient setting	Patients with symptoms of active infection (e.g., diarrhea, rash, respiratory symptoms, draining wounds, skin lesions) come at a time when the facility is less crowded
	Alert registration staff to place potentially infected patients in a private exam room upon arrival and if available and follow the procedures pertinent to the route of transmission
	If the purpose of the visit is nonurgent, patients are encouraged to reschedule the appointment until symptoms have resolved

Adapted from the CDC's, basic infection control and prevention plan for outpatient oncology settings [21]

ASCs by the Government Accountability Organization (GAO) in 2009. The report emphasized the unacceptable absence of health outcomes and process measure data available for ASCs. They concluded:

> The increasing volume of procedures and evidence of infection control lapses in ASCs create a compelling need for current and nationally representative data on HAIs in ASCs in order to reduce their risk. Because HAIs generally only occur after a patient has left an ASC, data on the occurrence of these infections—outcome data—are difficult to collect. But data on the implementation of CDC-recommended infection control practices—process data—in ASCs can be collected more easily and can provide critical information on why HAIs are occurring and what can be done to help prevent them [43].

The GAO went on to recommend that the Acting Secretary of DHHS develops and implements a written plan to use a data collection instrument and methodology to conduct recurring periodic surveys of randomly selected ASCs in order to collect data on infection control practices and target ICP strategies [43]. In 2013, the DHHS developed the *National Action Plan to Prevent Health Care-Associated Infections: Road Map to Elimination*. As part of Phase Two of the action plan, ASCs and end-stage renal disease facilities were selected as focus areas. As the DHHS plan is implemented over the next few decades, we are likely to witness transformational changes concerning regulations, mandatory reporting, and monitoring in outpatient settings.

Transmission-Based Precautions

Transmission-based precautions are intended to serve as an adjunct to standard precautions in patients with known or suspected colonization or infection of highly transmissible or epidemiologically important pathogens. Transmission-based precautions encompass three categories: contact precautions, droplet precautions, and airborne precautions.

Transmission of MDROs such as methicillin-resistant *Staphylococcus aureus* (MRSA), carbapenemase-producing *Enterobacteriaceae* (CRE), and *Clostridium difficile* is not confined to the inpatient setting. These organisms have the potential to be acquired in the outpatient setting as well. With

the rise of community-associated MRSA and *C. difficile*, some experts have hypothesized that outpatient care settings may be serving as silent reservoirs for these organisms. Indeed, environmental contamination and patient colonization with vancomycin-resistant *Enterococcus* (VRE) and MRSA have been reported in the outpatient setting [45, 46]. Although research is limited, the risk of infection transmission in the outpatient setting is thought to be lower than in the hospital owing to shorter contact time, fewer encounters, and exposure to lower inoculums of bacteria [47]. Consequently, the traditional approach to isolation in the outpatient setting has not been as aggressive as its inpatient counterpart. However, as more and more high-risk populations such as bone marrow and solid organ transplant recipients, and patients with febrile neutropenia are managed in the outpatient setting, traditional paradigms will need to be reevaluated. Risk of transmission of infectious pathogens will vary between outpatient settings depending on the patient population, facility design, and services provided.

In general, the CDC recommends that *each outpatient facility should evaluate the services they provide to determine specific needs and to assure that sufficient and appropriate personal protective equipment (PPE) is available for adherence to Standard Precautions* [15]. All HCWs at outpatient facilities should be educated regarding proper use of and selection of PPE. Comprehensive guidance on the selection and proper use of PPE is available in the CDC's *HICPAC 2007 Guideline for Isolation Precautions* [20].

The CDC has issued specific guidance for special settings. In 2011, they released recommendations pertaining to infection control and prevention in outpatient oncology settings [21]. Identifying potentially infected patients prior to arrival is recommended (see Table 6.6).

The CDC has also provided specific recommendations pertaining to contact precautions, droplet precautions, and airborne precautions in the outpatient oncology setting

Table 6.7 Contact precautions

Apply to patients with the following conditions:	Presence of stool incontinence (may include patients with norovirus, rotavirus, C. diff), draining wounds, uncontrolled secretions, pressure ulcers, presence of ostomy tubes and/or bags draining body fluids
	Presence of generalized rash or exanthems
Isolation	Stool incontinence, draining wounds and/or skin lesions that cannot be covered, or uncontrolled secretions
Hand hygiene	Perform hand hygiene before touching patient and prior to wearing gloves
	Perform hand hygiene after removal of PPE; note: use soap and water when hands are visibly soiled (e.g., blood, body fluids) or after caring for patients with known or suspected infectious diarrhea (e.g., *Clostridium difficile*, norovirus)
PPE use	Wear gloves when touching the patient and the patient's immediate environment or belongings
	Wear a gown if substantial contact with the patient or their environment is anticipated
Environmental cleaning	Clean/disinfect the exam room
Bathroom use	Instruct patients with known or suspected infectious diarrhea to use a separate bathroom, if available; clean/disinfect the bathroom before it can be used again (refer to section IV.F.5. for bathroom cleaning/disinfection)

Adapted from the CDC's, basic infection control and prevention plan for outpatient oncology settings [21]

Table 6.8 Respiratory etiquette

Key components of respiratory etiquette	Education of healthcare facility staff, patients, and visitors
	Posted signs, in language(s) appropriate to the population served, with instructions to patients and accompanying family members or friends
	Source control measures (e.g., covering the mouth/nose with a tissue when coughing and prompt disposal of used tissues, using surgical masks on the coughing person when tolerated and appropriate)
	Hand hygiene after contact with respiratory secretions
	Spatial separation, ideally >3 ft, of persons with respiratory infections in common waiting areas when possible

Adapted from the HICPAC 2007 guideline for isolation precautions: preventing transmission of infectious agents in healthcare settings [20]

(see Table 6.7). These recommendations may serve as a general guide for transmission-based precautions in the outpatient setting, though more recommendations tailored to the myriad of unique outpatient settings are needed.

Respiratory Hygiene and Cough Etiquette

Patients awaiting care in the outpatient setting often sit for long periods in common areas such as waiting rooms, which complicates the application of transmission-based precautions. Often times, patients with transmissible respiratory illnesses are awaiting a diagnosis and are not recognized immediately. This is especially risky for immunocompromised patients such as bone marrow or solid organ transplant recipients that may be sitting next to a patient with influenza, respiratory syncytial virus (RSV), measles, or varicella zoster. Transmission of *Mycobacterium tuberculosis* and measles has been reported in the outpatient setting [48, 49]. To minimize transmission or airborne and droplet infectious agents, patients must be screened for these infections at the outset of the patient encounter [20]. This is especially important for

patients with clinical signs including cough, rhinorrhea, and other respiratory secretions. The CDC's *2007 Guideline for Isolation Precautions: Preventing Transmission of Infectious Agents in Healthcare Settings* outlines the most important elements of cough etiquette, which should be implemented in outpatient settings [20] (see Table 6.8).

Patients with potentially transmissible airborne or droplet infectious diseases should be quickly separated, and appropriate transmission-based infection control measure should be implemented as outlined in the 2007 Guideline for Isolation Precautions: Preventing Transmission of Infectious Agents in Healthcare Settings [20] (see Tables 6.9 and 6.10).

Of note, implementation of contact precautions in the United States is undergoing a period of significant paradigm shift. Recently, the utility of isolating carriers of MRSA and resistant *Enterococcus* in the hospital setting has been called into question [50]. Many hospitals have changed longstanding infection prevention practices accordingly. As new evidence and protocols are deployed for inpatient infection control, these data and practices should be extrapolated to the outpatient setting, as well, when appropriate.

Environmental Cleaning

All outpatient healthcare facilities should develop protocols and procedures for the systematic cleaning and disinfection of environmental surfaces. High-contact patient care surfaces should be prioritized, including bedrails, doorknobs, bedside tables, commodes, sinks, surfaces, and any other surfaces in close proximity to the patient [20]. Facilities should be utilizing EPA-registered disinfectants and cleaning supplies best suited for their particular needs. Strict adherence to the manufacturer's recommendations regarding the usage of cleaning products should be followed. Particular infectious agents

Table 6.9 Droplet precautions

Apply to patients with known or suspected:	Respiratory viruses (e.g., influenza, parainfluenza virus, adenovirus, respiratory syncytial virus, human metapneumovirus, etc.)
	For first 24 h of antibiotic therapy: *Neisseria meningitidis*, group A streptococcus
	Bordetella pertussis
Isolation	Place the patient in an exam room with a closed door as soon as possible
	Prioritize patients who have excessive cough and sputum production
	If an exam room is not available, the patient is provided a facemask and placed in a separate area as far from other patients as possible while awaiting care
PPE	Wear a facemask, such as a procedure or surgical mask, for close contact with the patient; the facemask should be donned upon entering the exam room
	If substantial spraying of respiratory fluids is anticipated, gloves and gown as well as goggles (or face shield in place of goggles) should be worn
	Instruct patient to wear a facemask when exiting the exam room, avoid coming into close contact with other patients, and practice respiratory hygiene and cough etiquette
Hand hygiene	Perform hand hygiene before and after touching the patient and after contact with respiratory secretions and contaminated objects/materials; note: use soap and water when hands are visibly soiled (e.g., blood, body fluids)
Environmental cleaning	Clean and disinfect the exam room

Adapted from the CDC's, basic infection control and prevention plan for outpatient oncology settings [21]

Table 6.10 Airborne precautions

Apply to patient with known or suspected:	Active tuberculosis
	Measles
	Chickenpox (until lesions crusted over)
	Localized (in immunocompromised patient) or disseminated herpes (until lesions are crusted over)
Isolation	Have patient enter through a separate entrance to the facility (e.g., dedicated isolation entrance), if available, to avoid the reception and registration area
	Place the patient immediately in an airborne infection isolation room (AIIR)
	If an AIIR is not available:
	• Provide a facemask (e.g., procedure or surgical mask) to the patient and place the patient immediately in an exam room with a closed door
	• Instruct the patient to keep the facemask on while in the exam room, if possible, and to change the mask if it becomes wet
	• Initiate protocol to transfer patient to a healthcare facility that has the recommended infection-control capacity to properly manage the patient
PPE	Wear a fit-tested N-95 or higher-level disposable respirator, if available, when caring for the patient; the respirator should be donned prior to room entry and removed after exiting room
	If substantial spraying of respiratory fluids is anticipated, gloves and gown as well as goggles or face shield should be worn
Hand hygiene	Perform hand hygiene before and after touching the patient and after contact with respiratory secretions and/or body fluids and contaminated objects/materials; note: use soap and water when hands are visibly soiled (e.g., blood, body fluids)
Patient instructions	Instruct patient to wear a facemask when exiting the exam room, avoid coming into close contact with other patients, and practice respiratory hygiene and cough etiquette
Environmental cleaning	Once the patient leaves, the exam room should remain vacant for generally 1 h before anyone enters; however, adequate wait time may vary depending on the ventilation rate of the room and should be determined accordingly
	If staff must enter the room during the wait time, they are required to use respiratory protection

Adapted from the CDC's, basic infection control and prevention plan for outpatient oncology settings [21]

such as *C. difficile*, norovirus, rotavirus, and prions may be resistant to disinfectants and require specialized disinfectants. For detailed recommendations regarding the disinfection of surfaces, outpatient infection control programs should adhere to the Guidelines for Environmental Infection Control in Healthcare Facilities [51]. Adherence to environmental cleaning procedures and protocols should be monitored and reinforced (see Table 6.11).

Medical Devices

Manufacturers classify medical devices as either single use or multiuse. Single-use devices (SUDs) should never be reused, with the exception of those entities that have received special authorization from the Food and Drug Administration (FDA) [52]. In such cases, reprocessing of SUDs can only be performed by third party or hospital reprocessors that have explicit clearance from the FDA and are registered with FDA as reprocessing facilities [52]. Transmission of infection can occur through medical devices that are

Table 6.11 Cleaning and disinfection of environmental surfaces in outpatient settings

Establish policies and procedures for routine cleaning and disinfection of environmental surfaces in the facility
Policies and procedures should also address prompt and appropriate cleaning and decontamination of spills of blood or other potentially infectious materials
Select EPA-registered disinfectants or detergents/disinfectants with label claims for use in healthcare
Follow manufacturer's recommendations for use of cleaners and EPA-registered disinfectants (e.g., amount, dilution, contact time, safe use, and disposal)

Adapted from: Guide to infection prevention in outpatient settings: minimum expectations for safe care [15]

inadequately cleaned between patients before disinfection or sterilization (e.g., endoscopes, bronchoscopes, surgical instruments) or that have manufacturing defects that interfere with the effectiveness of reprocessing [20]. In the ambulatory care setting, the field of endoscopy makes up a significant proportion of the medical devices pertinent to this discussion. The number of outpatient gastroenterology procedures being performed in the United States is on the rise. In 2009, there were an estimated 11.5 million lower (i.e., colonoscopy, sigmoidoscopy), 6.9 million upper (i.e., esophagogastroduodenoscopy), and 228,000 biliary endoscopies performed in the United States culminating in an estimated total outpatient cost of $32.4 billion [53]. The estimated incidence of infection transmitted by GI endoscopic procedures is 1 in 1.8 million procedures [54]. Bronchoscopy also makes up a significant number of ambulatory procedures, estimated at nearly 500,000 per year [55]. The field of endoscopy continues to rapidly expand into urology, ENT, cardiology, and more. The true rate of infection associated with these procedures is difficult to assess given the absence of robust surveillance systems in the outpatient setting. Consequently, infections are typically identified in outbreak scenarios. Most pathogen transmission occurs due to a failure to adhere to established cleaning, disinfection, and sterilization guidelines. A study evaluating the infection control procedures across a random sample of 68 ambulatory care centers in three states identified reprocessing of reusable medical devices as one of the most common lapses in infection control, with nearly 30% of facilities failing to adhere to recommended practices regarding reprocessing of equipment [56]. Inappropriate reprocessing and reuse of single-devices (e.g., bite blocks and syringes used to flush the endoscope during endoscopy procedures) was also discovered in 6% of all ambulatory facilities in the study [56]. Reprocessing of medical devices is highly complex. For example, contamination of bronchoscopes has been linked to a myriad of causes including ineffective cleaning, contamination of instilled solutions, disinfectants

(inadequate activity, incorrect disinfectant, or contaminated disinfectant), recontamination after disinfection (e.g., rinsing with tap water, contaminated tap water filters), contaminated reprocessing equipment, and many other sources [57]. Biofilm production further inhibits the disinfection process [58]. Finally, the burden of contaminating infectious organisms can be massive. After a routine bronchoscopy, the instrument is contaminated with about 6.4×10^4 cfu/ml of bacteria [59].

When lapses in reprocessing of SUD or reusable medical devices occur, the consequences are not insignificant. In a review of infectious complications of endoscopy between 1966 and 2002, the authors identified 281 cases of transmission due to GI procedures and 96 cases due to bronchoscopy. Various pathogens were implicated in GI endoscopy including *Pseudomonas aeruginosa, Salmonella spp., Helicobacter pylori, Klebsiella pneumoniae, Enterobacter cloacae, Serratia marcescens, Clostridium difficile, Strongyloides stercoralis*, HBV, and HCV [60]. In a review of flexible bronchoscopy-associated infections occurring between 1977 and 2003, only 18 publications reporting true infection were identified with the most common pathogens being *M. tuberculosis, Serratia* spp., atypical mycobacterium, and *P. aeruginosa* [61]. Creutzfeldt-Jakob disease (CJD) and HIV have not been reported to be transmitted via endoscopy [60]. All cases were linked to breaches in reprocessing recommendations. However, it must be noted that outbreaks have been reported even when all reprocessing recommendations have been followed. After an outbreak of New Delhi metallo-β-lactamase-producing carbapenem-resistant *Escherichia coli* (CRE) associated with exposure to duodenoscopes was investigated, no breaches in the six-step reprocessing procedure were identified [62]. To control the outbreak, the facility changed its reprocessing procedure from automated high-level disinfection with ortho-phthalaldehyde to gas sterilization with ethylene oxide. Subsequently there were no cases of CRE identified. These findings suggest that sterilization, rather than high-level disinfection, was needed to fully mitigate the risk of transmission. The authors suggested that conducting testing for residual contamination after reprocessing might be warranted. Concerns over pathogen transmission occurring despite adherence to manufacturer reprocessing instructions prompted a special safety communication from the FDA in 2015 to raise awareness among HCP and reprocessing units that the complex design of ERCP endoscopes (also called duodenoscopes) may impede effective reprocessing and that meticulous cleaning of duodenoscopes prior to high-level disinfection should reduce the risk of transmitting infection but may not entirely eliminate it [63].

The reprocessing of reusable medical devices is not a simple matter. Flexible endoscopes used in procedures such as duodenoscopy, bronchoscopy, and colonoscopy are challenging to clean and disinfect owing to the long, thin internal channels and their inability to be steam sterilized [64]. Proper reprocessing requires an understanding of the internal structure of the device and attention to detail. Because endoscopes are expensive, they are often reused at a high frequency that increases the risk of breaches in cleaning and disinfection protocol. Furthermore, each model must be reprocessed by the unique specifications outlined by the manufacturer, and this is incompatible with a "one-size-fits-all" approach. Traditionally, the Spaulding Classification has defined the

Table 6.12 The Spaulding Classification

Category	Examples of instruments	Level of disinfection
Critical	Surgical instruments	Highest level of disinfection, must be sterile prior to use
	Cardiac and urinary catheters	
	Implants	
	Probes used in sterile body cavities	
	Objects that enter sterile tissue or the vascular system	
Semi-critical	Endoscopes used for upper endoscopy and colonoscopy	At minimum, high-level disinfection prior to use
	Respiratory therapy and anesthesia equipment	
	Laryngoscope blades	
	Esophageal manometry probes	
	Cystoscopes	
	Anorectal manometry catheters	
	Diaphragm fitting rings	
	Contact mucous membranes or non-intact skin	
Noncritical	Blood pressure cuffs	Low- or intermediate-level disinfection depending on the nature of contamination
	Bedpans	
	Crutches	
	Computers	
	May come in contact with intact skin but not mucous membranes	
Environmental surfaces	Floors, walls (surfaces typically not in direct contact with patients during delivery of care)	Simple cleaning or low-level disinfection

Adapted from the CDC's guideline for disinfection and sterilization in healthcare facilities, 2008 [66]

reprocessing of medical equipment (see Table 6.12) [65]. This approach is based on categorizing medical instruments as critical, semi-critical, and noncritical according to the degree of risk for infection involved in their use. Each category has a different degree of disinfection required. The goal of the highest level of disinfection is total sterility of the instrument. High-level disinfection is traditionally defined as the complete elimination of all microorganisms in or on an instrument, except for small numbers of bacterial spores [66].

More recently, the Spaulding Classification has come under scrutiny due to oversimplification of certain complexities among medical devices and fastidious organisms. For example, the method does not account for challenges reprocessing the complicated mechanical hardware within new endoscopes or inactivating certain types of infectious agents such as Creutzfeldt-Jakob disease (CJD). There is not universal agreement among professional organizations as to the optimal contact time for high-level disinfection [66].

Healthcare personnel involved in reprocessing of reusable medical devices should be properly trained, and their competency in carrying out their duties should be evaluated regularly [15]. This is especially important when new devices enter the medical environment, as well as new methods of reprocessing. Individual healthcare organizations should create policies and procedures that guide the proper handling and reprocessing of contaminated reusable medical devices pertinent to their facility, as outlined by the manufacturer's instructions. Infection control personnel should also be versed in the most up-to-date recommendations and guidelines regarding the cleaning and disinfection process of medical devices (see Table 6.13) [15, 20, 52, 58, 66, 67].

Antimicrobial Stewardship

Antibiotic use is thought to be the most important modifiable cause of antibiotic resistance [68]. Outpatient antimicrobial stewardship promotes the appropriate prescribing of antibiotics for non-hospitalized patients in clinics, offices, and emergency rooms [69]. The primary objective of stewardship programs is to promote compliance with clinical practice guidelines in order to optimize patient care and minimize the spread of antibiotic-resistant bacteria. A tremendous amount of antibiotic prescribing occurs in the outpatient setting. A study conducted to evaluate trends in antibiotic prescribing for adults in the United States from 1995 to 2002 revealed that 15.3–17.9% of all outpatient office visits resulted in an antibiotic prescription [70]. Outpatient healthcare providers often feel pressured by patients to prescribe antibiotics for conditions that are most likely viral in etiology. A study evaluating

Table 6.13 Cleaning and disinfection or sterilization of medical devices in outpatient settings

Key recommendations	Facilities should ensure that reusable medical devices (e.g., blood glucose meters and other point-of-care devices, surgical instruments, endoscopes) are cleaned and reprocessed appropriately prior to use on another patient
	Reusable medical devices should be cleaned and reprocessed (disinfection or sterilization) and maintained according to the manufacturer's instructions. If the manufacturer does not provide such instructions, the device may not be suitable for multi-patient use
	Assign responsibilities for reprocessing of medical devices to HCP with appropriate training:
	• Maintain copies of the manufacturer's instructions for reprocessing of devices in use at the facility; post instructions at locations where reprocessing is performed
	• Hands-on training on proper selection and use of PPE and recommended steps for reprocessing assigned devices should be provided upon hire (prior to being allowed to reprocess devices), annually, and when new devices are introduced or policies/procedures change
	○ HCP should be required to demonstrate competency with reprocessing procedures (i.e., correct technique is observed by trainer) following each training
	Assure HCP has access to and wears appropriate PPE when handling and reprocessing contaminated medical devices

Adapted from: Guide to infection prevention in outpatient settings: minimum expectations for safe care [15]

antibiotic prescribing for adults in ambulatory care in the United States from 2007 to 2009 concluded that of the rough 985 million outpatient office visits per year, >100 million visits resulted in an antibiotic prescription and over half of all antibiotic prescribing was unnecessary. The most common conditions associated with inappropriate treatment were acute respiratory infections like sinusitis and bronchitis [71].

Much progress is needed in the field of outpatient antimicrobial stewardship. Improving adherence to guidelines can improve antibiotic prescribing. For instance, it is estimated that a 10% decrease in inappropriate antibiotic prescribing in the outpatient setting could produce a 17% decrease in rates of *Clostridium difficile* infection [72]. Outpatient infection control programs should closely collaborate with their facility's Antibiotic Stewardship Program. Recently, the CDC has developed the "Get Smart: Know When Antibiotics Work" program to ensure that antibiotics are prescribed only when they are needed. The reader is directed to the CDC website for more information and resources [73].

Medical Waste

Some medical waste poses a public health risk and requires special processing with autoclaves or incinerators. Many ambulatory care facilities may not have an expert in infectious waste management at their facility. Ambulatory care facilities must comply with medical waste processing requirements pertaining to their particular city, county, and state, as well as federal regulations. A full discussion of this topic is beyond the scope of this chapter, but has been expounded upon in other texts [74]. A review by Herwaldt et al. [64] advised that outpatient facilities must:

- Define which items are noninfectious waste and which are infectious
- Develop protocols and procedures for separating infectious waste from noninfectious waste, labeling the infectious waste properly and transporting, storing, and disposing of infectious wastes safely
- Develop contingency plans for managing waste spills and inadvertent exposures of patients, visitors, or healthcare workers
- Develop programs to teach staff to handle infectious waste
- Identify ways to minimize infectious waste, e.g.:
  - Stop discarding noninfectious waste, such as wrappers and newspapers in infectious waste
  - Substitute products that do not require special modes of disposal (e.g., needleless intravenous systems) for those that must be discarded in the infectious waste (e.g., needles)
  - Substitute reusable items for the single-use items

Education of Healthcare Personnel

The education of HCP regarding infection control policies and procedures is vital to optimize patient safety. The frequent updates to guidelines and recommendations require that educational programs be longitudinal and that they incorporate regular competency evaluations. Individual healthcare organizations should develop programs that are tailored to the specific needs of the HCP. The CDC recommends that training should be provided upon orientation and anytime policies and procedures are updated or revised [15].

Risk Assessment

To assist with performing a self-assessment of outpatient infection prevention programs, the CDC has developed a checklist tool. This basic checklist can aid in ensuring that ambulatory facilities have appropriate infection prevention policies and procedures in place, as well as supplies to enable healthcare personnel (HCP) to provide safe care. The tool also provides a systematic approach to assessing HCP adherence to correct infection prevention practices [15].

Special Considerations

Clostridium difficile in the Outpatient Setting

Clostridium difficile infection (CDI) is the major cause of infectious diarrhea in the hospital setting; however, community-associated CDI (CA-CDI) is on the rise [75, 76]. *C. difficile* infection is defined as community acquired if symptom onset occurs in the community or within 48 h of admission to a hospital, after no hospitalization in the past 12 weeks [77]. It is estimated that CA-CDI actually represents one-third of all *C. difficile* cases. Traditional risk factors such as age and prior antibiotic exposure may be absent; indeed CA-CDI may affect low-risk hosts such as healthy peripartum women; antibiotic-naïve, young adults or children; and those lacking recent health care exposure [75]. One recent study of 984 patients found that 35.9% did not receive preceding antibiotics, 18% had no outpatient healthcare exposure, and 40.7% had low-level outpatient healthcare exposure [78]. While the primary means of transmission has traditionally been presumed to be person to person or environment to person via the fecal-oral route, recent studies utilizing whole-genome sequencing of isolates from the community setting demonstrated that 45% of all isolates were genetically unique [79].

In addition to overuse of antibiotics, one possible explanation for the increasing burden of CA-CDI is the rising burden of spores in the outpatient healthcare environment. Patients that are successfully treated for hospital-acquired CDI (HA-CDI) have been found to exhibit skin contamination and environmental shedding of *C. difficile* spores 1–4 weeks after therapy [80]. Furthermore, 80% of patients with HA-CDI are seen in the outpatient setting within 12 weeks of discharge [81]. Therefore, patients recovering from a recent CDI could pose a significant risk for transmission of spores during outpatient visits and the outpatient setting may be an underappreciated source of CA-CDI cases [81]. However, current guidelines do not recommend contact precautions for patients in whose diarrhea has resolved [82].

At this time, the best infection control approach to active or suspected CDI in the outpatient setting is unknown. Some experts suggest that patients at highest risk for transmission (i.e., patients on CDI therapy for ≤2 weeks, recent treatment for CDI in the past 2–12 weeks but not on current therapy) should be managed with enhanced precautions including wearing gloves when examining patients and cleaning high-touch surfaces with sporicidal disinfectants after visits [81]. Infection prevention programs should stay up to date with the most current recommendations to prevent *C. difficile* transmission in the outpatients setting, as this topic will likely evolve in the coming years [82].

Epidemic Keratoconjunctivitis

Epidemic keratoconjunctivitis (EKC) is a severe, acute infection of the eye caused by multiple serotypes of Adenovirus. Patients may be contagious even before symptoms arise and remain contagious for up to 2 weeks after symptoms resolve [83]. Viral particles are hardy and may remain viable on surfaces for up to 3 months [84]. For these reasons, EKC is highly contagious and is a frequent cause of epidemics worldwide [83, 85–88]. Outbreaks may last weeks to months, and transmission has occurred in both healthcare-associated and community-associated settings. Transmission may occur directly via contact with eye secretions or indirectly when an uninfected person is exposed to contaminated surfaces, hands, eye drops, or instruments. In the United States, outpatient ophthalmology clinics have been linked to numerous outbreak reports [89–92]. From 2008 to 2010, there were six healthcare-associated outbreaks reported to the CDC across four states, resulting in 411 cases of EKC. Transmission was linked to ophthalmologic examination [92]. Outbreaks have been linked to numerous ophthalmologic procedures such as slit-lamp examinations, contact lens placement, multiple patient visit, tonometry, contaminated solutions, and contact with HCWs that continue to work despite having active EKC [90–92].

Implementation of a formal infection control policy has been shown to reduce and control EKC outbreaks [86, 91]. To minimize the risk of EKC outbreaks, several key recommendations have been made in an article by Herwaldt et al. [64] including:

- HCP should wash hands before and after examining patients.
- HCP should wear gloves for possible contact with the conjunctiva.
- Equipment, including tonometers, should be cleaned and disinfected according to the manufacturer's recommendations and consensus guidelines.

- If a healthcare-associated outbreak is identified, all open ophthalmic solutions should be discarded, and the equipment and environment should be cleaned and disinfected thoroughly.
- During an outbreak, unit doses of ophthalmic solutions should be used.
- During an outbreak, patients with conjunctivitis should be examined in a separate room with designated equipment, supplies, and ophthalmic solutions.
- During an outbreak, elective procedures such as tonometry should be postponed.
- HCP who work in any outpatient area and who have adenovirus conjunctivitis should not work until the inflammation has resolved, which may take 14 or more days.

Ambulatory Surgery Centers

Ambulatory surgery centers are defined by CMS as distinct entities that exclusively provide surgical services to patients who do not require hospitalization and are not expected to need to stay in a surgical facility longer than 24 h [93]. The number of facilities of this type has experienced a meteoric rise in the past few decades, increasing by 54% between 2001 and 2010 to reach a total of >5300 US Medicare-certified ASCs [43]. There is a tremendous volume of care being provided in ASCs. In 2007, over six million procedures were performed in ASCs and at a cost of nearly three billion dollars to Medicare [43]. Greater than three quarters of all surgical procedures in the United States are performed in ASCs, and the spectrum of procedures is vast, including endoscopy, injections to treat chronic pain, cosmetic surgery, dental surgery, and more [3]. Numerous outbreaks have been linked to ambulatory surgical centers, indicating that infection control efforts need to be enhanced. From 2001 through 2011, there were 18 known outbreaks in ASCs in which two or more patients became infected with viral hepatitis associated with unsafe injection practices. Of these known outbreaks, approximately 100,000 patients were notified to seek testing for possible exposure to blood-borne pathogens, and a total of 358 of them were infected with viral hepatitis [94]. One such outbreak in 2007 occurring in an endoscopy clinic in Las Vegas, Nevada, resulted in the notification of >60,000 patients of possible exposure to blood-borne pathogens [38, 94]. A joint investigation by CDC, Southern Nevada Health District (SNHD), and the Nevada State Health Division (NSHD) concluded that hepatitis C transmission likely resulted from reuse of syringes and single-dose vials of propofol on multiple patients. It was also discovered that this Las Vegas clinic had not undergone a full state inspection to evaluate ASC compliance with Medicare health and safety standards in 7 years [56].

Table 6.14 Action plan to prevent HAIs in ASCs [95]

CMS is now requiring all states to use the infection control audit tool and case tracer method for ASC inspections [96]
ASCs cited for deficient practices are required to correct them; ASCs that fail to correct serious deficiencies risk termination of their participation in Medicare
CMS and CDC have provided in-depth infection control training sessions for surveyors, making CMS regional office physicians available to accompany surveyors on inspections and arranging consultations with experienced personnel when questions arise
CMS updated several ASC health and safety standards, effective May 2009
CMS committed to inspect one-third of all ASCs nationwide this year, including a nationally representative subsample for an updated analysis of infection control practices, as recommended by the GAO

Adapted from CDC's webpage, "Infection Control Assessment of Ambulatory Surgical Centers" [95]

As alluded to earlier (see section on "surveillance"), historically infection control in these facilities has not been well regulated, and little is known about actual infection rates and adherence to basic infection control practices. In order to gain insight into the infection control practices within ASCs, CMS piloted an infection control audit tool in 68 ASCs across three states (Maryland, Oklahoma, and North Carolina), to assess facility adherence to recommended practices [56]. Nearly 68% of facilities were found to have at least one lapse in infection control. The most common lapses included mishandling of blood glucose monitoring equipment (25/54; 46.3%), using single-dose medication vials on more than one patient (18/64; 28.1%), and failing to adhere to recommended practices regarding reprocessing of equipment (19/67; 28.4%), and environmental cleaning (12/64; 19%) [56].

In response to this disparity, the DHHS convened a task force in 2007 to develop an action plan to prevent HAIs in ASCs. The CDC has subsequently summarized the current action plan as follows (see Table 6.14):

Ambulatory Surgery Centers should take a proactive role in enhancing their infection control practices. In addition to tighter regulatory control and surveillance at the federal and state level, ASCs must stay up to date with the most current evidence-based guidelines to inform their local infection control programs. Self-audits should be performed on a regular basis using the infection control audit tool designed by CMS [96].

Dialysis Centers

End-stage renal disease (ESRD) is on the rise. According to the most recent data available from US Renal Data System, in 2013 the overall prevalence of ESRD patients in the United States was 661,648, up from ~190,000 in 1999 [97, 98]. While the yearly incidence seems to have plateaued, the prevalence is increasing by about 21,000 cases per year [98]. Nearly 90% of all dialysis patients receive hemodialysis (HD) at one of the nearly 6500 outpatient dialysis units in the United States [98]. This large volume of patients receiving HD in the outpatient setting poses a formidable challenge for infection control programs. The principal infection control problem in dialysis centers is transmission of blood-borne pathogens. Several factors predispose HD patients to infections with blood-borne pathogens, including the following [97]:

- Frequent contact with other patients and HCWs at dialysis centers increasing risk of person-to-person transmission of infectious agents
- Repeated contact with medical devices, equipment, and environmental surfaces in the healthcare setting
- Frequent vascular access for prolonged time periods via various modalities (arteriovenous or "AV" fistula, AV graft, catheters – tunneled and non-tunneled)
- Immunosuppression secondary to uremia, DM, and other comorbidities

Infection is particularly devastating in ESRD patients, conferring a higher risk of mortality than that of the general population. For example, a diagnosis of septicemia bears a cumulative mortality rate of 43% at 1 year, compared to 20% for the general population [99]. The type of HD access is an important factor when considering infection risk. In a systematic review in 2013, Ravani et al. concluded that central venous catheters were associated with the highest risk of fatal infection when compared to other types of vascular access (AV fistulas and grafts). AV fistulas were associated with the lowest risk of infection, followed by AV grafts [100]. Among patients initiating HD in 2013, 80.2% began using a catheter as their vascular access (changing minimally since 2005), and at 90 days, 68.3% were still using a catheter [98]. Consequently, practice guidelines recommend that AV fistulas be the preferred access for HD [97, 101, 102]. With that said, placement of a viable AV fistula is difficult or impossible in some cases, and not necessarily the best option for all patients [103]. Fortunately, between 2005 and 2013, the use of AV fistula at initiation of HD rose from 12 to 17.1% [98]. The most current data suggest that AV fistulas are the most common type of vascular access overall, achieving 61% prevalence [98].

Patients receiving HD at dialysis centers are at risk for transmission of viral hepatitis and HIV. Since the implementation of the first recommendations for the control of hepatitis B in dialysis centers in 1977, and the recommendations for hepatitis B vaccination for all HD patients and staff members in 1982 [104], overall rates of hepatitis B have decreased. From the period of 1976 to 1997, the incidence of HBV infection decreased from 3.0 to 0.05% among patients and from 2.6 to 0.05% among staff members [105]. More recently, the

Table 6.15 CDC health advisory recommendations to improve infection control practices to stop hepatitis C virus transmission in patients undergoing hemodialysis [107]

Evaluate infection control practices in each facility and ensure adherence to infection control standards

- CDC has checklists and audit tools (http://www.cdc.gov/dialysis/prevention-tools/index.html) that providers can use to assess their practices, identify gaps, and improve infection control practices to protect patients
- If gaps are identified, promptly address any issues to protect patients' health and safety (http://www.cdc.gov/dialysis/)

Take action to improve injection safety (http://www.cdc.gov/injectionsafety/), hand hygiene (http://www.cdc.gov/handhygiene/) and routine environmental disinfection procedures, as appropriate

Ensure staff are aware of and trained to implement infection control guidelines (http://www.cdc.gov/dialysis/guidelines/index.html) for hemodialysis settings. Facilities should provide regular (e.g., annual) training (http://www.cdc.gov/dialysis/clinician/index.html) of staff to ensure adherence to infection control recommendations

Follow CDC recommendations for HCV screening of hemodialysis patients and management of patients who test positive

Immediately report any case of new HCV infection among patients undergoing hemodialysis to the state or local health department

Inform patients if HCV transmission is suspected to have occurred within the facility, and explain steps being taken to address the problem

prevalence of hepatitis B surface antigen (HBsAg) positivity among US dialysis patients has improved and is estimated to be around 1%. The current prevalence of HCV is estimated at 7.8% [106].

Despite significant gains being made, outbreaks of viral hepatitis continue to plague dialysis centers in the United States. Recently, the CDC has been receiving an increasing number of reports of acute HCV infection among patients undergoing HD. From 2014 to 2015, the CDC was made aware of 36 cases of acute HCV infection in 19 different hemodialysis clinics in eight states. Investigation of the outbreaks revealed breaches in infection control practices including injection safety, environmental disinfection, and hand hygiene. This prompted the CDC to release an official health advisory alert (see Table 6.15).

To date, there have been no reported cases of person-to-person transmission of HIV at dialysis centers in the United States [97].

Infections are the second leading cause of mortality in dialysis patients. Bacteremia accounts for the majority of severe infections in this population and is most often associated with vascular access [97]. Infection caused by bacterial pathogens in HD patients can be classified as either exogenous (acquired from contaminated dialysis fluids or equipment) or endogenous (caused by invasion of bacteria present in or on the patient) [97]. Exogenous infections have been linked to inadequate dialyzer reprocessing procedures and inadequate treatment of municipal water used in dialysis [108, 109]. One such outbreak was found to be related to the use of contaminated water coupled with the malfunction and improper maintenance of dialysis machine waste handling option ports [109].

Updated federal infection control requirements for dialysis centers in the United States were developed in 2008 when CMS published the final rule on Conditions for Coverage for End-Stage Renal Disease in the Federal Register that integrated the CDC's Recommendations for Preventing Transmission of Infections among Chronic Hemodialysis Patients [93, 97]. In order for dialysis centers to remain certified and receive payments under Medicare, they must comply with the infection control requirements outlined by CMS. The DHHS recently spearheaded the *National Action Plan to Prevent Health Care-Associated Infections: Road Map to Elimination* campaign, Phase Two of which focuses on End-Stage Renal Disease Facilities [11]. The Steering Committee emphasized the need to maintain the HAI Action Plan as a "living document," aimed at "developing successor plans in collaboration with public and private stakeholders to incorporate advances in science and technology, shifts in the ways health care is delivered, changes in health care system processes and cultural norms, and other factors" [110]. Infection control programs must remain up to date on the most current infection control guidelines for dialysis centers. A compendium of the most current guidelines and recommendations along with additional resources can be found at the CDC's webpage devoted to dialysis safety [15, 101, 102, 107, 111].

Conclusions

As healthcare in the United States continues to evolve from the inpatient to the outpatient setting, and as healthcare has become more complex, outpatient infection control has become increasingly important. Infection prevention in the outpatient setting has not received the attention or resources afforded inpatient programs to date. However, high profile infection control lapses have led to greater awareness of the need for robust outpatient infection prevention programs. At this point, the most optimal program elements for all outpatient settings are not clear. However, basic infection prevention practices should be deployed and monitored.

References

1. Friedman C, Barnette M, Buck AS, et al. Requirements for infrastructure and essential activities of infection control and epidemiology in out-of-hospital settings: a consensus panel report. Association for professionals in infection control and epidemiology and society for healthcare epidemiology of America. Infect Control Hosp Epidemiol. 1999;20(10):695–705. doi:10.1086/501569.
2. Ashman J, Hing E, Talwalkar A. NCHS data brief: variation in physician office visit rates by patient characteristics and state, 2012. http://www.cdc.gov/nchs/data/databriefs/db212.htm. Updated 2015. Accessed 14 Jan 2016.
3. Barie PS. Infection control practices in ambulatory surgical centers. JAMA. 2010;303(22):2295–7. doi:10.1001/jama.2010.760.
4. Halpern MT, Yabroff KR. Prevalence of outpatient cancer treatment in the united states: estimates from the medical panel expenditures survey (MEPS). Cancer Investig. 2008;26(6):647–51. doi:10.1080/07357900801905519.
5. Williams DN, Rehm SJ, Tice AD, Bradley JS, Kind AC, Craig WA. Practice guidelines for community-based parenteral anti-infective therapy. ISDA practice guidelines committee. Clin Infect Dis. 1997;25(4):787–801.
6. American Hospital Association. Fast facts on US hospitals. http://www.aha.org/research/rc/stat-studies/fast-facts.shtml. Updated 2015. Accessed 14 Jan 2016. n.d.
7. Al-Tawfiq J, Tambyah PA. Healthcare associated infections (HAI) perspectives. J Infect Public Health. 7(4):339–44. doi:10.1016/j.jiph.2014.04.003.
8. Stelfox HT, Palmisani S, Scurlock C, Orav EJ, Bates DW. The "to err is human" report and the patient safety literature. Qual Saf Health Care. 2006;15(3):174–8. doi:10.1136/qshc.2006.017947.
9. Kohn L, Corrigan J, Donaldson M. To err is human: building a safer health system. Washington, DC: National Academy Press; 2000.
10. Magill SS, Edwards JR, Bamberg W, et al. Multistate point-prevalence survey of health care-associated infections. N Engl J Med NEJM. 2014;370(13):1198–208. doi:10.1056/NEJMoa1306801.
11. National action plan to prevent health care-associated infections. Road map to elimination. http://health.gov/hcq/prevent-hai-action-plan.asp. Updated 2016. Accessed 23 Jan 2016. n.d.
12. Maki DG, Crnich CJ. History forgotten is history relived: nosocomial infection control is also essential in the outpatient setting. Arch Intern Med. 165(22):2565–7. doi:10.1001/archinte.165.22.2565.
13. Outbreaks and patient notifications in outpatient settings, selected examples, 2010–2014. http://www.cdc.gov/HAI/settings/outpatient/outbreaks-patient-notifications.html. Updated 2015. Accessed 19 Jan 2016.
14. Multistate fungal meningitis outbreak investigation. http://www.cdc.gov/hai/outbreaks/infographic.html. Updated 2013. Accessed 19 Jan 2016.
15. Guide to infection prevention for outpatient settings: Minimum expectations for safe care. http://www.cdc.gov/HAI/settings/outpatient/outpatient-care-guidelines.html. Updated 2016. Accessed 19 Jan 2016.
16. Centers for Disease Control and Prevention. Summary of infection prevention practices in dental settings: basic expectations for safe care. Atlanta: US Department of Health and Human Services, Centers for Disease Control and Prevention, National Center for Chronic Disease Prevention and Health Promotion, Division of Oral Health; 2016. http://www.cdc.gov/oralhealth/infectioncontrol/pdf/safe-care.pdf. Updated 2016. Accessed 12 Apr 2016.
17. Clark P. Emergence of infection control surveillance in alternative health care settings. J Infus Nurs. 33(6):363–70. doi:10.1097/NAN.0b013e3181f85a5e.
18. Rhinehart E. Infection control in home care. Emerg Infect Dis. 7(2):208–11. doi:10.3201/eid0702.700208.
19. Wenzel RP, Edmond MB. Infection control: the case for horizontal rather than vertical interventional programs. Int J Infect Dis. 2010;14(Suppl 4):S3–5. doi:10.1016/j.ijid.2010.05.002.
20. Siegel J, Rhinehart E, Jackson M, Chiarello L. 2007 guideline for isolation precautions: preventing transmission of infectious agents in healthcare settings. 2007.
21. Basic infection control and prevention plan for outpatient oncology settings. http://www.cdc.gov/HAI/settings/outpatient/basic-infection-control-prevention-plan-2011/standard-precautions.html. Updated 2011. Accessed 23 Jan 2016.
22. Reybrouck G. Role of the hands in the spread of nosocomial infections. 1. J Hosp Infect. 1983;4(2):103–10.

23. Ellingson K, Haas JP, Aiello AE, et al. Strategies to prevent health-care-associated infections through hand hygiene. Infect Control Hosp Epidemiol. 2014;35(Suppl 2):S155–78.

24. Tyler SW. A course of lectures on the theory and practice of obstetrics. Lancet. 1856;68(1732):503–5. doi:10.1016/S0140-6736(02)60262-4. info:doi/10.1016/S0140-6736(02)60262-4

25. Harris AD, Samore MH, Nafziger R, DiRosario K, Roghmann MC, Carmeli Y. A survey on handwashing practices and opinions of healthcare workers. J Hosp Infect. 2000;45(4):318–21. doi:10.1053/jhin.2000.0781.

26. Mensah E, Murdoch IE, Binstead K, Rotheram C, Franks W. Hand hygiene in routine glaucoma clinics. Br J Ophthalmol. 2005;89(11):1541–2. doi:10.1136/bjo.2005.072538.

27. Shimokura G, Weber DJ, Miller WC, Wurtzel H, Alter MJ. Factors associated with personal protection equipment use and hand hygiene among hemodialysis staff. Am J Infect Control. 2006;34(3):100–7. doi:10.1016/j.ajic.2005.08.012.

28. Bittle MJ, LaMarche S. Engaging the patient as observer to promote hand hygiene compliance in ambulatory care. Jt Comm J Qual Patient Saf. 2009;35(10):519–25.

29. WHO guidelines on hand hygiene in health care, first global patient safety challenge clean care is safer care. 2009.

30. Boyce JM, Pittet D. Guideline for hand hygiene in health-care settings. Recommendations of the healthcare infection control practices advisory committee and the HICPAC/SHEA/APIC/IDSA hand hygiene task force. Society for healthcare epidemiology of America/association for professionals in infection control/infectious diseases society of America. MMWR. 2002;51(16):1–45. quiz CE1

31. Counard CA, Perz JF, Linchangco PC, et al. Acute hepatitis B outbreaks related to fingerstick blood glucose monitoring in two assisted living facilities. J Am Geriatr Soc. 2010;58(2):306–11. doi:10.1111/j.1532-5415.2009.02669.x.

32. Smith RM, Schaefer MK, Kainer MA, et al. Fungal infections associated with contaminated methylprednisolone injections. N Engl J Med. 2013;369(17):1598–609. doi:10.1056/NEJMoa1213978.

33. Transmission of hepatitis B virus among persons undergoing blood glucose monitoring in long-term-care facilities – Mississippi, North Carolina, and Los Angeles County, California, 2003–2004. Morbid Mortal Wkly Rep. 2005;54(9):220–223.

34. Taylor L, Greeley R, Dinitz-Sklar J, et al. Notes from the field: injection safety and vaccine administration errors at an employee influenza vaccination clinic – New Jersey, 2015. Morb Mortal Wkly Rep. 2015;64(49):1363–4. doi:10.15585/mmwr.mm6449a3.

35. Guh AY, Thompson ND, Schaefer MK, Patel PR, Perz JF. Patient notification for bloodborne pathogen testing due to unsafe injection practices in the US health care settings, 2001-2011. Med Care. 2012;50(9):785–91. doi:10.1097/MLR.0b013e31825517d4.

36. Ezzati M, Lopez AD, Rodgers A, Vander Hoorn S, Murray CJL. Selected major risk factors and global and regional burden of disease. Lancet. 2002;360(9343):1347–60. doi:10.1016/S0140-6736(02)11403-6.

37. Thompson ND, Perz JF, Moorman AC, Holmberg SD. Nonhospital health care-associated hepatitis B and C virus transmission: United states, 1998-2008. Ann Intern Med. 2009;150(1):33–9.

38. Acute hepatitis C virus infections attributed to unsafe injection practices at an endoscopy clinic – Nevada, 2007. Morbid Mortal Wkly Rep. 2008;57(19):513–517.

39. Comstock RD, Mallonee S, Fox JL, et al. A large nosocomial outbreak of hepatitis C and hepatitis B among patients receiving pain remediation treatments. Infect Control Hosp Epidemiol. 2004;25(7):576–83. doi:10.1086/502442.

40. Ford K. Survey of syringe and needle safety among student registered nurse anesthetists: are we making any progress? AANA J. 2013;81(1):37–42.

41. CDC injection safety. http://www.cdc.gov/injectionsafety/. Updated 2015. Accessed 5 Apr 2016.

42. Anderson DJ, Shimpi RA, McDonald JR, et al. Infectious complications following endoscopic retrograde cholangiopancreatography: an automated surveillance system for detecting postprocedure bacteremia. Am J Infect Control. 2008;36(8):592–4. doi:10.1016/j.ajic.2007.10.023.

43. Healthcare-associated infections: HHS action needed to obtain nationally representative data on risk in ambulatory surgical centers. 2009;GAO-09-213.

44. Edwards JR, Peterson KD, Mu Y, et al. National healthcare safety network (NHSN) report: data summary for 2006 through 2008, issued December 2009. Am J Infect Control. 2009;37(10):783–805. doi:10.1016/j.ajic.2009.10.001.

45. Johnston CP, Cooper L, Ruby W, Carroll KC, Cosgrove SE, Perl TM. Epidemiology of community-acquired methicillin-resistant Staphylococcus aureus skin infections among healthcare workers in an outpatient clinic. Infect Control Hosp Epidemiol. 2006;27(10):1133–6. doi:10.1086/507970.

46. Atta MG, Eustace JA, Song X, Perl TM, Scheel PJ. Outpatient vancomycin use and vancomycin-resistant enterococcal colonization in maintenance dialysis patients. Kidney Int. 2001;59(2):718–24. doi:10.1046/j.1523-1755.2001.059002718.x.

47. Nafziger DA, Lundstrom T, Chandra S, Massanari RM. Infection control in ambulatory care. Infect Dis Clin N Am. 1997;11(2):279–96.

48. Haley CE, McDonald RC, Rossi L, Jones WD, Haley RW, Luby JP. Tuberculosis epidemic among hospital personnel. Infect Control Hosp Epidemiol. 1989;10(5):204–10.

49. Atkinson WL, Markowitz LE, Adams NC, Seastrom GR. Transmission of measles in medical settings – United States, 1985-1989. Am J Med. 1991;91(3):320S–4S.

50. Morgan DJ, Kaye KS, Diekema DJ. Reconsidering isolation precautions for endemic methicillin-resistant staphylococcus aureus and vancomycin-resistant enterococcus. JAMA. 2014;312(14):1395–6. doi:10.1001/jama.2014.10142.

51. Sehulster L, RYW C. Guidelines for environmental infection control in health-care facilities. Recommendations of CDC and the healthcare infection control practices advisory committee (HICPAC). Morb Mortal Wkly Rep. 2003;52(10):1–42.

52. Guidance for industry and FDA staff – medical device user fee and modernization act of 2002, validation data in premarket notification submissions (510(k)s) for reprocessed single-use medical devices. http://www.fda.gov/MedicalDevices/DeviceRegulationandGuidance/GuidanceDocuments/ucm071434. Updated 2015. Accessed 5 Apr 2016.

53. Peery AF, Dellon ES, Lund J, et al. Burden of gastrointestinal disease in the United States: 2012 update. Gastroenterology. 2012;143(5):1179–87.e1. doi:10.1053/j.gastro.2012.08.002.

54. Schembre DB. Infectious complications associated with gastrointestinal endoscopy. Gastrointest Endosc Clin N Am. 2000;10(2):215–32.

55. Vital and health statistics from the Centers for Disease Control and Prevention/National Center for Health Statistics. Ambulatory and inpatient procedures in the united states, 1996. http://www.cdc.gov/nchs/data/series/sr_13/sr13_139.pdf. Updated 1996. Accessed 6 Apr 2016.

56. Schaefer MK, Jhung M, Dahl M, et al. Infection control assessment of ambulatory surgical centers. JAMA. 2010;303(22):2273–9. doi:10.1001/jama.2010.744.

57. Culver DA, Gordon SM, Mehta AC. Infection control in the bronchoscopy suite: a review of outbreaks and guidelines for prevention. Am J Respir Crit Care Med. 2003;167(8):1050–6. doi:10.1164/rccm.200208-797CC.

58. Alvarado CJ, Reichelderfer M. APIC guideline for infection prevention and control in flexible endoscopy. Association for professionals in infection control. Am J Infect Control. 2000;28(2):138–55.

59. Alfa MJ, Sitter DL. In-hospital evaluation of orthophthalaldehyde as a high level disinfectant for flexible endoscopes. J Hosp Infect. 1994;26(1):15–26.

60. Nelson DB. Infectious disease complications of GI endoscopy: part II, exogenous infections. Gastrointest Endosc. 2003;57(6):695–711. doi:10.1067/mge.2003.202.

61. Mehta AC, Prakash UBS, Garland R, et al. American college of chest physicians and American association for bronchology corrected consensus statement: prevention of flexible bronchoscopy-associated infection. Chest. 2005;128(3):1742–55. doi:10.1378/chest.128.3.1742.

62. Epstein L, Hunter JC, Arwady MA, et al. New delhi metallo-β-lactamase-producing carbapenem-resistant *escherichia coli* associated with exposure to duodenoscopes. JAMA. 2014;312(14):1447–55. doi:10.1001/jama.2014.12720.

63. Design of endoscopic retrograde cholangiopancreatography (ERCP) duodenoscopes may impede effective cleaning: FDA safety communication. http://www.fda.gov/MedicalDevices/Safety/AlertsandNotices/ucm434871.htm. Updated 2015. Accessed 7 Apr 2016.

64. Herwaldt LA, Smith SD, Carter CD. Infection control in the outpatient setting. Infect Control Hosp Epidemiol. 1998;19(1):41–74.

65. Disinfection, sterilization, and preservation. 4th ed. Philadelphia: Lea & Febiger; 1991.

66. Rutala WA, Weber DJ. Guideline for disinfection and sterilization in healthcare facilities. Centers for Disease Control and Prevention; 2008. http://www.cdc.gov/hicpac/pdf/guidelines/Disinfection_Nov_2008.pdf. Updated 2008. Accessed 6 Apr 2016.

67. Petersen BT, Chennat J, Cohen J, et al. Multisociety guideline on reprocessing flexible gastrointestinal endoscopes: 2011. Gastrointest Endosc. 2011;73(6):1075–84. doi:10.1016/j.gie.2011.03.1183.

68. CDC's antibiotic resistance threats in the United States. 2013. http://www.cdc.gov/drugresistance/pdf/ar-threats-2013-508.pdf. Updated 2013. Accessed 24 June 2015.

69. Centers for Disease Control and Prevention. Outpatient antibiotic stewardship. http://www.cdc.gov/getsmart/community/improving-prescribing/outpatient-stewardship.html. Updated 2015. Accessed 7 Apr 2016. n.d.

70. Roumie CL, Halasa NB, Grijalva CG, et al. Trends in antibiotic prescribing for adults in the united states – 1995 to 2002. J Gen Intern Med. 2005;20(8):697–702. doi:10.1111/j.1525-1497.2005.0148.x.

71. Shapiro DJ, Hicks LA, Pavia AT, Hersh AL. Antibiotic prescribing for adults in ambulatory care in the USA, 2007-09. J Antimicrob Chemother. 2014;69(1):234–40. doi:10.1093/jac/dkt301.

72. Wendt JM, Cohen JA, Mu Y, et al. Clostridium difficile infection among children across diverse US geographic locations. Pediatrics. 2014;133(4):651–8. doi:10.1542/peds.2013-3049.

73. Get smart: know when antibiotics work, centers for disease control and prevention. http://www.cdc.gov/getsmart/community/index.html. Updated 2015. Accessed 7 Apr 2016.

74. Hospital epidemiology and infection control. 3rd ed. Philadelphia: Lippincott Williams & Wilkins; 2004.

75. Gupta A, Khanna S. Community-acquired clostridium difficile infection: an increasing public health threat. Infect Drug Resist. 2014;7:63–72. doi:10.2147/IDR.S46780.

76. Khanna S, Pardi DS. The growing incidence and severity of clostridium difficile infection in inpatient and outpatient settings. Expert Rev Gastroenterol Hepatol. 2010;4(4):409–16. doi:10.1586/egh.10.48.

77. McDonald LC, Coignard B, Dubberke E, Song X, Horan T, Kutty PK. Recommendations for surveillance of clostridium difficile-associated disease. Infect Control Hosp Epidemiol. 2007;28(2):140–5. doi:10.1086/511798.

78. Chitnis AS, Holzbauer SM, Belflower RM, et al. Epidemiology of community-associated clostridium difficile infection, 2009 through 2011. JAMA Intern Med. 2013;173(14):1359–67. doi:10.1001/jamainternmed.2013.7056.

79. Eyre DW, Cule ML, Wilson DJ, et al. Diverse sources of *C. difficile* infection identified on whole-genome sequencing. N Engl J Med NEJM. 2013;369(13):1195–205. doi:10.1056/NEJMoa1216064.

80. Sethi AK, Al-Nassir W, Nerandzic MM, Bobulsky GS, Donskey CJ. Persistence of skin contamination and environmental shedding of clostridium difficile during and after treatment of *C. difficile* infection. Infect Control Hosp Epidemiol. 2010;31(1):21–7. doi:10.1086/649016.

81. Jury LA, Sitzlar B, Kundrapu S, et al. Outpatient healthcare settings and transmission of clostridium difficile. PLoS One 2013;8(7):e70175–e70175. doi:10.1371/journal.pone.0070175.

82. Cohen SH, Gerding DN, Johnson S, et al. Clinical practice guidelines for clostridium difficile infection in adults: 2010 update by the society for healthcare epidemiology of america (SHEA) and the infectious diseases society of america (IDSA). Infect Control Hosp Epidemiol. 2010;31(5):431–55. doi:10.1086/651706.

83. Meyer-Rüsenberg B, Loderstädt U, Richard G, Kaulfers P, Gesser C. Epidemic keratoconjunctivitis: the current situation and recommendations for prevention and treatment. Dtsch Arztebl Int. 2011;108(27):475–80. doi:10.3238/arztebl.2011.0475.

84. Kramer A, Schwebke I, Kampf G. How long do nosocomial pathogens persist on inanimate surfaces? A systematic review. BMC Infect Dis. 2006;6:130. doi:10.1186/1471-2334-6-130.

85. Ford E, Nelson KE, Warren D. Epidemiology of epidemic keratoconjunctivitis. Epidemiol Rev. 1987;9:244–61.

86. Buffington J, Chapman LE, Stobierski MG, et al. Epidemic keratoconjunctivitis in a chronic care facility: risk factors and measures for control. J Am Geriatr Soc. 1993;41(11):1177–81.

87. Cheung D, Bremner J, Chan JTK. Epidemic kerato-conjunctivitis – do outbreaks have to be epidemic? Eye. 2003;17(3):356–63. doi:10.1038/sj.eye.6700330.

88. Colón LE. Keratoconjunctivitis due to adenovirus type 8: report on a large outbreak. Ann Ophthalmol-Glaucoma. 1991;23(2):63–5.

89. Doyle TJ, King D, Cobb J, Miller D, Johnson B. An outbreak of epidemic keratoconjunctivitis at an outpatient ophthalmology clinic. Infect Dis Rep 2010;2(2):e17–e17. doi:10.4081/idr.2010.e17.

90. Jernigan JA, Lowry BS, Hayden FG, et al. Adenovirus type 8 epidemic keratoconjunctivitis in an eye clinic: risk factors and control. J Infect Dis. 1993;167(6):1307–13.

91. American OS. Surveillance and control of epidemic keratoconjunctivitis. Trans Am Ophthalmol Soc Ann Meet. 1996;94:539–87.

92. Adenovirus-associated epidemic keratoconjunctivitis outbreaks – four states, 2008–2010. Morbid Mortal Wkly Rep. 2013;62(32):637–641.

93. Medicare program: changes to the ambulatory surgical center payment system and CY 2009 payment rates: final rule. 2008;73(223):68714.

94. PATIENT SAFETY HHS has taken steps to address unsafe injection practices, but more action is needed. Report to the ranking member, subcommittee on health, committee on energy and commerce, house of representatives. United States Government Accountability Office (GAO). 2012;GAO 12–712.

95. Infection control assessment of ambulatory surgical centers, centers for disease control and prevention. http://www.cdc.gov/injectionsafety/pubs/IC-Assessment-Ambulatory-Surgical-Centers.html. Updated 2011. Accessed 12 Apr 2016.

96. Ambulatory surgical center (ASC) INFECTION CONTROL SURVEYOR WORKSHEET (rev: 142, issued: 07-17-15, effective: 07-17-15, implementation: 07-17-15), centers for medicare and medicaid. https://www.cms.gov/Regulations-and-Guidance/Guidance/Manuals/downloads/som107_exhibit_351.pdf. Updated 2015. Accessed 12 Apr 2016, 2016.

97. Recommendations for preventing transmission of infections among chronic hemodialysis patients. Morbid Mortal Wkly Rep. 2001;50(−5):1–43.

98. United States Renal Data System. 2015 USRDS annual data report: epidemiology of kidney disease in the United States. Bethesda: National Institutes of Health, National Institute of Diabetes and Digestive and Kidney Diseases; 2015.

99. Lafrance J, Rahme E, Lelorier J, Iqbal S. Vascular access-related infections: definitions, incidence rates, and risk factors. Am J Kidney Dis. 2008;52(5):982–93. doi:10.1053/j.ajkd.2008.06.014.

100. Ravani P, Palmer SC, Oliver MJ, et al. Associations between hemodialysis access type and clinical outcomes: a systematic review. J Am Soc Nephrol. 2013;24(3):465–73. doi:10.1681/ASN.2012070643.

101. Infection control requirements for dialysis facilities and clarification regarding guidance on parenteral medication vials. Morbid Mortal Wkly Rep. 2008;57(32):875–876.

102. Gilmore J. KDOQI clinical practice guidelines and clinical practice recommendations – 2006 updates. Nephrol Nurs J. 33(5):487–8.

103. Dember LM, Beck GJ, Allon M, et al. Effect of clopidogrel on early failure of arteriovenous fistulas for hemodialysis: a randomized controlled trial. JAMA. 2008;299(18):2164–71. doi:10.1001/jama.299.18.2164.

104. Recommendation of the immunization practices advisory committee (ACIP). Inactivated hepatitis B virus vaccine. Morbid Mortal Wkly Rep. 1982;31(24):317–22, 327.

105. National surveillance of dialysis-associated diseases in the United States, 1997. Semin Dial. 2000;13(2):75–85.

106. Finelli L, Miller JT, Tokars JI, Alter MJ, Arduino MJ. National surveillance of dialysis-associated diseases in the United States. Semin Dial. 2002;18(1):52–61. doi:10.1111/j.1525-139X.2005.18108.x.

107. Centers for Disease Control and Prevention. Health alert network. CDC urging dialysis providers and facilities to assess and improve infection control practices to stop hepatitis C virus transmission in patients undergoing hemodialysis. http://emergency.cdc.gov/han/han00386.asp. Updated 2016. Accessed 12 Apr 2016. n.d.

108. Vital signs: central line-associated blood stream infections – United States, 2001, 2008, and 2009. Morbid Mortal Wkly Rep. 2011;60(8):243–248.

109. Rao CY, Pachucki C, Cali S, et al. Contaminated product water as the source of phialemonium curvatum bloodstream infection among patients undergoing hemodialysis. Infect Control Hosp Epidemiol. 2009;30(9):840–7. doi:10.1086/605324.

110. Office of Disease Prevention and Health Promotion, Office of the Assistant Secretary for Health, Office of the Secretary, U.S. Department of Health and Human Services. National action plan to prevent health care-associated infections: road map to elimination. http://health.gov/hcq/prevent-hai-action-plan.asp. Updated 2016. Accessed 13 Apr 2016. n.d.

111. CDC. Dialysis safety. Guidelines and recommendations. http://www.cdc.gov/dialysis/guidelines/index.html. Updated 2016. Accessed 12 Apr 2016. n.d.

New Technologies for Infection Prevention

Michelle Doll, Michael P. Stevens, and Gonzalo Bearman

Introduction

Interest in technologies to assist infection prevention efforts is increasing. The basic science literature contains an abundance of novel ideas at varying stages of development. A few of these technologies have been developed beyond preclinical testing and have been used in the healthcare setting with the goal of reducing bioburden and interrupting the transmission paths of healthcare-associated organisms. New technologies are assisting in cleaning of surfaces and devices. Other technologies endeavor to insert bactericidal materials into healthcare center furnishings and garments. Additional technologies capable of tracking and monitoring have been developed to assess hand hygiene of healthcare workers. These products are attractive to infection prevention departments and hospital administrators given the difficulties inherent in achieving and maintaining desired staff

M. Doll (✉)
Department of Internal Medicine-Division of Infectious Diseases, VCU Medical Center, 1300 East Marshall Street, North Hospital, 2nd Floor, Room 2-100, P.O. Box 980019, Richmond, VA 23298, USA

Internal Medicine/Division of Infectious Diseases, Virginia Commonwealth University Medical Center, Richmond, VA, USA

Infectious Diseases/Epidemiology, Virginia Commonwealth University Health System, Richmond, VA, USA
e-mail: michelle.doll@vcuhealth.org

M.P. Stevens
Department of Internal Medicine, Division of Infectious Diseases, Virginia Commonwealth University Medical Center, 1300 East Marshall Street, North Hospital, 2nd Floor, Room 2-100, P.O. Box 980019, Richmond, VA 23298, USA

Infectious Diseases/Epidemiology, Virginia Commonwealth University Health System, Richmond, VA, USA
e-mail: michael.stevens@vcuhealth.org

G. Bearman
VCUHS Epidemiology and Infection Control, North Hospital, 2nd Floor, Room 2-073, 1300 East Marshall Street, Richmond, VA 23298-0019, USA
e-mail: gonzalo.bearman@vcuhealth.org

behaviors; they promise to bypass the human element and deliver automated infection prevention. Yet effectiveness of these often expensive interventions is uncertain, and incremental benefit over traditional infection prevention best practices may be scant. Nevertheless, as infection prevention programs are tasked with more activities than ever [1], they will continue to look for innovative strategies to improve the effectiveness of existing efforts.

Ultraviolet (UV) and Hydrogen Peroxide (HP) Room Disinfection Systems

Contamination of the inanimate hospital environment is an area of ongoing concern for the accumulation of bioburden and increased potential for transmission of organisms between patients. Variations in the effectiveness of the cleaning provided by environmental services staff have led to the development of technologies designed to complement human efforts and provide a more consistent and complete level of cleaning for patient rooms and other hospital areas. Extensive research has been done on the efficacy of these devices using various methodologies. However, true clinical benefit currently remains dubious, especially when traditional human cleaning practices can be optimized.

Touchless Device Killing Efficacy

Studies relating to the efficacy of HP and UV devices typically employ two different methodologies: (1) an "in vitro" assessment in which known quantities of bacteria inoculated onto carrier materials or biologic indicators are deliberately placed in a test space and (2) an "in vivo" assessment in which the real contamination in a room formerly inhabited by a patient is assessed by environmental cultures both before and after application of a device. Killing efficacy depends on the method employed to measure killing, the type of device, the time of application, the type of organisms, and a multitude of room features.

© Springer International Publishing AG 2018
G. Bearman et al. (eds.), *Infection Prevention*, DOI 10.1007/978-3-319-60980-5_7

In general, studies suggest that killing power of vaporized HP is slightly higher than for aerosolized HP and UV devices [2]. For example, several studies using vaporized hydrogen peroxide have reported killing rates for experimentally placed inoculum to be essentially complete, averaging >5–6 log reductions [3–7]. This is in contrast to aerosolized hydrogen peroxide devices, in which the particles are larger at 1–10 um and reported kill rates vary more widely by the type of device and experimental protocol [3, 8]. Direct comparisons between aerosolized hydrogen peroxide (aHP) devices and vaporized hydrogen peroxide (HPV) devices have been made. In one study, biologic indicators with a six-log load of bacteria were tested against each HP device; HPV was able to completely eradicate the experimentally placed bacteria, while aHP decreased the bacterial load by 10–79% [9]. Fu et al. also noted a difference in killing ability between the systems, with an HPV-based device achieving complete eradication of experimentally placed methicillin-resistant *Staphylococcus aureus* (MRSA), *Acinetobacter* (ACB), and *Clostridium difficile*, whereas the aHP device achieved variable and incomplete killing of these same organisms. The study team also noted that the distribution of aHP levels in the room was not uniform, potentially explaining gaps in coverage area and decreased effectiveness compared to HP vapors [3].

UV devices most often employ UVC or pulsed xenon, with wavelengths of 240–280 nm [10] and 200–230 nm [11], respectively. UVC devices have been reported to achieve two to four log reductions in experimentally placed bacteria, depending on the type of carrier or surface being inoculated and the placement arrangement within the room [12–14]. This is in contrast to pulsed-xenon UV devices which reportedly yield <1 log reductions in bacterial colonies [15]. Time required to run devices favors pulsed-xenon, however, with a recommended run time of 15–20 min total for a given room, compared to 20–40 min for UVC devices and up to several hours for HP devices. However, UVC could potentially be run on cycles shorter than currently recommended by manufacturers. A study by Nerandzic et al. compared a UVC device to pulsed-xenon UV device and found that they could achieve superior reductions in colony-forming units of experimentally placed *C. difficile*, vancomycin-resistant *Enterococcus* (VRE), and MRSA using a 10-min UVC run time compared to a normal pulsed-xenon UV run time [15]. This suggests that the UVC device protocol could be individualized for optimal feasibility in a given healthcare setting by striking a balance between killing efficacy and run time requirements. Furthermore, to achieve an equal level of killing with shorter time duration, Rutala et al. document that the use of a reflective paint allowed a UVC device to run less than 10 min while still achieving about a four log reduction similar to a 30–40-min cycle without the reflective coatings [16–18].

Building on the data accumulated from work with experimentally placed bacteria, several studies have undertaken extensive environmental sampling to determine the efficacy of these devices in cleaning actual patient rooms at the time of patient discharge. Several important observations have resulted: (1) percent reductions in site contamination tend to be equalized among different devices when measured in this way [11, 15, 19–21], (2) no device has the ability to completely eradicate residual bioburden from a real patient room at terminal cleaning [4, 11, 15, 19, 20, 22], and (3) certain structures and devices may be difficult for even touchless technologies to penetrate [23, 24].

Site contamination has been reported to decrease by around 70–90% when compared to a baseline dirty room [11, 15, 19–21] and 24–33% when compared to a room cleaned by standard methods when using a variety of UV and HP devices [22, 25]. Havill et al. found a much lower percent decrease of 51% for a UVC device compared to 91% from an HPV device in the same study [4]. Of note, two thirds of the environmental samples that UVC failed to decontaminate came from the patient bathroom. Anderson et al. also observed that the bathroom had decreased reductions in site contamination using a UVC device: 74% versus up to 98% for structures in the main room [19]. Timing does influence the efficacy of environmental decontamination; in a study by Ali et al., running HPV devices for shorter 2-h run times resulted in a higher percentage of low-level site contamination when compared to previously reported 3–4-h run times. They argue that the actual bioburden of these residually contaminated sites was quite low in terms of CFUs recovered, such that the remaining risk to future patients was also low [24]. Wong et al. also point out that UVC not only decreased the percentage of positive sites but also significantly decreased the remaining CFU bioburden of those sites that did remain positive [26]. There may be flexibility to balance the duration of device cycles with a desired level of cleaning effectiveness.

It is unknown how much of a decrease in residual contamination is needed to impact clinically important outcomes. Given that the purpose of these devices is disinfection and certainly not sterilization, there will always be some residual bioburden expected in patient rooms. It is also important to remember that regardless of device efficacy, patient rooms are recontaminated soon after receipt of a new patient [27]. Certain structures may be more susceptible to residual contamination. In the case of HP devices, these include complex structures such as Velcro [23] and furniture seating [24]. In the case of UV devices, shading such as the underside of tables and areas behind toilets is problematic [28, 29]. Also, heavy contamination with organic matter or bacterial colonies themselves impacts killing efficacy [30, 31]. Since the performance of touchless technologies is less variable than human workers, they will also likely experience the same limitations with every cycle run, leaving certain areas or structures consistently contaminated. It is up to individual institutions to be aware of the limitations of these technologies and to maintain a rigorous traditional cleaning program to complement touchless devices.

Touchless Device Efficacy in Clinical Outcomes

Clearly UV and HP devices are able to decrease the bioburden of the hospital environment further than with traditional cleaning alone. Yet to justify the time, cost, and effort required to implement touchless devices, this decrease in bioburden must translate into tangible patient outcomes. Several studies have attempted to demonstrate decreases in hospital-acquired infection rates among patients (Table 7.1). Manian et al. compared their *C. difficile* rates for 23 months pre-intervention with 12 months post-implementation of an HPV device in their 900-bed community hospital. While only capturing 54% of their *C. difficile* rooms at terminal discharge, they were employing the device in other rooms around the hospital and saw a significant reduction in *C. difficile* rates from 0.88 to 0.55 cases per 1000 patient days. However, no information regarding detailed trends in these rates were available as only yearly aggregated rates were reported [32]. Levin et al. also evaluated *C. difficile* rates before and after implementation of a pulsed-xenon UV device in their 140-bed community hospital. They captured 56% of their discharged rooms over a 1-year period. They also reported rates in yearly aggregates, finding a significant decrease from 0.95 cases per 1000 patient days in 2010 to 0.45 cases per 1000 patient days in 2011; rates had been stable in 2008–2010 at 0.92 per 1000 patient days [33]. Haas et al. also shared their experience in implementing a pulsed-xenon UV device in a 643-bed tertiary care center comparing 30 months pre-intervention with 22 months post-intervention. They retrospectively assessed rates of MRSA, VRE, multidrug-resistant gram-negative rods (MDR-GNRs), and *C. difficile* from clinical cultures in both time periods, finding significant reductions in each of these organisms in the period after device implementation. The device capture rate for their contact rooms was 76% [34].

Attempting to limit bias inherent to retrospective quasi-experimental designs, Passaretti et al. performed a prospective study of an HPV device on three units attempting to match them to three other high-risk units for comparison. They analyzed screening cultures for MRSA and VRE, as well as clinical cultures for MDR-GNRs and *C. difficile*. They found a trend toward decreased acquisition of all organisms in patients in the HPV units; only the decrease in VRE risk was statistically significant, despite the large number of room occupations analyzed ($N = 8813$) [35]. Finally, in a large, multicenter,

cluster-randomized, crossover trial, Anderson et al. compared manual cleaning with quaternary ammonium (reference arm), manual cleaning with bleach, and each of these manual methods + UVC device cleaning. The main outcome was a new diagnosis of an organism of interest by clinical culture in a patient who stayed >24 h in a room previously occupied by another patient with known colonization or infection history with the same organism of interest. This restrictive criterion was meant to capture presumed transmission of infection from an environmental source and provide strong justification for enhanced cleaning. All intervention arms showed a decreased risk of patient acquisition of the combined multidrug-resistant organisms of interest (MRSA, VRE, ACB, *C. difficile*). However, this decrease in relative rate was due exclusively to the significance of VRE reductions; MRSA decreases failed to reach statistical significance, and there was no difference, significant or not, found between arms using bleach + UVC or bleach alone for *C. difficile*. There were not enough ACB in the study for comparisons to be made [36].

The seemingly disappointing results from the well-designed studies of Passaretti et al. and Anderson et al. have not resulted in abatement of interest in touchless devices. Additional single-center quasi-experimental designs continue to appear in the literature to report modestly positive results after implementation of a given device in their institution [37–41]. The natural fluctuation of infection rates and the ability of a small change in case numbers to influence rates and statistical significance demand caution in interpreting such results. The study by Miller et al. is unique in its application of a pulsed-xenon UV device to cleaning protocols in a long-term care center. The device was used primarily to do weekly cleaning of common areas shared by residents; less frequently it was used for resident rooms after discharge [41]. As part of regional approaches to controlling MDROs, enhanced cleaning of long-term care facilities with touchless devices may be an advantageous strategy.

Outbreak Management

In addition to attempts to reduce hospital-acquired infections (HAIs) in endemic situations, touchless technologies have also been used in outbreak scenarios. Most frequently, HP devices have been used and have been successful in halting outbreaks from a variety of organisms. For example, MRSA polyclonal outbreaks [42] and hyperendemic rates [43] have been combated with hydrogen peroxide vapor and essentially eradicated. Numerous studies have reported a rapid recontamination rate after the use of touchless technologies [42, 44, 45]; however, Dryden et al. noted that MRSA environmental contamination levels remained at a lower post-intervention baseline. They attributed this to extensive concurrent decolonization efforts targeting staff

Table 7.1 Evidence for UV and HP device reductions in healthcare-associated acquisitions or infections

Author	Device type	Main outcomes	Study design	Main findings	Main limitations
Manian et al. [32]	HPV	Cdiff rates from clinical cultures	Quasi-experimental	Cdiff rates fell 0.88–0.55 per 1000 patient days, a 38% decrease	Bleach clean ×4 used in place of HPV in cases of room double occupancy
Levin et al. [33]	PX-UV	Cdiff rates from clinical cultures	Quasi-experimental	Cdiff rates fell 0.95–0.45 per 1000 patient days, a 53% decrease	Overall decrease in fluoroquinolone usage over the same time period, small center, rates of device usage not reported
Haas et al. [34]	PX-UV	Cdiff, MRSA, VRE, MDR GNRs rates from clinical cultures	Quasi-experimental	20% decrease in infections with MDROs from 2.67 to 2.14 per 1000 patient days, each individual MDRO was also significantly decreased	Multiple other interventions occurring at the same time
Passaretti et al. [35]	HPV	MRSA and VRE acquisition by screening swabs, MDR GNRs and Cdiff infections by clinical cultures	Prospective cohort with matched control units	64% decrease in acquisitions of organisms of interest combined, driven largely by VRE; trend toward decreases in other organisms	Variable compliance with screening cultures
Anderson et al. [36]	UVC	New MRSA, VRE, ACB, Cdiff from clinical cultures in patients linked by location to previously colonized room occupants	Cluster randomized, multicenter crossover study	Relative rate for all organisms of interest decreased significantly for only the UVC + quaternary ammonium cleaning group; rates trended down for all intervention arms. Combined outcome driven by VRE: no difference in MRSA and Cdiff in intervention arms and not enough ACB for comparisons	Limited sample size despite multicenter design due to restrictive inclusion criteria for analysis
Nagaraja et al. [37]	PX-UV	Cdiff rates from clinical cultures in an ICU subset from Haas et al. study above	Quasi-experimental	Cdiff rates in the ICUs fell from 1.83 cases per 1000 patient days to 0.55	Authors note clustering of cases on some units, such that the possibility of outbreak over endemic rates of Cdiff is raised
Napolitano et al. [40]	UVC	Clinical cultures for MRSA, VRE, ACB, Cdiff, *Klebsiella pneumoniae*	Quasi-experimental	All HAIs decreased from 3.7 cases per 1000 patient days to 2.4. Individual ACB, Cdiff, *Klebsiella* rates also fell significantly	Small sample size in terms of both time of study (6-month pilot) and beds ($N = 239$)
Horn et al. [39]	HPV	Cases of Cdiff infection, MRSA, VRE, ESBL	Quasi-experimental	All HAIS decreased by 47% in the 2-year post-intervention compared to the year before intervention; combined endpoint driven by Cdiff and ESBL	Dual intervention of increased hand hygiene and HPV
Miller et al. [41]	PX-UV	Cdiff rates from clinical cultures	Quasi-experimental	Cdiff rates decreased from 2.33 to 0.83 per 1000 patient days in long-term care center	Small single-center study with a dual stepped intervention of a Cdiff Multidisciplinary team
Vianna et al. [38]	PX-UV	Clinical cultures for MRSA, VRE, Cdiff	Quasi-experimental	All HAIs decreased from 1.51 cases per 1000 patient days to 1.07; this was driven by a decrease in VRE in the ICU and Cdiff in non-ICU areas	Small single-center study (126 beds)

C. diff Clostridium difficile, *MRSA* methicillin-resistant *Staphylococcus aureus*, *ACB Acinetobacter*, *VRE* vancomycin-resistant *Enterococcus*, *GNRs* gram-negative rods, *MDR* multidrug resistant, *MDROs* multidrug-resistant organisms, *HAI* hospital-acquired infection, *HPV* hydrogen peroxide vapor, *UVC* ultraviolet C, *PX-UV* pulsed-xenon ultraviolet, *ICU* intensive care unit and patients [42]. This illustrates the point that closure of a unit for decontamination may be very effective at aborting the active outbreak, but improvements in standard cleaning, hand hygiene, and other infection prevention initiatives remain important in maintaining these results. Barbut et al. also documented a sustained decrease in MRSA and *Acinetobacter* following an outbreak. Their response included closure and decontamination of an entire burn unit using an HP vapor device and then reopening the unit with incorporation of an infection control bundle that included preemptive isolation of patients, cohorting of infected or colonized patients, increased emphasis on hand hygiene, and regular use of the HP device for terminal discharge cleaning (Barbut) [46].

Most recontamination of units post-intervention are assumed to occur from newly admitted colonized patients. For example, Ray et al. describe their experience using an aerosolized HP device to control an *Acinetobacter* outbreak at a long-term care facility. They were able to successfully stop the outbreak, but noted rapid recontamination of the environment that was presumed to be due to high-risk colonized patients readmitted to the space. They were also able to identify a wound care cart that was a potential source linking infected patients [44]. In addition to colonized patients, occult environmental reservoirs that persist after touchless device interventions may also contribute to recontamination of wards. This may explain the difficulties that other groups have reported in controlling outbreaks due to *Acinetobacter*. Otter et al. were able to halt an outbreak in their 12-unit ICU, but noted subsequent recontamination with *Acinetobacter* that was genetically related to the strains infecting the previous patients; none of the current patients could be linked to the patients prior to the unit closure and decontamination intervention [47]. Alfandari et al. were able to identify a reservoir that was felt to be contributing to the propagation of an *Acinetobacter* outbreak in their ICU when Velcro on a shared blood pressure cuff yielded the same clone that infected 12 of their 14 case patients. This residual contamination had persisted despite decontamination with an HP device, and only removal of the cuff from the unit finally ended the outbreak [23]. HP vapor was used as an adjunct to multiple other interventions in protracted [48] and recurrent [49] *Acinetobacter* outbreaks at two centers in Europe. Both groups emphasize the need for a multifaceted approach to these outbreaks. In fact, Landelle et al. note that only by cohorting of both patients and staff on a separate unit were they able to finally end their 18-month battle with *Acinetobacter* [48]. Residual environmental reservoirs may contribute to ongoing transmission if general infection prevention principles are not meticulously applied. Thus touchless devices are not magic bullets; these devices provide a useful adjunct strategy to outbreak mediation, but require concomitant application of broadly reaching infection prevention bundles.

Other Applications of Touchless Technology

High-intensity narrow beam light at 405 nm has been used in a series of experiments by a group in the United Kingdom to reduce staphylococcal bioburden in burn units and an intensive care unit [50–52]. These devices use visible violet light to exert a bactericidal effect on organisms that is thought to occur due to excitation of bacterial intracellular porphyrins and resulting oxidative damage [52]. They have the benefit of safe continuous use in a room occupied by patients and/or staff. The violet light is combined with white light to exist as part of the normal light fixture of a patient room and is operated by a light switch. The device has demonstrated an ability to decrease bioburden in an occupied room with ongoing use. However, the studies were small including few occupied rooms and focused mainly on *Staphylococcus* species [50–52].

Apart from whole room cleaning, touchless devices have been employed specifically to clean mobile medical equipment [53] and unused medical supplies [54]. In the later study, each item had to be removed from drawers in the patient room and spread out to allow the HP vapor to access the items. However, the authors note that this effort would have the potential to save the institution $387,055 per year, because they otherwise discard all unused supplies from the rooms of isolation patients at discharge [54]. Another option for small-item touchless cleaning is a "nanoclave cabinet" consisting of a 129 × 94 × 89 cm box filled with UVC lamps that has been utilized to clean nonessential patient care items such as TV remotes and blood pressure cuffs in the test environment [55]. Lastly, a handheld device has been trialed on units for staff-driven decontamination of commonly touched objects such as keyboards, phones, and documents [56].

Challenges and Limitations of Touchless Devices

The existing literature on touchless devices for cleaning of the hospital environment is limited by non-standardized methods of evaluation of different devices and industry influence on study design and reporting of data. Robust study designs sufficiently powered to compare devices to optimized cleaning procedures are lacking with few exceptions. Even in the largely positive reports of device effectiveness, several shortcomings are evident such as the inability to penetrate all surfaces. Problem areas seem to include floor corners [24], heavily soiled areas [30, 31], and complex structures [23].

Touchless devices for room cleaning may have an important role in providing some consistency to terminal cleaning. However, rapid recontamination emphasizes the importance of standard and daily cleaning efforts to maintain a low overall bioburden in clinical areas. If the limitations of these devices are not fully understood by staff, they could actually compromise standard cleaning efforts by inducing a false sense of security; staff depending on the robot to clean could neglect important infection prevention practices. Education regarding the role of touchless devices as one of many important concomitant strategies for improving the environment of care is essential to preserve human participation in these efforts.

Antimicrobial Surfaces

Given the challenges involved in cleaning the hospital environment, there is substantial interest in self-disinfecting surfaces. While many materials remain in preclinical investigations of their antimicrobial effects, a few have been installed and assessed in the clinical environment. As with touchless devices, these technologies are difficult to compare between studies due to differing material compositions, culturing techniques, and timing of the study protocols [57]. In 2010, Casey et al. conducted a 10-week crossover study of 60–70% copper-containing materials implanted on high-touch surfaces. Surfaces were cultured weekly for aerobic colony counts and compared to control surfaces. After 5 weeks, the hospital switched the copper and control surfaces and repeated the experiment. The group found significant reductions in bacterial counts on all sampled sites and an overall 90% reduction in bacterial contamination of the copper alloy surfaces [58]. In contrast, Mikolay et al. applied a copper alloy to certain high-touch surfaces and then sampled them one to two times per week for 16 weeks in summer months and another 16 weeks in winter months; aerobic heterotrophic colony counts were compared between the copper alloy surfaces and control surfaces. The authors found a disappointing overall 33% reduction in bacterial load from the copper surfaces that was statistically significant only on door knob sites. The authors hypothesized that their cleaner may have obstructed the antimicrobial copper effects. Also, the exact composition percentage of copper in the study was not reported [59]. The amount of copper present in the material is known to be important in antimicrobial efficacy [57]. Sheets of 99.9% copper were installed in a clinic consultation room and compared to a regular room by a series of cultures every 6 weeks over 6 months. There was a 71% overall reduction in bacterial colony counts as well as significant reductions on all copper surfaces [60]. Prolonged exposure of organisms to copper raises concerns for the development of copper resistance. In a 24-week crossover study, Karpanen et al. also found significant reductions in aerobic colony counts on 8 of 14 surface types sampled comparing a copper alloy to standard surfaces. They also checked

for and found no evidence of resistance to copper in VRE, *Staphylococcus aureus*, and coliforms [61]. Duration of antimicrobial effect has been assessed in a longitudinal study that collected environmental samples for 23 months pre-intervention, and then 20 months post-intervention, in 16 rooms split between 3 hospitals. Copper alloys containing 70–99.9% copper were installed on 6 high-touch surfaces in 8 of the 16 rooms at month 23. The team found a sustained decrease in bacterial contamination of copper surfaces both compared to pre-intervention surfaces and to ongoing control surfaces [62].

Finally, copper surfaces have been evaluated for their ability to decrease HAI rates. Rivero et al. conducted a 13-month study comparing infection rates for central line-associated bloodstream infection (CLABSI), catheter-associated urinary tract infection (CAUTI), and ventilator-associated pneumonia (VAP) in a 14-room ICU in which 7 of 14 rooms had 99% copper materials installed on high-touch surfaces; they found no differences in HAIs in patients admitted for at least 24 h, though admitted they were likely underpowered to do so [63]. In contrast, Salgado et al. performed an 11-month study comparing eight copper rooms to eight standard rooms among three ICUs at three separate facilities and found a significant decrease in HAIs in copper rooms as well as a 66% reduction in environmental contamination of copper surfaces when compared to non-copper surfaces in control rooms [64]. HAI reduction has not been replicated in other studies to date.

Antimicrobial Fabrics

Textiles with antimicrobial properties have been developed and show promise in the laboratory setting in their ability to kill bacteria after a few hours of contact time [65]. In the clinical environment, silver appeared to limit the contamination with bacteria when 14 curtains were tested in an ICU over 6 months. The same area from each curtain was cultured monthly and few nosocomial pathogens were recovered. However, there is a lack of microbiologic data provided regarding the organisms that were recovered from each sampling exercise as the focus of the report was on results of laboratory testing of swatches of the same silver-impregnated textile. Furthermore, there were no control curtains used for comparisons in the testing done in the ICU [66]. A comparison to standard curtains was performed in a randomized controlled trial across two ICUS in which 15 curtains containing an antimicrobial metal-alloy and 15 standard curtains were cultured twice weekly for 4 weeks. The study found no difference in the amounts of organisms of interest between the two curtains with the exception of VRE. VRE was recovered eight times more often from the standard curtains. In addition, they observed a significant increase in the median length of time until first contamination from 2 days for standard curtains to 14 days for antimicrobial curtains [67].

Protection of industry advantage can limit the information available regarding the composition of antimicrobial scrubs. In one randomized controlled trial of healthcare worker scrub uniforms, standard scrubs were compared between two competing antimicrobial scrubs containing a "propriety antimicrobial chemicals." One of the scrubs also contained silver. Scrubs and skin of workers involved in direct patient care activities were cultured after an 8-h shift and found to be no different in terms of total bacterial colony counts and colony counts of various MDROs between the three groups [68]. Comparison between studies is thus further limited by uncertainty about what materials are being tested.

Boutin et al. performed a randomized controlled trial using a chitosan-based antimicrobial scrub and culturing staff skin and scrubs near the end of a 12-h shift. Similar to the findings of Burden et al., they found no difference in total bacteria or individual MDROs of interest between the chitosan scrubs and standard scrubs [69]. Another randomized controlled trial by Bearman et al. tested organosilane-based quaternary ammonium-impregnated scrubs against standard scrubs in ICU clinical staff, finding a reduction in MRSA at a single scrub site (abdominal area) at the end of the shift. MRSA colony counts were also lower on the leg cargo pockets at the beginning of shifts. There were no significant differences in VRE or GNRs [70]. Lastly, a veterinary clinic trialed a silver-impregnated scrub uniform and compared bacterial contamination to a standard scrub. They found a significant difference only at the beginning of the shift, prior to any animal care, in which fresh silver scrubs had less bacteria present than the standard scrubs; no differences existed at 4 and 8 h into the shift. They conclude that while the antimicrobial scrubs may be able to decrease contamination in storage, there are likely better ways to target infection prevention in the clinical setting [71].

Despite the apparent powerful bactericidal effects of self-disinfecting surfaces and fabrics in the laboratory, utilization in the clinical setting has been unable to produce the desired effects of decreasing environmental and healthcare worker contamination consistently in well-designed studies. Important differences in the environments and perhaps even the organisms of the laboratory versus the hospital may be to blame for the discrepancies. Caution is clearly required in interpreting the wealth of basic science data for infection prevention technologies that is available from the bench; it does not always translate to the bedside.

Hand Hygiene Technologies

Hand hygiene is arguably the simplest and most important of infection prevention measures, yet, ironically, it is often neglected by healthcare workers. Reasons for non-compliance with hand hygiene in the healthcare setting are most often related to inconvenience for the healthcare worker, perceived lack of an indication for hand hygiene, skin irritation, and forgetfulness [72]. Estimated compliance rates vary widely from below 10% to greater than 90% depending on the institution and method of assessment [73]. One reason for the wide variation in these estimates may be that compliance with hand hygiene is difficult to assess accurately.

Hand hygiene practices are potentially important to the overall bioburden of a given unit. If healthcare workers are consistently washing their hands, then environmental contamination would be less likely to be passed from location to location or patient to patient. Since enduring disinfection of the environment is problematic, hand hygiene represents an important compensation mechanism to reduce transmission risks from both patient source and environmental contamination risks.

Recent years have seen increasing interest in high-tech options to improve hand hygiene practices. Hand hygiene technologies have been employed in various hospitals and clinics, most often on the scale of a pilot targeting selected healthcare workers on one or a few selected units. The published experience with these hand hygiene monitoring and/or feedback technologies includes everything from product dispensation counters to complete monitoring networks using radio-frequency and infrared signals [74], wireless-based signals [75, 76], or video camera observation systems [77]. The implementation of these technologies is a challenge because they introduce additional complexity to the busy clinical environment with unproven benefits. Staff may be suspicious of the system capabilities and overall purpose, it can interfere with workflows, and the system may be financially costly [78]. While investing in cleaning technologies has a certain public relations benefit, it is not clear if that will extend to hand hygiene technologies. The public can generally understand that because sick people are in the hospital, the environment accumulates their germs, and cleaning is an ongoing battle. It is more difficult to justify the expenditure of thousands of dollars for a monitoring technology because healthcare workers cannot be bothered to consistently wash their hands.

Furthermore, the ability of hand hygiene technology to meet a healthcare system's goals is dependent on several prerequisites. If the overall goal is to increase the hand hygiene performance of healthcare workers, essentially changing behavior, in order to enhance patient safety, then several criteria must be met by the product and its implementation. First, the technology must provide feedback on performance to the user [77–80]. Second, the user must trust the technology to be accurate in its assessment. Third, the user must believe that the behavior is important. Fourth, the obstacles to using the technology cannot outweigh the benefit in terms of enhanced performance. Before adopting such a system, institutions will need to determine if they will be able to effectively implement the technology in the target groups and locations, to allow these criteria to be met. They will also need to assess the hand hygiene technology system to ensure that it is capable of providing the accuracy, ease of use, and feedback required to achieve staff buy-in. These crucial system attributes are summarized in Table 7.2.

Utility of Hand Hygiene Monitoring Systems

Accuracy of any hand hygiene monitoring method, whether high or low tech, is of paramount importance to convince healthcare workers that the data is meaningful; unfortunately, it is also a challenge for most available monitoring methods. Often, accuracy is not the goal of the product trial in the published literature; Ward et al. found that of the 40 articles on

Table 7.2 Conditions necessary for hand hygiene technologies to induce behavior change

Criteria	Details	Supporting evidence
Feedback: The system must provide feedback to the user on hand hygiene performance	Individual feedback controlled by the user is optimal	Armellino et al. [77]
		Conway et al. [78]
		Swodoba et al. [79]
	Real-time feedback is more actionable	Ellingson et al. [80]
Trust: The user must trust the technology to be accurate in its assessment	Inaccurate feedback will be dismissed as meaningless	Boyce et al. [81]
	Accurate capture of events must be achievable with limited disruption to clinical workflow	
Belief: The user must believe that the behavior is important, either for infection prevention or other reasons	Education on the importance of hand hygiene should be ongoing, though beliefs may be fixed	Pittet et al. [72]
	A desire to conform to social norms may compensate for lack of personal belief in hand hygiene benefits	
Usability: The effort required to use the technology cannot outweigh the benefit of enhanced personal performance	Interaction with the system must be easy to understand so that workers can use it with minimal training	Harrison et al. [83]
	Adoption of the technology cannot seriously compromise healthcare worker efficiency	McGuckin et al. [82]

hand hygiene technologies, only 20% included any data on accuracy [84]. It has been suggested that the accuracy of hand hygiene technologies may be better than the traditional "gold standard" method of direct observation of staff behavior due to less of the Hawthorne effect, the ability to collect more data, and increased objectivity of the data [85, 86]. However, most of this is in the context of counting systems that offer a global assessment of product usage on the floor and do not attempt to match hand hygiene events to individual healthcare workers [86, 87]. A radio-frequency-/infrared-based system was compared to direct observation in which individual entry and exit from a clinic room were used as opportunities and both the observer and the automated system recorded hand hygiene compliance [88]. The automated system was found to be superior in accuracy. However, the human observer was positioned at the far end of a clinic hallway, where vision to many of the unit's hand hygiene events was limited [88]. Another study comparing a monitoring network attempting to assign events to individual healthcare workers which was compared to direct observation found the compliance rates detected by the system lagging behind direct observation: 44% by human observers versus 22% by the technology. This study was done on an intermediate medical unit, and all staff and visitors to the floor were made to participate in the pilot [79].

Therefore, the compliance rate reported in studies must be interpreted with caution because it is essentially a surrogate marker for hand hygiene and defined by the user's ability to interact with the system. The extent to which this surrogate data is reflective of true hand hygiene behaviors depends on the situation. Pineles et al. tested a radiofrequency and infrared system in a controlled environment using volunteers educated on the system function and found that it appropriately credited the correct healthcare worker with hand hygiene between 75 and 88% of the time depending on the position of the worker and the badge. However, when they integrated this system into routine medical care on a ward, the system correctly attributed hand hygiene events to workers only 50–54% of the time [74]. While training may have been able to improve this system-measured marker of compliance, ongoing badge and body positioning efforts for system capture may not be compatible with clinical workflow on a high intensity unit. Furthermore, these results cast uncertainty on the reported compliance results from other studies of electronic monitoring systems. Increases in system-defined compliance may indicate improved hand hygiene practices, but it may be no more than staff improvement in their ability to trigger an electronic device.

In contrast, a wireless device was able to detect similar compliance when compared to direct observation in a study by Cheng et al. However, the comparison is limited by short periods of comparison and relatively few hand hygiene events occurring within the designated time frame. Of note, the compliance during monitoring was 90–95% and only 35.1% overall. The study attributes this to the Hawthorne effect [76]. However, both the system and the observer are usually not designed or specifically trained to assess if an indication for hand hygiene has been met. Thus healthcare workers may perform additional or extra hand hygiene for the benefit of an observer on the unit such as re-washing hands on exit of the room in the observer's line of vision despite having just performed hand hygiene in the room prior to exit. Furthermore, night and weekend hours are understudied in the hand hygiene literature, and it is unclear what factors might explain apparent noncompliance during these generally unobserved hours.

Video recordings have the added benefit of providing visual data to assist in accurately determining healthcare worker compliance with hand hygiene opportunities. In the most extensive studies using video recordings and external auditors, Armellino et al. collected 432,482 hand hygiene observations over 107 weeks in a medical ICU [77] and then performed a similar study in a surgical ICU over 68 weeks [89]. They saw a striking increase in compliance from 6.5 to 81.6% during the course of the study in the MICU. Interestingly, the increase only occurred after feedback on compliance rates, and education regarding hand hygiene was initiated; the installation of the system itself produced no change in measured hand hygiene compliance rates. The authors offer little specific explanation for the abysmal pre-feedback compliance rates except that "lack of knowledge of hand hygiene guidelines" or "remote video auditing monitoring rules" may be to blame [77]. If the latter were true, this could be another case where healthcare workers were learning to work with the system such that it could capture the hand hygiene that was already being performed, such as by ensuring these events took place in front of a camera. One the other hand, if the former, "lack of knowledge," were true, healthcare workers could have been performing selective hand hygiene only when they felt it were indicated. While some activities such as rounding in a patient's doorway or checking on the patient and/or patient monitoring equipment without touching anything may not truly require hand hygiene from an infection prevention standpoint, providers probably underestimate the extent of activities that require hand hygiene to occur.

Hand hygiene monitoring technologies have several important limitations that may impact their usefulness. This is particularly true if the intent is to use the systems in a real-world setting of a busy clinical ward with staff whose participation is not voluntary. However, there are several advantages in the amount of data the system can collect and the objectivity of the data. In addition, while these devices cannot determine if hand hygiene is specifically indicated when a healthcare worker crosses a patient threshold, they are useful in taking any assessment of appropriateness out of the equation. Healthcare workers should not be performing individual split-second risk assessments with every entry and exit to a patient room to determine whether or not they will perform hand hygiene in that instance. Hand hygiene technologies have the ability to completely automatize this decision-making process such that regardless of the intended task or duration of stay in the room, the workers know they must foam in and out every time they cross the threshold into the patient area. One other added benefit is to assist in identifying those few individuals who may have blatant disregard for hand hygiene requirements. Even if a system is not accurate, one can detect a compliance rate of essentially zero if all peers are measuring at 20–30%. There is modeling data to suggest that one healthcare worker consistently neglecting all hand hygiene may be more damaging in terms of potential transmission of infectious organisms than many healthcare workers who occasionally neglect the practice [90]. Thus while the systems are most likely to be accepted if they are used nonpunitively, serious ongoing breaches in infection prevention practices are important to detect and rectify.

Conclusion

The search for new technologies to assist in infection prevention will continue to intensify as programs strive to raise their standards and accomplish more with less human resources. However, clearly some skepticism is required in the evaluation of new technologies in a literature infused with industry agendas and weaker study designs with potential for bias. More technologies must be integrated into the real clinical environment in pragmatic research designs that can be sustainable in the long term. Under such circumstances, many of the products discussed here have the potential to be useful adjuncts to more traditional infection prevention efforts and may be important in providing some standardization to practices that until recently have depended on individual human behaviors.

References

1. Morgan DJ, Deloney VM, Bartlett A, et al. The expanding role of the hospital epidemiologist in 2014: a survey of the Society for Hospital Epidemiology of America (SHEA) research network. Infect Control Hosp Epidemiol. 2015;36:605–8.
2. Doll M, Morgan DJ, Anderson D, Bearman G. Touchless technologies for decontamination in the hospital: a review of hydrogen peroxide and UV devices. Curr Infect Dis Rep. 2015;17(9):498.
3. Fu TY, Gent P, Kumar V. Efficacy, efficiency and safety aspects of hydrogen peroxide vapour and aerosolized hydrogen peroxide room disinfection systems. J Hosp Infect. 2012;80:199–205.

4. Havill NL, Moore BA, Boyce JM. Comparison of the microbiological efficacy of hydrogen peroxide vapor and ultraviolet light processes for room decontamination. Infect Control Hosp Epidemiol. 2012;33:507–12.

5. Barbut F, Yezli S, Otter JA. Activity in vitro of hydrogen peroxide vapour against clostridium difficile spores. J Hosp Infect. 2012;80:85–7.

6. Galvin S, Boyle M, Russell RJ, et al. Evaluation of vaporized hydrogen peroxide, Citrox and pH neutral Ecasol for decontamination of an enclosed area: a pilot study. J Hosp Infect. 2012;80:67–70.

7. Lemmen S, Scheithauer S, Hafner H, Yezli S, Mohr M, Otter JA. Evaluation of hydrogen peroxide vapor for the inactivation of nosocomial pathogens on porous and nonporous surfaces. Am J Infect Control. 2015;43:82–5.

8. Steindl G, Fiedler A, Huhulescu S, Wewalka G, Allerberger F. Effect of airborne hydrogen peroxide on spores of Clostridium difficile. Wien Klin Wochenschr. 2014.

9. Holmdahl T, Lanbeck P, Wullt M, Walder MH. A head-to-head comparison of hydrogen peroxide vapor and aerosol room decontamination systems. Infect Control Hosp Epidemiol. 2011;32(9):831–6.

10. Otter JA, Yezli S, Perl TM, Barbut F, French GL. The role of 'no-touch' automated room disinfection systems in infection prevention and control. J Hosp Infect. 2013;83:1–13.

11. Ghantoji SS, Stibich M, Stachowiak J, et al. Non-inferiority of pulsed xenon UV light versus bleach for reducing environmental clostridium difficile contamination on high-touch surfaces in clostridium difficile infection isolation rooms. J Med Microbiol. 2015;64:191–4.

12. Rutala WA, Gergen MF, Weber DJ. Room decontamination with UV radiation. Infect Control Hosp Epidemiol. 2010;31(10):1025–9.

13. Boyce JM, Havill NL, Moore BA. Terminal decontamination of patient rooms using an automated mobile UV light unit. Infect Control Hosp Epidemiol. 2011;32(8):737–42.

14. Nerandzic MM, Cadnum JL, Pultz MJ, Donskey CJ. Evaluation of an automated ultraviolet radiation device for decontamination of Clostridium difficile and other healthcare-associated pathogens in hospital rooms. BMC Infect Dis. 2010;10:197. 2334-10-197

15. Nerandzic MM, Thota P, Sankar CT, et al. Evaluation of a pulsed xenon ultraviolet disinfection system for reduction of healthcare-associated pathogens in hospital rooms. Infect Control Hosp Epidemiol. 2015;36:192–7.

16. Rutala WA, Gergen MF, Tande BM, Weber DJ. Rapid hospital room decontamination using ultraviolet (UV) light with a nanostructured UV-reflective wall coating. Infect Control Hosp Epidemiol. 2013;34:527–9.

17. Rutala WA, Gergen MF, Tande BM, Weber DJ. Room decontamination using an ultraviolet-C device with short ultraviolet exposure time. Infect Control Hosp Epidemiol. 2014;35:1070–2.

18. Rutala WA, Weber DJ, Gergen MF, Tande BM, Sickbert-Bennett EE. Does coating all room surfaces with an ultraviolet C light-nanoreflective coating improve decontamination compared with coating only the walls? Infect Control Hosp Epidemiol. 2014;35:323–5.

19. Anderson D, Gergen MF, Smathers E, et al. Decontamination of targeted pathogens from patient rooms using an automated ultraviolet-C-emitting device. Infect Control Hosp Epidemiol. 2013;34:466–71.

20. Jinadatha C, Quezada R, Huber TW, Williams JB, Zeber JE, Copeland LA. Evaluation of a pulsed-xenon ultraviolet room disinfection device for impact on contamination levels of methicillin-resistant *Staphylococcus aureus*. BMC Infect Dis. 2014;14:187. 2334-14-187

21. Hosein I, Madeloso R, Nagaratnam W, Villamaria F, Stock E, Jinadatha C. Evaluation of a pulsed xenon ultraviolet light device for isolation room disinfection in a United Kingdom hospital. Am J Infect Control. 2016;44:e157.

22. Blazejewski C, Wallet F, Rouze A, et al. Efficiency of hydrogen peroxide in improving disinfection of ICU rooms. Crit Care. 2015;19:30.

23. Alfandari S, Gois J, Delannoy PY, et al. Management and control of a carbapenem-resistant Acinetobacter Baumannii outbreak in an intensive care unit. Med Mal Infect. 2014;44:229–31.

24. Ali S, Muzslay M, Bruce M, Jeanes A, Moore G, Wilson AP. Efficacy of two hydrogen peroxide vapour aerial decontamination systems for enhanced disinfection of methicillin-resistant *Staphylococcus aureus*, *Klebsiella pneumoniae* and clostridium difficile in single isolation rooms. J Hosp Infect. 2016;93:70–7.

25. Mitchell BG, Digney W, Locket P, Dancer SJ. Controlling methicillin-resistant *Staphylococcus aureus* (MRSA) in a hospital and the role of hydrogen peroxide decontamination: an interrupted time series analysis. BMJ Open. 2014;4:e004522. 2013-004522

26. Wong T, Woznow T, Petrie M, et al. Postdischarge decontamination of MRSA, VRE, and clostridium difficile isolation rooms using 2 commercially available automated ultraviolet-C-emitting devices. Am J Infect Control. 2016;44:416–20.

27. Hardy KJ, Gossain S, Henderson N, et al. Rapid recontamination with MRSA of the environment of an intensive care unit after decontamination with hydrogen peroxide vapour. J Hosp Infect. 2007;66:360–8.

28. Mahida N, Vaughan N, Boswell T. First UK evaluation of an automated ultraviolet-C room decontamination device (Tru-D). J Hosp Infect. 2013;84:332–5.

29. Beal A, Mahida N, Staniforth K, Vaughan N, Clarke M, Boswell T. First UK trial of Xenex PX-UV, an automated ultraviolet room decontamination device in a clinical haematology and bone marrow transplantation unit. J Hosp Infect. 2016.

30. Zhang A, Nerandzic MM, Kundrapu S, Donskey CJ. Does organic material on hospital surfaces reduce the effectiveness of hypochlorite and UV radiation for disinfection of clostridium difficile? Infect Control Hosp Epidemiol. 2013;34:1106–8.

31. Cadnum JL, Tomas ME, Sankar T, et al. Effect of variation in test methods on performance of ultraviolet-C radiation room decontamination. Infect Control Hosp Epidemiol. 2016;37:555–60.

32. Manian FA, Griesnauer S, Bryant A. Implementation of hospital-wide enhanced terminal cleaning of targeted patient rooms and its impact on endemic clostridium difficile infection rates. Am J Infect Control. 2013;41(6):537–41.

33. Levin J, Riley LS, Parrish C, English D, Ahn S. The effect of portable pulsed xenon ultraviolet light after terminal cleaning on hospital-associated clostridium difficile infection in a community hospital. Am J Infect Control. 2013;41:746–8.

34. Haas JP, Menz J, Dusza S, Montecalvo MA. Implementation and impact of ultraviolet environmental disinfection in an acute care setting. Am J Infect Control. 2014;42(6):586–90.

35. Passaretti CL, Otter JA, Reich NG, et al. An evaluation of environmental decontamination with hydrogen peroxide vapor for reducing the risk of patient acquisition of multidrug-resistant organisms. Clin Infect Dis. 2013;56:27–35.

36. Anderson D, Chen LF, Weber DJ, et al. The benefits of enhanced terminal room (BETR) disinfection study: a cluster randomized, multicenter crossover study with 2x2 factorial design to evaluate the impact of enhanced terminal room disinfection on acquisition and infection caused by multi-drug resistant organisms (MDRO). Oral abstract at: Infectious Diseases Society of America 2015 Annual conference; October 9, 2015; San Diego, CA.

37. Nagaraja A, Visintainer P, Haas JP, Menz J, Wormser GP, Montecalvo MA. Clostridium difficile infections before and during use of ultraviolet disinfection. Am J Infect Control. 2015;43:940.

38. Vianna PG, Dale CR Jr, Simmons S, Stibich M, Licitra CM. Impact of pulsed xenon ultraviolet light on hospital-acquired infection rates in a community hospital. Am J Infect Control. 2016;44:299–303.

39. Horn K, Otter JA. Hydrogen peroxide vapor room disinfection and hand hygiene improvements reduce clostridium difficile infection, methicillin-resistant *Staphylococcus aureus*, vancomycin-resistant enterococci, and extended-spectrum beta-lactamase. Am J Infect Control. 2015;43:1354–6.

40. Napolitano NA, Mahapatra T, Tang W. The effectiveness of UV-C radiation for facility-wide environmental disinfection to reduce health care-acquired infections. Am J Infect Control. 2015;43:1342–6.

41. Miller R, Simmons S, Dale C, Stachowiak J, Stibich M. Utilization and impact of a pulsed-xenon ultraviolet room disinfection system and multidisciplinary care team on clostridium difficile in a long-term acute care facility. Am J Infect Control. 2015;43:1350–3.

42. Dryden M, Parnaby R, Dailly S, et al. Hydrogen peroxide vapour decontamination in the control of a polyclonal methicillin-resistant *Staphylococcus aureus* outbreak on a surgical ward. J Hosp Infect. 2008;68:190–2.

43. French GL, Otter JA, Shannon KP, Adams NM, Watling D, Parks MJ. Tackling contamination of the hospital environment by methicillin-resistant *Staphylococcus aureus* (MRSA): a comparison between conventional terminal cleaning and hydrogen peroxide vapour decontamination. J Hosp Infect. 2004;57:31–7.

44. Ray A, Perez F, Beltramini AM, et al. Use of vaporized hydrogen peroxide decontamination during an outbreak of multidrug-resistant Acinetobacter Baumannii infection at a long-term acute care hospital. Infect Control Hosp Epidemiol. 2010;31(12):1236–41.

45. Best EL, Parnell P, Thirkell G, et al. Effectiveness of deep cleaning followed by hydrogen peroxide decontamination during high clostridium difficile infection incidence. J Hosp Infect. 2014;87:25–33.

46. Barbut F, Yezli S, Mimoun M, Pham J, Chaouat M, Otter JA. Reducing the spread of Acinetobacter baumannii and methicillin-resistant *Staphylococcus aureus* on a burns unit through the intervention of an infection control bundle. Burns. 2013;39:395–403.

47. Otter JA, Yezli S, Schouten MA, van Zanten AR, Houmes-Zielman G, Nohlmans-Paulssen MK. Hydrogen peroxide vapor decontamination of an intensive care unit to remove environmental reservoirs of multidrug-resistant gram-negative rods during an outbreak. Am J Infect Control. 2010;38:754–6.

48. Landelle C, Legrand P, Lesprit P, et al. Protracted outbreak of multidrug-resistant Acinetobacter baumannii after intercontinental transfer of colonized patients. Infect Control Hosp Epidemiol. 2013;34:119–24.

49. Chmielarczyk A, Higgins PG, Wojkowska-Mach J, et al. Control of an outbreak of Acinetobacter baumannii infections using vaporized hydrogen peroxide. J Hosp Infect. 2012;81:239–45.

50. Maclean M, Macgregor SJ, Anderson JG, et al. Environmental decontamination of a hospital isolation room using high-intensity narrow-spectrum light. J Hosp Infect. 2010;76:247–51.

51. Bache SE, Maclean M, MacGregor SJ, et al. Clinical studies of the high-intensity narrow-Spectrum light environmental decontamination system (HINS-light EDS), for continuous disinfection in the burn unit inpatient and outpatient settings. Burns. 2012;38:69–76.

52. Maclean M, McKenzie K, Anderson JG, Gettinby G, MacGregor SJ. 405 nm light technology for the Inactivation of pathogens and its potential role for environmental disinfection and infection control. J Hosp Infect. 2014;88:1–11.

53. Andersen BM, Rasch M, Hochlin K, Jensen FH, Wismar P, Fredriksen JE. Decontamination of rooms, medical equipment and ambulances using an aerosol of hydrogen peroxide disinfectant. J Hosp Infect. 2006;62:149–55.

54. Otter JA, Nowakowski E, Salkeld JA, et al. Saving costs through the decontamination of the packaging of unused medical supplies using hydrogen peroxide vapor. Infect Control Hosp Epidemiol. 2013;34:472–8.

55. Moore G, Ali S, Cloutman-Green EA, et al. Use of UV-C radiation to disinfect non-critical patient care items: a laboratory assessment of the Nanoclave cabinet. BMC Infect Dis. 2012;12:174.

56. Umezawa K, Asai S, Inokuchi S, Miyachi H. A comparative study of the bactericidal activity and daily disinfection housekeeping surfaces by a new portable pulsed UV radiation device. Curr Microbiol. 2012;64:581–7.

57. Weber DJ, Rutala WA. Self-disinfecting surfaces. Infect Control Hosp Epidemiol. 2012;33(1):10–3.

58. Casey AL, Adams D, Karpanen TJ, et al. Role of copper in reducing hospital environment contamination. J Hosp Infect. 2010;74:72–7.

59. Mikolay A, Huggett S, Tikana L, Grass G, Braun J, Nies DH. Survival of bacteria on metallic copper surfaces in a hospital trial. Appl Microbiol Biotechnol. 2010;87:1875–9.

60. Marais F, Mehtar S, Chalkley L. Antimicrobial efficacy of copper touch surfaces in reducing environmental bioburden in a South African community healthcare facility. J Hosp Infect. 2010;74:80–95.

61. Karpanen TJ, Casey AL, Lambert PA, et al. The antimicrobial efficacy of copper alloy furnishing in the clinical environment: a crossover study. Infect Control Hosp Epidemiol. 2012;33:3–9.

62. Schmidt MG, Attaway HH, Sharpe PA, et al. Sustained reduction of microbial burden on common hospital surfaces through introduction of copper. J Clin Microbiol. 2012;50:2217–23.

63. Rivero P, Brenner P, Nercelles P. Impact of copper in the reduction of hospital-acquired infections, mortality and antimicrobial costs in the adult intensive care unit. Rev Chil Infectol. 2014;31:274–9.

64. Salgado CD, Sepkowitz KA, John JF, et al. Copper surfaces reduce the rate of healthcare-acquired infections in the intensive care unit. Infect Control Hosp Epidemiol. 2013;34:479–86.

65. Irene G, Georgios P, Ioannis C, et al. Copper-coated textiles: armor against MDR nosocomial pathogens. Diagn Microbiol Infect Dis. 2016;85:205–9.

66. Kotsanas D, Wijesooriya WR, Sloane T, Stuart RL, Gillespie EE. The silver lining of disposable sporicidal privacy curtains in an intensive care unit. Am J Infect Control. 2014;42:366–70.

67. Schweizer M, Graham M, Ohl M, Heilmann K, Boyken L, Diekema D. Novel hospital curtains with antimicrobial properties: a randomized, controlled trial. Infect Control Hosp Epidemiol. 2012;33:1081–5.

68. Burden M, Keniston A, Frank MG, et al. Bacterial contamination of healthcare workers' uniforms: a randomized controlled trial of antimicrobial scrubs. J Hosp Med. 2013;8:380–5.

69. Boutin MA, Thom KA, Zhan M, Johnson JK. A randomized crossover trial to decrease bacterial contamination on hospital scrubs. Infect Control Hosp Epidemiol. 2014;35:1411–3.

70. Bearman GM, Rosato A, Elam K, et al. A crossover trial of antimicrobial scrubs to reduce methicillin-resistant *Staphylococcus aureus* burden on healthcare worker apparel. Infect Control Hosp Epidemiol. 2012;33:268–75.

71. Freeman AI, Halladay LJ, Cripps P. The effect of silver impregnation of surgical scrub suits on surface bacterial contamination. Vet J. 2012;192:489–93.

72. Pittet D. Improving adherence to hand hygiene practice: a multidisciplinary approach. Emerg Infect Dis. 2001;7:234–40.

73. Boyce JM, Pittet D, Healthcare Infection Control Practices Advisory Committee. Society for Healthcare Epidemiology of America. Association for Professionals in Infection Control. Infectious Diseases Society of America. Hand Hygiene Task Force. Guideline for hand hygiene in health-care settings: recommendations of the healthcare infection control practices advisory committee and the HICPAC/SHEA/APIC/IDSA hand hygiene task force. Infect Control Hosp Epidemiol. 2002;23:S3–40.

74. Pineles LL, Morgan DJ, Limper HM, et al. Accuracy of a radio-frequency identification (RFID) badge system to monitor hand hygiene behavior during routine clinical activities. Am J Infect Control. 2014;42:144–7.

75. Sahud AG, Bhanot N, Radhakrishnan A, Bajwa R, Manyam H, Post JC. An electronic hand hygiene surveillance device: a pilot study exploring surrogate markers for hand hygiene compliance. Infect Control Hosp Epidemiol. 2010;31:634–9.

76. Cheng VC, Tai JW, Ho SK, et al. Introduction of an electronic monitoring system for monitoring compliance with Moments 1 and 4 of the WHO "My 5 Moments for Hand Hygiene" methodology. BMC Infect Dis. 2011;11:151. 2334-11-151

77. Armellino D, Hussain E, Schilling ME, et al. Using high-technology to enforce low-technology safety measures: the use of third-party remote video auditing and real-time feedback in healthcare. Clin Infect Dis. 2012;54:1–7.

78. Conway LJ. Challenges in implementing electronic hand hygiene monitoring systems. Am J Infect Control. 2016;44:e7–e12.

79. Swoboda SM, Earsing K, Strauss K, Lane S, Lipsett PA. Electronic monitoring and voice prompts improve hand hygiene and decrease nosocomial infections in an intermediate care unit. Crit Care Med. 2004;32:358–63.

80. Ellingson K, Polgreen PM, Schneider A, et al. Healthcare personnel perceptions of hand hygiene monitoring technology. Infect Control Hosp Epidemiol. 2011;32:1091–6.

81. Boyce JM, Cooper T, Lunde A, Yin J, Arbogast J. Impact of an electronic hand hygiene monitoring system trial on hand hygiene compliance in a surgical intensive care unit (SICU and general medicine ward (GMW). Poster abstract at: Infectious Diseases Society of America 2012 Annual Conference; October 19, 2012; San Diego.

82. McGuckin M, Govednik J. A review of electronic hand hygiene monitoring: considerations for hospital management in data vcollection, healthcare worker supervision, and patient perception. J Healthc Manag. 2015;60:348–61.

83. Harrison R, Flood D, Duce D. Usability of mobile applications: literature review and rationale for a new usability model. J Interact Sci. 2013;1(1):1–16.

84. Ward MA, Schweizer ML, Polgreen PM, Gupta K, Reisinger HS, Perencevich EN. Automated and electronically assisted hand hygiene monitoring systems: a systematic review. Am J Infect Control. 2014;42:472–8.

85. Hagel S, Reischke J, Kesselmeier M, et al. Quantifying the Hawthorne effect in hand hygiene compliance through comparing direct observation with automated hand hygiene monitoring. Infect Control Hosp Epidemiol. 2015;36:957–62.

86. Morgan DJ, Pineles L, Shardell M, et al. Automated hand hygiene count devices may better measure compliance than human observation. Am J Infect Control. 2012;40:955–9.

87. Marra AR, Edmond MB. New technologies to monitor healthcare worker hand hygiene. Clin Microbiol Infect. 2014;20:29–33.

88. Sharma D, Thomas GW, Foster ED, et al. The precision of human-generated hand-hygiene observations: a comparison of human observation with an automated monitoring system. Infect Control Hosp Epidemiol. 2012;33:1259–61.

89. Armellino D, Trivedi M, Law I, et al. Replicating changes in hand hygiene in a surgical intensive care unit with remote video auditing and feedback. Am J Infect Control. 2013;41:925–7.

90. Temime L, Opatowski L, Pannet Y, Brun-Buisson C, Boelle PY, Guillemot D. Peripatetic health-care workers as potential super-spreaders. Proc Natl Acad Sci U S A. 2009;106:18420–5.

What Is the Role of Mobile No-Touch Disinfection Technology in Optimizing Healthcare Environmental Hygiene?

Philip C. Carling

Introduction

As a result of epidemiologic and microbiologic studies over the past decade, it has become increasingly evident that interventions to mitigate environmental surface pathogen contamination constitute an important component of healthcare-associated infection (HAI) prevention. It has now become widely appreciated that, "Cleaning of hard surfaces in hospital rooms is critical for reducing healthcare-associated infections" [1] (p. 598). Indeed, as noted by the directors of the Duke Prevention Epicenter Program, "the contaminated hospital environment has emerged as a key target area to prevent the spread of HAIs"[2] (p. 872).

Preliminary studies documenting patient zone surface contamination with healthcare-associated pathogens (HAPs) more than a decade ago raised concerns that cleaning practice should be improved [3]. It was not until actual cleaning practice was objectively monitored, initially using a covert visual monitoring system [4] and later with covertly applied fluorescent markers [5], that actual cleaning practice itself was objectively evaluated [6, 7]. The discovery that near-patient surfaces, also referred to as patient zone surfaces, in many acute care hospitals and other healthcare settings were not being disinfection cleaned according to hospital policies [7], along with the landmark study by Huang et al. [8] which quantified the risk of MRSA and VRE acquisition posed by occupying a room previously occupied by a patient colonized or infected by these pathogens that the clear risk of suboptimal disinfection cleaning became widely appreciated. Eight similar studies have now confirmed an average 120% increased risk of the subsequent occupant becoming colonized or infected with MRSA, VRE, *Clostridium difficile* (CD), *Pseudomonas*, and *Acinetobacter* [9].

Shortly after confirming the sensitivity and specificity of covert use of fluorescent markers to objectively and reproducibly identify opportunities to improve terminal cleaning thoroughness, process improvement interventions based on structured educational activities and direct performance feedback to environmental services (EVS) staff were shown to be highly effective in improving cleaning thoroughness [10]. Published reports have now confirmed the effectiveness of such programs in more than 120 hospitals in the United States, Canada, and Australia [7]. In the study hospitals, not only has cleaning improved as demonstrated by the thoroughness of disinfection scores (proportion of objects cleaned relative to objects expected to be cleaned by hospital policy or TDC) increasing from approximately 40–60% to 80–90% or higher as a result of similar programmatic intervention, there has also been excellent sustainability of the results over at least 3 years where ongoing programs have been evaluated [11–13].

Several studies have now confirmed that improved environmental cleaning decreases HAP contamination of surfaces [4, 14, 15]. Although the complexity and cost of studies to evaluate the impact of decreased patient zone HAP contamination on acquisition has limited such undertakings, two landmark studies found similar statistically significant results. The 2006 study by Hayden confirmed a 66% ($p < 0.001$) reduction in VRE acquisition as a result of a 75% improvement in thoroughness of disinfection cleaning [4]. A more recent study by Datta found a 50% ($p < 0.001$) reduction in MRSA acquisition and a 28% reduction ($p < 0.02$) in VRE acquisition as a result of an 80% improvement in environmental cleaning [14]. The latter study also confirmed significantly decreased prior room occupant transmission for both pathogens during the intervention period. These studies clearly show that direct patient safety benefits can be realized by improving the thoroughness of patient zone surface disinfection cleaning.

P.C. Carling (✉)
Department of Infectious Diseases, Boston University School of Medicine and Carney Hospital, 2100 Dorchester Avenue, Boston, MA 02124, USA
e-mail: pcarling@comcast.net

© Springer International Publishing AG 2018
G. Bearman et al. (eds.), *Infection Prevention*, DOI 10.1007/978-3-319-60980-5_8

Fig. 8.1 Vertical and
horizontal approaches to
preventing healthcare-
associated infections
(Reprinted from, Philip [7],
with permission from
Elsevier)

Vertical approaches reduce risk of infections due to specific
pathogens:

> Active surveillance testing to identify asymptomatic carriers
>
> Contact precautions for patients colonized or infected with
> specific organisms
>
> Decolonization of patients colonized or infected with specific
> organisms

Horizontal approaches reduce risk of a broad range of infections and
are not pathogen specific:

> Standard precautions (e.g. hand hygiene)
>
> Universal use of gloves or gloves and gowns
>
> Universal decolonization (e.g. chlorhexidine gluconate bathing)
>
> Antimicrobial stewardship
>
> Environmental cleaning and disinfection

Unfortunately, the complexity of the interrelated factors necessary to optimize the safety of surfaces in the patient zone remains an evolving challenge [7, 16]. Furthermore, defining how the impact of various surface cleaning interventions and optimized hand hygiene practice can be validated to develop clinically grounded implementation guidance has yet to be substantially realized [7]. In this context, it is important to recognize that environmental hygiene represents a critical element of what Wenzel and Edmonds defined as "horizontal interventions" that are central to mitigating a wide range of HAIs [17]. These approaches aim to reduce the risk of infections caused by a broad range of pathogens by implementing standard practices that are effective regardless of patient-specific conditions (Fig. 8.1). In contrast to the horizontal interventions, "vertical interventions" are pathogen and/or condition specific. They remain important in defined settings and become most cost-effective when the indications for their use are clearly defined. While vertical and horizontal approaches are not mutually exclusive, there is evolving evidence that, in endemic situations, horizontal interventions represent a best use of HAI prevention resources [17]. Indeed, recent well-designed studies of horizontal interventions such as chlorhexidine bathing and decolonization as well as expanded use of contact precautions in intensive care units appear to have significant potential for HAI reduction, at least in certain settings [17].

In order to facilitate discussion of the many elements necessary to optimize healthcare hygienic cleaning, it is useful to put these interventions into a defined construct of HAI prevention activities. As noted in Fig. 8.2, hygienic cleaning and hand hygiene as well as interventions related to instrument reprocessing, air quality, water quality, and physical setting design are all horizontal interventions [7]. All of these horizontal inter-

ventions represent elements of "healthcare hygienic practice." While these elements have traditionally been discussed independently, their effectiveness in clinical settings is substantially interrelated, particularly environmental hygiene and hand hygiene, as will be discussed below. The term "environmental hygiene" with respect to healthcare can be defined as "cleaning activities directed at removing and/or killing potentially harmful pathogens capable of being transmitted directly from surfaces or indirectly to susceptible individuals or other surfaces." As such it consists of both the physical cleaning of surfaces as well as surface disinfection cleaning (Fig. 8.2). While liquid chemistries are well established as the most clinically useful approach to surface disinfection, innovative approaches which may have the potential for complementing traditional liquid chemistry have been developed over the past several years.

No-Touch Disinfection Technologies

Prior to 2005, ultraviolet (UV) radiation devices had been used for disinfection of endocavity ultrasound transducers and ventilation ducts [18] and hydrogen peroxide (HP) as a liquid disinfectant. The first detailed evaluation of the use of HP vapor to disinfect multiple patient rooms was reported in 2004 [19]. The documentation of suboptimal near-patient surface cleaning [3, 16] prompted more extensive evaluation of HP systems and the development of UV no-touch disinfection systems (NTDS) [20] Both these technologies can only be used in closed spaces, such as vacated patient rooms or dedicated equipment closets. Currently there are two somewhat different forms of each technology [18, 20, 21]. Hydrogen peroxide vapor (HPV), the earlier technology, utilizes a generated vapor, 30–35% aqueous H_2O_2, which is

Fig. 8.2 Horizontal
healthcare hygienic practices

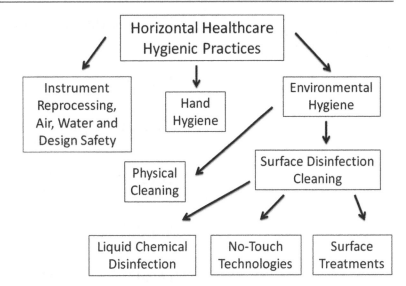

characterized by small particle generation [20]. Dry mist HP is pressure generated and combines 5–6% H_2O_2 with <50 ppm silver cations. UV-C technology utilizes a continuous mercury bulb generated high-intensity light focused on a wave length of 250 nm which is capable of damaging mitochondrial DNA [18]. Pulsed xenon UV technology utilizes pulses of high-intensity xenon-generated UV light [22].

Methods

PubMed was used to search the terms disinfection cleaning, hydrogen peroxide environmental disinfection, ultraviolet environmental decontamination, or environmental hygiene, between 2000 and 2016. Studies which were published in English in peer review journals were reviewed. Abstracts, conference proceedings, and review articles were not part of the evaluation process. Articles were also identified by hand-searching references in the reviewed articles. No financial support was received for this review. The review was performed in accordance with PRISMA recommendations [23].

In order to facilitate discussion of the studies that over the past decade have investigated both the in vitro potency and potential clinical roles of these NTDS, studies related to each system will be categorized using the CDC evidentiary hierarchy proposed by McDonald and Arduino in 2013 [24] (Fig. 8.3). Given the availability of Level I and III studies utilizing healthcare-associated pathogens, the limited number of Level II studies looking at simple (nonpathogen) heterotrophic bioburden reduction was not reviewed. Furthermore, this analysis of NTDS will relate exclusively to large (non-handheld) portable technology for which at least two clinical (Level IV or V) studies have been published in a peer-reviewed medical journal through December, 2015.

Hydrogen Peroxide No-Touch Systems

Level I HP Studies: Laboratory Demonstration of Meaningful Pathogen Bioburden Reduction (In Vitro Studies)

Both the HP vapor system (Bioquil) and the vaporized HP system (Steris) have shown a >6 $\log^{10}$ reduction (LR) of all vegetative bacteria and microbacterial pathogens evaluated as well as *C. difficile* spores [20]. Recent studies with a range of human viruses have confirmed HPV to be broadly viricidal [25]. While viricidal effectiveness does not appear to be impacted by high titers, studies have yet to determine the impact of organic load such as fecal material on viricidal efficacy [26]. Microbicidal efficacy is adversely impacted by both pathogen load and organic soil, but the impact has been incompletely quantified [27]. Given the fact that HP systems have been designed to be used only after surfaces are cleaned effectively prior to treatment, it is conceptually possible that the efficacy of these systems would be compromised in clinical settings where the thoroughness of disinfection cleaning is suboptimal. A recent report found that HPV decontamination was effective in killing both *C. difficile* spores and vegetative bacteria seeded onto cotton material, but potency and dose effectiveness needed to be evaluated further [25].

Level III HPV Studies: Demonstrate In-Use Pathogen Reduction of Clinical Relevance (In Situ Studies)

As noted in Table 8.1, nine studies have evaluated the impact of HPV technology on healthcare pathogen environmental contamination since 2004 [19, 28–35]. One of the studies employed a two-arm design, and the other eight evaluated the same clinical surfaces before and after HPV treatment. Rooms previously occupied by methicillin-resistant *Staph-*

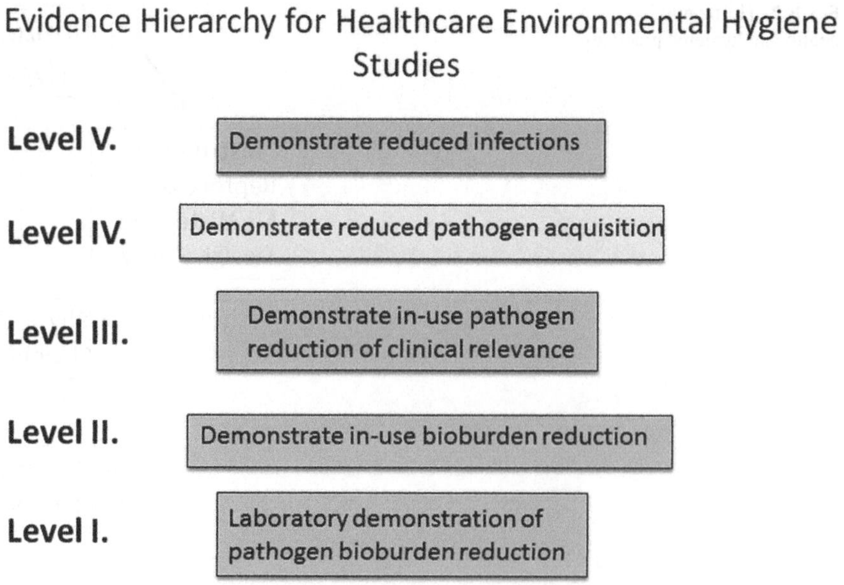

Fig. 8.3 Evidence hierarchy for healthcare environmental hygiene studies (Adapted from McDonald and Arduino [24])

Evidence Hierarchy for Healthcare Environmental Hygiene Studies

Level V. — Demonstrate reduced infections

Level IV. — Demonstrate reduced pathogen acquisition

Level III. — Demonstrate in-use pathogen reduction of clinical relevance

Level II. — Demonstrate in-use bioburden reduction

Level I. — Laboratory demonstration of pathogen bioburden reduction

ylococcus aureus (MRSA)-colonized or infected patients [6] or patients treated for *C. difficile* infection (CDI) [3] *Acinetobacter* (Ab) [1] were evaluated. Although not always quantified, all studies involved multiple rooms and 3–30 surfaces per room. The rate of pre-cleaning of surfaces contaminated with MRSA ranged widely (78%, 60%, 28%, 12%), possibly as a reflection of differences in the size of the areas cultured. As noted in Table 8.1, HPV treatment reduced or limited healthcare-associated pathogen (HAP) environmental contamination substantially in seven studies. In two studies, borderline significant [34] and nonsignificant [33] reduction of target pathogens were noted. In the only study which compared HPV to bleach, the intervention did decrease CD environmental contamination in rooms from 12% of surfaces following bleach cleaning to 2% with HPV treatment (*p* 0.005) [31].

Level IV HPV Studies: Demonstrate Reduced Pathogen Acquisition

As noted in Table 8.2, there has been only one study to evaluate the impact of an HPV program to decrease HAP acquisition [33]. Passaretti et al. used weekly screening cultures to measure MRSA and VRE acquisition in three surgical intensive care units compared with three control units during a 30-month study. While VRE acquisition decreased significantly from 8.1 to 1.7% of at-risk patients (*p* < 0.01), MRSA acquisition decreased nonsignificantly from 2.8 to 0.9% (*p* = 0.30). The findings of the study are particularly difficult to interpret given the fact that chlorhexidine bathing and "multiple" HAI prevention interventions were initiated during the course of the study and may have had an impact on the findings.

Level V HPV Studies: Demonstration of Reduced Infections

As noted in Table 8.3, three studies have evaluated the addition of HPV treatment to routine disinfection cleaning with bleach on healthcare-associated CDI (HA-CDI) rates during intervention periods between 3 and 11 months [30, 33, 34] and three others evaluated MDR Ab, VRE and "pathogen rates" [36–38]. Unlike other studies discussed below, the pre-intervention HA-CDI rate of 8.8/10,000 PTD in the study by Manian was similar to that seen in many acute care hospitals. While the addition of HPV in this report was associated with a significant decrease in HA-CDI from 8.8 to 5.5/10,000 PTD (*p* < 0.001), the fact that just prior to the addition of the HPV intervention program 21% of the rooms had undergone four serial cycles of bleach cleaning and the fact that only 53% of eligible rooms received HPV treatment suggests that the modest improvement in HA-CDI may have been multifactorial. Although not discussed by the authors, the substantial increase in piperacillin–tazobactam use might have also had a favorable impact on HA-CDI rates during the intervention period. HO-CDI rates in the other two studies of 27 and 28/10,000 PTD were quite high [30, 33]. While the two studies in settings with very high HA-CDI rates observed a decrease in incidence in cases following implementation of the HPV programs, the statistical significance of the change was borderline (*p* = 0.05) in the report by Boyce [30] and not statistically significant in the report by Passaretti [33] (*p* = 0.19). Fishner evaluated VRE colonization/infection noting that it was lower during a 28-month study of HPV use than during the preceding 55 months, but multiple other interventions were implemented during the HPV study period [36]. While Chmielarczyk in 2012 reported that over-

Table 8.1 Level III hydrogen peroxide vapor technology studies

Author year	Nature of study	Prior room occupant	Rooms studied	Surfaces per room	Intervention	Outcome
French (2004) [19]	2 arm B/A Detergent B/A HPV	MRSA C/I	10 control	12	Control arm – P/P cultures in 10 rooms cleaned with detergent	Control arm −78% surface MRSA +, after detergent cleaning 74% +
			6 HPV		HPV arm – P/P cultures in 9 rooms given HPV Tx	HPV arm 72% surface MRSA +, post-HPV Tx. – 1%
Otter (2007) [28]	Before cleaning, after cleaning, after HPV	MRSA	12	15	Cultures done before cleaning, after cleaning with QAC, and after HPV Tx	Surface sites with MRSA decreased significantly from 60% to 40% and 3% following each intervention. VRE decreased similarly from 30% to 10% to 0%
Hardy (2007) [29]	Before, after cleaning, after HPV	NA	Multiple ICU rooms	3	Cultures over 3 months pre-intervention after routine cleaning compared to HPV Tx	Just before the intervention after standard cleaning 17% of sites showed MRSA. Following HPV Tx. no sites were positive
Boyce (2008) [30]	Observational B/A HPV	CD	18	Multiple	"Intensive" HPV decontamination of CD patient rooms on 5 "high-incidence" wards	Pretreatment surface contamination rate of 25% fell to 0 immediately after HPV Tx
Barbut (2009) [31]	Two-arm comparison	CD	30	12–13	CD D/C rooms were randomized to 0.5% bleach (5000 ppm available chlorine) cleaning vs. HPV Tx	Contamination decreased by 50% after bleach and 91% after HPV treatment (p 0.005)
Otter (2010) [32]	Single culture B/A decontamination activity	MDR-GNB	ICU	Multiple sites combined	Pooled site cultures done before and after HPV Tx. decontamination of an ICU	46% of areas were + for GNB (only two for MDR *Enterobacter*) before treatment and none after HPV Tx
Passaretti (2013) [33]	Observational B/A HPV	CD	12	18	Proportion of surfaces with MRSA, CD VRE, or MDRG-GNB before and after HPV Tx. compared	Proportion of surfaces contaminated before and after HPV Tx. were not significantly different
		MRSA				
		VRE				
		MDR-GNB				
Manian (2011) [34]	Observational B/A HPV	MRSA and/or Ab	Multiple	9–30	Room surface cultures before and after HPV Tx .	MRSA and AB room surface contamination was low but decreased after HPV Tx. for both organisms (p 0.04)
Dryden (2008) [35]	Observational B/A HPV	MRSA	Single ward	Not stated	Room surface cultures before and after HPV Tx	MRSA contamination of surfaces decreased from 28% before to 10% after HPV Tx. but was not significant (p 0.2)

all MDR Ab incidence density decreased dramatically during an HPV intervention program, the impact of a "combination of rigorous infection control measures" most probably impacted the observed change in Ab rates [37]. Horn in 2015 attributed decreased rates of several HAPs to an HPV program during which an average of only two rooms a day in the 270-bed hospital received HPV treatments [38]. Given the limited nature of the intervention and the observation that hand hygiene increased very significantly during the inter-

vention period, it would appear difficult to attribute the changes substantially to the HPV program.

Summary of Hydrogen Peroxide Vapor Disinfection Studies

Extensive testing of HPV environmental disinfection systems has confirmed in vitro (Level I) effectiveness in killing all tested vegetative microorganisms, viruses, and spores evaluated. While incompletely quantified, the obser-

Table 8.2 Level IV hydrogen peroxide vapor technology studies

Author year	Endemic setting	Clinical outcome	Pre-int mo.	Post-int. mo.	Outcome	Confounder evaluated
Passaretti (2013)	Endemic	Rectal VRE nasal MRSA	12 months	18 months 3 units HPV on D/C 3 units studied	VRE acquisition decreased from 8.19% to 1.7% ($p < 0.01$). MRSA acquisition decreased from 2.8% to 0.9 (p 0.3)	A dedicated HPV team led to 71% of eligible rooms being treated
						Multiple infection control interventions implemented during 30 months period including CHG bathing

vation that high titers of microbes/spores as well as organic material can decrease the potency of HP disinfection reinforces the importance of cleaning of environmental surfaces prior to HP treatment. The impact of HPV treatments on environmental pathogen contamination in clinical settings (Level III) has been evaluated in nine reports over the past 12 years (Table 8.1). Although most studies reported substantial or complete resolution of environmental contamination after HPV treatment, two studies failed to show a significant decrease in the proportion of surfaces still contaminated with the target organism during the HPV treatment program [33, 35]. While not directly evaluated in the latter report, the documentation by Hardy and Dryden that HPV-treated surfaces can quickly become recontaminated [29] raises the possibility that the findings of the study by Passaretti may have been adversely impacted by recontamination during the study, particularly since 30% of eligible rooms did not receive HPV treatment. The only study which objectively measured actual acquisition during an ICU admission (Level IV) observed significantly decreased VRE ($p < 0.01$) but not MRSA ($p = 0.30$) acquisition [33]. While these findings could have been a reflection of different routes of acquisition, it is of note that Datta in 2011, in the only other large study to analyze the impact of an environmental disinfection intervention on HAP acquisition, observed a highly significant ($p < 0.001$) decrease in MRSA with only borderline significant ($p < 0.02$) decrease in VRE acquisition in response to objectively improved standardized ICU disinfection cleaning [14]. Six studies evaluated clinical outcomes (Level V) before and after implementing HPV programs (Table 8.3). In the single study that reported a highly significant impact on HA-CDI, the actual endemic HA-CDI rate only fell slightly from 8.8 to 5.5/10,000 PTD. As discussed above, improving environmental hygiene and hand hygiene precluded accurate assessment of the HPV technology and may have substantially impacted two of the reports evaluating clinical outcomes following the implementation of HPV programs [36, 37].

Ultraviolet No-Touch Systems

Level I Studies: Laboratory Demonstration of Pathogen Bioburden (In Vitro Studies) Reduction

Eight studies have evaluated the in situ effectiveness of UV-C systems, and one study evaluated PX-UV technology for killing CD spores, MRSA, and VRE [22, 39–45]. One study each also evaluated the potency of UV-C against *A. baumannii*, and one study evaluated *Aspergillus* species (Table 8.4). All studies used 3–6 log ^{10} organisms dried onto stainless steel or *Formica* discs which were then exposed to varying doses of UV light for 10–90 min. Between one and ten strains of test organisms were evaluated in each study. No study which evaluated multiple strains disclosed any significant difference in sensitivity to UV light between strains of the same pathogen.

UV-C – As summarized in Table 8.4, each of the seven studies evaluating UV-C technology found three to four LR reduction of vegetative bacteria with UV intensity settings between 12,000 and 36,000 uWs/cm^2 and exposure times between 15 and 73 min. Similar exposure led to a two to three LR of CD spores. Mahida reported that an exposure time (distance not documented) of 60–90 min led to a greater than four LR of VRE, AB, and *Aspergillus* sp. [43]. Havill documented only a 1.7–3.0 LR of CD spores exposed to high-dose UV-C for 73 min [42]. Using a 10-min exposure, Nerandzic found a somewhat decreased potency against vegetative bacteria but a substantial decrease in CD killing with only a one LR at a 4 ft exposure distance [22]. Several studies found that shading had a significantly adverse impact on killing, particularly for *C. difficile* spores [39, 40, 43]. Even at short distances (20 in.) LR fell from 2–3 to 1.0 as a result of shading in the 2010 study by Nerandzic [40]. Similarly shading decreased LR from 4 to 2.4 despite very high intensity (39,000 uWs/cm²) and a long exposure time (50 min) in the 2010 study by Rutala [39], while the study by Zhang documented significantly decreased killing UV-C of CD spores with dilute (10%) calf serum and "heavy" organic

Table 8.3 Level V hydrogen peroxide vapor technology studies

Author year	Endemic setting	Clinical outcome	Pre-int mo.	Post-int. mo.	Outcome	Confounder evaluated
Manian (2013) [34]	Yes	HA-CDI	24 months bleach	11 months enhanced bleach (4 cycles) or HPV	HA-CDI rate of 8.8 decreased to 5.5 during the intervention period ($p < 0.0001$)	Patient days (stable)
						HH (stable)
						Isolation precaution compliance (stable)
						Antimicrobial use – Zosyn increased while clindamycin and cephalosporin use decreased
						Personnel – HPV technicians one or more
Boyce (2008) [30]	No	HA-CDII	9 months bleach	9 months	HA-CDI rates before intervention on 5 units were between 10 and 30 cases/10,000 PTD (mean28) which decreased to 2.5–20/10,000 PTD (Mean 1.3) ($P = 0.05$)	No significant difference in antimicrobial use, but linear regression analysis showed a significant correlation with third-generation cephalosporin use
						No changes in IC P/P
						No differences in HH or CP
						No difference in NAP – 1 prevalence
Passaretti (2013) [33]	No	HA-CDI	12 months non-bleach	3 months	HA-CDI incidence decreased HPV Tx. units decreased from 27/10,000 PTD to 10/10,000 PTD but was not significant ($p = 0.19$)	See Passaretti (Table ___)
Chmielarczyk (2012) [37]	No	MDR Ab	18	12	Incidence density resolved from 24/1000 PTD to zero during the program	A combination of infection prevention initiatives was implemented (Not described in detail)
Horn (2015) [38]	Yes	Pathogen "rate"/1000/PTD	12	12.	Rates (not defined) decreased significantly for CD, VRE, and MDRO-GNB but not for MRSA	Hand hygiene improved significantly from 78% before to 89% during the intervention with HPV Tx. ($p < 0.001$)
Fishner (2016) [36]	No	VRE	55	28	Modeling analysis showed decreased VRE infection/ colonization	Increased active surveillance and isolation practices
						The use of cleaning improved from 60% at baseline to >79% during study period ($p < 0.001$)
						Increased educational interventions

Table 8.4 Level I ultraviolet technology studies

Author year	Device	Pathogen (strains tested)	Inoculum log10	Distance	Dosage uWs/cm²	Duration (minutes)	Log10 reduction (LR)	Log10 reduction shaded
Rutala (2010) [39]	UV-C	MRSA [10]	4.9	NS	12,000	15	4.3	3.9
		VRE [10]	4.4	NS	12,000	15	3.9	3.2
		AB [10]	4.6	NS	12,000	15	4.2	3.8
		CD [10]	4.1	NS	36,000	50	4	2.4
Nerandzic (2010) [40]	UV-C	CD [3]	3–5	20″–10.5′	22,000	45	2.3	
		MRSA [3]	3–5	20″–10.5′	22,000	45	3	
		VRE 3	3–5	20″–10.5′	22,000	45	3.5	
		CD	3–5	20″	22,000	45		1.0
Boyce (2011) [41]	UV-C	CD	5	NS	22,000	NS	1.7–2.9	
Havill (2012) [42]	UV-C	CD	6	NS	22,000	73	2.2	
Mahida (2013) [43]	UV-C	VRE	NS	NS	22,000	60–90	>4	(3.5)
		AB	NS	NS	22,000	60–90	>4	(3.0)
		Aspergillus	NS	NS	22,000	60–90	>4	(1.0)
Nerandzic (2014) [44]	UV-C (2 machines)	CD [2]	5	4′	NS	40	3	
		MRSA [2]	5	4′	NS	40	4	
		VRE [2]	5	4′	NS	40	5	
		CD [2]	6	4′		10	<1	
		MRSA [2]	6	4′		10	3	
		VRE [2]	6	4′		10	4	
Nerandzic (2015) [22]	PX – UV	CD [2]	3–5	4′	NS	10	0.5	
		MRSA [2]	3–5	4′	NS	10	1.85	
		VRE [2]	3–5	4′	NS	10	0.6	
	PX- UV	CD [2]	5	6″, 4′, 10′	NS	10	1.8, 0.5, 0.25	
		MRSA [2]	5	6″, 4′, 10′	NS	10	33, 1.8, 0.7	
		VRE [2]	5	6″, 4′, 10′	NS	10	2.5, 0.5, <0.2	
	UV-C	CD	5	4′	NS	10	1.0	
		MRSA	5	4′	NS	10	3.0	
		VRE	5	4′	NS	10	3.5	
Zhang (2013) [45]	UV-C	CD [7]	6	10.5′	22,000	45	4.5	
		CD	6 + 10% calf serum	10.5′	22,000	45	3.0	
		CD [3]	6 + 5% calf serum	10.5′	22,000	45	3.5	
		CD [5]	6+ light organic load	10.5′	22,000	45	4.5	
		CD	6+ moderate organic load	10.5′	22,000	45	<4.5 (*P* = 0.01)	

loads (*p* < 0.001 and *p* = 0.01) [45]. Lesser amounts of organic material led to no loss in LR compared to controls. To date there have been no additional studies using full-strength human serum, blood, or fecal material to further evaluate these preliminary findings. Although only evaluated by Mahida, it is of note that shading greatly decreased the LR of *Aspergillus* sp. using an exposure time of 60–90 min [43]. Given the importance of fungal pathogens in high-risk patient areas, it will be important to further evaluate UV-C's efficacy against these pathogens.

PX-UV – Only one published study, by Nerandzic, has evaluated the potency of this type of UV disinfection system in comparison to UV-C [22]. The authors found only limited (0.6–2) LR for MRSA and VRE at 4 ft and <1 LR for CD spores at 4 and 10 ft. Furthermore, at a distance of 6 in., LR for MRSA was only 3.3, for VRE 2.5 and CD 1.8. In addition, this study also showed that the dramatic adverse impact of distance from the unit which was greater for CD spores than for MRSA and VRE.

Level III UV Studies: Objectively Demonstrate Clinical Relevance (In Situ Studies)

As outlined in Table 8.5, there have been eight studies evaluating the impact of UV technology on healthcare-associated pathogen environmental contamination since 2010 (UV-C – 3, PX-UV-5) [15, 22, 39, 40, 45–49].

UV-C – The three studies evaluating pathogen bioburden reduction with UV-C evaluated individual rooms primarily occupied by MRSA-infected or colonized patients or CD-treated patients prior to and following UV treatment. In 2010, Rutala found only 9.5% of ten surfaces still contaminated with MRSA after UV-C treatment in comparison to 20% prior to routine cleaning ($P < 0.001$) [39]. Similar results were noted for VRE but not described. Contaminated CDI patient rooms were not studied and a vegetative microbicidal, not sporicidal, UV cycle of 15 min was utilized. Similar results were noted by Nerandzic for MRSA and VRE with a borderline significant decrease in CD contamination using a 45 min "sporicidal" UV treatment cycle [40]. In 2013, Sitzlar and associates described a three-phase clinical intervention which compared terminal cleaning following educational interventions, the addition of a UV-C cycle to standard terminal disinfection with bleach, and the use of a special team for daily and terminal cleaning of CD-infected patient rooms [15]. While the addition of UV-C treatment during phase III decreased residual contamination in comparison to phase II, 35% of surfaces remained CD culture positive after UV-C treatment. Subsequently with a dedicated cleaning team intervention utilizing daily cleaning, residual *C. difficile* contamination was eliminated from the study rooms during the final 2 months of the program.

PX-UV – Two of the five PX-UV studies utilized a two-arm evaluation of environmental pathogen reduction in treated rooms vs. routinely disinfected rooms [47, 49]. The other three studies were uncontrolled measurements of pathogen prevalence on between 5 and 11 surfaces before and after treatment in the same rooms. Two studies utilized rooms previously occupied by patients treated for CDI, two studies MRSA-colonized or infected patients, and one VRE study colonized or infected patients. All but one of these studies performed environmental cultures only for the pathogen associated with the prior room occupant. As noted in Table 8.5, outcomes reported by the authors varied between studies. Stibich evaluated VRE contamination but failed to find a significant difference in the treated vs. routinely cleaned rooms [46]. A study by Ghantoji compared PX-UV to bleach disinfection for CDI patient rooms and noted no significant difference between the interventions [49]. Jinadatha documented a borderline significant decrease in MRSA colony counts per site before and after treatment but no clear difference in the number of contaminated sites [48]. Nerandzic compared bleach disinfection to PX-UV treat-

ment in CDI-associated contaminated rooms and found no difference in the proportion of sites still contaminated with *C. difficile* spores following either treatment [22].

Level V UV Studies: Demonstrate Decreased Infections

Over the past 3 years, there have been five published studies which evaluated the clinical impact of NTDT UV technologies (UV-C, 1; PX-UV, 3) [50–54]. As outlined in Table 8.6, all studies were uncontrolled retrospective before and after (quasi-experimental) in design. Of the three CDI studies, two were in epidemic setting with rates of 23.3 and 18.3/10,000 PTD [53, 54]and one in a high-level endemic setting with a rate of 9.22/10,000 PTD [50]. Several of the studies inconsistently noted possible confounders whose impact on observed outcomes was not directly evaluated. The specific limitations of these studies will be discussed in a subsequent portion of this review.

UV-C – In the single study evaluating the clinical impact of a UV-C disinfection intervention program, Napolitano compared "overall HAI rates" during a 6 month pre-intervention period followed by a 5-month evaluation period [52]. Average HAI incidence decreased minimally from 3.7 to 2.4/1000 PTD. Although HA-CDI decreased from 12.3 to 6.6/10,000 PTD, no impact on either MRSA or VRE infections was noted. During the study, 70–100% of available discharge rooms were treated by three UV system technicians.

PX-UV – In 2013, Levin described the use of a PX-UV system on 73% of patient rooms previously occupied by individuals treated for CDI [50]. A single machine was used to deliver three cycles for 7 min each, two in the patient room and one in the bathroom. Pre-intervention the HO-CDI rate had been stable at 9.22/10,000 PTD for 30 months. Following intervention, the rate decreased moderately to 4.5/10,000 PTD during the following 12 months ($p = 0.01$). Haas evaluated overall HAI rates comparing 30 months before and 22 months after intervention using a PX-UV system on 76% of contact precaution patient rooms [51]. The authors note that they also had implemented "multiple" other infection prevention interventions during the study period (not described). The overall HAI rate decreased minimally but significantly from 2.7 to 2.1/1000 PTD. In 2015, Miller reported a decrease in HO-CDI from 23.3 to 19.3/10,000 PTD following "improved emphasis on environmental hygiene." The rate subsequently fell further to 8.3/1000 PTD during a 12-month period following the addition of a PX-UV program [53]. In 2015 Nagaraja reported that the implementation of a PX-UV program decreased the incidence of HA-CDI from 18.3 to 5.5/10,000 PTD ($P < 0.001$) in the intensive care unit but did not significantly impact the overall HO-CDI rate for the hospital [54].

Table 8.5 Level III ultraviolet technology studies

Author year	System	Nature of study	Prior room occupant	Rooms studied	Surfaces per room	Intervention	Outcome
Rutala (2010) [39]	UV-C	Observational P/P	MRSA	NS	10	UV-C treatment 15 min before cleaning	MRSA-positive sites decreased from 81/4000 (20%) to 4/400 (0.5%) ($p < 0.001$). Similar results were noted for VRE (data not shown)
Nerandzic (2010) [40]	UV-C	Same room P/PTX	MRSA I/C (59 rooms) CDI treated (7 rooms)	66	4	No pre-cleaning	MRSA 10% of surfaces before and 0.8% of surfaces after UV-C TX. ($p < 0.0001$)
						UV-C treatment 20–45 min depending on size of room	VRE 2.7% positive before and 0.38 % after TX. (p 0.07)
							CD 3.4% before 0.38% after TX. (p 0.02)
Sitzlar (2013) [15]	UV-C	Observational P/P	CDI	20–25	Multiple standard sites	Four phases	Addition of UV-C treatment decreased but did not eliminate CD from 35% of surfaces. During final phase increased daily cleaning eliminated CD from tested surfaces
						Baseline, terminal cleaning	
						Education and positive feedback; terminal UV-C added, special team cleaning	
Stibich (2011) [46]	PX-UV	Observational P/P	VRE I/C	12	11	Routine cleaning with QAC followed by PX-UV Tx – 3 positions 4 min each	No significant impact of PX-UV on VRE contamination in comparison to standard cleaning with QAC (p 0.13)
Jinadatha (2014) [47]	PX – 4 V	Two arms	MRSA I/C	10 per arm	5	Control arm – 1:10 bleach routine cleaning	MRSA contamination was found on 86% of sites prior to intervention and 76 the two study arms manual cleaning decreased contamination to 16% in the control arm and 8% in the treatment arm (p 0.23)
						Intervention arm – 1:10 bleach for visible soil plus PX – UV 15 min	
Nerandzic (2015) [22]	PX-UV	Observational P/P	CDI	16	7	Cultures for CD, MRSA, and VRE before cleaning and after routine bleach cleaning + PX-UV-C 25 min cycles <3 sect from cultured sites	While CD + sites decreased by 50% (p 0.34), the difference was not significant and may have been in part due to bleach cleaning
Jinadatha (2015) [48]	PX-UV	Observational P/P	MRSA	14 confirmed >1 site + MRSA	5	PX-UV 3 locations for 5 min	Mean colony count per site decreased from 5.7 to 4.3 after treatment ($p < 0.01$)
Ghantoji (2015) [49]	PX-UV	Two arms	CDI treated	15 per arm	5	Intervention arm: activated HP for visible soil + PX-UV 3 locations each <3′ for unit for 5 min each	35–40% of surfaces + for CD pre-intervention in both arms. Both methods equal in reducing positive cultures

Table 8.6 Level V ultraviolet technology studies

Author year	System	Endemic setting	Clinical outcome	Pre-int. Mo.	Post-int. mo.	Outcome	Confounder noted
Levin (2013) [50]	PX-UV	High-level endemic	HA-CDI	36	12	Pre-intervention HA-CDI of 9.22 decreased to 4.5/10,000 PTD (p 0.002)	CA-CDCI (stable)
							Intervention use – 56% of CDI rooms
							Hospital PTD (stable)
							MCCMI (stable)
							Quinolone use (stable)
Haas (2014) [51]	PX-UV	Yes	HAI	30	22	HAI average incidence decreased 21% from 2.7 to 2.11/1000 PTD	76% of CD rooms treated. Multiple infection control interventions implemented serially during the >4 years studied. Cleaning thoroughness monitored but not reported
Napolitano (2015) [52]	UV-C	Yes	HAI (not defined)	5	6	HAI incidence 3.7/1000 PTD before to 2.4 after program but no impact noted on MRSA and VRE rates	Personnel added – 3 UV-C technicians
Miller (2015) [53]	PX-UV	No	HA-CDI	12	12	HA-CDI decreased from 23.3 baseline to 19.3/10,000 PTD with increased focus on EH. Following additional PX-UV, the rate declined to 8.3/10,000 PTD over the next 12 months	Hand hygiene did not change over time
Nagaraja (2015) [54]	PX-UV	No	HA-CDI	12 months	12 months	Hospital-wide HA-CDI pre-intervention rate of 10.6/10,000 PTD fell to 8.6 (not significant), but the ICU rate decreased from 18.3 to 5.5 ($p < 0.001$)	Admission CDI incidence increased 18% during the intervention phase
							New ES coping contract implemented 3 months before intervention. Fifty percent of CDI rooms treated

Summary of UV Disinfection Studies

As outlined in Table 8.4, Level I studies of UV technology have clearly defined the relative microbicidal potency of both UV-C and PX-UV systems. The most recent studies have confirmed the substantial and significant adverse impact of both shading and distance from the light source with UV technologies. While reflective paint [53] and modifications in light source placement within the rooms as well as cycle duration modification might affect these limitations, these possibilities await further investigation. Taken together, the in vitro studies of UV-C technology document that the effectiveness of the tested machines increased moderately with greater light intensity and duration of exposure. Conversely, potency decreased moderately to substantially with shading, especially for CD spores. While UV-C LR for vegetative pathogens was consistently in the three to four range with direct exposure, impact on CD spores was clearly less and varied quite widely (<1, 1.0, 1.7, 2.2, 2.3, 2.9, 3.0, 4.0). Although only evaluated in the 2014 study by Nerandzic using two machines, the wide range in CD spore LR suggests that there may be significant differences in the potency of different UV-C machines. Furthermore, it is of note that the only study that found a four LR of CD spores used a very high dosage of UV light (36,000 uWs/cm^2) and a long exposure time (90 min) [39].

The only published Level I study of P-UV by Nerandzic, et al. raises serious concerns regarding the potency of the technology when tested against log 10^5 vegetative organisms and spores and compared to UV-C treatment [44]. The authors also found a particularly striking fall off in PX-UV LR with increasing distance from the light source. Killing was similar to UV-C at 6 in., about half as potent at 4 ft and minimal at 10 ft from the light source. Although LR for VRE was similar to MRSA in the UV-C studies cited, VRE was found to be less sensitive to PX-UV in this study. Although the UV-C studies by Rutala and Nerandzic described a significant impact of UV treatment with fairly short treatment cycles (45 and 15 min, respectively), it is of note that precleaning was not performed in either study [39, 40]. While it might be suggested that such modeling could relate to settings where routine terminal disinfection cleaning is not being performed thoroughly, the study design, for this reason, likely overestimated the relative impact of the UV-C treatment in the clinical setting where 40–60% of surfaces were cleaned during terminal cleaning in nonperformance optimized hospital settings [7].

With respect to the impact of UV-C systems on in situ patient room contamination (Level III), Rutala (2010) found that treatment reduced MRSA surface contamination prior to disinfection cleaning [39]. Using a similar study design, Nerandzic, with a 20–45 a minute UV-C treatment cycle, noted both MRSA and VRE contamination were decreased but surfaces had a low prevalence of pretreatment contamination (MRSA – 10%, VRE – 2.7%) [40]. Treatment employing a PX-UV system in a heavily MRSA-contaminated environment was found by Jinadatha to be equivalent to cleaning with bleach [47]. The two studies evaluating the impact of PX-UV on surface contamination with *C. difficile* and VRE found equivalence but no advantage in comparison to bleach cleaning [22, 49]. While the Sitzlar study found that adding UV-C to routine daily cleaning was associated with a decrease in *C. difficile* contamination, 35% of surfaces remained contaminated after treatment in the setting of low-level thoroughness of routine daily cleaning. Subsequently daily cleaning by a dedicated team eliminated *C. difficile* environmental contamination from patient room surfaces during the final 2 months of the study [15].

Since 2013, five Level V studies have retrospectively evaluated the impact of UV treatment in acute care hospitals (HAI rates, 2; HO-CDI, 3) [50–54]. None of the three studies of PX-UV evaluating patient room MRSA, VRE, or CD found a substantial impact on pathogen contamination in comparison to "standard" (not objectively measured) disinfection cleaning [51, 53, 54]. Given the fact that the improvement in the studies with very high rates of HA-CDI may have substantially reflected a regression to the mean phenomenon and that two of the studies in endemic settings employed multiple other infection control interventions during the study, it becomes quite difficult to draw clini-cally generalizable conclusions regarding the clinical relevance of these studies. While the UV-C study of endemic HAI rates by Napolitano found that a decrease from 3.7 to 2.4/1000 PTD in association with implementing a UV-C disinfection program was consistent with an effect of the program, the finding that neither MRSA nor VRE HAI rates decreased is difficult to explain [52]. Intrinsic study design limitations that further compromise evaluation of the clinical relevance of these Level III and V studies will be discussed below.

Assessment of the Limitation of Published Clinical Studies

Level III Studies

Given the well-documented finding that environmental surface contamination with HAPs including MRSA, VRE, CD, Ab, and GNB is substantially and quantitatively impacted by disinfectant cleaning, it is of particular note that only one Level III study used an objective monitoring system to quantify the thoroughness of disinfection cleaning against which the NTDT system was being evaluated [22]. Since no Level III study utilized a sham machine control, it is quite conceivable that the thoroughness level of disinfection cleaning either increased or decreased during the intervention phase of the study. While the three studies of UV-C technology studies and seven of the nine HPV studies evaluated uncleaned rooms, the relevance of the findings of these studies is difficult to relate to a clinical setting where complete bioburden elimination was realized for 40% of surfaces objectively cleaned with a quaternary ammonium compound and 77% of surfaces cleaned with a novel sporicidal disinfectant in a clinical setting [55].

Level IV and V Studies

In the context of the intrinsic limitations of quasi-experimental studies [57], and given the limited and often incomplete assessment of evaluable confounders in these 11 reports, it is quite plausible that confounders had an impact on the veracity of what appeared to be an effect of the tested technology. Table 8.7 presents a summary of the manner in which confounders related to disinfection cleaning intervention studies were and were not analyzed in the Level V studies. In the analysis which follows, if a specific confounder was considered but not objectively quantified or specifically evaluated, it was categorized as a "limited" assessment in Table. As outlined, 8 factors were recognized in at least one of the 11 Level V reports as representing significant quantifiable con-

Table 8.7 Confounder evaluation pre-/post-intervention in 11 level V NTDT studies 2004–2016

Confounder	Objectively evaluated	Limited evaluation	Not evaluated
Changes in infection prevention interventions	7/11 (64%)	2/11 (18%)	2/11 (18%)
Compliance with planned intervention use	6/11 (55%)	3/11 (27%)	2/11 (18%)
Admission incidence density	3/11 (27%)		8/11 (73%)
Hand hygiene compliance	3/11 (27%)		8/11 (73%)
Isolation practice compliance	2/11 (18%)		9/11 (82%)
Thoroughness of disinfection cleaning	2/11 (18%)		9/11 (82%)
Antibiotic use trends	1/11 (9%)	2/11 (18%)	8/11 (73%)
Case mix	1/11 (9%)		10/11 (91%)

founders with potential impact on measured outcomes. Of the 11 studies, 64% described changes in infection control practice between pre- and post-intervention periods. While two of the studies describing this confounder noted no changes in their programs, in five (71%) of the reports interventions were described by the authors as "multiple" (2), "several initiatives" (1), a "multidisciplinary intervention" (1), and an "intervention bundle" (1). Although these enhancements to routine infection prevention and environmental cleaning practices were described in varying detail, the authors clearly believed the enhancements were substantive, yet none of the discussion portions of the manuscripts considered the substantial possibility that such broadly improved infection prevention activities may have impacted the outcomes they attributed to the NTDT program. Evaluation of compliance with the use of the planned NTDT intervention was reported for 6 of 11 (55%) of studies. In these studies, use of the NTDT program averaged 66% (range 53–93%). Hand hygiene compliance was objectively evaluated in three studies (27%). A significant improvement was noted in one study ($p < 0.001$) [38] and was without change in the other two. None of the eight other studies considered or evaluated hand hygiene as a confounder. Given the known impact of the thoroughness of disinfection cleaning on HAP acquisition [4, 14, 16], it is of note that 9 of 11 (82%) studies failed to consider the probability that routine thoroughness of disinfection cleaning could have impacted the objective clinical evaluation of the NTDTS. Although one report describing the use of nonstandardized fluorescent marker monitoring found that thoroughness of cleaning had improved significantly from 60 to 78% in association with an HPV program intervention ($p < 0.001$), the relevance of this observation

was not discussed by the authors [35]. The other study which evaluated the thoroughness of cleaning used a standardized fluorescent marking system but did not describe the results of the monitoring [36]. While the impact of changes in antibiotic use was thoroughly evaluated in one study [29] and to a limited degree in two other studies, no consideration of the potential impact of changes in antibiotic use on the index HAI prevalence was evaluated in the remaining eight studies (83%). As noted in Table 8.7, only a limited number of studies considered other relevant confounders, including admission incidence density, isolation practice compliance, and case mix.

While the phenomenon of regression to the mean is an intrinsic limitation of single site quasi-experimental evaluations of NTDTs, the fact that 5 of 11 studies (45%) were described as interventions implemented to address specific pathogen "outbreaks" and 3 others were associated with very high pre-intervention rates of HO-CDI substantially limits the generalizability of the findings of these reports. In addition, the use of overall HAI rates in three studies likely affected the analysis of the apparent impact of NTDTs since urinary tract infections and many surgical site infection rates would not have been substantially impacted by the effectiveness of environmental hygiene practices.

Conclusions

Despite the substantial antimicrobial potency of HPV on both vegetative pathogens and spores, it is concerning that in the five clinical (Level III, IV, V) studies published over the past 12 years, consistent clinical effectiveness commensurate with the potency of the technology has not been clearly confirmed. While several of the nine studies evaluating the impact of HPV on surface pathogen contamination observed an impact on contamination, two of the studies did not [33, 35]. Despite the implementation of a dedicated technician-supported HPV program as well as a broad-based environmental hygiene initiative, it is of note that an extensive and well-controlled program documented only a modest decrease in VRE acquisition but not in MRSA acquisition [33]. While the six Level V studies of HPV observed what may have, in part, been a response to the HPV program, the limitations of study design and the limited evaluation of the impact of confounders as well as intrinsic design limitations preclude defining a role for the routine use of this technology in endemic HAI settings based on published reports.

Level I in vitro studies of UV technology have clearly documented both the effectiveness and limitations of UV-C and PX-UV. Given the particular challenge of killing CD spores with UV systems, it is unfortunate that none of the three studies evaluating a program's impact on HO-CDI were in other than epidemic or high-level endemic settings [50, 53, 54]. Given the limited measureable impact of the UV programs described as well as limitations in study design and oversights in confounder analysis, it must be concluded that the published literature in this area has yet to provide clear support for the use of UV technology in clinical settings.

Taken together, the fact that less than one third of confounders were objectively evaluated, the fact that most (64%) of studies implemented a broad range of activities to improve infection prevention interventions along with the NTDT program, and the fact that 8 of 11 (83%) studies were carried out in outbreak or high-rate HAI settings, all limit the feasibility of defining a role for these technologies in clinical practice, particularly in endemic settings.

Recommendations for Future Studies of Environmental Hygiene Interventions

In light of this review of both study design limitations and the relatively inconsistent clinical impact of the NTDT studies reported to date, it is evident that further studies of these technologies will be needed before their role in HAI prevention can be objectively defined. While advanced-level study design would be most valuable [24] given the complexity and cost of such studies, the importance of optimizing quasi-experimental studies must be considered. Given the fact that some intrinsic limitations of such studies are unavoidable even with the use of interrupted time series design, crossover studies, and multisite studies which intrinsically have the potential for significantly nullifying undefined confounders, well-designed studies which directly and objectively compare environmental hygiene interventions could prove to be very informative [7, 16, 56, 58]. Aside from the elements noted in Table 8.8, unique issues such as selection bias, physical plant alterations, and changes in personnel resources will need to be evaluated as potential confounders in future clinical studies of NTDT. Study design issues specifically related to Level III studies would include environmental culturing methods which are standardized and optimally sensitive [59] as well as assuring expedient culturing before and after the intervention to minimize the possibility of recontamination of tested surfaces. In reporting the results of all Level III, IV, and V studies, it will be important to optimize and allow for assessment of generalizability of the findings by clearly defining the study setting, openly discuss observations related to confounder monitoring results, and consider the relevance of potential confounders which were not able to be evaluated. Finally, reports of such studies should discuss both the justification for and the specific limitations of the study's quasi-experimental design [60]. Developing such studies with careful attention to the design elements noted

Table 8.8 Suggested elements for clinical studies of NTDT

Aspect of the study	Issue	Rationale
Design	Endemic setting	Minimize the potential for regression to the mean errors
	Single intervention	The need to minimize the impact of major confounders
	Adequate duration of pre-/post-intervention analysis	Minimum of several months during which potential confounders are objectively quantified
	Minimize or eliminate performance bias	The impact of the Hawthorne or novelty effect can be particularly problematic
	Quantify completeness of intervention use	Significant confounder
	Minimize room/patient unit selection bias	Possible confounder
Ongoing confounder analysis	Minimize changes in infection prevention initiatives	Significant confounder
	Objective analysis of thoroughness of routine disinfection cleaning	Significant confounder
	Antibiotic use trends	Significant confounder
	Hand hygiene compliance trends	Significant confounder
	Isolation precaution compliance trends	Significant confounder
	Monitor case mix trends	Possible confounder
	Monitor for target HAP admission incidence density trends	Possible confounder
	Monitor for introduction of new laboratory testing which could impact data	Possible confounder
	Monitor for increased or decreased frequency of testing which could impact data	Possible confounder
	Evaluate potential changes in HAI definitions which could impact data	Possible confounder

could provide clear, objective outcomes with substantial potential for moving all elements of hygienic practice (Fig. 8.2) toward a solidly evidence-based foundation for optimizing patient and healthcare worker safety across the entire spectrum of patient care.

References

1. Han JH, Sullivan N, Leas BF, Pegues DA, Kaczmarck JL, Umscheid CA. Cleaning hospital room surfaces to prevent healthcare-associated infections. Ann Intern Med. 2015;163:598–607.
2. Knelson LP, Williams DA, Gergen MF, Rutala WA, Weber DJ, et al. A comparison of environmental contamination by patients infected or colonized with methicillin-resistant Staphylococcus aureus or vancomycin-resistant enterococci: a multicenter study. Infect Control Hosp Epidemiol. 2014;35(7):872–5.
3. Dancer SJ. How do we assess hospital cleaning? A proposal for microbiological standards for surface hygiene in hospitals. J Hosp Infect. 2004;56:10–5.
4. Hayden MK, Bonten MJ, Blom DW, Lyle EA, van de Vijver DA, Weinstein RA. Reduction in acquisition of vancomycin-resistant enterococcus after enforcement of routine environmental cleaning measures. Clin Infect Dis. 2006;42(11):1552–60.
5. Carling PC, Briggs J, Hylander D, Perkins J. Evaluation of patient area cleaning in 3 hospitals using a novel targeting methodology. Am J Infect Control. 2006;34:513–9.
6. Carling PC, Parry MF, Von Beheren SM. Identifying opportunities to enhance environmental cleaning in 23 acute care hospitals. Infect Control Hosp Epidemiol. 2008;29(1):1–7.
7. Carling PC. Optimizing healthcare environmental hygiene. Infect Dis Clin N Am. 2016;30(3):639–60.
8. Huang S, Datta R, Platt R. Risk of acquiring antibiotic-resistant bacteria from prior room occupants. Arch Intern Med. 2006;166:1945–51.
9. Carling PC, Bartley JM. Evaluating hygienic cleaning in healthcare settings: what you do not know can harm your patients. Am J Infect Control. 2010;38:S41–50.
10. Carling PC, Parry MM, Rupp ME, Po JL, Dick B, Von Beheren S. Improving cleaning of the environment surrounding patients in 36 acute care hospitals. Infect Control Hosp Epidemiol. 2008b;29(11):1035–41.
11. Carling PC, Eck EK. Achieving sustained improvement in environmental hygiene using coordinated benchmarking in 12 hospitals. Abstracts of the SHEA Fifth Decennial Meeting; Atlanta, GA. March 18–22, 2010.
12. Carling PC, Herwaldt LA, VonBeheren S. The Iowa disinfection cleaning project: opportunities, successes and challenges of a structured intervention project in 56 hospitals. Presented at the Iowa Association for Infection Prevention Annual Meeting, 10 May 2012.
13. Holmer L, Russell D, Steger P, Creed J, Speer R, Lakhanpal A. Sustainability of an environmental cleaning program in California small and critical access hospitals. Abstract presented at the annual meeting of the Association for Infection Control Professionals. San Diego, CA, May 2014.
14. Datta R, Platt R, Yokoe DS, Huang SS. Environmental cleaning intervention and risk of acquiring multidrug-resistant organisms from prior room occupants. Arch Intern Med. 2011;171(6):491–4.
15. Sitzlar B, Deshparade A, Fentelli D, Kundnapu S, Sethi AK, Donskey CJ. An environmental disinfection odyssey: evaluation of dequential interventions to improve disinfection of Clostridium Difficile patient rooms. Infect Control Hosp Epidemiol. 2013;34(5):459–65.
16. Carling PC, Huang SS. Improving healthcare environmental cleaning and disinfection: current and evolving issues. Infect Control Hosp Epidemiol. 2013;34(5):507–13.
17. Septimus E, Weinstein A, Perl T, Goldmann D, Yokoe S. Approaches for preventing healthcare-associated infections: go long or go wide? Infect Control Hosp Epidemiol. 2014;35(7):797–801.
18. Qureshi Z, Yassin M. Role of ultraviolet (UV) disinfection in infection control and environmental cleaning. Infect Disord – Drug Targets. 2013;13:191–5.
19. French G, Otter J, Shannon K, Adams N, Watling D, Parks M. Tackling contamination of the hospital environment by methicillin-resistant Staphylococcus aureus (MRSA): a comparison between conventional terminal cleaning and hydrogen peroxide vapour decontamination. J Hosp Infect. 2004;57:31–7.
20. Otter JA, Yezli S, Perl TM, Barbut F, French GL. The role of "no-touch" automated room disinfection systems in infection prevention and control. J Hosp Infect. 2013;83:1–13.
21. Rutala W, Weber D. Are room decontamination units needed to prevent transmission of environmental pathogens? Infect Control Hosp Epidemiol. 2011;32(8):743–7.
22. Nerandzic MM, Thota P, Sandar CT, et al. Evaluation of a pulsed xenon ultraviolet disinfection system for reduction of healthcare-associated pathogens in hospital rooms. Infect Control Hosp Epidemiol. 2015;36:192–7.
23. PRISMA – Transparant reporting of systemic reviews and meta-analysis. 2015. Accessed at: http://www.prisma-statement.org/Extensions/Protocols.aspx. 18 Sept 2016.
24. McDonald LC, Arduino M. Climbing the evidentiary hierarchy for environmental infection control. Clin Infect Dis. 2013;56(1):36–9.
25. Lemmen S, Scheithauer S, Hafner H, Yezli S, Mohr M, Otter J. Evaluation of hydrogen peroxide vapor for the inactivation of nosocomial pathogens on porous and nonporous surfaces. Am J Infect Control. 2015;43:82–5.
26. Goyal S, Chander Y, Otter J. Evaluating the virucidal efficacy of hydrogen peroxide vapour. J Hosp Infect. 2014;86:255–9.
27. Pottage T, Richardson C, Parks S, Walker JT, Bennett AM. Evaluation of hydrogen peroxide gaseous disinfection systems to decontaminate viruses. J Hosp Infect. 2010;74:55–61.
28. Otter JA, Cummins M, Ahmad F, van Tonder C, Drabu JY. Assessing the biological efficacy and rate of recontamination following hydrogen peroxide vapour decontamination. J Hosp Infect. 2007;67:182–8.
29. Hardy KJ, Gossain S, Henderson N, Drugan C, Oppenheim BA, Gao F, Hawkey PM. Rapid recontamination with MRSA of the environment of an intensive care unit after decontamination with hydrogen peroxide vapour. J Hosp Infect. 2007;66(4):360–8.
30. Boyce JM, Havill NL, Otter JA, et al. Impact of hydrogen vapor room decontamination on clostridium difficile environmental contamination and transmission in a healthcare setting. Infect Control Hosp Epidemiol. 2008;29(8):723–9.
31. Barbut F, Menuet D, Verachten M, Girou E. Comparison of the efficacy of a hydrogen peroxide dry-mist disinfection system and sodium hypochlorite solution for eradication of Clostridium difficile spores. Infect Control Hosp Epidemiol. 2009;30:507–14.
32. Otter J, Yezli S, Schouten MA, van Zanten A, Zielman GH, Nohlmans-Paulssen M. Hydrogen peroxide vapor decontamination of an intensive care unit to remove environmental reservoirs of multidrug-resistant gram-negative rods during an outbreak. Am J Infect Control. 2010;38:754–6.
33. Passaretti CL, Otter JA, Reich NG, et al. An evaluation of environmental decontamination with hydrogen peroxide vapor for reducing the risk of patient acquisition of multidrug-resistant organisms. Clin Infect Dis. 2013;56:627–35.
34. Manian FA, Griesenauer S, Senkel D, Setzer J, Doll SA, Perry AM, Wiechens M. Isolation of Acinetobacter baumannii complex and methicillin resistant Staphylococcus aureus from hospital rooms following terminal cleaning and disinfection: can we do better? Infect Control Hosp Epidemiol. 2011;32(7):667–72.
35. Dryden M, Parnaby R, Dailly S, et al. Hydrogen peroxide vapour decontamination in the control of a polyclonal methicillin-resistant Staphylococcus aureus outbreak on a surgical ward. J Hosp Infect. 2008;68:1990–2.
36. Fishner D, Pang L, Salmon S, Lin R, Teo C, Tambyah P, Jureen R, Cook A, Otter J. A successful vancomycin-resistant reduction bundle at a Singapore Hospital. Infect Control Hosp Epidemiol. 2016;37(1):107–9.

37. Chmielarczyk PG, Higgins J, Wojkowska-Mach E, Synowiec E, Zander E, et al. Control of an outbreak of Acinetobacter baumannii infections using vaporized hydrogen peroxide. J Hosp Infect. 2012;81:239–45.
38. Horn K, Otter JA. Hydrogen peroxide vapor room disinfection and hand hygiene improvements reduce Clostridium difficile infection, methicillin-resistant *Staphylococcus aureus*, vancomycin-resistant enterococci and extended-spectrum B-lactamase. Am J Infect Control. 2015;43:1354–6.
39. Rutala WA, Gergen MF, Weber DJ. Room contamination with UV radiation. Inhfect Control Hosp Epidemiol. 2010;31(10):1025–9.
40. Nerandzic MM, Cadnum JL, Pultz MJ, DOnskey CJ. Evaluation of an automated ultraviolet radiation device for decontamination of Clostridium difficile and other healthcare-associated pathogens in hospital rooms. BMC Infect Dis. 2010;10:197–2334. 10-97
41. Boyce JM, Havill NL, Moore BA. Terminal decontamination of patient rooms using an automated mobile UV light unit. Infect Control Hosp Epidemiol. 2011;32(8):732–42.
42. Havill N, Moore B, Boyce J. Comparison of the microbiological efficacy of hydrogen peroxide vapor and ultraviolet light processes for room decontamination. Infect Control Hosp Epidemiol. 2012;33(5):507–12.
43. Mahida N, Vaughan N, Boswell T. First UK evaluation of an automated ultraviolet-C room decontamination device (Tu-D™). J Hosp Infect. 2013;84:332–5.
44. Nerandzic MM, Fisher CW, Donskey CJ. Sorting through the wealth of options: comparative evaluation of two ultraviolet disinfection systems. PLoS One. 2014;9:e107444.
45. Zhang A, Nerandzic MM, Kundrapu S, Donskey CJ. Does organic material on hospital surfaces reduce the effectiveness of hypochlorite and UV radiation for disinfection of Clostridium difficile? Infect Control Hosp Epidemiol. 2013;34:1106–8.
46. Stibich M, Stachowiak J, Tanner B, Berkheiser M, Moore L, Raad I, Chemaly R. Evaluation of a pulsed-xenon ultraviolet room disinfection device for impact on hospital operations and microbial reduction. Infect Control Hosp Epidemiol. 2011;32(3):286–8.
47. Jinadatha C, Quezada R, Huber TW, Williams JB, Zeber JE, Copeland LA. Evaluation of a pulsed-xenon ultraviolet room disinfection device for impact on contamination levels of methicillin-resistant *Staphylococcus aureus*. BMC Infect Dis. 2014;14:187–2334.
48. Jinadatha C, Villamaria FC, Restrepo MI, Nagaraja GM, Liao I, Stock EM, et al. Is the pulsed xenon ultraviolet light no-touch disinfection system effective on methicillin-resistant *Staphylococcus*

aureus in the absence of manual cleaning? Am J Infect Control. 2015;43:878–81.
49. Ghantojii SS, Stibich M, Stachowiak J, et al. Non-inferiority of pulsed xenon UV light versus bleach for reducing environmental clostridium difficile contamination on high-touch surfaces in clostridium difficile infection isolation rooms. J Med Microbiol. 2015;64:191–4.
50. Napolitano N, Mahapatra T, Tang W. The effectiveness of UV-C radiation for facility-wide environmental disinfection to reduce healthcare-acquired infections. Am J Infect Control. 2015;43:1342–6.
51. Levin J, Riley LS, Parrish C, English D, Ahn S. The effect of portable pulsed xenon ultraviolet light after terminal cleaning on hospital-associated Clostridium difficile infection a community hospital. Am J Infect Control. 2013;41:746–8.
52. Haas JP, Menz J, Dusza S, Montecalvo MA. Implementation and impact of ultraviolet environmental disinfection in an acute care setting. Am J Infect Control. 2014;42(6):586–90.
53. Miller R, Simmons S, Dale C, Stachowiak J, Stibich M. Utilization and impact of a pulsed-xenon ultraviolet room disinfection system and multidisciplinary care team on Clostridium difficile in a long-term acute care facility. Am J Infect Control. 2015;43:1350–3.
54. Nagaraja A, Visintainer P, Haas JP, Menz J, Wormeser GP, Montecalvo MA. Clostridium difficile infections before and during use of ultraviolet disinfection. Am J Infect Control. 2015;43:940–5.
55. Carling PC, Perkins J, Ferguson J, Thomasse A. Evaluating a new paradigm for company surface disinfection in clinical practice. Infect Control Hosp Epidemiol. 2014;35(11):1349–55.
56. Rutala WA, Gergen MF, Tande MF, Weber DJ. Rapid hospital room decontamination using ultraviolet (UV) light with a nanostructured UV-reflective wall coating. Infect Control Hosp Epidemiol. 2013;34:527–9.
57. Schweizer ML, Braun, Milstone AM. Research methods in healthcare epidemiology and antimicrobial stewardship-quasi-experimental designs. Infect Control Hosp Epidemiol. 2016;41:1–6.
58. Dancer SJ. Dos and don'ts for hospital cleaning. CurrOpin Infect Dis. 2016;29(4):41523.
59. Carling PC, Kaye K. *Acinetobacter baumannii* environmental epidemiology: do culture methods impact findings? Abstract presented at the annual meeting of the Society for Hospital Epidemiology of America. Orlando FL, May 2015.
60. Schwizer ML, Braun BI, Milstone AM. Research methods in healthcare research design. Infect Control Hosp Epidemiol. 2016;37(10):1135–40.

Universal MRSA/Staphylococcal Decolonization for Hospitalized Patients

Edward J. Septimus

Introduction

Hospital-acquired infections (HAIs) burden patients, complicate treatments, prolong hospital stays, increase costs, and can be life-threatening. Up to 15% of patients develop an infection while hospitalized. The recent Centers for Disease Control and Prevention (CDC) report "Antibiotic Resistance Threats in the United States, 2013" highlights that at least two million Americans acquire serious infections from microorganisms resistant to one or more antimicrobial agents each year including methicillin-resistant *Staphylococcus aureus* (MRSA), resulting in 23,000 deaths annually. That CDC report recommends attempting to prevent these infections through appropriate use of antibiotics and adherence to infection prevention practices [1]. HAIs are now the 5th leading cause of death in U.S. acute-care hospitals [2]. The substantial human suffering and financial burden of these infections is significant. Recent reports have estimated that US healthcare system costs attributable to HAIs range from $9.8 billion to $45 billion per year [3]. Beyond direct financial costs, HAIs also contribute significantly to increased patient length-of-stay (LOS) in the hospital resulting in both operational cost loss, and patient dissatisfaction.

In the last several years, major changes in US healthcare have had an impact on HAI prevention. First we now know a significant percentage of HAIs are preventable using evidence-based strategies [4]. Second there are now coordinated efforts among federal agencies aimed at HAI prevention, including public reporting of hospital-specific HAI rates and linking hospital-specific HAI performance measures to financial reimbursement in order to stimulate HAI prevention efforts [5]. Since 2011 hospitals have been required to report to the CDC's National Healthcare Safety Network (NHSN) all of their central-line associated-bloodstream infections (CLABSIs) among intensive care unit (ICU) patients in order to qualify for annual payment updates. Five additional required data are now being reported through NHSN to CMS including MRSA bloodstream infections. In addition, invasive healthcare-associated (HA) MRSA infections has been identified as a focus area in Healthy People 2020 [6].

MRSA infections have significantly increased in most countries in the last decade. MRSA is one of the most common causes of HAIs in most hospitals and the incidence of community-acquired MRSA has also increased dramatically. *S. aureus* is the most common pathogen to cause HA pneumonia and surgical site infections [2]. In a recent report, 47.9% of *S. aureus* HAI were MRSA [7]. In addition, MRSA infections are associated with worse outcomes and higher costs compared to methicillin sensitive *S. aureus* (MSSA). [8].

The primary human reservoir for *S. aureus* is the anterior nares. Between 15% and 30% of all U.S. adults are nasally colonized with methicillin-susceptible *S. aureus* (MSSA) and 1–2% are nasally colonized with MRSA [9, 10]. Hospitalized patients and long-term care facility residents are even more likely to be colonized with MRSA. Up to 58% of long-term care facility residents are colonized with MRSA [11, 12]. *S. aureus* colonization at other body sites including the pharynx, groin, perianal region or axilla is also associated with development of *S. aureus* infections. This is most common among high risk groups such as ICU patients, men who have sex with men and HIV infected patients [9, 13].

Endogenous infections occur when a colonizing isolate enters a different body site on the same person and causes an infection. These infection sites include open cuts or wounds, surgical sites, and device sites. Patients who are nasally colonized with *S. aureus* are more than twice as likely to develop a *S. aureus* infection compared with non-colonized patients. [14] Bacterial colonization can be categorized as persistent carriage, intermittent carriage, or noncarriage. Among *S. aureus* nasal carriers, approximately 40% are persistently

E.J. Septimus (✉)
Infection Prevention and Epidemiology, Clinical Services Group, HCA, Nashville, TN, USA

Internal Medicine, Texas A&M Health Science Center College of Medicine, 4257 Albans, Houston, TX 77005, USA
e-mail: eseptimus@gmail.com

© Springer International Publishing AG 2018
G. Bearman et al. (eds.), *Infection Prevention*, DOI 10.1007/978-3-319-60980-5_9

colonized and 60% are intermittently colonized [15]. Those who are persistently colonized with *S. aureus* have a higher risk of infection compared with intermittent carriers or non-carriers [16]. Persistent *S. aureus* carriers also have been found to carry a greater quantity of *S. aureus* in their noses (measured in log_{10} colony forming units [CFUs]) compared with intermittent carriers [17]. Average *S. aureus* bacterial loads among nasal carriers tend to range between 1.8 and 2.9 log_{10} CFUs. One study found that this load increased among MRSA carriers when patients received antibiotics that did not have activity against MRSA (e.g., beta-lactams, fluoroquinolones) [18]. Another study found that higher log counts of MRSA in the nose were associated with colonization at other body sites. Additionally, log counts for each body site correlated with log counts for all other cultured sites. That study found that mean extranasal MRSA loads ranged from 0.87 log_{10} CFUs in the axilla to 1.65 log_{10} CFUs in the perineum to 1.70 log_{10} CFUs in the groin [19]. It has also been established that the odds of developing an infection increase as more body sites are colonized [20]. Some decolonizing agents claim to completely eliminate bacterial load from their application sites, while others only claim to decrease the load. Yet, there is little data on what level the bacterial load must be reduced to in order to prevent transmission and infections.

In contrast to endogenous infections, exogenous infections occur due to transmission from person-to-person via direct or indirect contact by hands of healthcare workers and shared hospital environments such as bed rails. Carriers with high bacterial loads or colonized at multiple sites are not only at higher risk of infection but are more likely to transmit the bacteria to their environments [21].

Decolonization strategies aim to prevent transmission and infection. Some decolonization can decrease the bioburden of microorganisms on the patient, the environment, and the hands of healthcare personnel. The two most common methods of decolonization are application of antimicrobial ointment alone to the nose or combined with an antimicrobial body washes to the skin usually with CHG. This approach has been shown to reduce infections in specific subsets of patients [22, 23].

Decolonization is the most effective among patient populations who are only at risk of infection for a short period of time. These include populations such as surgical patients who only need to be decolonized for the time period that it takes the surgical wound to heal, and ICU patients who are at much lower risk once they are discharged from the ICU. This window of time is important because of concern regarding both recolonization and resistance to colonizing agents. Thus, patient populations who are only at risk for short periods of time can achieve short-term success with decolonization [24], since studies have found that patients tend to become recolonized within weeks or months of being decol-

onized [25]. In fact, recolonization rates at 1 year approached 50% for healthcare workers and 75% for patients on peritoneal dialysis [26].

Over the last decade, the general approaches to healthcare-associated infection (HAI) prevention have taken two conceptually different paths: (Table 9.1) (1) vertical approaches that aim to reduce colonization, infection, and transmission of specific pathogens including MRSA, largely through use of active surveillance testing (AST) to identify carriers, followed by implementation of measures aimed at preventing transmission from carriers to other patients including targeted decolonization, and (2) horizontal approaches that aim to reduce the risk of infections due to a broad array of pathogens through implementation of standardized practices that do not depend on patient-specific conditions. Examples of horizontal infection prevention strategies include minimizing the unnecessary use of invasive medical devices, enhancing hand hygiene, improving environmental cleaning, antimicrobial stewardship, and CHG bathing. This has led investigators to ask whether a horizontal approach including universal decolonization is more effective than a vertical approach or targeted decolonization [27]. This chapter will explore the evidence comparing a vertical approach versus a horizontal approach(universal decolonization) in reducing MRSA infections in hospitalized patients.

Nasal Topical Decolonization Strategies (Vertical)

Nasal mupirocin has emerged as the most widely used topical antibacterial agent. Mupirocin is a topical antibacterial agent produced from *Pseudomonas fluorescens* that inhibits bacterial protein synthesis by reversibly binding to bacterial isoleucyl-tRNA-synthetase. It has excellent activity against staphylococci and most streptococci [28]. Mupirocin exists in two formulations: a nasal ointment in petrolatum and a generic topical ointment in a polyethylene glycol vehicle.

Table 9.1 Vertical and horizontal approaches

Vertical (pathogen specific)
Active surveillance (e.g. for MRSA, VRE, gram-negative MDROs)
Contact precautions (e.g. for MRSA/VRE/gram-negative MDRO colonization or infection)
Targeted decolonization (e.g. MRSA)
Horizontal (reduces infections not pathogen specific)
Standard precautions (hand hygiene, universal gloving)
Environmental cleaning
Bundles of care (e.g. CLABSI, Ventilator, Surgical care improvement project)
CHG bathing
Antimicrobial stewardship

Modified from Ref. [27]

Both have been used for nasal decolonization. Side effects are uncommon mostly limited to local site reaction such as stuffy nose, or burning/stinging of the nose. Mupirocin is applied to the anterior nares two times/day for 5 days. Perl et al. reported nasal colonization of *S. aureus* was eliminated in 83.4% of patients who received mupirocin, as compared with 27.4% of patients who received placebo (*P* < 0.001). Nasal colonization of *S. aureus* was eliminated from 81.3% of carriers (*P* < 0.001) who received three to five doses of mupirocin and from 93.3% of carriers who received six or more doses of mupirocin [29].

In a recent systemic review, Ammerlaan et al. reviewed 23 clinical trial including 12 that looked at topically applied antibiotics. They concluded short-term nasal application of mupirocin is the most effective treatment for eradicating MRSA carriage with an estimated success rate of 90% at 1 week after treatment and approximately 60% after a longer follow-up [30].

Several studies have demonstrated that mupirocin alone is highly effective in eradicating nasal colonization with *S. aureus* resulting in decreased infections in patients in intensive care, hemodialysis, in surgical settings, and long-term care [31–34]. Mody et al. published a double-blind randomized study looking at the efficacy of intranasal mupirocin versus placebo in reducing colonization and preventing infections in two long term care centers. Twice-daily treatment was given for 2 weeks with follow-up to 6 months. After treatment, mupirocin eradicated colonization in 93% of residents compared to only 15% in placebo group (*p* = 0.001). At 90 days after treatment, 61% of residents in the mupirocin group remained decolonized. The authors concluded that mupirocin was effective in decolonizing persistent carriers in long-term care and showed a trend towards reduction of infections [35].

A meta-analysis found that decolonization with mupirocin alone or in combination with agents such as CHG, decreased the odds of *S. aureus* infection by approximately 60% among dialysis patients [31]. This was due to a reduction in both exit-site infections and catheter-related bloodstream infections among both hemodialysis patients and peritoneal dialysis patients.

In a Cochrane review, the authors sought to determine if the use of mupirocin nasal ointment in patients identified as *S. aureus* carriers reduced *S. aureus* infections. Only randomized controlled trials comparing mupirocin with no treatment or placebo or alternative nasal treatment were included. They found mupirocin ointment resulted in a significant reduction in *S. aureus* infections (RR 0.55, 95% CI 0.43–0.70) [34].

However, mupirocin resistance to *S. aureus* has now been identified in several studies especially with widespread use over prolonged periods [36]. A study found the use of mupirocin, especially when mupirocin is repeatedly applied to exit sites to prevent infections in chronic dialysis patients, was associated with increasing risk of *S. aureus* high-level mupirocin resistance (HL-MR) exit-site infections [37].

There are two phenotypes of mupirocin resistance: low-level mupirocin resistance with minimum inhibitory concentrations (MICs) from 8 to 64 µg/mL, and high-level mupirocin resistance with MICs ≥512 µg/mL [38]. Caffrey et al. reported risk factors associated with mupirocin resistance to MRSA. They identified 40 mupirocin resistant cases and 270 matched controls and performed an adjusted conditional logistic regression model. They found three independent risk factors: exposure to mupirocin in the year prior to the culture date (OR 9.84; 95% CI 2.93–33.09), *Pseudomonas aeruginosa* infection in the year before the culture-related admission (4.85; 1.20–19.61), and cefepime use in the year prior to culture (2.80; 1.03–7.58). In sensitivity analysis, prior mupirocin exposure was associated with both low-level and high-level mupirocin resistance. This study highlighted the strong association between previous mupirocin exposure and subsequent mupirocin resistance to MRSA [39]. More importantly, studies have shown that high-level mupirocin resistance to *S. aureus* results in decolonization failure. The association with low-level mupirocin resistance and outcomes of mupirocin decolonization is unclear. Walker et al. [40] published a prospective evaluation to determine the efficacy of nasal mupirocin ointment in reducing colonization with mupirocin-susceptible, methicillin-resistant *S. aureus* (MS MRSA) as well as mupirocin-resistant MRSA both low-level (LL-MR MRSA) and high-level (HL-MR MRSA). All patients were treated twice daily with 2% topical mupirocin ointment for 5 days. Treated patients had post-treatment cultures at day 3 and weeks 1, 2, and 4. Post-treatment nares cultures on day 3 were negative for 78.5%, 80%, and 27.7% of patients with MS MRSA, LL-MR MRSA, and HLMR MRSA respectively. However, at the 1–4-week follow-up, the sustained decolonization for patients with HL-MR MRSA and LL-MR MRSA was low (25% each) compared to 91% in patients colonized with MS MRSA. This result suggests that mupirocin in LL-MR MRSA probably temporally suppresses growth, but does not result in sustained decolonization. Post-treatment cultures were usually the same genotype and susceptibility phenotypes as the patient's baseline culture. This appears to reflect treatment failure rather than exogenous recolonization. In a recently published analysis from the REDUCE trial, the odds of mupirocin resistance was no greater in the intervention period versus baseline across all arms. However, given the wide confidence intervals this results should be interpreted with caution [41].

In contrast to unrestrictive use, short-term use of nasal mupirocin as part of perioperative prophylaxis to prevent surgical site infections due to S. aureus has not been associated with increased mupirocin resistance. Perl et al. treated over 2000 patients and performed mupirocin susceptibility testing on 1021 S. aureus isolates and only 6 isolates (0.6%) were resistant [29]. Fawley et al. described the results of repeated point-prevalence for 4 years to determine if mupirocin resistance had emerged in surgical units using a 5-day peri-operative prophylaxis with nasal mupirocin. They found no evidence of sustained emergence or spread of mupirocin resistance. No HL-MR strains were identified [42]. Finally in a Dutch hospital more than 20,000 patients received mupirocin prophylaxis who were undergoing major cardiothoracic surgery. No mupirocin resistance emerged [32].

Although mupirocin has emerged as the topical agent of choice for elimination of S. aureus nasal carriage, there is growing evidence of increasing mupirocin resistance and treatment failures, especially with widespread use over long periods of time.

Recently there has been increase attention to the use of nasal 5–10% povidone-iodine. Povidone-iodine (PI) is a complex of polyvinylpyrrolidine and tri-iodine ions that has been widely used as an antiseptic on skin, wounds, and mucous membranes. PI has broad activity against grampositive and gram-negative bacteria. Specifically, PI has good activity against S. aureus, including MRSA. Hill and Casewell evaluated the in vitro activity of 5% PI as a possible alternative to mupirocin for the elimination of nasal carriage of S. aureus. The results suggested PI may have a role in the prevention of colonization and infection due to MRSA, including mupirocin-resistant strains [43].

Phillips et al. conducted a prospective, open label trial of twice daily application of nasal mupirocin ointment for 5 days before surgery compared to two applications of a 5% PI solution in each nostril within 2 h of surgical incision in patients undergoing arthroplasty or spine fusion surgery. Both groups also received CHG bath with 2% cloths the night before and the morning of surgery. In the per protocol analysis, S. aureus deep surgical site infections(SSI) developed in 5 of 763 surgical procedures in the mupirocin group and 0 of 776 surgical procedures in the PI group (P = 0.03) In addition, if the preoperative nasal culture grew S. aureus a second nasal culture was obtained within 1–3 days after surgery. The proportion of postoperative negative nasal cultures was 92% (78 of 85 patients) in the mupirocin group versus only 54% (45 of 84 patients) in the PI group. Unfortunately, the authors could not perform multivariate analysis due to small sample size, and patients were not followed after discharge to identify late infections [44].

In a second study, Bebko and colleagues recently published a preoperative decontamination protocol to reduce SSIs in orthopedic patients undergoing elective hardware implantations. This was a quasi-experimental, retrospective, nonrandomized trial comparing a bundle intervention to historical controls. The intervention consisted of application of 2% CHG and oral CHG the night before and morning of surgery plus intranasal PI solution the morning of surgery. Patients were followed for 30 days postoperatively for SSI. The SSI was significantly lower in the intervention group 1.1% vs. 3.8% in the control group (P = 0.02). This was a retrospective quasi-experimental nonrandomized trial, patients were only followed for 30 days, and information regarding MRSA carrier status of patients before and after decontamination was not collected; therefore the study did not allow evaluation of the effect of nasal decolonization vs other interventions [45]. Although nasal PI may be a potential alternative to nasal mupirocin for prevention of SSIs, more studies are needed. Nasal PI has not been studied in other clinical settings.

Chlorhexidene Bathing (Horizontal)

Chlorhexidine is a topical antiseptic solution that has been used worldwide since the 1950s. Chlorhexidine gluconate is a water-soluble, cationic biguanide that binds to the negatively charged bacterial cell wall, altering the bacterial cell osmotic equilibrium. CHG has broad-spectrum activity against gram-positive and gram-negative bacteria as well as yeast. CHG has an excellent safety record. Adverse events associated with CHG include mild skin irritation and rare serious allergic reactions.

CHG efficacy has been documented for diverse indications such as hand washing, procedure skin preparation, vaginal antisepsis, and oral care for prevention of VAP, treatment of gingivitis, and body washes to prevent infections. Chlorhexidine is commercially available at a variety of concentrations (0.5–4%) and formulations (with and without isopropyl alcohol or ethanol), and certain chlorhexidine-containing products are available over the counter. This section will focus on use of CHG bathing to prevent MRSA HAIs.

Recently, multiple studies have evaluated CHG bathing to reduce bacterial skin burden among patients in the ICU in an effort to reduce HAIs. CHG bathing has been shown to decrease the bioburden of microorganisms on the patient, the environment, and the hands of healthcare personnel [46]. Bleasdale et al. observed a 60% reduction in BSI among MICU patients who were bathed with 2% CHG cloths daily versus soap and water. [47] Popovich et al. also compared CHG bathing with soap and water in another MICU and also reported a significant reduction in BSIs including S aureus [48]. During 2013, four randomized cluster trials were published evaluating the effectiveness of CHG bathing in preventing HAIs or MDRO acquisition among ICU patients.

Climo et al. performed a multi-center cluster-crossover study and reported that daily 2% CHG cloth bathing in the ICU resulted in a 23% reduction of VRE/MRSA acquisition and a 28% reduction in BSIs [13]. Using a similar study design, Milstone et al. reported that 2% CHG cloth bathing was associated with a significant reduction in bloodstream infections among pediatric ICU patients compared to standard bathing [49]. Huang et al. compared three approaches to MRSA prevention among patients in 74 adult ICUs (the REDUCE MRSA study): Arm 1 MRSA screening and isolation, Arm 2 targeted decolonization: screening, isolation, and decolonization of MRSA carriers with chlorhexidine bathing and nasal mupirocin, and Arm 3 universal decolonization: no screening, all patients decolonized with CHG cloth bathing and nasal mupirocin. The investigators found that universal decolonization of all ICU patients was associated with the largest reduction in all-cause bloodstream infection (44%; $P < 0.001$) and MRSA clinical culture rates (37%; $P = 0.01$) [23]. In a secondary analysis, CHG bathing was also shown to reduce blood culture contamination by 45% ($P = 0.02$) confirming earlier studies [50]. A European study demonstrated that improved hand hygiene plus universal CHG cloth bathing reduced acquisition of MDROs including MRSA and showed that in a setting where high levels of adherence to hand hygiene and CHG bathing were sustained, the addition of active surveillance testing (either rapid or conventional testing) and isolation of carriers did not further reduce MDRO acquisition rates [51]. There is very little evidence on the use of CHG bathing in non-critical settings. Kassakian et al. did study the effectiveness of daily CHG bathing in a non-ICU setting to reduce MRSA and VRE HAIs, compared with daily bathing with soap and water. This was a quasi-experimental before and after trial. Daily CHG bathing was associated with a reduced HAI risk, using a composite endpoint of MRSA and VRE HAIs, in a general medical inpatient population [52].

Decolonization Prior to Surgery

In the recent Vital Sign report 44.4% of *S. aureus* SSIs were MRSA [7]. Decolonization has been found to reduce the incidence of gram-positive surgical site infections (SSIs) after some types of surgery [22]. This is because SSIs are often endogenous, spreading from one body site (e.g. nose, skin) to the surgical wound of the same patient. Multiple studies have demonstrated that the genotypes (via pulsed field gel electrophoresis [PFGE]) of *S. aureus* colonizing and infecting isolates are identical in 75–85% of surgical patients [29, 53]. There is strong evidence that nasal and skin decolonization (nasal mupirocin plus CHG bathing) prior to cardiac and orthopedic surgery is effective at preventing SSIs caused by gram-positive organisms. Two systemic literature reviews

and meta-analyses of published studies found a protective effect of mupirocin decolonization against surgical site infections, especially among non-general surgery such as cardiac, orthopedic, and neurosurgery [33]. A meta-analysis of 17 randomized controlled trials or quasi-experimental studies that included cardiac and orthopedic surgery patients evaluated the effectiveness preoperative decolonization [22]. The meta-analysis found that decolonization was significantly protective against gram-positive SSIs, specifically *S. aureus* SSIs. A recent pragmatic quasi-experimental study implemented a bundle in 20 hospitals in order to prevent complex *S. aureus* SSIs after cardiac surgery and hip and knee arthroplasty [54]. The bundle included CHG bathing for all patients, screening for MRSA and MSSA nasal colonization, nasal mupirocin decolonization for *S. aureus* carriers, and both vancomycin and cefazolin perioperative prophylaxis for MRSA carriers. The mean rate of complex *S. aureus* SSIs significantly decreased from 36 per 10,000 operations during the baseline period to 21 per 10,000 operations during the intervention period (rate ratio [RR] = 0.58; 95% CI: 0.37, 0.92).

Universal Decolonization Versus Targeted Decolonization

Both targeted decolonization and universal decolonization strategies have been shown to decrease cross-transmission and infection due to MRSA. Currently, there is debate as to whether decolonization regimens should only be performed among patients who are colonized with pathogens that are sensitive to the decolonizing agents (e.g. *S. aureus* including MRSA) or if all high-risk patients should receive decolonizing agents without being screened for colonization. Universal decolonization, decolonizing all high-risk patients regardless of colonization status, only requires healthcare workers to provide the decolonizing agents to the patients without the labor and complexity of screening. Targeted decolonization requires the collection of a screening swab and laboratory testing before decolonization. This usually entails nasal screening for *S. aureus* colonization. Targeted decolonization is considered by some the preferred standard because antimicrobial agents would only be used in patients who need them, which may prevent antimicrobial resistance. However, this strategy would not identify patients who are *S. aureus* colonized at extranasal body sites, would not decolonize patients with false negative results, and would not decolonize patients who are colonized with other pathogens such as the skin commensal organism CNS or other multidrug resistant organisms.

Depending on the patient populations, different laboratory tests may be appropriate for screening. If fast results are needed, real-time polymerase chain reaction (PCR) can be used to test nasal swabs for both MRSA and MSSA within 1 h [55]. However, PCR is more costly than both chromogenic agar (test time at least 1–2 days) and standard culture (test time approximately 2–3 days) [56]. Fast results may be needed in the pre-operative clinic, so that patients can be sent home with mupirocin and CHG as needed. Slower methods could be used for dialysis patient populations who have frequent contact with the healthcare system and thus could obtain their decolonizing agents at their next healthcare visit. However, any type of screening is likely to be more expensive and certainly utilizes more healthcare worker time compared with universal decolonization [57–59].

Meta-analyses of decolonization studies among surgical and non-surgical populations found that both universal and targeted decolonization strategies resulted in similar protection against *S. aureus* infections [22, 60]. The only multicenter study that compared universal and targeted decolonization head-to-head found that in the ICU, universal decolonization was superior to targeted decolonization at reducing the number of bloodstream infections caused by any pathogen including skin commensal organisms. The reduction in MRSA bloodstream infections was not significantly different between the universal and targeted decolonization groups, however, there was a trend toward a larger reduction among the universal decolonization group [23]. However, this study also found a 37% reduction is MRSA clinical cultures ($P = 0.01$). Universal decolonization has been shown to have other potential benefits, such as reducing rates of CLABSI, overall BSIs, and environmental contamination with and acquisition of VRE [46–48]. Thus, universal decolonization is effective at reducing the total number of positive cultures and infections including MRSA in both surgical and non-surgical patients.

The patient population must also be factored into the decision of targeted versus universal decolonization. Given the evolving epidemiology of MDROs and the complexity of managing epidemiologically important pathogens across the continuum of care we must ensure reliable performance of basic infection prevention practices known to reduce transmission of all MDROs and the infections they cause. Applying evidence-based horizontal strategies such as universal decolonization in settings where benefits have been demonstrated and cost effective should be implemented. Vertical approaches such as active surveillance testing should be considered when epidemiologically important pathogens are newly emerging or rare to a given institution or to control outbreaks. Universal decolonization may be preferred in ICU settings in which there is concern over both endogenous infection and exogenous patient-to-patient transmission. In the ICU setting, missed colonization sites or false negative tests could result in the spread of pathogens from one patient to another. Conversely, targeted decolonization may be preferred for pre-operative and dialysis settings where endogenous infections are the main concern. There are even differences in the pre-operative setting. Targeted decolonization may be feasible for elective procedures but not for urgent procedures such as emergency coronary artery bypass graft. A compromise between the two types of decolonization prior to surgery, would be to attempt targeted decolonization, but, if a patient presented to surgery with unknown results, that patients could be treated as colonized and receive a dose of mupirocin and a CHG bath prior to surgery and finish the 3–5 days of mupirocin after surgery [53]. Current guidelines suggest decolonization as a special approach during MRSA outbreak or to combat endemic MRSA when other strategies have failed. Decolonization can be targeted to MRSA colonized persons or applied universally to populations deemed to be at high risk for infection [61].

The primary concern regarding universal decolonization is the emergence of resistance to the decolonizing agents. Mupirocin resistance has been reviewed earlier. Most studies of short-term, target mupirocin use have not seen significant emergence of mupirocin. Resistance to CHG has been rare. However, increased use of decolonizing agents could lead to selection for resistant strains. One study found that patients with persistent *S. aureus* carriage after decolonization were statistically more likely to be colonized with *S. aureus* isolates with combined low-level mupirocin resistance and genotypic chlorhexidine resistance before decolonization compared with patients who were successfully decolonized [62]. Another study showed that decolonization with chlorhexidine in the ICU led to selection of a non-epidemic MRSA strain (ST239) that had reduced susceptibilities to chlorhexidine [63]. Finally, in a recent publication Hetem and colleagues developed a mathematical model of mupirocin resistance comparing a targeted strategy of applying mupirocin and CHG in *S. aureus* carriers only versus universal decolonization in the prevention of SSIs. Based on their results, they conclude that there is a similar low risk of mupirocin resistance for *S. aureus* in the setting of targeted or universal decolonization and treating all surgical patients with mupirocin and CHG preoperatively eliminated the need for preoperative testing and simplifies implementation. The downside of this approach would be to expose 70% of patients who are not *S. aureus* carriers and are unlikely to benefit from this intervention [64]. Implementation of universal decolonization should be done with caution with monitoring for mupirocin and CHG resistance.

Lastly there are a limited studies looking at the cost effectiveness strategies to prevent MRSA infections. A series of economic computer models found that screening and nasal decolonization are cost effective in some patient populations but not others. Murthy et al. evaluated a bundled intervention that included PCR screening for MRSA prior to surgery, decolonization of MRSA positive patients with mupirocin and CHG, and contact isolation for MRSA positive patients.

They found that this was not strongly cost-effective, meaning that the costs avoided through reducing MRSA infections did not completely offset the costs of screening. However, this model was based on data from a hospital in Geneva, which is known for its low rates of MRSA [65]. Conversely, using data inputs from the United States, multiple studies found that MRSA screening and decolonization prior to cardiac, vascular or orthopedic surgery or heart-lung transplant was cost-effective from both the third party payer perspective and the hospital perspective [24, 57, 58, 66–68]. Additionally, other economic models have found MRSA screening and decolonization to be cost effective among hemodialysis patients, ICU patients and all hospitalized patients [59, 69–72]. Recently Robotham and colleagues evaluated the costs and benefits of universal MRSA screening in English National Health Services(NHS) hospitals. They found that at current MRSA prevalence, that screening of all admissions was not cost effective [73]. However, screening of high-risk specialties might be an option such as admission to nephrology, hematology and oncology, orthopedic and cardiac surgery. In contrast two different studies performed cost analyses of universal decolonization in the ICU setting and found it to be the most cost effective strategy [72, 74]. One economic model compared seven different strategies to prevent MRSA transmission and infection in ICUs and found that the strategies that included decolonization were less expensive and more effective than other strategies [59]. Universal decolonization was found to be cost-effective by preventing 44% of cases of MRSA colonization and 45% of cases of MRSA infection.

Conclusion

Given the evolving epidemiology of MDROs and the complexity of managing the multiplicity of epidemiologically important pathogens across different healthcare settings including MRSA, ensuring adherence to evidence-based strategies to prevent HAIs prevention strategies is critical. Apply horizontal strategies such as universal decolonization in settings where benefits are likely and cost-effective; and use active surveillance testing for MDROs including MRSA and other vertical approaches selectively when epidemiologically important pathogens are newly emerging, to control out breaks of specific pathogens, or pre-operative screening in orthopedic and cardiovascular surgery and other high-risk populations.

There is growing evidence that in endemic settings in the ICU, vertical strategies that involve active surveillance testing for MRSA, isolation, and targeted decolonization are not as effective as horizontal approaches utilizing hand hygiene and universal decolonization using CHG bathing with or without intranasal mupirocin. In addition, several studies have shown this is also the most cost-effective strategy. Evidence for universal decolonization with CHG bathing in non-critical care is unresolved. The results of the recently completed ABATE Trial (Active Bathing to Eliminate Infection Trial), a 2-arm cluster randomized trial in non-critical care comparing usual bathing with CHG bathing and intranasal mupirocin for MRSA positive patients, will hopefully answer this important question [75].

References

1. Prevention CfDCa. Antibiotic resistance threats in the United States. 2013. http://www.cdc.gov/drugresistance/threat-report-2013/pdf/ar-threats-2013-508.pdf. Accessed 7 Mar 2016.
2. Magill SS, Edwards JR, Bamberg W, et al. Multistate point-prevalence survey of health care-associated infections. N Engl J Med. 2014;370:1198–208.
3. Zimlichman E, Henderson D, Tamir O, et al. Health care-associated infections: a meta-analysis of costs and financial impact on the US health care system. JAMA Intern Med. 2013;173:2039–46.
4. Umscheid CA, Mitchell MD, Doshi JA, et al. Estimating the proportion of healthcare-associated infections that are reasonably preventable and the related mortality and costs. Infect Control Hosp Epidemiol. 2011;32:101–14.
5. Services. CfMaM. Medicare.gov HospitalCompare. http://www.medicare.gov/hospitalcompare/search.html. Accessed 5 Mar 2016.
6. Healthcare-Associated Infections – Healthy People. http://healthy-people.gov/2020/topicsobjectives2020/overview.aspx?topicId=17. Accessed 24 Jan 2016.
7. Weiner LM, Fridkin SK, Aponte-Torres Z, et al. Vital signs: preventing antibiotic-resistant infections in hospitals-United States, 2014. MMWR Morb Mortal Wkly Rep. 2016;65:235–41.
8. Cosgrove SE, Qi Y, Kaye KS, Harbarth S, Karchmer AW, Carmeli Y. The impact of methicillin resistance in Staphylococcus aureus bacteremia on patient outcomes: mortality, length of stay, and hospital charges. Infect Control Hosp Epidemiol. 2005;26:166–74.
9. den Heijer CD, van Bijnen EM, Paget WJ, et al. Prevalence and resistance of commensal Staphylococcus aureus, including meticillin-resistant S aureus, in nine European countries: a cross-sectional study. Lancet Infect Dis. 2013;13:409–15.
10. Graham PL 3rd, Lin SX, Larson EL. A U.S. population-based survey of Staphylococcus aureus colonization. Ann Intern Med. 2006;144:318–25.
11. Lim CJ, Cheng AC, Kennon J, et al. Prevalence of multidrug-resistant organisms and risk factors for carriage in long-term care facilities: a nested case-control study. J Antimicrob Chemother. 2014;69:1972–80.
12. Evans ME, Kralovic SM, Simbartl LA, et al. Nationwide reduction of health care-associated methicillin-resistant Staphylococcus aureus infections in veterans affairs long-term care facilities. Am J Infect Control. 2014;42:60–2.
13. Climo MW, Yokoe DS, Warren DK, et al. Effect of daily chlorhexidine bathing on hospital-acquired infection. N Engl J Med. 2013;368:533–42.
14. Wertheim HF, Melles DC, Vos MC, et al. The role of nasal carriage in Staphylococcus aureus infections. Lancet Infect Dis. 2005;5:751–62.
15. VandenBergh MF, Yzerman EP, van Belkum A, et al. Follow-up of Staphylococcus aureus nasal carriage after 8 years: redefining the persistent carrier state. J Clin Microbiol. 1999;37:3133–40.

16. Nouwen JL, Fieren MW, Snijders S, et al. Persistent (not intermittent) nasal carriage of *Staphylococcus aureus* is the determinant of CPD-related infections. Kidney Int. 2005;67:1084–92.

17. Nouwen JL, Ott A, Kluytmans-Vandenbergh MF, et al. Predicting the *Staphylococcus aureus* nasal carrier state: derivation and validation of a "culture rule". Clin Infect Dis. 2004;39:806–11.

18. Cheng VC, Li IW, Wu AK, et al. Effect of antibiotics on the bacterial load of meticillin-resistant *Staphylococcus aureus* colonisation in anterior nares. J Hosp Infect. 2008;70:27–34.

19. Mermel LA, Cartony JM, Covington P, et al. Methicillin-resistant *Staphylococcus aureus* colonization at different body sites: a prospective, quantitative analysis. J Clin Microbiol. 2011;49:1119–21.

20. Sim BL, McBryde E, Street AC, Marshall C. Multiple site surveillance cultures as a predictor of methicillin-resistant *Staphylococcus aureus* infections. Infect Control Hosp Epidemiol. 2013;34:818–24.

21. Bhalla A, Aron DC, Donskey CJ. *Staphylococcus aureus* intestinal colonization is associated with increased frequencu of S aureus on skin of hospitalized patients. BMC Infect Dis. 2007;7:105.

22. Schweizer M, Perencevich E, McDanel J, et al. Effectiveness of a bundled intervention of decolonization and prophylaxis to decrease Gram positive surgical site infections after cardiac or orthopedic surgery: systematic review and meta-analysis. BMJ. 2013;346:f2743.

23. Huang SS, Septimus E, Kleinman K, et al. Targeted versus universal decolonization to prevent ICU infection. N Engl J Med. 2013;368:2255–65.

24. Lee BY, Wiringa AE, Bailey RR, et al. Screening cardiac surgery patients for MRSA: an economic computer model. Am J Manag Care. 2010;16:e163–73.

25. Immerman I, Ramos NL, Katz GM, et al. The persistence of *Staphylococcus aureus* decolonization after mupirocin and topical chlorhexidine: implications for patients requiring multiple or delayed procedures. J Arthroplast. 2012;27:870–6.

26. Loeb MB, Main C, Eady A, Walker-Dilks C. Antimicrobial drugs for treating methicillin-resistant *Staphylococcus aureus* colonization. Cochrane Database Syst Rev. 2003; doi:10.1002/14651858. cd003340:CD003340.

27. Wenzel RP, Edmond MB. Infection control: the case for horizontal rather than vertical interventional programs. Int J Infect Dis. 2010;14(Suppl 4):S3–5.

28. Ward A, Campoli-Richards DM. Mupirocin. A review of its antibacterial activity, pharmacokinetic properties and therapeutic use. Drugs. 1986;32:425–44.

29. Perl TM, Cullen JJ, Wenzel RP, et al. Intranasal mupirocin to prevent postoperative *Staphylococcus aureus* infections. N Engl J Med. 2002;346:1871–7.

30. Ammerlaan HS, Kluytmans JA, Wertheim HF, Nouwen JL, Bonten MJ. Eradication of methicillin-resistant *Staphylococcus aureus* carriage: a systematic review. Clin Infect Dis. 2009;48:922–30.

31. Tacconelli E, Carmeli Y, Aizer A, et al. Mupirocin prophylaxis to prevent *Staphylococcus aureus* infection in patients undergoing dialysis: a meta-analysis. Clin Infect Dis. 2003;37:1629–38.

32. van Rijen MM, Bonten M, Wenzel RP, Kluytmans JA. Intranasal mupirocin for reduction of *Staphylococcus aureus* infections in surgical patients with nasal carriage: a systematic review. J Antimicrob Chemother. 2008;61:254–61.

33. Kallen AJ, Wilson CT, Larson RJ. Perioperative intranasal mupirocin for the prevention of surgical-site infections: systematic review of the literature and meta-analysis. Infect Control Hosp Epidemiol. 2005;26:916–22.

34. van Rijen M, Bonten M, Wenzel R, Kluytmans J. Mupirocin ointment for preventing *Staphylococcus aureus* infections in nasal carriers. Cochrane Database Syst Rev. 2008; doi:10.1002/14651858. CD006216.pub2:CD006216.

35. Mody L, Kauffman CA, McNeil SA, et al. Mupirocin-based decolonization of *Staphylococcus aureus* carriers in residents of 2 long-term care facilities: a randomized, double-blind, placebo-controlled trial. Clin Infect Dis. 2003;37:1467–74.

36. Perez-Fontan M, Rosales M, Rodriguez-Carmona A, et al. Mupirocin resistance after long-term use for *Staphylococcus aureus* colonization in patients undergoing chronic peritoneal dialysis. Am J Kidney Dis. 2002;39:337–41.

37. Annigeri R, Conly J, Vas S, Dedier H, et al. Emergence of mupirocin-resistant *Staphylococcus aureus* in chronic peritoneal dialysis patients using mupirocin prophylaxis to prevent exit-site infection. Perit Dial Int J Int Soc Perit Dial. 2001;21:554–9.

38. Eltringham I. Mupirocin resistance and methicillin-resistant *Staphylococcus aureus* (MRSA). J Hosp Infect. 1997;35:1–8.

39. Caffrey AR, Quilliam BJ, LaPlante KL. Risk factors associated with mupirocin resistance in meticillin-resistant *Staphylococcus aureus*. J Hosp Infect. 2010;76:206–10.

40. Walker ES, Vasquez JE, Dula R, Bullock H, Sarubbi FA. Mupirocin-resistant, methicillin-resistant *Staphylococcus aureus*: does mupirocin remain effective? Infect Control Hosp Epidemiol. 2003;24:342–6.

41. Hayden MK, Lolans K, Haffenreffer K, et al. Chlorhexidine (CHG) and mupirocin susceptibility of methicillin-resistant *Staphylococcus aureus* (MRSA) isolates in the REDUCE-MRSA trial. J Clin Microbiol. 2016;54:2735–42

42. Fawley WN, Parnell P, Hall J, Wilcox MH. Surveillance for mupirocin resistance following introduction of routine peri-operative prophylaxis with nasal mupirocin. J Hosp Infect. 2006;62:327–32.

43. Hill RL, Casewell MW. The in-vitro activity of povidone-iodinecream against *Staphylococcus aureus* and its bioavailability in nasal secretions. J Hosp Infect. 2000;45:198–205.

44. Phillips M, Rosenberg A, Shopsin B, et al. Preventing surgical site infections: a randomized, open-label trial of nasal mupirocin ointment and nasal povidone-iodine solution. Infect Control Hosp Epidemiol. 2014;35:826–32.

45. Bebko SP, Green DM, Awad SS. Effect of a preoperative decontamination protocol on surgical site infections in patients undergoing elective orthopedic surgery with hardware implantation. JAMA Surg. 2015;150:390–5.

46. Vernon MO, Hayden MK, Trick WE, et al. Chlorhexidine gluconate to cleanse patients in a medical intensive care unit: the effectiveness of source control to reduce the bioburden of vancomycin-resistant enterococci. Arch Intern Med. 2006;166:306–12.

47. Bleasdale SC, Trick WE, Gonzalez IM, et al. Effectiveness of chlorhexidine bathing to reduce catheter-associated bloodstream infections in medical intensive care unit patients. Arch Intern Med. 2007;167:2073–9.

48. Popovich KJ, Hota B, Hayes R, et al. Effectiveness of routine patient cleansing with chlorhexidene gluconate for infection prevention in the medical intensive care unit. Infect Control Hosp Epidemiol. 2009;30:959–63.

49. Milstone AM, Elward A, Song X, et al. Daily chlorhexidine bathing to reduce bacteraemia in critically ill children: a multicentre, cluster-randomised, crossover trial. Lancet. 2013;381:1099–106.

50. Septimus EJ, Hayden MK, Kleinman K, et al. Does chlorhexidine bathing in adult intensive care units reduce blood culture contamination? A pragmatic cluster-randomized trial. Infect Control Hosp Epidemiol. 2014;35(Suppl 3):S17–22.

51. Derde LP, Cooper BS, Goossens H, et al. Interventions to reduce colonisation and transmission of antimicrobial-resistant bacteria in intensive care units: an interrupted time series study and cluster randomised trial. Lancet Infect Dis. 2014;14:31–9.

52. Kassakian SZ, Mermel LA, Jefferson JA, et al. Impact of chlorhexidene bathing on hospital-acquired infections among general medical patients. Infect Control Hosp Epidemiol. 2011;32:238–43.

53. Bode LG, Kluytmans JA, Wertheim HF, et al. Preventing surgical-site infections in nasal carriers of *Staphylococcus aureus*. N Engl J Med. 2010;362:9–17.

54. Schweizer ML, Hsiu-Yin C, Septimus E, et al. Association of a bundled intervention with surgical site infections among patients undergoing cardiac, hip, or knee surgery. JAMA. 2015;313:2162–71.

55. Patel PA, Schora DM, Peterson KE, et al. Performance of the Cepheid Xpert(R) SA nasal complete PCR assay compared to culture for detection of methicillin-sensitive and methicillin-resistant *Staphylococcus aureus* colonization. Diag Microbiol Infect Dis. 2014;80:32–4.

56. Jeyaratnam D, Whitty CJ, Phillips K, et al. Impact of rapid screening tests on acquisition of meticillin resistant *Staphylococcus aureus*: cluster randomised crossover trial. BMJ. 2008;336:927–30.

57. Courville XF, Tomek IM, Kirkland KB, et al. Cost-effectiveness of preoperative nasal mupirocin treatment in preventing surgical site infection in patients undergoing total hip and knee arthroplasty: a cost-effectiveness analysis. Infect Control Hosp Epidemiol. 2012;33:152–9.

58. Young LS, Winston LG. Preoperative use of mupirocin for the prevention of healthcare-associated *Staphylococcus aureus* infections: a cost-effectiveness analysis. Infect Control Hosp Epidemiol. 2006;27:1304–12.

59. Gidengil CA, Gay C, Huang SS, et al. Cost-effectiveness of strategies to prevent methicillin-resistant *Staphylococcus aureus* transmission and infection in an intensive care unit. Infect Control Hosp Epidemiol. 2015;36:17–27.

60. Nair R, Perencevich EN, Blevins AE, et al. Clinical effectiveness of mupirocin for preventing Staphlylococcus aureus infections in nonsurgical settings: a meta-analysis. Clin Infedt Dis. 2016;62:618–30.

61. Calfee DP, Salgado CD, Milstone AM, et al. Strategies to prevent methicillin-resistant *Staphylococcus aureus* transmission and infection in acute care hospitals: 2014 update. Infect Control Hosp Epidemiol. 2014;35:S108–32.

62. Lee AS, Macedo-Vinas M, Francois P, et al. Impact of combined low-level mupirocin and genotypic chlorhexidine resistance on persistent methicillin-resistant *Staphylococcus aureus* carriage after decolonization therapy: a case-control study. Clin Infect Dis. 2011;52:1422–30.

63. Batra R, Cooper BS, Whiteley C, et al. Efficacy and limitation of a chlorhexidine-based decolonization strategy in preventing transmission of methicillin-resistant *Staphylococcus aureus* in an intensive care unit. Clin Infect Dis. 2010;50:210–7.

64. Hetem DJ, Bootsma MCJ, Bonten JM. Preventionb of surgical site infections: decontamination with mupirocin based preoperative screening for *Staphylococcus aureus* carriers or universal decontamonation? Clin Infect Dis. 2016;62:631–6.

65. Murthy A, De Angelis G, Pittet D, et al. Cost-effectiveness of universal MRSA screening on admission to surgery. Clin Microbiol Infect. 2010;16:1747–53.

66. Lee BY, Tsui BY, Bailey RR, et al. Should vascular surgery patients be screened preoperatively for methicillin-resistant *Staphylococcus aureus*? Infect Control Hosp Epidemiol. 2009;30:1158–65.

67. Clancy CJ, Bartsch SM, Nguyen MH, et al. A computer simulation model of the cost-effectiveness of routine *Staphylococcus aureus* screening and decolonization among lung and heart-lung transplant recipients. Eur J Clin Microb Infect Dis. 2014;33:1053–61.

68. Lee BY, Wiringa AE, Bailey RR, et al. The economic effect of screening orthopedic surgery patients preoperatively for methicillin-resistant *Staphylococcus aureus*. Infect Control Hosp Epidemiol. 2010;31:1130–8.

69. Lee BY, Song Y, McGlone SM, et al. The economic value of screening haemodialysis patients for methicillin-resistant *Staphylococcus aureus* in the USA. Clin Microbiol Infect. 2011;17:1717–26.

70. Nelson RE, Samore MH, Smith KJ, et al. Cost-effectiveness of adding decolonization to a surveillance strategy of screening and isolation for methicillin-resistant *Staphylococcus aureus* carriers. Clin Microbiol Infect. 2010;16:1740–6.

71. Bloom BS, Fendrick AM, Chernew ME, Patel P. Clinical and economic effects of mupirocin calcium on preventing *Staphylococcus aureus* infection in hemodialysis patients: a decision analysis. Am J Kidney Dis. 1996;27:687–94.

72. Huang SS, Septimus E, Avery TR, Lee GM, Hickok J, Weinstein RA, Moody J, Hayden MK, Perlin JB, Platt R, Ray GT. 2014Cost savings of universal decolonization to prevent intensive care unit infection: implications of the REDUCE MRSA trial. Infect Control Hosp Epidemiol. 2014;35(Suppl 3):S23–31.

73. Robotham JV, Deeny SR, Fuller SR, et al. Cost effectiveness of national mandatory screening of all admissions to English National Health Service hospitals for meticillin-resistant Staphylococcal aureus: a mathematical modelling study. Lancet Infect Dis. 2016:348–59.

74. Ziakas PD, Zacharioudakis IM, Zervou FN, Mylonakis E. Methicillin-resistant *Staphylococcus aureus* prevention strategies in the ICU: a clinical decision analysis. Crit Care Med. 2015;43:382–93.

75. Active Bathing to Eliminate Infection (ABATE Infection) Trial. https://clinicaltrials.gov/ct2/show/NCT02063867. Last accessed 27 Mar 2016.

Staphylococcal Decolonization in Surgery Patients

Andrew D. Ludwig and E. Patchen Dellinger

Introduction

Incidence and Sites of Colonization

Staphylococcus aureus is a commensal skin bacterium found on approximately 30% of adults in developed nations [1–3]. Its primary site of colonization is thought to be the keratinized epithelium of the anterior nares, from which it can seed additional external sites, such as the pharynx and the skin of the hands, axillae, and perineum [4]. When multiple sites are cultured, the anterior nares are most often colonized and carry a 93% sensitivity in detecting colonization [5]. Decolonization of the anterior nares leads to a decrease in the rate of colonization of other external sites of colonization [6, 7].

Type of Carriage

Historically, nasal carriers of *S. aureus* have been divided into three classifications: persistent carriers of a single strain (20% of the population), intermittent carriers of changing strains (60%), and noncarriers (20%) [1, 4]. The determination of carriage type appears to be based on both host and pathogen factors. When inoculated with multiple strains, persistent carriers were recolonized by only their original strain, while noncarriers eliminated all strains [8]. About 6% of individuals are carriers of multiple concomitant strains [9]. Based on cross-sectional surveys, the prevalence of nasal carriage in the community is about 35%, comprising both persistent and intermittent carriers [1, 10–12]. Some populations of patients have a significantly higher carriage rate, such as those with insulin-dependent diabetes mellitus, chronic ambulatory peritoneal dialysis (CAPD), intravenous drug abuse, liver dysfunction, and HIV [1, 8].

A.D. Ludwig • E.P. Dellinger (✉)
Department of Surgery, University of Washington Medical Center, 1959 NE Pacific St, Seattle, WA 98195, USA
e-mail: ludwiga@uw.edu; patch@uw.edu

Nasal carriage of *S. aureus* is an independent risk factor for clinically significant *S. aureus* infections of the bloodstream, skin and soft tissues, and surgical wounds [1, 13–16]. Carriage of methicillin-resistant *S. aureus* (MRSA) bears a higher risk than methicillin-sensitive *S. aureus* (MSSA) for nosocomial infection and a higher rate of morbidity and mortality in ICU patients [17, 18]. The association between nasal carriage of *S. aureus* and SSI has been studied extensively among general, thoracic, and orthopedic surgery patients. These efforts have determined that preoperative colonization with *S. aureus* carries an increased risk of surgical site infection (SSI) [13, 19]. Prospective studies have determined that the same strain colonizing the nares is found in infected surgical sites 75–85% of the time [16, 20, 21]. This association has led to the hypothesis that nasal decolonization of *S. aureus* may present an opportunity to decrease the rates of SSI.

Incidence of Surgical Site Infection (SSI), *S. aureus* SSI, and Association with Colonization

Based on a recent Centers for Disease Control and Prevention (CDC) survey, SSIs account for 21.8% of all nosocomial infections, and among surgical patients, SSIs are the most common nosocomial infection, accounting for 38% of hospital-acquired infections in this group [22]. A recent systematic review of SSI in the literature found an overall incidence of 3.7%, among operated patients with *S. aureus* implicated in 49% of cases [23], making it the most common cause of SSI. This finding is shared by many other large databases. *S. aureus* is responsible for 20% of SSI among hospitals that report to the CDC NNIS system [24] and up to 37% of community hospitals [25].

The CDC have published criteria for defining SSI which classifies infections as superficial incisional, deep incisional, and organ space infections. According to these criteria, superficial incisional SSI involves the skin and subcutaneous tissue; deep incisional SSI involves the deep soft tissue, including fascia and muscle; while organ space infections involve anatomy deep to the incision that was manipulated during surgery [26]. Regardless of classification, an infection is attributed to surgical intervention if it is related to the incision and occurs within 30 days of surgery if no implant was placed or within 90 days if an implant was placed.

Burden and Cost of Treating SSI

Surgical site infections portend a worse prognosis for patients, a longer duration of hospitalization, and a greater financial cost. Each SSI increases length of stay by 7–10 days, increases cost by $3000–$29,000 per patient, and increases mortality risk 2- to 11-fold [25, 27, 28]. Even compared to other types of infection, patients who undergo invasive surgery and have an *S. aureus* infection suffer additional burdens. An analysis of the Nationwide Inpatient Sample database revealed an additional 7.3 hospital days, $22,000 in charges, and 1.7-fold increased absolute risk of in-hospital mortality for those surgical patients with an *S. aureus* infection compared to those with other types of infections [29]. Antibiotic resistance increases these figures further. Patients who develop a MRSA SSI accrue an additional $14,000 in-hospital costs and 3.4 times higher 90-day mortality rates compared to those with a MSSA SSI [30]. Because of the significant clinical and financial impact of *S. aureus* surgical site infection, the high rate of nasal colonization, and the literature supporting the link between colonization and infection, a large amount of research has been devoted to developing effective screening and decolonization programs.

Screening

Screening for *S. aureus* nasal colonization has traditionally involved nasal swab and culture technique. Those that screen positive are then treated with topical intranasal medication to eradicate colonization prior to surgery, and eradication may be demonstrated with repeat testing prior to operating. Another strategy involves universal treatment of all patients without screening. When considering methods of decolonization, there are several important factors. The method must be safe, effective, rapid, cost-effective, and produce prolonged decolonization. Given these principles, several agents have been proposed and studied in the literature.

Methods of Decolonization

Mupirocin

Mupirocin (pseudomonic acid) has been used as a topical agent for nasal decolonization of *S. aureus* since the 1980s [31]. It is a potent and rapid agent for decolonization, clearing

>80% of patients immediately after application [6, 32, 33]. Long-term efficacy is persistent clearance rates of 50% at 6 months and 1 year [33, 34]. When healthcare workers were treated with mupirocin, it was found to decrease the rate of *S. aureus* hand colonization from 58% in placebo-treated participants to 3% in mupirocin-treated individuals [33].

Historic Controls

Initial investigations into the effectiveness of mupirocin to reduce the rate of SSI used historic control groups. In one of the largest such studies, Kluytmans et al. compared 983 cardiac surgery patients receiving preoperative mupirocin with 1003 historic controls and found a reduction in SSI from 7.3 to 2.8% [35]. It should be noted that the control group also experienced a decrease in the rate of SSI, indicating that there were unmeasured variables responsible for at least some of the reduction seen in both groups. In a study of consecutive cardiac surgery patients before and after the introduction of intranasal mupirocin treatment, Cimochowski et al. found that decolonization significantly decreased wound sternal infection rate by 66%, from 2.7 to 0.9% [36].

Randomized Controlled Trials

Despite the findings in these early studies, randomized controlled trials in unselected patient populations have failed to demonstrate a statistically significant decrease in SSI among patients preoperatively receiving mupirocin compared to placebo.

In the Mupirocin and Risk of *S. aureus* (MARS) study, Perl et al. investigated the effect of intranasal mupirocin in a randomized, placebo-controlled study of over 4000 elective general, cardiothoracic, oncologic-gynecologic, and neurosurgical patients [20]. The authors found that twice daily mupirocin up to 5 days before surgery eliminated *S. aureus* colonization in 83% of carriers and significantly reduced *S. aureus* nosocomial infections in nasal carriers. Overall nosocomial infections, overall SSI rate, and *S. aureus* SSI rate were all reduced following mupirocin treatment, though not to a statistically significant degree. However, among patients who were colonized preoperatively, *S. aureus* infections were reduced by 51% ($p = 0.02$). Among those carriers who developed *S. aureus* infections, 85% had identical strains in their nares and their infected sites, and rates of MRSA and mupirocin resistance were low (less than 1%).

In a randomized controlled trial of 614 orthopedic surgical patients, Kalmeijer et al. found a carriage rate of about 30%. Similar to the MARS study, mupirocin eradicated colonization in 83% of carriers. Among carriers who developed a *S. aureus* infection, the same strain was found in the nares and infected area of 84% of patients. Also like the MARS study, mupirocin lowered but did not significantly reduce the rate of overall SSI or *S. aureus* SSI [21]. In a pooled analysis of these two studies, Kluytmans et al. found a nearly significant reduction in *S. aureus* SSI among carriers ($p = 0.06$, pooled OR = 0.58, 95% CI 0.33–1.02) and a significant reduction in overall nosocomial infections in carriers (p = 0.01, RR 0.49, 95% CI 0.29–0.83) [7]. This analysis also revealed that 26 carriers would need to be treated to prevent one nosocomial S. aureus infection.

The prior two studies randomized both carriers and noncarriers to receive mupirocin treatment, and, as expected, a significant reduction in infections was seen only in the S. aureus carriers. Konvalinka et al. conducted a randomized controlled trial on the effect of mupirocin on cardiac surgery patients who were S. aureus carriers. The patients were screened by nasal swab and culture and then carriers were randomized to receive intranasal mupirocin or placebo. A total of 263 patients were enrolled after positive screening by nasal swab. Treatment with mupirocin eliminated S. aureus carriage in 81.5% of patients compared to a reduction of 46.5% in those treated with placebo (p < 0.0001). The authors found an overall wound infection rate of 13.8% in the treatment arm and 8.6% in the placebo arm (p = 0.27) with 3.8% of mupirocin-treated patients developing a S. aureus infection compared to 3.2% of patients treated with placebo (p = 1.0) [32]. So despite a significant reduction in nasal carriage, this patient population did not experience a significant reduction in overall SSI, S. aureus SSI, or nosocomial S. aureus infection. Furthermore, S. aureus colonization at the time of surgery was not found to be an independent predictor of SSI in multivariate regression analysis. Subgroup analysis of superficial and deep space infections was too limited for meaningful conclusions to be drawn. The authors concluded that due to the low rate of SSI in their patient population, the study size was too low to detect a difference in SSI rates, which is a common theme among randomized controlled trials on this topic.

In a Cochrane review and meta-analysis of nine randomized controlled trials encompassing 3396 patients, van Rijen et al. found a statistically significant reduction in the rate of S. aureus infection in patients treated with intranasal mupirocin (RR 0.55, 95% CI 0.43–0.70). A subgroup analysis of surgical trials found a significant reduction in the rate of nosocomial S. aureus infection associated with mupirocin use (RR 0.55, 95% CI 0.34–0.89). When looking specifically at surgical site infections caused by S. aureus, no significant reduction in infection rate was found (RR 0.63, 95% CI 0.38–1.04) likely due to low numbers [37]. This conclusion is echoed by a previous meta-analysis of four randomized controlled trials consisting of 686 mupirocin-treated surgical patients with S. aureus nasal carriage. This analysis did find a statistically significant reduction in the rate of overall S. aureus infection (RR 0.55, 95% CI 0.34–0.89, p = 0.02), but no such difference was found when examining S. aureus SSI (RR 0.64, 95% CI 0.38–1.06) [38]. All four of these trials were included in the later Cochrane analysis.

In another focused review of mupirocin prophylaxis in surgical patients, Kallen et al. conducted a meta-analysis of three RCTs and four single-institution before-after trials including both general surgery patients and cardiothoracic, orthopedic, and neurosurgery patients [39]. These authors found a significant reduction in the risk of overall surgical site infections in both RCTs (7.6% vs. 6.0%, RR 0.80, 95%CI 0.58–1.10) and in before-after trials (4.1% vs. 1.7%, RR 0.40, 95%CI 0.29–0.56) but only in the "non-general" surgery patient populations. Combining these two types of studies resulted in a population too heterogeneous for meaningful results. Because of the analyses conducted by the primary studies, no summary statistics could be performed on the rate of S. aureus infections as opposed to overall SSI.

More recently, a randomized controlled trial was conducted in the Netherlands by Bode et al. using PCR to rapidly screen and identify S. aureus nasal carriers at hospital admission [40]. Carriers were then treated with twice daily mupirocin ointment and daily chlorhexidine soap for 5 days, and treatment was continued even if surgery was performed during the initial treatment timeframe. The screening was carried out on 6771 patients from 2005 to 2007 and identified 1251 nasal carriers (18.4%), of whom 917 were included in an intent-to-treat analysis and 808 underwent surgery. If still hospitalized, inpatients were re-treated at 3 and 6 weeks after initial treatment, and the patients were followed until 6 weeks after hospital discharge. All S. aureus in this study were MSSA. The effect of combined nasal and skin decontamination resulted in a decrease in S. aureus surgical site infection from 7.7 to 3.4% (RR 0.42, 95%CI 0.23–0.75) and reduced the risk of deep space infection from 4.4 to 0.9% (RR 0.21, 95%CI 0.07–0.62). Superficial surgical site infections were also reduced in the study population, though not to a statistically significant degree (3.5% vs. 1.6%, RR 0.45, 95%CI 0.18–1.11). A comparison of S. aureus strains obtained from the nasal passages with those isolated from surgical site infections revealed that endogenous S. aureus infection was significantly less likely in the treatment population, though there was no effect seen the risk of exogenous S. aureus infections nor in overall hospital-acquired S. aureus infection.

Taken together, the high-quality studies that have been published to date on the use of intranasal mupirocin with or without chlorhexidine body wash as a means of S. aureus SSI prophylaxis do not reveal consistent findings of mupirocin treatment reducing the risk of SSI. However, some conclusions can be drawn from these analyses. Firstly, as expected, mupirocin treatment only benefits those with nasal colonization. Secondly, it appears that cardiac and orthopedic surgical patients benefit more from preoperative S. aureus decolonization than general surgery patients.

Mupirocin Resistance

In some institutions, mupirocin resistance, particularly among MRSA isolates, has emerged as a significant problem and has been correlated with an increased use of mupirocin [41, 42]. In a review of intranasal mupirocin use for MRSA decolonization in multiple healthcare settings, Poovelikunnel et al. concluded that indiscriminate use of mupirocin in both colonized and uncolonized patients could lead to an increasing prevalence of mupirocin resistance [43]. In the studies reviewed above, resistance was found to be low in elective surgical patients who received short preoperative courses of mupirocin [20, 35, 36]. In a 4-year study of routine empiric mupirocin prophylaxis in orthopedic and vascular surgical patients, Fawley et al. found no trend toward increasing prevalence of mupirocin resistance [44].

Povidone-Iodine

Because of the risk of mupirocin resistance, alternative treatments for nasal decolonization have been proposed. One such agent is povidone-iodine, which produces a bactericidal effect by disrupting protein and nucleic acid structure and synthesis. In a study of universal decontamination among elective orthopedic patients undergoing hardware implantation, Bebko et al. found a significant reduction in overall SSI using chlorhexidine washcloths and oral rinse along with intranasal povidone-iodine as compared to historical controls who received no decontamination [45]. Interestingly, the nasal treatment was applied only on the morning of the surgery, and therefore compliance could be assured.

In a randomized open-label comparison between nasal mupirocin and nasal povidone-iodine of over 1800 orthopedic patients undergoing arthroplasty or spine fusion, Phillips et al. found a reduced rate of deep SSI with povidone-iodine use in their per-protocol analysis, which excluded those participants who did not receive the full course their prescribed prophylaxis [46]. The difference in rates of deep SSI did not reach statistical significance in the intent-to-treat analysis. Importantly, in this study, the control participants received mupirocin twice daily for 5 days before the operation, whereas the treatment group received two applications of povidone-iodine within 2 h of the surgical incision. As in the prior study, the implication of receiving a short course of monitored prophylaxis has clear advantages with respect to patient compliance, even if the two treatments are equivalent in their prevention of SSI. In fact, in this randomized trial, about three times as many patients failed to complete at least seven doses of mupirocin as failed to receive the two doses of povidone-iodine. Regarding the role of mupirocin resistance, the authors detected resistance in 4 of 219 (1.8%) preoperative S. aureus isolates, but no deep S. aureus SSI occurred in these subjects. The authors also found that mupi-rocin was more effective than povidone-iodine at clearing nasal S. aureus colonization based on postoperative nasal cultures and spa typing. This is most likely due to the ability of mupirocin to eradicate colonization, while povidone-iodine probably suppresses S. aureus activity only for the duration of the surgery.

Another advantage of povidone-iodine over mupirocin is the significant cost savings associated with intranasal treatment because of both the reduced cost per dose and the reduced number of doses needed. Torres et al. compared a screen-and-treat algorithm targeted at eradicating MRSA colonization with a universal povidone-iodine prophylaxis strategy [47]. In this retrospective analysis of 1853 patients undergoing total hip or knee arthroplasty, the authors studied a cohort of patients screened for MRSA – and treated with 5 days of mupirocin if colonization was found – compared to a cohort of patients universally treated with one dose of povidone-iodine immediately before surgery. The authors found no significant difference in SSI rates between the cohorts. The screened population had a 4.8% incidence MRSA colonization, while the unscreened population had a 4.7% incidence of prior documented MRSA colonization or infection. However there was a significant difference in out-of-pocket cost, with MRSA screening and mupirocin treatment costing a mean of $110.47 per patient, whereas the universal povidone-iodine treatment cost a mean of $16.42 per patient.

Nasal Chlorhexidine

Chlorhexidine gluconate has been used extensively for topical decolonization of the skin in surgical patients; however it has also been used for nasal and oropharyngeal decolonization as well. In a randomized controlled trial of 991 elective cardiac surgery patients conducted in the Netherlands from 2003 to 2005, Segers et al. studied the effect of four-times-daily nasal and oropharyngeal chlorhexidine treatment from hospital admission until the day after surgery [48]. The authors found a significant reduction in the risk of overall nosocomial infection in chlorhexidine-treated patients (26.2% vs. 19.8%, ARR 6.4%, $p = 0.002$). On subgroup analysis, the risk of both deep and deep sternal infections were also significantly reduced (5.1% vs. 1.9%, p = 0.002; 3.0% vs. 1.0%, $p = 0.001$, respectively). Interestingly, lower respiratory tract infection rates and bacteremia rates were also lower in the group treated with chlorhexidine. However, neither overall SSI nor superficial SSI rates were significantly reduced in the treatment group, a finding that is shared with many studies of mupirocin decolonization. The authors also found a significant reduction in the length of hospital stay among those treated with chlorhexidine, from 10.3 to 9.5 days (ARR 0.8 days, 95%CI 0.24–1.88).

Photodisinfection

Photodisinfection of the nares is another approach that has been studied for decolonization. In combination with chlorhexidine wipes, photodisinfection in the preoperative area was found to decrease surgical site infection among 3068 elective cardiac, orthopedic, spinal, vascular, thoracic, and neurosurgical patients. However this study was limited by the use of a single-center observational study design, a historic control population, and a significant lag time between control and experimental groups [49]. Clearly further study is needed to determine the utility and efficacy of photodisinfection for *S. aureus* decolonization in surgical patients.

Perioperative Antibiotics

Timing and dose of perioperative systemic prophylactic antibiotic is critical and does reduce the risk of SSI [50–52]. As discussed above, despite correct timing and dosage of perioperative antibiotics, nasal carriers of *S. aureus* still retain a higher risk of *S. aureus* SSI over noncarriers. Specific systemic antibiotic treatments have been studied prospectively for their ability to decolonize nasal *S. aureus* carriers. In particular rifampin, either alone or in combination with novobiocin or trimethoprim-sulfamethoxazole, has been studied in randomized controlled fashion and found to be effective at decolonization [53, 54]. However emerging resistance to rifampin limits its usefulness for large-scale decolonization programs. Combining topical agents with systemic antibiotics has also been attempted. In a randomized trial of hemodialysis patients, Yu et al. found that rifampin and intranasal bacitracin was more effective at nasal decolonization than rifampin alone. In the same study, the authors determined the combination was also more effective than vancomycin, which itself was no more effective at nasal decolonization than no treatment [55]. Unfortunately no published studies have looked specifically at nasal decolonization with systemic antibiotics in surgical patients.

Body Wash

Because *S. aureus* and many other commensal and potentially pathogenic bacteria colonize the skin of surgical patients, the use of preoperative antimicrobial body washes is an appealing strategy to decrease SSI. In fact, showering or bathing with antiseptic agents such as chlorhexidine, povidone-iodine, or triclosan soap has been shown to decrease the burden of endogenous flora on the skin [56, 57]. Unfortunately large randomized trials, specifically of chlorhexidine preparations for all surgical patients, have

failed to demonstrate a reduction in SSI rates when compared to perioperative bathing with detergent alone [58–60].

Timing of Decolonization

If decolonization is chosen for surgical cases, it is important that it be done in close conjunction with the operative procedure. Mody has shown that recolonization is common at 90 days [61]. In another prospective study of decolonization for MRSA before orthopedic procedures, the authors confirmed decolonization and then patients were "admitted for operation within three months of a negative screen." Intravenous prophylaxis was cefuroxime. MRSA SSIs were statistically significantly more frequent in patients with a history of MRSA colonization who had been decolonized [62]. This presumably occurred because those patients had become recolonized with MRSA during the interval between decolonization and operation and were treated with an ineffective prophylactic antibiotic.

Cost-Effectiveness of Decolonization

The cost-effectiveness of treating *S. aureus* colonization depends on the cost of the prophylactic treatment; the cost of the prevented infection (both inpatient and outpatient costs); indirect costs; the costs of screening, if implemented; and the frequency of both colonization and infection. Because the cost associated with the most common decolonization treatments is low and the cost of a nosocomial infection is so high, most studies have determined that decolonization is cost-effective. Bloom et al. examined the cost-effectiveness of two treatment strategies in hemodialysis patients – a screen-and-treat program and a universal treatment program without screen. Assuming that 75% of *S. aureus* infections are attributable to nasal colonization and that eliminating colonization will reduce the number of infections by about 50%, the authors found an annual savings of $784,000 per thousand dialysis patients if patients were screened by culture and only carriers were treated. This saving was improved to $1,117,000 per thousand patients if all patients are treated for 3 days without screening [63].

Regarding surgical patients and prevention of surgical site infections, Vandenbergh et al. studied the cost-effectiveness of universal perioperative mupirocin in cardiothoracic surgery patients based on a prior intervention study using historical controls. As expected, postoperative costs were dramatically higher in patients with a SSI. Given an incidence of SSI of 7.3% in the control group and 2.8% in the mupirocin group, the use of mupirocin resulted in a cost savings of $16,633 per infection prevented [64].

A more recent study from the Netherlands found a similarly significant reduction in costs among cardiothoracic and orthopedic patients. The authors examined a subgroup of surgical patients who participated in a multicenter randomized controlled trial of hospitalized patients with *S. aureus* nasal carriage. This trial was discussed above and had previously shown a significant decrease in healthcare-associated *S. aureus* infections in patients receiving mupirocin nasal ointment and chlorhexidine gluconate medicated soap compared to placebo [40]. In the analysis of cost-effectiveness, the authors found that mupirocin and chlorhexidine treatment of nasal carriers resulted in an average savings of €1911 per patient, with cardiac patients saving €2841 and orthopedic patients saving €955 [65]. The number of patients needed to screen to prevent an SSI was 250, while the number of carriers needed to treat was 23. Although the colonized patients were treated with 5 days of nasal mupirocin, in one of the busiest hospitals in the study, 90% of the surgical patients were admitted the day before operation and received only one or two decolonization treatments before the operation (Jan Kluytmans, personal communication, September 2011).

An analysis of cost-effectiveness based on a culture-and-treat strategy in surgical patients found a savings of about $1.5 million per 10,000 patients screened based on a carriage rate of 31% and a risk reduction of 48% [66]. These rate estimates are in line with those derived in the above studies and systematic reviews in surgical patients.

MRSA Screening and Decolonization

Methicillin-resistant *S. aureus* colonization represents a special consideration when determining screening and decolonization methods. In the United States, a national survey from 2001 to 2004 demonstrated a decrease in the prevalence of MSSA colonization and an increase in the prevalence of MRSA colonization [3]. As mentioned above, MRSA colonization bears a higher risk than MSSA for nosocomial infection and a higher rate of morbidity and mortality in ICU patients [17, 18]. In addition, patients who develop a MRSA SSI have both a higher 90-day mortality rate and higher hospital costs compared to those with a MSSA SSI [30]. This risk is further heightened in patients who undergo hardware implantation. However, methods of decolonization have shown less success among MRSA carriers than MSSA carriers.

A randomized controlled trial of combined intranasal mupirocin, chlorhexidine gluconate body wash, and rifampin and doxycycline systemic treatment for MRSA colonization decolonized 74% of patient at 3 months and 54% at 8 months compared to no treatment. Mupirocin resistance appeared in 5% of follow-up isolates [67]. In a retrospective cohort analysis of MRSA carriers decolonized with mupirocin and chlorhexidine or povidone-iodine nasal and body wash, only 39% of patients were successfully decolonized. The nosocomial infection rate was significantly lower among those successfully decolonized [68]. A systematic review of randomized controlled trials of MRSA decolonization methods found insufficient evidence to support any topical or systemic antimicrobial treatment for eradicating MRSA carriage [69]. When looking only at surgical patients, the effect of MRSA decolonization is similarly contentious. In a prospective interventional cohort study of universal MRSA real-time PCR (RT-PCR) screening and 5 days of intranasal mupirocin and chlorhexidine body wash among surgical patients, there was no significant decrease in nosocomial or surgical site infections. There was, however, a low level of MRSA colonization at admission (5.1%) and a low overall rate of surgical site infection (0.6%) in this study population [70].

When deciding whether to screen and decolonize, especially for major clean operations where the primary pathogen is *S. aureus*, it makes the most sense to target both MSSA and MRSA. Infection with either for an arthroplasty, spinal fusion, open heart procedure, or vascular prosthesis is a disastrous complication. The Bode trial showed benefit when MSSA was the only *S. aureus* type found on screening [40]. In a multi-institutional study of patients having cardiac or orthopedic surgery performed in 20 hospitals in 9 US states, the investigators followed an algorithm that attempted to screen all patients. If no *S. aureus* were found, then standard protocols were followed. If either MSSA or MRSA were found, then decolonization was performed. Patients with MSSA received standard intravenous prophylaxis, while those with MRSA received both vancomycin and a cephalosporin. Patients who could not be screened were treated as MRSA positive. Those patients who were unscreened or whose screening results were unknown at the time of surgery received decolonization treatment and were assumed to be MRSA positive. Mupirocin was continued until screening results were known, and mupirocin was discontinued for those with negative results. If sites were analyzed according to adherence to the protocol, *S. aureus* infection rates were three times lower when the protocol was adhered to than when it was partially adhered to or not adhered to [71].

In addition to topical treatment for MRSA decolonization, patients known to be colonized with MRSA prior to surgery should receive perioperative antibiotic prophylaxis directed at MRSA. Perioperative antibiotic selection for patients colonized by *S. aureus* is especially important and should be based on whether MRSA or MSSA colonization is present. In a report of perioperative prophylaxis among cardiac surgery patients, MSSA SSIs were more common among those who received vancomycin compared to cefazolin prophylaxis [72]. This finding was echoed in a retrospective study of vancomycin or beta-lactam prophylaxis in nearly 23,000 clean cardiac and orthopedic surgery procedures from the Australian Surveillance Data (VICNISS). For these procedures, the risk of SSI with MSSA was nearly threefold higher if vancomycin prophylaxis was administered, whereas the risk of MRSA SSI was doubled if beta-lactam prophylaxis was used instead [73]. These two studies highlight the importance of accurately determining *S. aureus* carriage (MRSA or MSSA) and administering appropriate prophylaxis. Clinical practice guidelines further support this conclusion. A joint committee consisting of members of the American Society of Health-System Pharmacists (ASHP), the Infectious Diseases Society of America (IDSA), the Surgical Infection Society (SIS), and the Society for Healthcare Epidemiology of America (SHEA) recommends vancomycin plus a cephalosporin for SSI prophylaxis among patients known to be colonized with MRSA undergoing cardiac, thoracic, general, and neurosurgical procedures [74].

Conclusion and Summary of Recommendations

Patients colonized with *S. aureus* carry an increased risk of nosocomial and surgical site infections with the same organism. Carriage of MRSA is more difficult to eradicate, further increases the risk of infection, and makes treatment of infection more difficult, but MSSA is not benign. Programs aimed at screening and decolonizing patients prior to surgery have had varying degrees of success, depending on the endemic incidence of colonization, the type of organism, and the type of surgery. The benefit of decolonization has been most conclusively demonstrated in cardiothoracic and orthopedic surgery patients where surgical site and hardware infection is more problematic but is likely beneficial in other clean operations with placement of prostheses such as spinal operations and incisional hernia repairs with mesh. Results from trials of decolonization in general surgery patients have had variable success, largely due to limited sample size and an overall low incidence of staphylococcal SSI. In general, decolonization has a greater effect on the prevention of deep space surgical site infection compared to superficial or wound infections.

Strategies for decolonization have focused on universal treatment for all patients or screen-and-treat programs aimed at rapid detection of colonization and treatment of carriers. This latter approach also affords the opportunity to demonstrate decolonization prior to surgery, if necessary. Both methods have proven to be cost-effective in a variety of surgical patient populations given the relatively low cost of preoperative decolonization compared to the burden of treating a surgical site infection.

The optimal decolonization strategy depends on the incidence of colonization in the patient population, the speed and cost of detection of carriage, and the cost and compliance associated with treatment. As the cost and delay for RT-PCR decreases over time, this will likely be the best method for rapid detection. Conceivably, this screening could be accomplished at the outpatient preoperative clinic visit and a decolonization regimen prescribed at the end of the visit for those patients who are found to be colonized.

References

1. Kluytmans J, VanBelkum A, Verburgh H. Nasal carriage of *Staphylococcus aureus*: epidemiology, underlying mechanisms, and associated risks. Clin Microbiol Rev. 1997;10(3):505–20.
2. Wertheim HF, Melles DC, Vos MC, et al. The role of nasal carriage in *Staphylococcus aureus* infections. Lancet Infect Dis. 2005;5(12):751–62. doi:10.1016/S1473-3099(05)70295-4.
3. Gorwitz RJ, Kruszon-Moran D, McAllister SK, et al. Changes in the prevalence of nasal colonization with _Staphylococcus aureus_ in the United States, 2001–2004. J Infect Dis. 2008;197(0022–1899 (Print)):1226–34. doi:10.1086/533494.
4. Williams RE. Healthy carriage of *Staphylococcus aureus*: its prevalence and importance. Bacteriol Rev. 1963;27(96):56–71.
5. Sanford MD, Widmer AF, Bale MJ, Jones RN, Wenzel RP. Efficient detection and long-term persistence of the carriage of methicillin-resistant *Staphylococcus aureus*. Clin Infect Dis. 1994;19(6):1123–8. http://www.ncbi.nlm.nih.gov/pubmed/7888543
6. Doebbeling BN, Breneman DL, Neu HC, et al. Elimination of *Staphylococcus aureus* nasal carriage in health care workers: analysis of six clinical trials with calcium mupirocin ointment: 466–474.
7. Kluytmans JAJW, Wertheim HFL. Nasal carriage of *Staphylococcus aureus* and prevention of nosocomial infections. Infection. 2005;33(1):3–8. doi:10.1007/s15010-005-4012-9.
8. Nouwen J, Boelens H, van Belkum A, Verbrugh H. Human factor in *Staphylococcus aureus* nasal carriage. Infect Immun. 2004;72(11):6685–8. doi:10.1128/IAI.72.11.6685-6688.2004.
9. Cespedes C, Said-Salim B, Miller M, et al. The clonality of *Staphylococcus aureus* nasal carriage. J Infect Dis. 2005;191(3):444–52.
10. Shopsin B, Mathema B, Martinez J, et al. Prevalence of methicillin-resistant and methicillin-susceptible *Staphylococcus aureus* in the community. J Infect Dis. 2000;182(0022–1899 (Print)):359–62. doi:10.1086/315695.
11. Kenner J, O'Connor T, Piantanida N, et al. Rates of carriage of methicillin-resistant and methicillin-susceptible *Staphylococcus aureus* in an outpatient population. Infect Control Hosp Epidemiol. 2003;24(6):439–44. doi:10.1086/502229.
12. Bischoff WE, Wallis ML, Tucker KB, Reboussin BA, Sherertz RJ. *Staphylococcus aureus* nasal carriage in a student community: prevalence, clonal relationships, and risk factors. Infect Control Hosp Epidemiol. 2004;25(6):485–91. doi:10.1086/502427.
13. Kluytmans JA, Mouton JW, Ijzerman EP, et al. Nasal carriage of _Staphylococcus aureus_ as a major risk factor for wound infections after cardiac surgery. J Infect Dis. 1995;171(0022-1899 SB-AIM SB-IM):216–9.
14. Kalmeijer MD, van Nieuwland-Bollen E, Bogaers-Hofman D, de Baere GA. Nasal carriage of *Staphylococcus aureus* is a major risk factor for surgical-site infections in orthopedic surgery. Infect Control Hosp Epidemiol. 2000;21(5):319–23. doi:10.1086/501763.
15. Wertheim HFL, Vos MC, Ott A, et al. Risk and outcome of nosocomial *Staphylococcus aureus* bacteraemia in nasal carriers versus non-carriers. Lancet. 2004;364(9435):703–5. doi:10.1016/S0140-6736(04)16897-9.

16. von Eiff C, Becker K, Machka K, Stammer H, Peters G. Nasal carriage as a source of *Staphylococcus aureus* bacteremia. Study group. N Engl J Med. 2001;344(1):11–6. doi:10.1056/NEJM200101043440102.

17. Pujol M, Peña C, Pallares R, et al. Nosocomial *Staphylococcus aureus* bacteremia among nasal carriers of methicillin-resistant and methicillin-susceptible strains. Am J Med. 1996;100(5):509–16. doi:10.1016/S0002-9343(96)00014-9.

18. Safdar N, Bradley EA. The risk of infection after nasal colonization with *Staphylococcus aureus*. Am J Med. 2008;121(4):310–5. doi:10.1016/j.amjmed.2007.07.034.

19. Perl TM, Golub JE. New approaches to reduce *Staphylococcus aureus* nosocomial infection rates: treating *S. aureus* nasal carriage. Ann Pharmacother. 1998;32(1060–0280 SB-IM):S7–16.

20. Perl TM, Cullen JJ, Wenzel RP, et al. Intranasal mupirocin to prevent postoperative *Staphylococcus aureus* infections. N Engl J Med. 2002;346(24):1871–7. doi:10.1056/NEJMoa003069.

21. Kalmeijer MD, Coertjens H, van Nieuwland-Bollen PM, et al. Surgical site infections in orthopedic surgery: the effect of mupirocin nasal ointment in a double-blind, randomized, placebo-controlled study. Clin Infect Dis. 2002;35(4):353–8. doi:10.1086/341025.

22. Magill SS, Edwards JR, Bamberg W, et al. Multistate point-prevalence survey of health care-associated infections. N Engl J Med. 2014;370(13):1198–208. doi:10.1056/NEJMoa1306801.

23. Korol E, Johnston K, Waser N, et al. A systematic review of risk factors associated with surgical site infections among surgical patients. PLoS One. 2013;8(12):1–9. doi:10.1371/journal.pone.0083743.

24. Favero MS, Gaynes RP, Horan TC, et al. National Nosocomial Infections Surveillance (NNIS) report, data summary from October 1986–April 1996, issued May 1996. Am J Infect Control. 1996;24(5):380–8. doi:10.1016/S0196-6553(96)90026-7.

25. Anderson DJ, Kirkland KB, Kaye KS, et al. Underresourced hospital infection control and prevention programs: penny wise, pound foolish? Infect Control Hosp Epidemiol. 2007;28:767–73. doi:10.1086/518518.

26. Horan TC, Gaynes RP, Martone WJ, Jarvis WR, Emori TG. CDC definitions of nosocomial surgical site infections, 1992: a modification of CDC definitions of surgical wound infections. Infect Control Hosp Epidemiol. 1992;13(10):606–8.

27. Cruse PJ, Foord R. The epidemiology of wound infection. A 10-year prospective study of 62,939 wounds. Surg Clin North Am. 1980;60(1):27–40.

28. Kirkland KB, Briggs JP, Trivette SL, Wilkinson WE, Sexton DJ. The impact of surgical-site infections in the 1990s: attributable mortality, excess length of hospitalization, and extra costs. Infect Control Hosp Epidemiol. 1999;20(11):725–30. doi:10.1086/501572.

29. Noskin GA, Rubin RJ, Schentag JJ, et al. The burden of *Staphylococcus aureus* infections on hospitals in the United States: an analysis of the 2000 and 2001 nationwide inpatient sample database. Arch Intern Med. 2011;165(15):1756–61. doi:10.1001/archinte.165.15.1756.

30. Engemann JJ, Carmeli Y, Cosgrove SE, et al. Adverse clinical and economic outcomes attributable to methicillin resistance among patients with *Staphylococcus aureus* surgical site infection. Clin Infect Dis. 2003;36:27710.

31. Casewell MW, Hill RL. The carrier state: methicillin-resistant *Staphylococcus aureus*. J Antimicrob Chemother. 1986;18(Suppl A):1–12. http://www.ncbi.nlm.nih.gov/pubmed/3091562

32. Konvalinka A, Errett L, Fong IW. Impact of treating *Staphylococcus aureus* nasal carriers on wound infections in cardiac surgery. J Hosp Infect. 2006;64(2):162–8. doi:10.1016/j.jhin.2006.06.010.

33. Reagan DR, Doebbeling BN, Pfaller MA, et al. Elimination of coincident *Staphylococcus aureus* nasal and hand carriage with intranasal application of mupirocin calcium ointment. Ann Intern Med. 1991;114(2):101–6. http://www.ncbi.nlm.nih.gov/pubmed/1898585

34. Doebbeling BN, Breneman DL, Neu HC, et al. Elimination of *Staphylococcus aureus* nasal carriage in health care workers: analysis of six clinical trials with calcium mupirocin ointment. The Mupirocin Collaborative Study Group. Clin Infect Dis. 1993;17(3):466–74. http://www.ncbi.nlm.nih.gov/pubmed/8218691

35. Kluytmans JA, Mouton JW, VandenBergh MF, et al. Reduction of surgical-site infections in cardiothoracic surgery by elimination of nasal carriage of *Staphylococcus aureus*. Infect Control Hosp Epidemiol. 1996;17(12):780–5. http://www.ncbi.nlm.nih.gov/pubmed/8985763

36. Cimochowski GE, Harostock MD, Brown R, Bernardi M, Alonzo N, Coyle K. Intranasal mupirocin reduces sternal wound infection after open heart surgery in diabetics and nondiabetics. Ann Thorac Surg. 2001;71(5):1572–9. doi:10.1016/S0003-4975(01)02519-X.

37. van Rijen M, Bonten M, Wenzel R, Kluytmans J. Mupirocin ointment for preventing *Staphylococcus aureus* infections in nasal carriers (review). 2009;(1).

38. van Rijen MML, Bonten M, Wenzel RP, Kluytmans J a JW. Intranasal mupirocin for reduction of *Staphylococcus aureus* infections in surgical patients with nasal carriage: a systematic review. J Antimicrob Chemother. 2008;61(2):254–61. doi:10.1093/jac/dkm480.

39. Kallen AJ, Wilson CT, Larson RJ. Perioperative intranasal mupirocin for the prevention of surgical-site infections: systematic review of the literature and meta-analysis. Infect Control Hosp Epidemiol. 2005;26(12):916–22. doi:10.1086/505453.

40. Bode LGM, Kluytmans JAJW, Wertheim HFL, et al. Preventing surgical-site infections in nasal carriers of *Staphylococcus aureus*. N Engl J Med. 2010;362(1):9–17. doi:10.1056/NEJMoa0808939.

41. Miller MA, Dascal A, Portnoy J, Mendelson J. Development of mupirocin resistance among methicillin-resistant *Staphylococcus aureus* after widespread use of nasal mupirocin ointment. Infect Control Hosp Epidemiol. 1996;17(12):811–3. http://www.ncbi.nlm.nih.gov/pubmed/8985769

42. Lee AS, MacEdo-Vinas M, Franois P, et al. Impact of combined low-level mupirocin and genotypic chlorhexidine resistance on persistent methicillin-resistant *Staphylococcus aureus* carriage after decolonization therapy: a case-control study. Clin Infect Dis. 2011;52(12):1422–30. doi:10.1093/cid/cir233.

43. Poovelikunnel T, Gethin G, Humphreys H. Mupirocin resistance: clinical implications and potential alternatives for the eradication of MRSA. J Antimicrob Chemother. 2015;70:2681. (July):dkv169. doi:10.1093/jac/dkv169.

44. Fawley WN, Parnell P, Hall J, Wilcox MH. Surveillance for mupirocin resistance following introduction of routine peri-operative prophylaxis with nasal mupirocin. J Hosp Infect. 2006;62(3):327–32. doi:10.1016/j.jhin.2005.09.022.

45. Bebko SP, Green DM, Awad SS. Effect of a preoperative decontamination protocol on surgical site infections in patients undergoing elective orthopedic surgery with hardware implantation. JAMA Surg. 2015;77030(5):390–5. doi:10.1001/jamasurg.2014.3480.

46. Phillips M, Rosenberg A, Shopsin B, et al. Preventing surgical site infections: a randomized, open-label trial of nasal mupirocin ointment and nasal povidone-iodine solution. Infect Control Hosp Epidemiol. 2014;35(7):826–32. doi:10.1086/676872.

47. Torres EG, Lindmair-Snell JM, Langan JW, Burnikel BG. Is preoperative nasal povidone-iodine as efficient and cost-effective as standard methicillin-resistant *Staphylococcus aureus* screening protocol in total joint arthroplasty? J Arthroplast. 2016;31(1):215–8. doi:10.1016/j.arth.2015.09.030.

48. Segers P, Speekenbrink RG, Ubbink DT, van Ogtrop ML, de Mol BA. Prevention of nosocomial infection in cardiac surgery by decontamination of the nasopharynx and oropharynx with chlorhexidine gluconate: a randomized controlled trial. JAMA. 2006;296(1538–3598 (Electronic)):2460–6. doi:10.1097/sa.0b013e318149f702.

49. Bryce E, Wong T, Forrester L, et al. Nasal photodisinfection and chlorhexidine wipes decrease surgical site infections: a historical control study and propensity analysis. J Hosp Infect. 2014;88(2):89–95. doi:10.1016/j.jhin.2014.06.017.

50. Page CP, Bohnen JM, Fletcher JR, McManus AT, Solomkin JS, Wittmann DH. Antimicrobial prophylaxis for surgical wounds. Guidelines for clinical care. Arch Surg. 1993;128(1):79–88.

51. Classen DC, Evans RS, Pestotnik SL, Horn SD, Menlove RL, Burke JP. The timing of prophylactic administration of antibiotics and the risk of surgical-wound infection. N Engl J Med. 1992;326(5):281–6. doi:10.1056/NEJM199201303260501.

52. Steinberg JP, Braun BI, Hellinger WC, et al. Timing of antimicrobial prophylaxis and the risk of surgical site infections. Ann Surg. 2009;250(1):10–6. doi:10.1097/SLA.0b013e3181ad5fca.

53. Zimmerman SW, Ahrens E, Johnson CA, et al. Randomized controlled trial of prophylactic rifampin for peritoneal dialysis-related infections. Am J Kidney Dis. 1991;18(2):225–31.

54. Walsh TJ, Standiford HC, Reboli AEC, et al. Randomized double-blinded trial of rifampin with either novobiocin or trimethoprim-sulfamethoxazole against methicillin- resistant *Staphylococcus aureus* colonization: prevention of antimicrobial resistance and effect of host factors on outcome. Antimicrob Agents Chemother. 1993;37(6):1334–42. http://aac.asm.org/content/37/6/1334.full.pdf

55. Yu VL, Goetz A, Wagener M, et al. *Staphylococcus aureus* nasal carriage and infection in patients on hemodialysis. Efficacy of antibiotic prophylaxis. N Engl J Med. 1986;315(2):91–6. doi:10.1056/NEJM198607103150204.

56. Garibaldi RA. Prevention of intraoperative wound contamination with chlorhexidine shower and scrub. J Hosp Infect. 1988;11(SUPPL. B):5–9. doi:10.1016/0195-6701(88)90149-1.

57. Hayek LJ, Emerson JM, Gardner AM. A placebo-controlled trial of the effect of two preoperative baths or showers with chlorhexidine detergent on postoperative wound infection rates. J Hosp Infect. 1987;10(2):165–72. http://www.ncbi.nlm.nih.gov/pubmed/2889770

58. Rotter ML, Larsen SO, Cooke EM, et al. A comparison of the effects of preoperative whole-body bathing with detergent alone and with detergent containing chlorhexidine gluconate on the frequency of wound infections after clean surgery. J Hosp Infect. 1988;11(4):310–20. doi:10.1016/0195-6701(88)90083-7.

59. Leigh DA, Stronge JL, Marriner J, Sedgwick J. Total body bathing with "Hibiscrub" (chlorhexidine) in surgical patients: a controlled trial. J Hosp Infect. 1983;4(3):229–35. doi:10.1016/0195-6701(83)90023-3.

60. Lynch W, Davey PG, Malek M, Byrne DJ, Napier A. Cost-effectiveness analysis of the use of chlorhexidine detergent in preoperative whole-body disinfection in wound infection prophylaxis. J Hosp Infect. 1992;21(3):179–91. doi:10.1016/0195-6701(92)90074-V.

61. Mody L, Kauffman CA, McNeil SA, Galecki AT, Bradley SF. Mupirocin-based decolonization of *Staphylococcus aureus* carriers in residents of 2 long-term care facilities: a randomized, double-blind, placebo-controlled trial. Clin Infect Dis. 2003;37(11):1467–74. doi:10.1086/379325.

62. Murphy E, Spencer SJ, Young D, Jones B, Blyth MJG. MRSA colonisation and subsequent risk of infection despite effective eradication in orthopaedic elective surgery. J Bone Jt Surg Br. 2011;93(4):548–51. doi:10.1302/0301-620X.93B4.24969.

63. Bloom BS, Fendrick AM, Chernew ME, Patel P. Clinical and economic effects of mupirocin calcium on preventing *Staphylococcus aureus* infection in hemodialysis patients: a decision analysis. Am J Kidney Dis. 1996;27(0272–6386 SB-IM):687–94.

64. VandenBergh MF, Kluytmans JA, van Hout BA, et al. Cost-effectiveness of perioperative mupirocin nasal ointment in cardiothoracic surgery. Infect Control Hosp Epidemiol. 1996;17(12):786–92. http://www.ncbi.nlm.nih.gov/pubmed/8985764

65. Van Rijen MML, LGM B, Baak DA, Kluytmans JAJW. Reduced costs for *Staphylococcus aureus* carriers treated prophylactically with mupirocin and chlorhexidine in cardiothoracic and orthopaedic surgery. PLoS One. 2012;7(8):1–6. doi:10.1371/journal.pone.0043065.

66. Young LS, Winston LG. Preoperative use of mupirocin for the prevention of healthcare-associated *Staphylococcus aureus* infections: a cost-effectiveness analysis. Infect Control Hosp Epidemiol. 2006;27(12):1304–12. doi:10.1086/509837.

67. Simor AE, Phillips E, McGeer A, et al. Randomized controlled trial of chlorhexidine gluconate for washing, intranasal mupirocin, and rifampin and doxycycline versus no treatment for the eradication of methicillin-resistant *Staphylococcus aureus* colonization. Clin Infect Dis. 2007;44(2):178–85. doi:10.1086/510392.

68. Sai N, Laurent C, Strale H, Denis O, Byl B. Efficacy of the decolonization of methicillin-resistant *Staphylococcus aureus* carriers in clinical practice. Antimicrob Resist Infect Control. 2015;4:56. doi:10.1186/s13756-015-0096-x.

69. Loeb MB, Main C, Eady A, Walker-Dilks C. Antimicrobial drugs for treating methicillin-resistant *Staphylococcus aureus* colonization. Cochrane Database Syst Rev. 2003;4:CD003340. doi:10.1002/14651858.CD003340.

70. Harbarth S, Fankhauser C, Schrenzel J, et al. Universal screening for methicillin-resistant *Staphylococcus aureus* at hospital admission and nosocomial infection in surgical patients. JAMA. 2008;299(10):1149–57. doi:10.1001/jama.299.10.1149.

71. Schweizer ML, Chiang H-Y, Septimus E, et al. Association of a bundled intervention with surgical site infections among patients undergoing cardiac, hip, or knee surgery. JAMA. 2015;313(21):2162. doi:10.1001/jama.2015.5387.

72. Finkelstein R, Rabino G, Mashiah T, et al. Vancomycin versus cefazolin prophylaxis for cardiac surgery in the setting of a high prevalence of methicillin-resistant staphylococcal infections. J Thorac Cardiovasc Surg. 2002;123(2):326–32. doi:10.1067/mtc.2002.119698.

73. Bull AL, Worth LJ, Richards MJ. Impact of vancomycin surgical antibiotic prophylaxis on the development of methicillin-sensitive *Staphylococcus aureus* surgical site infections. Ann Surg. 2012;256(6):1. doi:10.1097/SLA.0b013e31825fa398.

74. Bratzler DW, Dellinger EP, Olsen KM, et al. Clinical practice guidelines for antimicrobial prophylaxis in surgery. Am J Health Syst Pharm. 2013;70(3):195–283. doi:10.2146/ajhp120568.

The Surgical Care Improvement Project Redux: Should CMS Revive Process of Care Measures for Prevention of Surgical Site Infections?

11

Deborah S. Yokoe

The Genesis of the Surgical Care Improvement Project

Many surgical procedures are performed each day in the USA; in 2006 approximately 46 million procedures were performed in inpatient hospital settings [1] and an additional 32 million were performed in ambulatory settings [2]. Surgical site infections (SSIs) are currently one of the most common types of infections associated with care that patients receive in healthcare facilities [3]. Approximately 300,000 SSIs occur each year in the USA [4] although this is likely to be an underestimate because of the challenges around complete ascertainment of these infections, especially for SSIs that are diagnosed after hospital discharge or are sequelae of procedures performed in the ambulatory setting. Estimates of average attributable costs of SSI range from $10,433 to $25,546 per infection (2005 and 2002 dollars, respectively), with substantially higher costs associated with some types of surgery [5–7]. The considerable impact of SSI on national healthcare costs is incontrovertible.

In August of 2002, the Centers for Medicare and Medicaid Services (CMS) and the Centers for Disease Control and Prevention (CDC) established the Surgical Infection Project (SIP) with the goal of improving SSI outcomes by increasing adherence to evidence-based use of perioperative antimicrobial prophylaxis (AMP) [8]. A SIP multidisciplinary expert panel selected these three performance measures for national surveillance and quality improvement:

1. The proportion of patients who have parenteral antimicrobial prophylaxis initiated within 1 h before the surgical incision

2. The proportion of patients who are provided a prophylactic antimicrobial agent that is consistent with currently published guidelines
3. The proportion of patients whose prophylactic antimicrobial therapy is discontinued within 24 h after the end of surgery

The SIP expert panel chose to focus on subgroups of surgical procedures with clear evidence-based benefits of AMP including coronary artery bypass graft and other cardiac surgeries excluding transplantation, vascular surgery, colorectal surgery, hip and knee arthroplasty, and abdominal and vaginal hysterectomy. In 2003, this national initiative evolved into the Surgical Care Improvement Project (SCIP) [9, 10], an extension of SIP supported by multiple agencies and organizations that continued to focus on the three AMP measures described above as well as three additional SSI prevention processes:

4. No hair removal or hair removal with clippers or a depilatory agent (i.e., avoidance of shaving) at the surgical site
5. Control of blood glucose during the immediate postoperative period for patients undergoing cardiac surgery (i.e., glucose of ≤200 mg/dL at 6AM on postoperative days 1 and 2)
6. Maintenance of perioperative normothermia among patients with anesthesia duration of at least 60 min

Because the overall goal of the SCIP was to reduce preventable surgical morbidity and mortality, some additional process measures focused on improving non-SSI outcomes were also included:

7. Surgery patients on beta-blocker therapy prior to arrival who received a beta-blocker during the perioperative period
8. Surgery patients who received appropriate venous thromboembolism prophylaxis within 24 h prior to surgery to 24 h after surgery
9. Surgery patients with urinary catheters removed on postoperative day 1 or postoperative day 2

D.S. Yokoe (✉)
Department of Medicine, Brigham and Women's Hospital and Harvard Medical School, 181 Longwood Avenue, Boston, MA 02115, USA
e-mail: dyokoe@bwh.harvard.edu

© Springer International Publishing AG 2018
G. Bearman et al. (eds.), *Infection Prevention*, DOI 10.1007/978-3-319-60980-5_11

Table 11.1 Surgical Care Improvement Project (SCIP) measures

SCIP performance measure	Performance measure description
SCIP Inf-1	Prophylactic antibiotic started within 1 h prior to surgical incision
SCIP Inf-2	Received prophylactic antibiotic consistent with recommendations
SCIP Inf-3	Prophylactic antibiotics discontinued within 24 h after surgery end time
SCIP Inf-4	Cardiac surgery patients with controlled postoperative blood glucose
SCIP Inf-6	Surgery patients with appropriate hair removal
SCIP Inf-9	Urinary catheter removed on postoperative day 1 or postoperative day 2 with day of surgery being day zero
SCIP Inf-10	Surgery patients with perioperative temperature management
SCIP Card-2	Surgery patients on beta-blocker therapy prior to arrival who received a beta-blocker during the perioperative period
SCIP VTE-2	Surgery patients who received appropriate venous thromboembolism prophylaxis within 24 h prior to surgery to 24 h after surgery

These SCIP measures (Table 11.1) were supported by a number of quality improvement organizations and endorsed by the National Quality Forum.

CMS and The Joint Commission provided the infrastructure for voluntary reporting of SCIP measures by hospitals. As part of the Deficit Reduction Act of 2005, CMS was required to collect hospital-reported performance measures and to make this information available to the public [11]. Although reporting of SCIP measure adherence by hospitals to CMS continued to be voluntary, hospitals that did not report these process measures did not receive their annual 2% CMS market basket reimbursement updates. Hospital-specific SCIP adherence rates were also made accessible to the public on the CMS Hospital Compare website [12]. The Patient Protection and Affordable Care Act of 2010 further accelerated implementation of the CMS Value-Based Purchasing (VBP) and Hospital-Acquired Conditions (HAC) Reduction programs, pay-for-performance programs with substantial potential to impact hospitals' Medicare reimbursement levels [13, 14]. Adherence to the SCIP measures along with other quality metrics was used to determine hospitals' VBP scores starting in 2013.

Evidence to Support the SCIP Measures

Perioperative Antimicrobial Prophylaxis

The evidence to support the impact of appropriate choice of antimicrobial agent(s) used for antimicrobial prophylaxis (AMP) and the importance of the timing of the start of AMP

administration have been summarized in other publications including the "Clinical practice guidelines for antimicrobial prophylaxis in surgery" that was jointly developed by the American Society of Health-System Pharmacists (ASHP), the Infectious Diseases Society of America (IDSA), the Surgical Infection Society (SIS), and the Society for Healthcare Epidemiology of America (SHEA) [15].

1. Choice of AMP Agent(s)

The antimicrobial agent(s) selected for SSI prophylaxis should have activity against the most common SSI organisms associated with the specific surgical procedure. In addition, fundamental AMP principles include using an antimicrobial agent with the narrowest spectrum of activity required for SSI prevention in order to minimize the risk of adverse consequences resulting from impact on the patient's native microbial flora, including the emergence of multidrug-resistant organisms and infection due to *Clostridium difficile*. Overall, the most common organisms associated with SSI following clean procedures continue to be *Staphylococcus aureus* and coagulase-negative staphylococci [16], and therefore recommended AMP regimens for most surgical procedures include an antistaphylococcal agent such as cefazolin. Because organisms that lead to SSI are those that are likely to contaminate the operative bed during the course of the procedure, procedure-specific AMP regimens recommended by SCIP also include agents with activity against other organisms that most commonly contaminate the operative field (e.g., antistaphylococcal, Gram-negative, and anaerobic coverage for colon surgery to cover bowel flora) [15].

2. Timing of the Start of AMP Administration

In order to optimize the impact of AMP, serum and tissue concentrations exceeding the minimal inhibitory concentrations of the agent(s) being used should be achieved prior to the initial surgical incision (i.e., before contamination occurs). Support for the importance of the SCIP recommendation to begin administering the first dose of the AMP agent(s) within 60 min prior to the initial surgical incision (or within 120 min before incision for antimicrobial agents with longer infusion times such as vancomycin and fluoroquinolones) is mainly based on observational study data, including the study by Classen et al. that assessed SSI outcomes for patients who underwent a variety of surgical procedures and found SSI rates to be significantly lower for patients who received AMP starting within 2 h before surgical incision compared to any time after incision (0.59% vs. 3.3%) [17]. When the results were stratified according to the timing of the start of prophylaxis administration in relation to incision time, a statistically significant trend was observed demonstrating increasing risk of SSI with each successive hour that the start of AMP was delayed. Although some studies have demonstrated lower SSI rates associated with shorter time intervals between the start of AMP and start of surgery (e.g., within 30 min prior to incision) [18, 19], the generalizability of those results is unresolved.

3. Minimize the Duration of AMP

Studies assessing the impact of varying durations of AMP strongly indicate that continuation of AMP after incision closure is not associated with added benefit compared with receipt of AMP limited to the procedure duration. Prolonged AMP administration, however, has been associated with adverse consequences including the emergence of resistant organisms [20] and increased risk for *Clostridium difficile* infection [21]. Although minimizing the duration of AMP is unlikely to impact patients' SSI risk, adherence to this antimicrobial stewardship-focused recommendation is important to reduce the risk of unintended adverse consequences associated with unnecessary exposure to antimicrobial agents.

Hair Removal Technique

There is limited high-quality data addressing the impact of hair removal or hair removal techniques on SSI risk. Theoretically, shaving using razors may lead to microabrasions of the skin that can increase the bioburden of microorganisms and therefore the risk for subsequent development of SSI. A Cochrane systematic review [22] demonstrated no significant difference in SSI risk between patients who were shaved and those who had no hair removal (relative risk of 1.75, 95% confidence interval 0.93–3.28) but did find a significantly higher risk of SSI associated with shaving compared with hair removal using clippers (relative risk of 2.03, 95% confidence interval 1.14–3.61). Although the evidence is limited, these results have been used to support the SCIP recommendation for no hair removal or, if hair removal is needed to perform the procedure, to avoid use of razors.

Perioperative Glucose Control

Although SCIP measures focus on blood glucose control in patients undergoing cardiac surgery during the immediate postoperative period [23, 24], beneficial impact of glucose control has also been demonstrated for patients undergoing other types of operative procedures [25–29]. Both the SHEA/IDSA "Strategies to prevent surgical site infections in acute care hospitals: 2014 update" [30] and the recently revised Healthcare Infection Control Practices Advisory Committee (HICPAC) "Guideline for prevention of surgical site infections, 2017" [31] recommend perioperative glycemic control for diabetic and nondiabetic patients undergoing cardiac and

noncardiac procedures. Guideline recommendations regarding blood glucose target levels typically range from <180 to <200. Studies comparing these blood glucose targets to stricter glucose targets (e.g., 80–100 mg/dL or 80–130 mg/dL) suggest that tighter glucose control does not significantly improve SSI risk compared to standard glucose control [32, 33].

Normothermia

High-quality, randomized controlled trial results suggest that maintenance of perioperative normothermia reduces SSI risk for a variety of surgical procedures [34, 35]. The most effective strategies and temperature targets needed to optimize benefit are unclear based on existing literature although some practice guidelines [30, 36] recommend maintaining a temperature of $\geq 36°$ or $\geq 35.5°$.

Did the SCIP Improve SSI Outcomes?

Despite evidence-based support for the beneficial impact of individual SCIP measures on SSI risk and despite national data demonstrating improved adherence to SCIP measures over time, a clear association between adherence to SCIP measures and improvements in SSI outcomes has been difficult to demonstrate [37, 38]. A retrospective cohort study from an inpatient administrative database (Premier, Inc's Perspective Database) that included information from discharges between July 1, 2006, and March 31, 2008, for over 400,000 patients used administrative data to identify surgical patients with probable SSI using an algorithm based on discharge diagnosis codes. The investigators assessed the association between risk of SSI and adherence to individual and composite SCIP measures [39]. Although adherence measured through a global all-or-none composite infection-prevention score was associated with a lower probability of developing a postoperative infection, adherence to individual SCIP measures was not significantly associated with SSI risk. Limitations of this study included dependence on International Classification of Diseases, Ninth Revision, Clinical Modification (ICD-9-CM) codes to identify patients with SSI and restriction of these discharge codes to the hospitalizations when the surgical procedures took place (i.e., no readmission data); this may have substantially limited SSI ascertainment since many SSIs are diagnosed after hospital discharge [40]. A retrospective cohort study by Hawn et al. used National Veteran's Affairs SCIP adherence data and SSI outcomes collected through the Veteran's Affairs Surgical Quality Improvement Program to assess the relationship between SCIP adherence and SSI risk. They found that although adherence to all SCIP measures significantly improved between 2006 and 2009, risk-adjusted SSI rates remained unchanged, and SCIP adherence was not associated with lower SSI risk at the hospital level [41].

Why Is It So Challenging to Demonstrate a Significant Impact on SSI Risk?

There are a number of possible reasons for the apparent limited impact of improvements in adherence to SCIP measures on national SSI rates.

1. Some SCIP measures were not designed to impact SSI risk.

As discussed, the goal of the SCIP program was to improve postoperative outcomes, and several of the SCIP measures are focused on non-SSI complications. For example, limiting the duration of AMP would not be expected to reduce an individual patient's SSI risk. The goal was instead to prevent the emergence of multidrug-resistant organisms and other complications of unnecessary exposure to antimicrobial agents through improved antimicrobial stewardship. Other SCIP measures are focused on preventing cardiac and venous thromboembolism-associated complications and catheter-associated urinary tract infections.

2. Adherence to many of the SCIP measures quickly became "topped off."

Hospitals attained high adherence to many of the SCIP measures shortly after SCIP implementation, and by 2009 national adherence rates exceeded 90% for all SCIP measures [12]. Because of this, further incremental improvements in adherence rates were unlikely to result in substantial improvements in SSI outcomes [42].

3. Reported adherence may not always reflect true practice.

Because CMS relied on self-reporting of SCIP adherence rates by hospitals with minimal data validation and because of pressure on hospitals to demonstrate good performance on publicly reported measures, the potential exists for "gaming" the system by inflating self-reported adherence rates.

4. SCIP recommendations may not be nuanced enough to impact outcomes.

Although AMP has been shown to reduce SSI risk for a wide variety of surgical procedures, it is possible that the specific aspects of AMP that are highlighted by SCIP were not nuanced enough to optimize impact. For example, although a menu of AMP choices for procedure categories was provided by the SCIP [43], a hospital's specific distribution of antimi-

crobial resistance (i.e., the hospital's "antibiogram") may suggest the need for broader or differing coverage than that recommended by the SCIP technical expert panel.

The effectiveness of AMP also depends on achieving adequate antimicrobial concentrations throughout the period of risk when the surgical incision is open. In order to achieve this, weight-based dosing may be required for some antimicrobial agents, including commonly used antimicrobials such as cefazolin and vancomycin. In addition, re-dosing of AMP agents for long surgical procedures is likely to be important for sustaining the protective effect of AMP during the period of risk [15]. Data from some studies suggest that repeat dosing of AMP agents for procedures lasting more than approximately two half-lives of the agent(s) is associated with lower SSI risk compared to procedures without re-dosing [18].

5. SCIP recommendations may constitute minimal requirements, but additional SSI prevention strategies may be needed for further improvements in outcomes.

The practices highlighted by SCIP may reflect minimum requirements for SSI prevention, but optimizing SSI prevention may require adherence to one or more additional interventions. Some of these interventions are discussed below (Table 11.2).

Preoperative Skin Preparation Using a Long-Acting Antiseptic Agent Plus Alcohol

A systematic review by Kamel et al. [44] included data from five randomized controlled trials, two cohort studies, and two case-control studies, including a randomized controlled trial [45] that compared the impact of chlorhexidine-alcohol versus povidone-iodine for preoperative skin preparation prior to clean-contaminated surgical procedures and demonstrated significantly lower SSI risk for patients randomized to receive skin preparation with chlorhexidine-alcohol. The overall conclusion of this systematic review was that conclusive evidence demonstrating the benefit of one

Table 11.2 Examples of supplemental surgical site infection prevention strategies

Use an antiseptic that includes a long-acting agent plus alcohol for preoperative skin preparation
Administer preoperative oral antimicrobial prophylaxis to patients undergoing colorectal surgery
Use hemodynamic goal-directed therapy
Use supplemental oxygenation for patients with normal pulmonary function who undergo general anesthesia with endotracheal intubation
Screen patients for *Staphylococcus aureus* (SA) carriage and decolonize SA carriers for selected surgical procedures
Implement surgical site infection prevention bundles

skin preparation agent over another was lacking but that this should be a high priority topic for further research. A Cochrane systematic review and meta-analysis evaluating the impact of preoperative skin antiseptics on SSI prevention following clean procedures also concluded that there was insufficient evidence to recommend the use of one preoperative skin preparation agent over another, but in a mixed treatment comparison, meta-analysis found that alcohol-containing products had the highest probability of being effective [46].

Administering Preoperative Oral Antimicrobial Prophylaxis to Patients Undergoing Colorectal Surgery

For patients undergoing colorectal surgery, the utility of preoperative oral antimicrobial agents with or without preoperative mechanical bowel preparation remains controversial. Interpreting the results of studies on this topic is challenging because of lack of clarity around the impact of the interaction between mechanical bowel preparation and oral antimicrobial prophylaxis on SSI risk. The results of a Cochrane systematic review and meta-analysis showed no significant difference in SSI risk between patients who did and did not receive mechanical bowel preparation prior to colorectal surgery [47], supporting the NICE surgical site infection guideline recommendation to not use mechanical bowel preparation routinely as a strategy to reduce the risk of surgical site infection for colorectal surgery [36]. Despite this, preoperative mechanical bowel preparation is still commonly favored by colorectal surgeons [48]. Among patients who undergo mechanical bowel preparation, receipt of preoperative oral antimicrobial agents, usually consisting of oral neomycin plus erythromycin or metronidazole given two or three times during the day prior to surgery, has been associated with significant reductions in SSI risk following colorectal surgery [49, 50]. Most studies demonstrating improved SSI outcomes associated with oral antimicrobial prophylaxis also utilized mechanical bowel preparations, making it difficult to extrapolate results to patients who receive oral AMP without mechanical bowel preparation prior to colorectal surgery. Overall, study results suggest a benefit to preoperative oral antimicrobial prophylaxis when provided in conjunction with mechanical bowel preparation.

Hemodynamic Goal-Directed Therapy

A systematic review and meta-analysis by Dalfino et al. [51] evaluated the impact of hemodynamic goal-directed therapy on SSI risk. Goal-directed therapy was defined as perioperative monitoring and manipulation of hemodynamic parameters to reach normal or supraoptimal values by fluid infusion alone or in combination with inotropic therapy within 8 h after surgery. In this meta-analysis of 18 randomized controlled trials, standard therapy was associated with significantly higher SSI risk compared with goal-directed therapy

(odds ratio of 5.8, 95% confidence interval 0.46–0.74). Hemodynamic goal-directed therapy is a component of "Enhanced Recovery After Surgery" protocols (see below).

Supplemental Oxygenation

Although studies evaluating the impact of supplemental oxygenation on SSI risk have had varying results, overall they provide support for the benefit of administering increased fraction of inspired oxygen ($FiO2$) both intraoperatively and post-extubation in the immediate postoperative period for patients with normal pulmonary function who undergo general anesthesia with endotracheal intubation. Benefit was seen in studies in which normothermia and adequate volume replacement were monitored and maintained [52, 53, 54], suggesting the importance of optimizing parameters needed to ensure tissue oxygen delivery in order to maximize the impact of supplemental oxygenation on SSI prevention.

Preoperative *Staphylococcus aureus* Screening and Decolonization

A number of recent studies have assessed the impact of a variety of strategies that include *Staphylococcus aureus* (SA) decolonization, including a randomized controlled trial performed in the Netherlands in which patients were screened for SA carriage on hospital admission and patients found to be SA carriers were then randomized to receive either 5 days of intranasal mupirocin and chlorhexidine bathing or placebo. In this study, SA carriers who received intranasal mupirocin and chlorhexidine bathing had significantly lower SSI risk [55]. A systematic review and meta-analysis evaluating studies that assessed the effectiveness of nasal SA decolonization and inclusion of a glycopeptide for AMP on SSI risk for patients undergoing cardiac surgery and orthopedic total joint replacement surgery concluded that a bundled intervention including nasal decolonization for all SA carriers and glycopeptide prophylaxis for methicillin-resistant SA (MRSA) carriers may decrease rates of SSI caused by SA or other Gram-positive bacteria [56]. A subsequent prospective, observational multicenter study involving patients who underwent cardiac surgery and hip or knee replacement procedures demonstrated that a bundled intervention that included preoperative SA screening, decolonization of SA carriers with intranasal mupirocin and topical chlorhexidine, and targeted addition of vancomycin to cefazolin or cefuroxime AMP for MRSA carriers was associated with a significantly lower deep incisional and organ/space SSI risk (rate ratio 0.58, 95% confidence interval 0.37–0.92) [57].

SSI Prevention Bundles

During recent years, there has been increasing interest in using bundled protocols to prevent healthcare-associated infections. A "bundle" is usually defined as a grouping of evidence-based practices that individually improve care.

Central line-associated bloodstream infection (CLABSI) prevention bundles, for example, have been shown to result in significant improvements in CLABSI outcomes [58]. Some examples of SSI prevention bundles that merit attention are discussed below.

1. Surgical Safety Checklist

Haynes et al. in collaboration with the World Health Organization evaluated a Surgical Safety Checklist in a multinational, multicenter observational study. Their checklist consisted of questions assessing adherence to practices aimed at preventing surgical complications. The checklist questions were administered at three perioperative time points (before induction of anesthesia, before skin incision, and before patient left the operating room). Implementation of the checklist was associated with significant improvements in SSI and mortality rates in a before-after comparison [59].

2. Other SSI Prevention Bundles

A variety of other SSI prevention bundles have been evaluated. These typically include SCIP-recommended practices in addition to varying combinations of supplemental practices including many of those discussed above. A systematic review and meta-analysis by Tanner et al. assessed the impact of SSI prevention bundles for colorectal surgery using results from 13 studies and concluded that the use of evidence-based surgical care bundles significantly reduced the risk of SSI compared with standard care (risk ratio of 0.55, 95% confidence interval of 0.39–0.77) [60].

3. Enhanced Recovery After Surgery

The use of a bundle of perioperative practices aimed at improving surgical recovery following colorectal procedures referred to as Enhanced Recovery After Surgery (ERAS) has been gaining support in the surgical community based on a growing body of literature suggesting beneficial impact of ERAS bundles on postoperative outcomes, including SSI [61–64]. ERAS protocols typically include administration of a carbohydrate beverage prior to surgery, avoidance of sedatives, goal-directed fluid administration, multimodal pain control minimizing the use of narcotics, and postoperative immediate diet and mobilization. ERAS protocols have been implemented with and without additional bundles of practices specifically aimed at SSI prevention. For example, a study by Keenan et al. evaluated sequential implementation of an ERAS pathway followed by a SSI prevention bundle and found that introduction of the ERAS pathway alone resulted in reduced length of stay and improved superficial

and organ/space SSI rates, while subsequent addition of an SSI bundle that included mechanical bowel preparation with oral antibiotics, preoperative chlorhexidine cleansing of patient, chlorhexidine-alcohol preoperative skin preparation, standardized AMP, maintenance of euglycemia and normothermia, fascial wound protectors, gown and glove change prior to fascial and skin closure, and a dedicated wound closure tray led to further significant reductions in SSI and sepsis rates [65].

The impact of SSI bundles likely depends on adherence to bundle elements, and some studies demonstrated that the number of bundle processes that were adhered to correlated with patients' SSI risk, suggesting an additive effect for each SSI prevention element [66].

Change of Focus from Process to Outcome Measures Used for Pay for Performance

Over the past several years, CMS's approach to assessing the quality of care provided by hospitals has undergone a major shift in focus from process to outcome measures. In the area of SSI prevention, the shift toward focus on SSI outcomes was reflected by a change in CMS reimbursement practices implemented in October of 2008 in which CMS ceased additional payment for hospital-acquired conditions not present on admission (POA), including some specific types of SSI [67]. Beginning in 2012, acute care hospitals were required to either report SSI outcomes following abdominal hysterectomy and colon surgery in addition to other healthcare-associated infection outcomes to CMS as part of the Hospital Inpatient Quality Reporting Program or receive a 2% penalty on Medicare reimbursement. As part of the CMS HAC Reduction program, beginning in fiscal year 2016, CMS reimbursement was tied to hospital performance around SSI and other healthcare-associated infection outcomes. Hospitals with HAC scores that fall within the lowest-performing quartile are subject to a 1% loss in total Medicare inpatient prospective payment system (IPPS) reimbursement [68].

Metrics used to determine a hospital's VBP score are divided into domains that include clinical process of care (including the SCIP measures), patient experience, and outcome measures (including SSI outcomes following colon surgery and abdominal hysterectomy procedures). In fiscal year 2013, process of care measures accounted for 70% of a hospital's VBP score, but by fiscal year 2016, process of care measures accounted for only 20% of VBP scores compared to a 40% weight for outcome measures. Starting in fiscal year 2017, VBP will no longer include SCIP process of care measures. By fiscal year 2017, a hospital's VBP performance will have the potential to result in forfeit of up to a 2% withhold in Medicare IPPS base operating payments.

Limitations of SSI Outcome Measures for Pay for Performance

Although judging the performance of hospitals based on SSI outcomes makes intuitive sense since the goal of quality improvement efforts is ultimately to prevent postoperative complications, utilizing SSI outcomes as pay-for-performance metrics has led to a number of major challenges.

SSI Surveillance Relies on Subjective Interpretation of Medical Information and Is Vulnerable to Gaming

There are a number of studies that demonstrate substantial variation in the completeness of SSI data reported by hospitals [69, 70]. Even when using standardized CDC National Healthcare Safety Network (NHSN) surveillance definitions [71], application of SSI surveillance definitions requires some subjective interpretation of clinical information. For example, assessing the presence of "purulent drainage," a criterion for both deep incisional and organ/space SSIs, requires both highly subjective interpretation of the quality of drainage material and documentation in the medical record. Some SSI criteria also depend on provider practices that may vary between hospitals; for example, facilities that are more aggressive about aspirating and culturing postoperative intra-abdominal fluid collections are more likely to fulfill microbiology-based SSI criteria.

Ascertainment of SSI diagnosed after hospital discharge can be particularly challenging, especially for postoperative infections diagnosed and treated solely in the ambulatory setting or SSI diagnosed and treated at healthcare facilities other than the hospital where the original surgical procedure took place. The proportion of patients with SSI who are readmitted to the same hospital where the index surgery took place can vary considerably among healthcare facilities, and this can impact the completeness of SSI ascertainment and relative ranking of hospitals based on SSI outcomes [72].

Surveillance Bias and Accessibility to Data

The completeness of hospitals' SSI ascertainment is highly dependent on the intensity of resources focused on SSI surveillance. Healthcare facilities with robust electronic health records or surveillance processes that effectively utilize automated medical data will be more likely to capture information that can be used to determine the presence of postoperative infections. These hospitals are therefore likely to report more SSI events than healthcare facilities with limited access to electronic health data and can be erroneously characterized and penalized as poor performers. Variability in infection preventionist access to electronic surveillance systems is reflected in the finding by Stone et al. that only 34.3% of NHSN facilities reported using an electronic surveillance system for identifying healthcare-associated infections [73]. In addition, SSI surveillance is resource intensive, requiring review of a broad range of clinical information in order to apply surveillance definitions, and the effort available for surveillance can vary substantially between facilities, affecting the completeness of SSI ascertainment [74].

Using SSI Outcomes to Judge the Performance of Hospitals Requires Adequate Risk Adjustment

In order to meaningfully compare hospitals' SSI outcomes, adequate risk adjustment is critically important in order to take account of intrinsic differences in patient risk factors that are not modifiable through improvements in hospitals' practices. Currently, the standardized infection ratio for complex SSI used for CMS submission utilizes only a small number of variables for SSI risk adjustment. For example, for patients undergoing colon surgery and abdominal hysterectomy procedures, only age, gender, body mass index, American Society of Anesthesiologists (ASA) score, presence or absence of diabetes, and wound closure technique are included in the logistic regression model used for risk adjustment [75]. Other potentially important risk factors including medical comorbidities that increase SSI risk (e.g., active malignancies) are not currently taken into account, and hospitals with more complex patient populations at higher intrinsic risk for SSI may be more likely to receive lower performance rankings and to incur financial penalties. The possibility of inadequate risk adjustment was highlighted in a recent study examining Medicare fiscal year 2015 payments that found that major teaching hospitals were four times more likely to receive the HAC Reduction penalty compared to nonteaching hospitals [76].

Outcome Measures Are Challenging to Apply to Small-Volume Hospitals

Because SSIs are relatively rare events and because of limitations in the stability and reliability of SSI outcome measures for hospitals that perform relatively few surgical procedures, SSI data for all hospitals with <1 expected SSI per year based on procedure volume are excluded from metrics contributing to that hospital's HAC score and ranking. Based on CMS Hospital Compare data, this meant that SSI outcome measures from over 30% of hospitals performing colon surgery and over 60% of hospitals performing abdominal hysterectomy procedures were excluded from metrics used to determine those hospitals' HAC scores during the performance period of April 2014 through March 2015 [77]. This is problematic for a number of reasons. First, it means absence of SSI performance measures for a large proportion of hospitals that perform the targeted surgical procedures. Secondly, there is evidence that hospitals that perform a lower volume of surgical procedures may have higher postoperative complication rates [78–80]; this means that the hospitals that are most likely to benefit from SSI-related quality improvement efforts are excluded from submitting SSI metrics and that some larger-volume hospitals may consequently receive undeserved financial penalties. The study by Kahn et al. described above found that hospitals with 400 or more beds were almost twice as likely to receive the HAC penalty and more than twice as likely to be penalized under VBP compared to hospitals with fewer than 100 beds [76].

The limitations of using SSI outcome measures for inter-hospital comparisons are underscored by studies that suggest that hospitals' performance around healthcare-associated infection metrics may not adequately reflect the quality of care provided. A study by Rajaram et al. evaluated hospitals that were penalized based on HAC Reduction program performance data used for fiscal year 2015 assessments and examined the association between those hospitals' HAC scores and other quality metrics. The investigators found that hospitals that were penalized under the HAC program were more likely to have quality accreditations, to offer advanced services, to be major teaching institutions, and to have better performance on other process and outcome measures, suggesting a disconnect between hospitals' HAC scores and the quality of care provided [81].

Going Forward: Back to the Future?

CMS incentives and penalties have the potential to exert powerful motivating forces on hospital decision-makers and can result in major changes in prioritization of hospital resources. For this reason, thoughtful alignment of incentives and penalties with performance metrics that are likely to promote adherence to processes that result in improved patient outcomes is critically important. As discussed above, CMS is in the process of transitioning from using process measures to outcome measures as pay-for-performance SSI metrics. Limitations around the ability to standardize application of SSI surveillance definitions and methods and to adequately risk adjust SSI outcomes may unfairly penalize some high-performing hospitals with robust surveillance processes or complex, intrinsically high-risk patients and excludes low-volume hospitals from evaluation. For these

reasons, investing research into improving our ability to perform adequate SSI outcome risk adjustment is essential.

Until these challenges are resolved, it may also be worth considering shifting the focus of pay-for-performance programs back toward SSI process measures. In order to optimize the impact of SSI process of care measures, it will be important to choose processes that are evidence-based and that augment fundamental SSI prevention practices already in place at most hospitals, to consider procedure-specific modifications of recommendations, and to take into consideration the additive effects of bundled approaches to SSI prevention.

Importantly, our ability to prevent SSI is limited by gaps in our understanding about which perioperative practices, individually or in combination, are most likely to impact SSI risk. We also have limited insight into about how best to implement and sustain adherence to those practices that have been shown to be effective. In order to optimize national efforts to improve surgical outcomes, it will be essential to allocate adequate financial resources to support high-quality SSI prevention research.

References

1. DeFrances CJ, Lucas CA, Buie VC, Golosinskiy A. 2006 National Hospital Discharge Survey. National health statistics reports; no 5. (2008); Available at: http://www.cdc.gov/nchs/data/nhsr/nhsr005.pdf. Accessed 2 Feb 2016.
2. Cullen KA, Hall MJ, Golosinskiy A. Ambulatory Surgery in the United States, 2006. National health statistics reports; no 11. Revised. (2009); Available at: http://www.cdc.gov/nchs/data/nhsr/nhsr011.pdf. Accessed 2 Feb 2016.
3. Magill SS, Edwards JR, Bamberg W, et al. Multistate point-prevalence survey of healthcare-associated infections. New Engl J Med. 2014;370:1198–208.
4. Umscheid CA, Mitchell MD, Doshi JA, Agarwal R, Williams K, Brennan PJ. Estimating the proportion of healthcare-associated infections that are reasonably preventable and the related mortality and costs. Infect Control Hosp Epidemiol. 2011;32(2):101–14.
5. Scott RD. The direct medical costs of healthcare-associated infections in U.S. hospitals and the benefits of prevention. Centers for Disease Control and Prevention (2009); Available at: http://www.cdc.gov/hai/pdfs/hai/scott_costpaper.pdf Accessed 29 Feb 2016.
6. Stone PW, Braccia D, Larson E. Systematic review of economic analyses of health care associated infections. Am J Infect Control. 2005;33(9):501–9.
7. Zimlichman E, Henderson D, Tamir O, et al. Health care-associated infections: a meta-analysis of costs and financial impact on the US health care system. JAMA Intern Med. 2013;173(22):2039–46.
8. Bratzler DW, Houck PM. Antimicrobial prophylaxis for surgery: an advisory statement from the National Surgical Infection Prevention Project. Clin Infect Dis. 2004;38:1706–15.
9. Bratzler DW, Hunt DR. The surgical infection prevention and surgical care improvement projects: national initiatives to improve outcomes for patients having surgery. Clin Infect Dis. 2006;43:322–30.
10. Dellinger EP, Hausmann SM, Bratzler DW, et al. Hospitals collaborate to decrease surgical site infections. Am J Surg. 2005;190:9–15.

11. U.S. Government Printing Office. The deficit reduction act of 2005. Available at: https://www.gpo.gov/fdsys/pkg/PLAW-109publ171/html/PLAW-109publ171.htm Accessed 26 Feb 2016.

12. Centers for Medicare & Medicaid Services. Hospital compare. Available at: https://www.cms.gov/medicare/quality-initiatives-patient-assessment-instruments/hospitalqualityinits/hospitalcompare.html. Accessed 26 Feb 2016.

13. Centers for Medicare & Medicaid Services. Medicare program: hospital inpatient prospective payment systems for acute care hospitals and the long-term care hospital prospective payment system and fiscal year 2013 rates; hospitals' resident caps for graduate medical education payment purposes; quality reporting requirements for specific providers and for ambulatory surgical centers. Final rule. Fed Regist. 2012;77(170):53257–750.

14. Centers for Medicare & Medicaid Services. Medicare program; hospital inpatient value-based purchasing program. Final rule. Fed Regist. 2011;76(88):26490–547.

15. Bratzler DW, Dellinger EP, Olsen KM, et al. Clinical practice guidelines for antimicrobial prophylaxis in surgery. Am J Health-System Pharm. 2013;70(3):195–283.

16. Sievert DM, Ricks P, Edwards JR, et al. Antimicrobial-resistant pathogens associated with healthcare-associated infections: summary of data reported to the National Healthcare Safety Network at the Centers for Disease Control and Prevention, 2009–2010. Infect Control Hosp Epidemiol. 2013;34(1):1–14.

17. Classen DC, Evans RS, Pestotnik SL, et al. The timing of prophylactic administration of antibiotics and the risk of surgical-wound infection. New Engl J Med. 1992;326:281–6.

18. Steinberg JP, Braun BI, Hellinger WC, et al. Timing of antimicrobial prophylaxis and the risk of surgical site infections: results from the trial to reduce antimicrobial prophylaxis errors. Ann Surg. 2009;205(1):10–6.

19. van Kasteren ME, Mannien J, Ott A, et al. Antibiotic prophylaxis and the risk of surgical site infections following total hip arthroplasty: timely administration is the most important factor. Clin Infect Dis. 2007;44(7):921–7.

20. Harbath S, Samore MH, Lichtenberg D, Carmeli Y. Prolonged antibiotic prophylaxis after cardiovascular surgery and its effect on surgical site infections and antimicrobial resistance. Circulation. 2000;101:2916–21.

21. Coakley BA, Sussman ES, Wolfson TS, et al. Postoperative antibiotics correlate with worse outcomes after appendectomy for nonperforated appendicitis. J A Coll Surg. 2011;213(6):778–83.

22. Tanner J, Norrie P, Melen K. Preoperative hair removal to reduce surgical site infection. (2011). Cochrane Database of Systematic Reviews issue 11: CD004122.

23. Furnary AP, Zerr KJ, Grunkemeier GL, Starr A. Continuous intravenous insulin infusion reduces the incidence of deep sternal wound infection in diabetic patients after cardiac surgical procedures. Ann Thorac Surg. 1999;67:352–60.

24. Carr JM, Sellke FW, Fey M, et al. Implementing tight glucose control after coronary artery bypass surgery. Ann Thorac Surg. 2005;80:902–9.

25. Dronge AS, Perkal MF, Kancir S, Concato J, Aslan M, Rosenthal RA. Long-term glycemic control and postoperative infectious complications. Arch Surg. 2006;141(4):375–80.

26. Golden SH, Peart-Vigilance C, Kao WH, Brancati FL. Perioperative glycemic control and the risk of infectious complications in a cohort of adults with diabetes. Diabetes Care. 1999;22(9):1408–14.

27. Olsen MA, Nepple JJ, Riew KD, et al. Risk factors for surgical site infection following orthopaedic spinal operations. J Bone Joint Surg Am. 2008;90(1):62–9.

28. Kwon S, Thompson R, Dellinger P, Yanez D, Farrohki E, Flum D. Importance of perioperative glycemic control in general surgery: a report from the surgical care and outcomes assessment program. Ann Surg. 2013;257(1):8–14.

29. Umpierrez GE, Smiley D, Jacobs S, et al. Randomized study of basal-bolus insulin therapy in the inpatient management of patients with type 2 diabetes undergoing general surgery (RABBIT 2 surgery). Diabetes Care. 2011;34(2):256–61.

30. Anderson DJ, Podgorny K, Berríos-Torres SI, et al. Strategies to prevent surgical site infections in acute care hospitals: 2014 update. Infect Control Hosp Epidemiol. 2014;35(suppl 2):S66–88.

31. Berríos-Torres SI, Umscheid CA, Bratzler DW, et al. Centers for Disease Control and Prevention guideline for the prevention of surgical site infection, 2017. JAMA Surg. 2017; [published online May 3, 2017]. JAMASurg. doi:10.1001/jamasurg.2017.0904

32. Gandhi GY, Nuttall GA, Abel MD, et al. Intensive intraoperative insulin therap versus conventional glucose management during cardiac surgery: a randomized trial. Ann Intern Med. 2007;146(4):233–43.

33. Chan RP, Galas FR, Hajjar LA, et al. Intensive perioperative glucose control does not improve outcomes of patients submitted to open-heart surgery: a randomized controlled trial. Clinics (Sao Paulo). 2009;64(1):51–60.

34. Kurz A, Sessler DI, Lenhardt R. Study of wound infection and temperature group. Perioperative normothermia to reduce the incidence of surgical wound infection and shorten hospitalization. N Engl J Med. 1996;334(19):1209–15.

35. Melling AC, Ali B, Scott EM, Leaper DJ. Effects of preoperative warming on the incidence of wound infection after clean surgery: a randomised controlled trial. Lancet. 2001;358(9285):876–80.

36. National Institute for Health and Clinical Excellence (NICE). Surgical site infection: prevention and treatment of surgical site infection. London: NICE, (2008). http:www.nice.org.uk/nicemedia/pdf/CG74NICEGuideline.pdf. Accessed Feb 26 2016.

37. Nguyen N, Yegiyants S, Kaloostian C, Abbas MA, Difronzo LA. The surgical care improvement Project (SCIP) initiative to reduce infection in elective colorectal surgery: which performance measures affect outcome? Am Surg. 2008;74(10):1012–6.

38. Hawn MT, Itani KM, Gray SH, Vick CC, Henderson W, Houston TK. Association of timely administration of prophylactic antibiotics for major surgical procedures and surgical site infection. J Am Coll Surg. 2008;206(5):814–9.

39. Stulberg JJ, Delaney CP, Neuhauser DV, Aron DC, Fu P, Koroukian SM. Adherence to surgical care improvement Project measures and the association with postoperative infections. JAMA. 2010;303(24):2479–85.

40. Sands K, Vineyard G, Platt R. Surgical site infections occurring after hospital discharge. J Infect Dis. 1996;173(4):963–70.

41. Hawn MT, Vick CC, Richman J, Holman W, Deierhoi RJ, Graham LA, Henderson WG, KMF I. Surgical site infection prevention: time to move beyond the surgical care improvement program. Ann Surg. 2011;254:494–501.

42. Bratzler DW. Surgical care improvement project performance measures: good but not perfect. Clin Infect Dis. 2013;56(3):428–9.

43. The Joint Commission. Specifications manual for national hospital inpatient quality measures. Available at: http://www.jointcommission.org/specifications_manual_for_national_hospital_inpatient_quality_measures.aspx. Accessed 26 Feb 2016.

44. Kamel C, McGahan L, Polisena J, et al. Preoperative skin antiseptic preparations for preventing surgical site infections: a systematic review. Infect Control Hosp Epidemiol. 2012;33:608–17.

45. Darouiche RO, Wall MJ, Itani KM, et al. Chlorhexidine-alcohol versus povidone-iodine for surgical-site antisepsis. NEJM. 2010;362:18–26.

46. Dumville JC, McFarlane E, Edwards P, Lipp A, Holmes A. Preoperative skin antiseptics for preventing surgical wound infections after clean surgery. Cochrane Database Syst Rev 2013; Issue 3. Art. No.: CD003949. doi:10.1002/14651858.CD003949.pub3

47. Guenaga KF, Matos D, Wille-Jorgensen P. Mechanical bowel preparation for elective colorectal surgery. Cochrane Database Syst Rev. 2011;9:CD001544.

48. Englesbe MJ, Brooks L, Kubus J, et al. A statewide assessment of surgical site infection following colectomy: the role of oral antibiotics. Ann Surg. 2010;252(3):514–9.

49. Englesbe; Nelson RL, Gladman E, Barbateskovic M. Antimicrobial prophylaxis for colorectal surgery. Cochrane Database of Syst Rev 2014; Issue 5. Art. No.: CD001181. doi: 10.1002/14651858. CD001181.pub4

50. Deierhoi RJ, Dawes LG, Vick C, Itani KMF, Hawn MT. Choice of intravenous antibiotic prophylaxis for colorectal surgery does matter. J Am Coll Surg. 2013;217:763–9.

51. Dalfino L, Giglio MT, Puntillo F, et al. Haemodynamic goal-directed therapy and postoperative infections: earlier is better. A systematic review and meta-analysis. Crit Care. 2011;153:R154.

52. Belda FJ, Aguilera L, Garcia de la Asuncion J, et al. Supplemental perioperative oxygen and the risk of surgical wound infection: a randomized controlled trial. JAMA. 2005;294(16):2035–2042.

53. Bickel A, Gurevits M, Vamos R, et al. Perioperative hyperoxygenation and wound site infection following surgery for acute appendicitis: a randomized, prospective, controlled trial. Arch Surg. 2011;146(4):464–470.

54. Robert Greif, Ozan Akça, Ernst-Peter Horn, Andrea Kurz, Daniel I. Sessler, (2000) Supplemental Perioperative Oxygen to Reduce the Incidence of Surgical-Wound Infection. New England Journal of Medicine 342 (3):161–167.

55. Bode LG, Kluytmans JA, Wertheim HF, et al. Preventing surgical-site infections in nasal carriers of *Staphylococcus aureus*. New Engl J Med. 2010;362:9–17.

56. Schweizer M, Perencevich E, McDanel J, et al. Effectiveness of a bundled intervention of decolonization and prophylaxis to decrease Gram positive surgical site infections after cardiac or orthopedic surgery: systematic review and meta-analysis. BMJ. 2013;346:f2743.

57. Schweizer ML, et al. Association of a bundled intervention with surgical site infections among patients undergoing cardiac, hip or knee surgery. JAMA. 2015;313(21):2162–71.

58. Pronovost P, Needham D, Berenholtz S, et al. An intervention to decrease catheter-related bloodstream infections in the ICU. N Engl J Med. 2006;355:2725–32.

59. Haynes AB, Weiser TG, Berry WR, et al. A surgical safety checklist to reduce morbidity and mortality in a global population. New Engl J Med. 2009;360:491–9.

60. Tanner J, Padley W, Assadian O, Leaper D, Kiernan M, Edmiston C. Do surgical care bundles reduce the risk of surgical site infections in patients undergoing colorectal surgery? A systematic review and cohort meta-analysis of 8,515 patients. Surgery. 2015;158:66–77.

61. Gustafsson UO, Scott MJ, Schwenk W, et al. Guidelines for perioperative care in elective colonic surgery: enhanced recovery after surgery (ERAS(R)) Society recommendations. World J Surg. 2013;37:259–84.

62. Getzeiler CV, Rotramel A, Wilson C, et al. Prospective study of colorectal enhanced recovery after surgery in a community hospital. JAMA Surg. 2014;149:955–61.

63. Nicholson A, Lowe MC, Parker J, et al. Systematic review and meta-analysis of enhanced recovery programmes in surgical patients. Br J Surg. 2014;101:172–88.

64. Zhuang CL, Ye XZ, Zhang XC, et al. Enhanced recovery after surgery programs versus traditional care for colorectal surgery: a meta-analysis of randomized controlled trials. Dis Colon Rectum. 2013;56:667–78.

65. Keenan JE, Speicher PJ, Nussbaum DP, Abdelgadir Adam M, Miller TM, Mantyh CR, Thacker JKM. Improving outcomes in colorectal surgery by sequential implementation of multiple standardized care programs. J Am Coll Surg. 2015;221:404–14.

66. Waits SA, Fritze D, Banarjee M, et al. Developing an argument for bundled interventions to reduce surgical site infection in colorectal surgery. Surgery. 2014;155(4):602–6.

67. Centers for Medicare & Medicaid. Hospital-acquired conditions. Available at: http://www.cms.gov/Medicare/Medicare-Fee-for-Service-Payment/HospitalAcqCond/Hospital-Acquired_Conditions.html Accessed 29 Feb 2016.

68. Centers for Medicare & Medicaid Services. Medicare program; hospital inpatient prospective payment systems for acute care hospitals and the long-term care hospital prospective payment system and fiscal year 2015 rates; quality reporting requirements for specific providers; reasonable compensation equivalents for physician services in excluded hospitals and certain teaching hospitals; provider administrative appeals and judicial review; enforcement provisions for organ transplant centers; and electronic health record (EHR) incentive program. Final rule. Fed Register. 2014;79(163):49853–50536.

69. Calderwood MS, Ma A, Khan YM, et al. Use of Medicare diagnosis and procedure codes to improve detection of surgical site infections following hip arthroplasty, knee arthroplasty, and vascular surgery. Infect Control Hosp Epidemiol. 2012;33(1):40–9.

70. Yokoe DS, Khan Y, Olsen MA, et al. Enhanced surgical site infection surveillance following hysterectomy, vascular, and colorectal surgery. Infect Control Hosp Epidemiol. 2012;33(8):768–73.

71. Centers for Disease Control and Prevention. National healthcare safety network. Surgical site infection (SSI) event. Available at: www.cdc.gov/nhsn/pdfs/pscmanual/9pscssicurrent.pdf. Accessed 28 Feb 2016.

72. Yokoe DS, Avery TR, Platt R, Huang SS. Reporting surgical site infections following total hip and knee arthroplasty: impact of limiting surveillance to the operative hospital. Clin Infect Dis. 2013;57(9):1282–8.

73. Stone PW, Pogorzelska-Maziarz M, Herzig CT, et al. State of infection prevention in US hospitals enrolled in the National Healthcare Safety Network. Am J Infect Control. 2014;42(2):94–9.

74. Talbot TR, et al. Public reporting of healthcare-associated infection data: recommendations from the healthcare infection control practices advisory committee. Ann Intern Med. 2013;159:631–5.

75. Centers for Disease Control and Prevention. National Healthcare Safety Network. The NHSN Standardized Infection Ratio (SIR). (2017). Available at: https://www.cdc.gov/nhsn/pdfs/ps-analysis-resources/nhsn-sir-guide.pdf Accessed 17 Jul 2017.

76. Kahn CN, Ault T, Potetz L, Walke T, Chambers JH, Burch S. Assessing Medicare's hospital pay-for-performance programs and whether they are achieving their goals. Health Aff. 2015;34(8):1281–8.

77. Centers for Medicare & Medicaid Services. Hospital compare datasets. Available at: https://data.medicare.gov/data/hospital-compare Accessed 26 Feb 2016.

78. Katz JN, Losina E, Barrett J, Phillips CB, Mahomed NN, Lew RA, et al. Association between hospital and surgeon procedure volume and outcomes of total hip replacement in the United States Medicare population. J Bone Joint Surg Am. 2001;83-A(11):1622–9.

79. Birkmeyer JD, Siewers AE, Finlayson EV, Stukel TA, Lucas FL, Batista I, et al. Hospital volume and surgical mortality in the United States. N Engl J Med. 2002;346(15):1128–37.

80. Guebbels EL, Wille JC, Nagelkerke NJ, Vandenbroucke-Grauls CM, Grobbee DE, de Boer AS. Hospital-related determinants for surgical-site infection following hip arthroplasty. Infect Control Hosp Epidemiol. 2005;26(5):435–41.

81. Rajaram R, Chung JW, Kinnier CV, Barnard C, Mohanty S, Pavey ES, McHugh MC, Bilimoria KY. Hospital characteristics associated with penalties in the Center for Medicare & Medicaid services hospital-acquired condition reduction program. JAMA. 2015;314(4):375–83.

Healthcare Worker Apparel and Infection Prevention

Salma Muhammad Abbas and Gonzalo Bearman

Healthcare Worker (HCW) Apparel and Infection Prevention

HCW attire is considered an important component of professionalism [1]. Traditionally, items of clothing such as lab coats and scrubs have been worn by HCWs for identification by hospital staff and patients. These garments also provide protection against infections caused by organisms such as methicillin-resistant *Staphylococcus aureus* (MRSA), *Enterobacteriaceae*, *Acinetobacter* spp., Ebola, respiratory viruses, as well as blood-borne viruses such as HIV, hepatitis B, and hepatitis C by preventing exposure to blood and body fluids [2]. According to one study, nasal carriage rates of MRSA among HCWs may range from 0.3 to 12%, and colonized individuals may spread these infections to others [3]. While the role of HCW apparel as a vehicle for the spread of infections is not completely understood, a growing body of evidence suggests that contaminated soft surfaces such as curtains, upholstery, and apparel are implicated in the transmission of infectious diseases [2].

Hospital Policies Regarding HCW Attire

Hospital policies pertaining to HCW attire address the general appearance of employees and provide guidelines for dress code appropriate for settings such as procedure areas and operating rooms [1]. Most of these outline detailed instructions regarding the use of items such as masks, head

S.M. Abbas
Infectious Diseases, Virginia Commonwealth University, Richmond, VA, USA
e-mail: Salma.muhammadabbas@vcuhealth.org

G. Bearman (✉)
VCUHS Epidemiology and Infection Control, North Hospital, 2nd Floor, Room 2-073, 1300 East Marshall Street, Richmond, VA 23298-0019, USA
e-mail: gonzalo.bearman@vcuhealth.org

covers, scrubs, footwear, and jewelry and are in agreement with the Association of Perioperative Nursing (AORN) standards [1]. Attire outside sterile procedure areas is not as well-defined at most facilities and practices vary across centers. Several facilities support the use of white coats, while others adopt measures such as "bare below the elbows" (BBE).

White Coats, Scrubs, and Uniforms

Some institutions mandate the use of lab coats and uniforms for certain HCWs in favor of projecting a professional image. Over recent years, these have been linked to the spread of multidrug-resistant organisms (MDROs). Microorganisms are capable of surviving in moisture and protein-rich soil or dirt that contaminates HCW apparel [2]. According to one study, 23% of lab coats were found to be contaminated with methicillin-sensitive *S. aureus* (MSSA) and 18% with MRSA [4]. In another study, samples were collected from uniforms of 135 HCWs including nurses and physicians, 58% of whom had reported changing uniforms every day. Potentially pathogenic bacteria were cultured from 60% of the uniforms [5]. In a study carried out by Munoz-Price and colleagues, cultures were obtained from the hands and apparel of HCWs working in five intensive care units. Microorganisms were isolated from 103 hands which constituted 86% of the total number cultured. These included *Staphylococcus aureus*, *Acinetobacter* spp., enterococci, and skin flora. Bacterial growth on hands was more likely to be associated with contamination of lab coats when compared to growth on scrubs [6]. Krueger et al. compared the bacterial profile of 30 pairs of scrubs worn continuously by on-call residents with unworn scrubs. Eighty-nine percent of post-call samples tested positive compared to 41% of unworn scrubs. Coagulase-negative *Staphylococcus* (CoNS), *Micrococcus*, MSSA, and gram-positive rods were isolated from post-call scrubs, while CoNS, gram-positive rods, and *Streptococcus viridans* were cultured from unworn scrubs [7].

G. Bearman et al. (eds.), *Infection Prevention*, DOI 10.1007/978-3-319-60980-5_12

Neckties

Multiple studies have examined the potential for neckties to be contaminated with bacteria during patient interactions. Organisms such as *Staphylococcus aureus*, bacillus, and gram-negative bacilli have been isolated from ties [8, 9]. According to a study, 20% of doctors' ties were colonized with *Staphylococcus aureus* and 70% admitted to have never washed the ties [8].

Bare Below the Elbows (BBE) Strategy

The Society for Healthcare Epidemiology of America (SHEA) defines BBE as wearing short sleeves and eliminating jewelry, wristwatches, and neckties from the attire of HCWs in an attempt to minimize the risk of transmitting infections [1]. This strategy has been implemented by multiple centers in the USA and nationwide in the UK. Multiple studies have been conducted to determine the effectiveness of this strategy for infection prevention, with conflicting results. According to a prospective, randomized controlled trial, the rates of *Staphylococcus aureus* contamination of garments and skin at wrists were similar among physicians wearing white coats or short-sleeved apparel following an 8-h work shift [10]. In addition, two other studies were unable to establish a significant difference in bacterial contamination when comparing the BBE attire with controls [11, 12]. A study conducted by Farrington et al. reported an advantage of this strategy while examining wrist disinfection rates after use of an alcohol handwash when compared to non-BBE apparel [13]. In view of these conflicting results, further trials are warranted to explore this strategy further.

Laundering

Laundering practices for HCW apparel vary across institutions. Some offer laundering facilities for lab coats, scrubs, and uniforms on-site. HCWs may use these or opt to launder items of clothing themselves. It is crucial for industrial laundering setups to clean as well as disinfect textiles contaminated with microorganisms [14]. These facilities are generally considered sufficient to render garments bacteria-free but several studies have indicated that clean laundry may be recontaminated due to improper handling. In a study conducted by Fijan and colleagues, rotavirus RNA was isolated from hospital laundry rinse water, laundered garments, environmental textiles, and hands of laundry workers following standard washing. This highlights the importance of regular education of workers regarding hygiene and regulation of disinfecting procedures with special focus on areas such as

sorting, ironing, folding, and packing of laundered textiles to prevent the transmission of infections through industrial laundering [14].

While these facilities have been linked to the transmission of infections, washing clothes at home may also be associated with the spread of infections. According to one study, artificially contaminated apparel was not free of bacteria at the end of a wash at home [15]. This is supported by other studies which whereby *Staphylococcus aureus*, *Acinetobacter*, and *Gordonia bronchialis* were isolated from domestically laundered apparel [16, 17]. Of note, not many studies have been conducted to evaluate the process of domestic washing or to compare this with professional hospital laundering.

Outbreaks Related to HCW Apparel

A recent study linked an outbreak of *Gordonia bronchialis* sternal infections to an anesthesia nurse's scrubs. Four different strains of *G. bronchialis* were isolated from her hands, scrubs, and axillae as well as her roommate. Following disposal of the washing machine used for laundry at home, repeat cultures from her scrubs, axillae, and hands were negative, and no further *G. bronchialis* sternal infections were identified [17].

Innovations in Textiles

Textiles impregnated with antimicrobials and those with fluid-repellant properties have been on the market for a long time but their use has not been widely implemented in infection control programs [2]. In a recent crossover trial to assess the effectiveness of antimicrobial scrubs, a four to seven mean log reduction in MRSA carriage was noted in the antimicrobial scrub group but no differences were noted for the burden of vancomycin-resistant enterococci or gram-negative rods [18]. Experts recommend combining hydrophobic repellency with this technology to optimize efforts dedicated to infection prevention through innovations in HCW apparel [2].

Patients' Perceptions Regarding HCW Attire

Several studies have been carried out to determine the perceptions and preferences of patients regarding HCW attire. Most studies revealed an inclination toward formal apparel when compared to casual dressing or wearing scrubs, and some of these indicated that attire preferences were unlikely to impact clinical encounters in terms of patient satisfaction

[19–26]. In contrast, multiple studies assessing perceptions regarding white coats revealed a patient preference for these with some studies indicating a higher level of trust in physicians wearing white coats [19, 21, 27–29]. With regard to BBE, most studies have indicated that patients do not favor this policy [19, 20, 25, 30, 31]. Following education, older patients were found to have a predilection for short-sleeved shirts, while younger patients preferred scrubs for choice of BBE attire [19]. Several studies addressing the inclusion of neckties in HCW attire revealed that these items were not considered a necessary component of physicians' apparel, and patients did not expect physicians to wear them [8, 31, 32]. According to a cross-sectional descriptive study, patients indicated daily laundering of clothes as the most important feature of HCW attire [27]. Patient perceptions are crucial in clinical interactions and must be taken into account when formulating policies pertaining to HCW apparel. Patient education is of paramount importance when changes such as BBE or mandating white coats are considered.

Proposed Approach for HCW Attire

The best choice for HCW attire is one that promotes a professional image while minimizing the transmission of infections [1]. Several studies have been conducted to determine the optimal approach to HCW apparel but no consensus has been reached, and this remains an area of ongoing debate. Current SHEA guidelines for HCW attire have been summarized in Table 12.1 [1]. Some experts recommend augmenting infection control strategies such as handwashing with introduction of strategies such as BBE attire in view of biological plausibility. The role of this approach has not been established in the realm of infection prevention but it is a cost-effective measure, unlikely to cause harm and may be considered for these reasons [1]. For facilities that opt for white coats, HCWs must be provided with two or more coats. Experts recommend laundering of such items of clothing daily if possible and at least once a weak. On-site professional laundering should ideally be available to employees at minimal cost. If domestically washed, the use of hot water and bleach is recommended. Additionally, institutions should make arrangements for hooks to enable HCWs to remove white coats prior to patient encounters to minimize contamination of these. With reference to items of clothing such as neckties, there is evidence to suggest that contamination may occur during patient interactions, and if worn, these must not come in contact with patients or their surroundings. There is, however, paucity of data to support elimination of neckties from HCW attire. Some studies support the use of a plastic apron to prevent bacterial contamination of the front of apparel worn by HCWs, and this may be a consideration for those wearing neckties [33]. Similarly, items such as jewelry,

Table 12.1 Current guidelines for HCW attire [1]

Component of HCW attire	Recommendations
White coats	HCWs must be provided with two or more coats
	Hooks should be available in areas close to patients' rooms to enable physicians to remove white coats prior to contact with patients or their surroundings
Neckties	Must be secured to prevent contact with patients or their surroundings
BBE	Use supported by biologic plausibility
	Exact impact on infection prevention unknown
	May be used as an adjunct to other infection control measures such as handwashing
	Scrubs or short-sleeved shirts may be used
Laundering	Ideally, items of daily wear should be laundered daily or at least once a week
	May be laundered at on-site facilities or at home
	If washed at home, hot water and bleach must be used
Footwear	Closed toes with small heels and nonskid soles
Personal items such as jewelry and pagers	Must be disinfected if contaminated

watches, cell phones, and pagers should be secured to prevent contact with patients and their surroundings; if contaminated, these must be disinfected. Items such as stethoscopes must be disinfected after use and patients in contact isolation must have designated medical equipment. The use of identification badges is strongly recommended and these must be clearly visible when worn [1]. In terms of protecting feet from contamination with blood and hazardous materials and preventing falls among HCWs, footwear with closed toes, low heels, and nonskid soles is recommended. Individual centers may differ in preferences, and therefore, consultation with HCWs and patients to determine their perceptions is critical in the process of formulating policies. HCW attire remains as area of scrutiny in the realm of infection prevention, and further studies are required to better characterize the best approach in this regard.

References

1. Bearman G, Bryant K, Leekha S, Mayer J, Munoz-Price LS, Murthy R, Palmore T, Rupp ME, White J. Healthcare personnel attire in non-operating-room settings. Infect Control Hosp Epidemiol. 2014;35(2):107–21.
2. Mitchell A, Spencer M, Edminston C Jr. Role of healthcare apparel and other healthcare textiles in the transmission of pathogens: a review of the literature. J Hosp Infect. 2015;90(4):285–92. doi:10.1016/j.jhin.2015.02.017.

3. Dulon M, Peters C, Schablon A, Nienhaus A. MRSA carriage among healthcare workers in non-outbreak settings in Europe and the United States: a systematic review. BMC Infect Dis. 2014; doi:10.1186/1471-2334-14-363.

4. Treakle AM, Thom KA, Furuno JP, Strauss SM, Harris AD, Perenvcevich EN. Bacterial contamination of healthcare workers' whitecoats. Am J Infect Control. 2009;37:101–5.

5. Wiener-Well Y, Galuty M, Rudensky B, Schlesinger Y, Attias D, Yinnon AM. Nursing and physician attire as possible source of nosocomial infections. Am J Infect Control. 2011;39:555–9.

6. Munoz-Price LS, Arheart KL, Mills JP, Clearly T, DePascale D, Jimenez A, Fajardo-Aquino Y, Coro G, Birnbach DJ, Lubarsky DA. Associations between bacterial contamination of health care workers' hands and contamination of white coats and scrubs. Am J Infect Control. 2012;40:e245–8.

7. Kreuger CA, Murray CK, Mende K, Guymon CH, Gerlinger TL. The bacterial contamination of surgical scrubs. Am J Orthop (Belle Mead NJ). 2012;41(5):E69–73.

8. Ditchburne I. Should doctors wear ties? J Hosp Infect. 2006;63:227–8.

9. Steinlechner C, Wilding G, Cumberland N. Microbes on ties: do they correlate with wound infection. Ann R Coll Surg. 2002;84:307–9.

10. Burden M, Cervantes L, Weed D, Keniston A, Price CS, Albert RK. Newly cleaned physician uniforms and infrequently washed white coats have similar rates of bacterial contamination after an 8-hour workday: a randomized controlled trial. J Hosp Med. 2011;6(4):177–82.

11. Burger A, Wijewardena C, Clayson S, Greatorex RA. Bare below elbows: does this policy affect handwashing efficacy and reduce bacterial colonisation? Ann R Coll Surg Engl. 2011;93:13–6.

12. Willis-Owen CA, Subramanian P, Kumari P, Houlihan-Burne D. Effects of 'bare below the elbows' policy on hand contamination of 92 hospital doctors in a district general hospital. J Hosp Infect. 2010;75:116–9.

13. Farrington RM, Rabindran J, Crocker G, Ali R, Pollard N, Dalton HR. 'Bare below the elbows' and quality of hand washing: a randomised comparison study. J Hosp Infect. 2010;74:86–8.

14. Fijan S, Poljsak-Prijatelj M, Steyer A, Koren S, Cencic A, Sostar-Turk S. Rotaviral RNA found in wastewaters from hospital laundry. Int J Hyg Environ Health. 2006;209:97–102.

15. Callaghan I. Bacterial contamination of nurses' uniforms: a study. Nurs Stand. 1998;13(1):37–42.

16. Home laundering can leave bacteria on uniforms. OR Manag. 2011;27(11):5. https://www.ncbi.nlm.nih.gov/pubmed/?term=Home+laundering+can+leave+bacteria+on+uniforms.+OR+Manag.+2011%3B27(11)%3A5.

17. Wright SN, Gerry JS, Busowski MT, Klocho AY, McNulty SG, Brown SA, Sieger BE, Ken MP, Wallace MR. Gordonia bronchialis sternal wound infection in 3 patients following open heart surgery: intraoperative transmission from a healthcare worker. Infect Control Hosp Epidemiol. 2012;33:1238–41.

18. Bearman G, Rosato A, Elam K, Sanogo K, Stevens MP, Sessler CN, Wenzel RP. A crossover trial of antimicrobial scrubs to reduce methicillin-resistant *Staphylococcus aureus* burden on healthcare worker apparel. Infect Control Hosp Epidemiol. 2012;33(3):268–75.

19. Ardolino A, Williams LA, Crook TB, Taylor HP. Bare below the elbows: what do patients think? J Hosp Infect. 2009;71:291–3.

20. Bond L, Clamp PJ, Gray K, Van Dam V. Patients' perceptions of doctors' clothing: should we really be 'bare below the elbow'? J Laryngol Otol. 2010;124:963–6.

21. Gallagher J, Waldron LF, Stack J, Barragry J. Dress and address: patient preferences regarding doctor's style of dress and patient interaction. Ir Med J. 2008;101:211–3.

22. Gonzalez del Rey JA, Paul RI. Preferences of parents for pediatric emergency physicians' attire. Pediatr Emerg Care. 1995;11:361–4.

23. Monkhouse SJ, Collis SA, Dunn JJ, Bunni J. Patients' attitudes to surgical dress: a descriptive study in a district general hospital. J Hosp Infect. 2008;69:408–9.

24. Cha A, Hecht BR, Nelson K, Hopkins MP. Resident physician attire: does it make a difference to our patients? Am J Obstet Gynecol. 2004;190:1484–8.

25. Toquero L, Abournarzouk O, Owers C, Chiang R, Thiagarajah S, Amin S. Bare below the elbows – the patient's perspective. Qual Patient Saf. 2011;2(4) WMC001401. Available at: http://www.webmedcentral.com/article_view/1401.

26. Niederhauser A, Turner MD, Chauhan SP, Magann EF, Morrison JC. Physician attire in the military setting: does it make a difference to our patients? Mil Milead. 2009;174:817–20.

27. Gherardi G, Cameron J, West A, Crossley M. Are we dressed to impress? A descriptive survey assessing patients' preference of doctors' attire in the hospital setting. Clin Med. 2009;9:519–24.

28. Hennessy N, Harrison DA, Aitkenhead AR. The effect of the anaesthetist's attire on patient attitudes. The influence of dress on patient perception of the anaesthetist's prestige. Anaesthesia. 1993;48:219–22.

29. Ikusaka M, Kamegai M, Sunaga T, et al. Patients' attitude toward consultations by a physician without a white coat in Japan. Intern Med. 1993;38:533–6.

30. Shelton CL, Raistrick C, Warburton K, Siddiqui KH. Can changes in clinical attire reduce likelihood of cross-infection without jeopardising the doctor-patient relationship? J Hosp Infect. 2010;74:22–9.

31. Baxter JA, Dale O, Morritt A, Pollock JC. Bare below the elbows: professionalism vs infection risk. Bull R Coll Surg Engl. 2010;92:248–251.

32. Palazzo S, Hocken DB. Patients' perspectives on how doctors dress. J Hosp Infect. 2010;74:30–4.

33. Wilson JA, Loveday HP, Hoffman PN, Pratt RJ. Uniform: an evidence review of the microbiological significance of uniforms and uniform policy in the prevention and control of healthcare-associated infections. Report to the Department of Health (England). J Hosp Infect. 2007;66(4):301–7.

Antimicrobial Textiles and Infection Prevention: Clothing and the Inanimate Environment

13

Rachel H. McQueen and Briana Ehnes

Introduction

Textiles are ubiquitous and an essential part of human society. Within the hospital environment textiles have many functions, such as the clothing worn by patients and healthcare workers, the towels and cloths used to contain and mop up fluids, drapes used to isolate and maintain sterility during surgery, furnishings such as upholstered chairs as well as curtains, carpets and also bedding. As part of the inanimate environment textiles could act as a potential source of infection [1, 2]. This is because microorganisms can be transferred from an infected patient, a healthcare worker, or some environmental source; persist within the textile then to be transferred to a susceptible individual. Frequent and effective laundering is the most common and most effective strategy for reducing microbial burden on textiles [3]. However, not all textiles in the hospital setting are frequently laundered (e.g. privacy curtains) or easily laundered (e.g. upholstery on chairs). As well, within a typical work shift (8–12 h), the microbial load on a healthcare workers' clothing could become significant [4], and thus the transmission of pathogenic microorganisms may be possible. A possible solution to the problem of relying solely on cleaning involves integrating biocidal textiles into the hospital environment in order to reduce the microbial burden to levels low enough to reduce the rate of hospital-acquired infections (HAIs) [1]. The purpose of this chapter is to review the literature pertaining to contamination of hospital textiles by potentially pathogenic microorganisms and the related transmission of HAIs, describe the antimicrobials agents incorporated in textiles, describe the in vitro standard test methods used to assess antimicrobial efficacy, and evaluate the effectiveness of antimicrobial-treated textiles in the hospital environment.

R.H. McQueen (✉) • B. Ehnes
Department of Human Ecology, University of Alberta,
116th Street and 89th Avenue, Edmonton, AB T6G 2N1, Canada
e-mail: rachel.mcqueen@ualberta.ca; ehnes@ualberta.ca

Textiles in Healthcare

Many textiles are utilized in a healthcare setting, including bedding (pillows, bed linens, blankets), patient gowns, towels, surgical gowns, scrub suits, lab coats, splash aprons, and privacy drapes. Healthcare-related textiles are functional and intended to provide some of all of the following functions: a protective function (e.g. surgical gowns), to ensure privacy (drapes, patient gowns), be absorbent (e.g. towels) or add a level of comfort (e.g. bedding). Hospital textiles fall under two broad categories, reusable and disposable. Reusable or multiple-use textiles tend to be woven structures composed of cotton or polyester or blends of these fibres. Other fibres and fabric structures can be present as well, for example, in compression garments, knitted fabrics composed of nylon/spandex and liquid impermeable aprons, which are typically a composite material with a polyurethane or PVC laminate film over a knit backing. Disposable or single-use textiles tend to be non-woven structures, which may include cellulose fibres (i.e. wood pulp) or synthetic fibres such as polypropylene, polyester and nylon. Disposable textiles vary widely in their functions and properties, but the majority are intended to be single-use items. They also tend to be less durable than reusable textiles, although some types of synthetic non-wovens can have high tensile strength. Multiple-use hospital textiles should be durable to the high wash/dry temperatures and chemical treatments (e.g. bleach) necessary to ensure removal of human-based soils and eradication of microorganisms. Any treatments that have been applied to the textile during or after construction in order to have specific (or more desirable) properties (e.g. stain repellency, antimicrobial) must also remain durable during use and to laundering.

The Role of Textiles in Hospital-Acquired Infections (HAIs)

Amongst the many routes of exposure to infectious agents, with the person-to-person route for transmission of HAI being the most common [5, 6], the inanimate environment, which includes textiles, plays a significant role. Clothing, worn by healthcare workers such as scrubs, white coats, and gowns, have been shown to harbour potentially pathogenic bacteria [7–9]; both the person's own microflora could become a source of transmission [10], but more concerning is the transmission of infected patient via healthcare workers clothing to other patients [2]. As well, hospital privacy curtains, bedding, towels, and drapes have been identified as textiles that have the potential to harbour harmful bacteria [11–14].

Privacy curtains have been found to frequently be contaminated with potential hospital pathogens such as vancomycin-resistant enterococci (VRE), methicillin-resistant *Staphylococcus aureus* (MRSA) and *Clostridium difficile* [11, 14]. Since curtains are touched by healthcare personnel before, during and after performing patient care, often before the worker has had time to wash their hands, it is likely that contaminated curtains can be a source of transmission of infective agents [11, 15]. Furthermore, compared with many other hospital textiles, privacy curtains are infrequently changed, difficult to clean and often only dealt with when visibly soiled [11]. Even after only one week of use, 92.3% of new curtains had evidence of contamination [11]. In an in vitro study, polyester fabric (used privacy curtains) was found to harbour harmful bacteria such as staphylococci and enterococci, which could survive for days and even months after drying on commonly used hospital fabrics. The authors reported that the viability of the enterococci on the fabrics tended to be much longer than on other common hospital surfaces [16].

Within the hospital ward, the process of making beds can release considerable amounts of microorganisms into the air which could be breathed in by staff or patients, as well as contaminate surrounding surfaces which may be transmitted later. For example, in one study high levels of MRSA were detected during and immediately after bed-making in the air, as well as being detected on the floor, on bed sheets, over-bed tables and on clothing [17].

Hospital linens and clothing have reportedly become contaminated due to poor-quality hygiene practices within hospital laundry facilities, as "clean" linen trolleys were not being cleaned frequently enough. Coagulase-negative staphylococci (human origin), and *Bacillus* spp., moulds (environmental origin) were found to have transferred to the freshly laundered linens [5]. Other cases where "clean" laundry has been implicated in transmission of infection are: an infection amongst infants connected to the presence of *Streptococcus pyogenes* on hospital laundry and, in particular, the vests given to newborns after birth [18]; an outbreak of *Bacillus cereus* in Japan in which laundered towels were the suspected source of contamination [12]; and another *Bacillus cereus* infection in which hospital linens and the washing machine were both highly contaminated

with bacteria [19]. In these cases, the contamination likely came from the washing machine itself, all from hospital laundries. Another case reported that a washing machine located in the home of a nurse anaesthetist was the cause of *Gordonia bronchialis* infections within three patients following open heart surgery [20].

In one hospital in the Netherlands, a case study was reported where pillows were implicated in the spread of HAIs as *Acinetobacter* spp. were allowed to flourish as a result of the lower washing temperature required of the feather pillows [13]. Replacing feather pillows with synthetic pillows that could be washed and dried at a higher temperature controlled the outbreak. Another study examined a mucormycosis outbreak at a Louisiana hospital following the death of five paediatric patients. It was suspected the outbreak was caused by hospital linen that had been contaminated after the laundering process [21]. These studies recognize the importance of proper laundering techniques in preventing outbreaks and HAIs as "clean" linen may still carry some microbial burden. Although the risk of infection is considered to be quite small for the majority of patients, the risk lies in the fact that many patients in these studies were already immunocompromised, increasing the opportunity for a HAI to take hold [21].

Hospital textiles being traced to HAIs occurring within hospital staff as a result of contaminated laundry has been suggested as the likely route of contamination in many case studies [3]. For example, transmission of scabies amongst laundry employees was traced to improper handling of infected hospital bed linens [22]; one housekeeping staff member likely acquired *Microsporum canis* through handling contaminated bed linens [23]; in another, following an outbreak of *Salmonella hadar* food poisoning occurring to patients in a nursing home, a subsequent outbreak 7–10 days later occurred within laundry workers infected via soiled bed linens [24]. Following standard precautions such as wearing protective clothing (gloves, apron) while handling dirty linen and hand washing is therefore vital for laundry workers.

Healthcare worker's uniforms have been postulated as a source of microbial contamination and spread of infection [25]. One study showed that the white coats of attendees on wards resulted in a significant proportion of *Staphylococcus aureus* being present [8], and in another the white coats of medical students showed high levels of bacterial contamination in sites of frequent contact (i.e. sleeve cuff and pockets) [26]. These studies suggest that the white coat could be an important vector for patient-to-patient transmission. Other clothing, such as hospital gowns, surgical scrubs and nurse uniforms, have been shown to pick up bacteria during patient contact [2, 4, 7, 27, 28]. In a survey of 160 healthcare professionals [25], even though 90% of respondents were aware that their uniforms (including scrubs and/or a white coat) were potentially contaminated with hospital pathogens, white coats were not laundered regularly. As well, not all uniforms were laundered using hot water (which is more effective at reducing microbial burden than laundering at low temperatures). These findings suggest that personal practices of healthcare workers in maintaining the cleanliness of their uniforms may impact the transmission of pathogens within a hospital setting. Furthermore, home laundering, while still commonly employed for nonoperative garments, is not recommended by AORN due to the potential for contamination to occur from home washing machines. Also, the laundering conditions at home may not meet the necessary "mechanical, thermal, or chemical measures" to reduce antimicrobial levels in soiled surgical attire [29].

Despite the hypothesis that contaminated uniforms become a vector for the transmission of pathogens, a literature review by Wilson, Loveday, Hoffman and Pratt concluded that no studies demonstrated the transfer of microorganisms from uniforms to patients in the clinical setting [30]. Nonetheless, the fact remains that potentially pathogenic microorganisms can survive within textiles for a considerable length of time in a dry state [16, 31]. The best course of action is to regularly launder uniforms and other hospital textiles following recommended practices and preferably in a healthcare-accredited laundry facility [29]. Furthermore, healthcare worker uniforms (such as scrubs and white coats) should not be treated as personal protective equipment (PPE), and proper PPE (such as gloves and plastic aprons) should be donned whenever possible [30]. Due to the fact that textiles can harbour microorganisms and the imperfect nature of personal and industrial hygiene practices, incorporating antimicrobials into hospital textiles is one suggested solution to reduce HAIs.

Antimicrobials in Textiles

Antimicrobials incorporated into textiles and other inanimate objects (e.g. plastics, foams, etc.) work as a biocide (i.e. killing microorganisms) or inhibiting their growth within the object. Most antimicrobial agents act by either damaging the cell wall, altering the cell membrane permeability, denaturing proteins or inhibiting or altering essential functions of the microorganisms' metabolic pathways [42]. Antimicrobials are typically added to a textile product or other inanimate product to (i) protect the product from degradation, staining or odour during its useful life and (ii) to reduce microbiological colonization with human pathogens. However, the US Environmental Protection Agency (EPA) and other regulatory bodies in many other countries consider the reduction of pathogens to be a health-related claim and as such no antimicrobials in textiles can specifically be marketed as reducing human pathogens. This does not, however, preclude antimicrobials from being incorporated into healthcare-related

textiles. If they are intended for healthcare applications, a number of requirements need to be met for the antimicrobial textile to be used in healthcare: the antimicrobial should be wide spectrum against bacteria, fungi and viruses; be effective against antibiotic-resistant strains of bacteria and not enable development of resistance microorganisms; remain effective for the duration of the textiles lifetime; and be durable to commercial launderings. As well, they should not cause skin irritation or be hazardous for humans following dermal exposure [32].

For synthetic textile fibres and plastics, the antimicrobial active agent can be imbedded into the fibre in the liquid polymer stage prior to fibre spinning. Synthetic (e.g. polyester) and natural fibres (e.g. cotton) can also have antimicrobial agents added at the fabric finishing stage. The former process typically denotes better durability of the antimicrobial into the textiles. Common antimicrobial agents used in textiles are triclosan, noble metals (e.g. silver, copper) and their ions, metal oxides, polyhexamethylene biguanides (PHMB), quaternary ammonium compounds (QAC) and N-halamines.

Triclosan

For decades, triclosan (5-chloro-2-(2,4-dichlorophenoxy)-phenol) has been added to a number of consumer products such as hand soap, toothpaste, mouthwash, food storage containers, toys and clothing. Triclosan inhibits an enzyme necessary for synthesizing fatty acids needed for building cell membranes and for cell division within microorganisms [33], and thus there has been concerns that due to the similarity in its mode of action to antibiotics, it may induce antibiotic-resistant strains [34]. Indeed resistant strains have been noted under laboratory conditions [35, 36].

Triclosan has been widely used in synthetic textiles and other products such as plastics as it can be incorporated in the polymer melt stage leading to better durability over the lifetime of the product. Windler et al. [37] estimated that about 5–15% of the total global production of triclosan is used for textiles, which they calculated to be about 75–210 metric tonnes. In comparison to other common antimicrobials used in textiles (i.e. silver, QAC, zinc pyrithione), a much higher proportion of triclosan is used due to the higher concentration needed for sustained antimicrobial activity [37]. Recently, triclosan is coming under increased scrutiny as it has been shown to accumulate within the environment and have adverse effects on aquatic life, as well as a potential risk as an endocrine disrupter, and found to be distributed in human tissues [37, 38]. The bioaccumulation in the Great Lakes has led to it being banned from soap in Minnesota by 2017 and recommendations that it also be banned in consumer products in Canada labelled as a chemical of "high concern" [39]. In a comprehensive review of five most common textile antimicrobials, Windler et al. [37] ranked triclosan to have the highest potential for a negative impact on the environment and human health.

Metallic Compounds

Metallic compounds such as silver and copper have been used for their bactericidal properties for centuries. Both silver and copper coins have been used in ancient times to purify water [40] and are still used today in water purification. Silver has been used in medicine as treatments of wound infection and incorporated into medical devices, such as catheters, due to the broad-spectrum antimicrobial activity, including antibiotic-resistant strains and therefore has been seen as having potential to control biofilms [41]. The metals must be in their ionized form (e.g. Ag^+, Cu^{2+}) to be effective against microbes, with the metal ions binding to intracellular proteins and subsequently inactivating them [42].

Silver and silver ions are the most common type of antimicrobial active agent utilized in textiles [43]. The forms of silver incorporated into textiles can differ and range from metallic silver, silver salts, silver-polymer composites, silver-impregnated zeolites, or silver nanoparticles [38]. The concentration of silver in textiles can also vary considerably with concentrations ranging from as low as 1 to ~3000 mg/kg (ppm) [44]. The wide application rate relates to the different forms silver can take. For example, application rates for nanosilver metal are considerably lower than application rates for silver zeolites [37]. Commercial textile products which had silver nanoparticles were found to exhibit much higher in vitro antimicrobial activity than other products where the silver was present in other forms (e.g. silver wires) [44].

Compared with silver, copper is used far less extensively as an antimicrobial in textiles. Copper oxide is the main active agent for any antimicrobial-treated copper textile and can be applied to cellulose and synthetic fibres [45]. Notably, copper alloys and polymeric surfaces containing copper oxide are the only antimicrobial solid surface that has gained EPA registration to make public health claims [46]. To receive this registration, manufacturers of copper products must show that their product kills 99.9% of Gram-positive and Gram-negative bacteria within 2 h of inoculation and continuously kills 99.9% of bacteria after multiple reinoculations as well as wet and dry abrasion "wear" cycles [46]. Therefore, in many hospitals, copper is replacing stainless steel in applications such as bed rails, door handles and other frequently touched hard surfaces. No copper-impregnated textiles have received such EPA registration, so public health claims about copper textiles cannot yet be made. There is compelling evidence that copper-treated textiles

would also be beneficial in healthcare settings as various strains of bacteria, viruses and fungi have been found to be reduced by 99.9% within relatively short time frames (i.e. ranging from 20 min to 4 h) by copper oxide-treated textiles [45].

Titanium dioxide is a strong photocatalytic material as it is comes into contact with UV light "the active oxygen species are released following the relaxation of electrons to the ground state from the excited singlet state, resulting in an antimicrobial effect due to the emission of light" [47]. In one study the outermost layer of a surgical facemask was treated with a mixture of silver nitrate and TiO_2 nanoparticles and evaluated for antimicrobial resistance against a strain of *Escherichia coli* and a strain of *Staphylococcus aureus*. The authors reported in vitro antimicrobial activity of 100% reduction with no viable colony counts present after 48 h incubation. Prior to antimicrobial testing, the facemasks were activated under UV radiation [48]. TiO_2-treated textiles have been found to not exhibit any antimicrobial activity without UV radiation and may potentially degrade the textile under UV radiation [49]. Therefore, with the exception of drapes and bedding in wards exposed to natural sunlight through windows, the suitability of using TiO_2 as the active agent in indoor applications such as most healthcare settings is questionable.

Quaternary Ammonium Compounds

Quaternary ammonium compounds (QACs) are cationic surfactants that are useful disinfectants in healthcare for both clinical use on skin and mucous membranes and for disinfecting hard surfaces [50]. As a hospital disinfectant QACs are used and registered with the EPA as being tuberculocides (i.e. kills *Mycobacterium tuberculosis*) [51]. QACs are membrane-active agents and damage the cell membrane, denature proteins and disrupt the cell structure [50]. In antimicrobial-treated textiles, the main type of QAC used are long-chained (12–18 carbon atoms) with a dominant compound being a linear alkyl ammonium QAC based on silane quaternary ammonium compounds [37]. The estimated metric tonnes of QAC used in antimicrobial-treated textiles are greater than other common textile antimicrobial products (i.e. silver, triclosan, zinc pyrithione) but overall, antimicrobial textiles make up a small component compared to the total consumption of QACs [37]. Durability of a QAC applied to 65% polyester/35% cotton fabrics (typical of that worn by healthcare workers) in an in vitro study was poor following multiple washings, as efficacy against *S. aureus* became less notable as washing increased and no activity against *Klebsiella pneumonia* was evident by about ten washes [52].

Polybiguanides

Polyhexamethylene biguanide (PHMB) is a polymeric antimicrobial compound that can have 8–15 biguanide units per molecule with an average of 11 [42, 53]. It is a broad-spectrum antimicrobial with low toxicity and as such has been used as a disinfectant for years. PHMB has been applied in the food industry, as swimming pool sanitizers, and contact lens solutions [42, 50]. In textile applications it is usually bound to cellulose fibres. In healthcare it has been successfully used in wound dressings in order to lower microbial burden [54, 55]. It kills microbes as the positively charged biguanide groups are attracted to the negatively charged bacterial cell wall and causing cell lysis by destroying the integrity of the bacterial cell [50, 54]. In vitro activity of PHMB was shown to be high (i.e. 94.11–99.9% reduction in *Staphylococcus aureus* and *Klebsiella pneumoniae*) up to 25 laundering cycles in polyester/cotton clothing typical of that worn by healthcare workers [52]. However, the antimicrobial efficacy of PHMB has been found to be inhibited when cotton fabrics are dyed with anionic reactive dyes [56].

N-Halamines

N-Halamines are compounds that contain amine, amide and imide bonds and are well known to be potent broad-spectrum biocides. N-Halamines have been used in water disinfection for swimming pools. Of the types of antimicrobials which can be incorporated into textiles, N-halamines are able to rapidly kill a wide range of microorganisms without causing resistant strains [57]. The mechanism of N-halamines are described as "the direct transfer of oxidative halogen (Cl+ or Br+) from the N-halamine nitrogen to the cell wall of the organism by direct contact followed by oxidation, rather than dissociation of X+ into water followed by diffusion over to the cell" [58]. N-Halamines have been incorporated to many textile fibres, including cotton, polyester, polypropylene, acrylic and nylon [57, 59–61]. Along with the rapid kill times [62], another advantage of N-halamines for their application in healthcare is their ability to be regenerated with chlorine bleach since the bleaching process is a routine part when laundering hospital linens. Although despite its success in the laboratory, the commercial applications of N-halamine-treated textiles are limited. This may result in part due to the undesirable residual chlorine on the surface resulting in staining and odour [42].

Test Methods for Assessing Antimicrobial Efficacy

Various standard test methods set by specific testing groups exist which assess the antimicrobial activity of textiles. These methods can be described as qualitative (where visual assessment of bacterial growth on agar are made) or quantitative test methods (where colony-forming units are counted). All test methods typically involve the textile to come into contact with a test microorganism for a set period of time, typically 18 or 24 h, but can be shorter such as 1–4 h. Diffusion tests, such as the AATCC 147 and JIS L 1902 "halo method," are qualitative test methods that are similar to the disc diffusion antibiotic sensitivity tests. A strip of fabric is placed in contact with agar that has been streaked with test microorganisms. Following incubation growth is examined underneath and surrounding the fabric. The size of the no growth area can be an indication of the potency of the antimicrobial or the rate at which the active agent is released from the fabric [42]. Several limitations exist, such as the inability to compare across different products, and the high nutrient component and presence of moisture are not realistic conditions for most textile applications [63]. Nonetheless, the qualitative methods are generally quick to administer and are useful for screening antimicrobial activity before quantitative tests are undertaken.

Quantitative methods range from absorption tests where a set amount of inoculum is directly applied to a test and control fabric (e.g. AATCC 100), or the control and test fabrics are individually placed directly in flasks of bacterial suspensions and shaken (e.g. ASTM E2149). The concentrations of the bacteria in colony-forming units are calculated at "time zero" and after a specific amount of contact time (e.g. 18 or 24 h). Antimicrobial activity is expressed as percentage of reduction (e.g. AATCC 100) or a log reduction (e.g. ISO 20743). Appropriate controls are included where possible, which typically include a fabric that has gone through the same finishing processes to ensure activity is due to the active agent rather than any other finishing process. A blank control of just inoculum is also recommended as per the ASTM E2149 test.

In the ISO 20743 test method, a set of control fabric samples are used to not only to show that there is no antimicrobial activity on the control fabric but is included in the calculation of the antibacterial activity value (A):

$$A = \left(\log C_t - \log C_0 \right) - \left(\log T_t - \log T_0 \right) = F - G$$

where A is the antibacterial activity value, F is the growth value on the control specimen, G is the growth value on the antibacterial testing specimen, T_t is the average number of bacteria obtained from three antimicrobial testing specimens after the specified (18 h or 24 h) of incubation, T_0 is the average number of bacteria obtained from three antimicrobial testing specimens immediately after transfer, C_t is the average number of bacteria obtained from three control specimens after the specified (18 h or 24 h) of incubation and C_0 is the average number of bacteria obtained from three control specimens immediately after transfer. Strong antimicrobial activity is when $A \geq 3$ and significant antimicrobial activity is when $2 \leq A \leq 3$ [64]. This indicator of what denotes significant antimicrobial activity is not typically provided in other test standards.

Within the ISO 20743 standard, three different methods can be conducted: the absorption method, the transfer method and the printing method. The absorption method is similar to the AATCC 100 test method in that the bacterial suspension is pipetted directly onto the fabric to be sorbed by the textile. The transfer method involves fabric specimens being pressed against inoculated agar for 60 s before being placed in an empty flask and incubated fabric face up at 37 °C in a humidity chamber for 24 h. The transfer method is less commonly used but is useful for fabrics which resist wetting [65]. The printing method requires specialized equipment in which bacteria are collected onto a membrane filter which is then used to "print" the bacteria onto a test specimen. Incubation at 20 °C and 70% relative humidity is carried out for up to 4 h.

Many limitations of the current in vitro test methods exist, such as they tend not to be realistic of real life circumstances, where reinoculation of microorganisms onto textiles would occur constantly. The length of time it takes for the antimicrobial textile to kill microorganisms is much longer in vitro than required for inherently sterile textile products. The ASTM E2149 test method in particular has been described as being non-realistic and typically shows no correlation between it and other quantitative tests [66]. The ISO 20743 printing method more closely represents conditions of use as humidity, and nutrient requirements are much less than those in the other standard methods. As well, incubation time is shorter, and incubation temperature is lower which reflects conditions more likely to be encountered in a hospital environment for airborne contamination or transfer (e.g. contaminated hands onto clothing). Despite it being more realistic, it has not been commonly used which might be due to the complexity of the method and equipment required for the procedure.

Evidence of Antimicrobial Activity in Hospital Textiles

For many commercial products, there is no certainty that the antimicrobial will indeed offer the protection it purports to have during use. This may be due to poor-quality control at the site of manufacture resulting in poor retention of the antimicrobial agent on the fabric, or the concentration of the antimicrobial applied to the fabric is below the minimum inhibitory concentration (MIC) for the challenge microorganisms. Many in vitro studies evaluating commercially available antimicrobial-treated textiles found that antimicrobial activity may not always be evident [44, 67, 68]. Of four reportedly antimicrobial-treated commercial products (QAC, silver, triclosan and one unknown antimicrobial), only two exhibited any antimicrobial activity against a strain of *S. aureus* (i.e. silver and the unknown) [67]. Variability in the efficacy of silver within eight commercially available textiles (socks, t-shirts, trousers) was noted against Gram-negative *Klebsiella pneumoniae*. This related to both variability in the quantity of silver present on the textile items and the form (e.g. silver wires throughout) [44]. Similar variability has been noted in other studies as well (e.g. [68]).

Even when in vitro testing shows the antimicrobial to be effective this may not correspond to antimicrobial efficacy in vivo [69]. This may be due to the conditions in use being quite different from in vitro laboratory tests (i.e. much higher moisture and nutrient content in vitro). This lack of certainty about whether an antimicrobial will actually inhibit growth of microorganisms during use raises important concerns for the use of antimicrobial textiles in healthcare where antimicrobial activity may be assumed. This concern has also been raised by Alvarez et al. [70] who argue that when public health claims can be made on the product label based on in vitro efficacy against human pathogens (as is the case with EPA approval of many copper products), this may create a public health concern as the public may believe the products reduce cross-contamination of microorganisms. Therefore, clinical data showing a reduction of HAIs due to antimicrobial-treated products is needed.

Bacterial Contamination of Antimicrobial-Treated Textiles Compared to a Control

Very few in situ studies have been conducted evaluating the effectiveness of an antimicrobial-treated product in reducing bacterial colonization [71–75], and still fewer with a focus on evaluating the effect of antimicrobial treatments on HAIs [76, 79, 80]. Furthermore, where studies have been implemented in this area, then a reduction from control garments/products has not always been shown [74, 75].

A randomized controlled double-blind study evaluating antimicrobial-treated hospital curtains was carried out in ICU units within an Iowa hospital. The antimicrobial treatment was by PurThread Technologies and described as a "complex element compound" (CEC) in which the active agent was a silver compound integrated into the fibre during fibre spinning. Although both types of curtains (standard and CEC experimental curtains) were found to be contaminated with potentially pathogenic microorganisms during the study, the CEC curtains were significantly lower in contamination than the standard curtains up to 10 days. After 10 days (up to 4 weeks), the CEC curtains did not differ from the standard curtains [72].

In another study, two outpatient units of a major NHS hospital in the UK were refurbished with either multiple products treated with the BioCote® silver technology (e.g. door furniture/safety rails, wall tiling, electrical switches, cubical curtains, water taps, furniture fabric) (Suite A) or non-BioCote®-treated materials (Suite B) [73]. The trial involved swabbing surfaces for total aerobic bacterial counts four times during a 4-month period (12 months following refurbishment). Surfaces in the treated Suite A ranged from 62 to 98% lower than surfaces in the non-treated Suite B. The fabric samples included in the study typically had lower levels of bacterial contamination than many of the other surfaces. This was likely due to these items being less frequently touched (e.g. curtains) compared with other objects (e.g. door handles, light switches), as well as being drier (e.g. compared with tiles near sinks). But the difference between bacterial contamination of the textile products in the treated suite compared with the untreated suite was less at a 70% reduction than for the untreated/treated hard surface objects. The authors also found that untreated surfaces within the treated suite were on average 43% lower than similar surfaces in the untreated suite, concluding that lower bacterial burden on many surfaces due to the treated objects resulted in lower levels of cross-contamination to untreated surfaces. This study is unique in that multiple objects and surfaces were impregnated with a bioactive agent and shows promise for reducing the likelihood of cross-contamination and the spread of infection. However, the authors did not state whether the research personnel swabbing samples were blinded to the suite treatment, nor did they indicate when environmental swabbing occurred in relation to room cleaning.

Another study evaluated the performance of antimicrobial-treated polyester fibres blended with untreated cotton. The treatment was described as "sodium aluminosilicate associated with silver and copper according to the BactiSTOP® process" [77], and the study included a regular cotton fabric with no antimicrobial finish as the control. A treated and control swatch (20 × 20 cm) were sewn onto either the left or right side of nurse uniforms ($n = 12$). The garments were sterilized before wear and then worn for 8–12 h in ICU or surgical units. The authors found that for heavily contaminated garments (i.e. >75 CFU/25 m²), there was a 50% reduction in bacterial counts per 25 cm² on the treated fabric compared with the untreated. However, since a complete reduction of bacteria did not occur, then cross-infection from the treated textile to a patient could still potentially occur.

Two trials evaluating the bacterial colonization of healthcare workers uniforms did not find the antimicrobial treatments to reduce colony counts. One prospective, randomized controlled trial was conducted comparing two antimicrobial-treated hospital scrubs with a control to determine whether there was a reduction in bacterial colony counts on the scrubs and wrists of healthcare workers after an 8-h shift [74]. A total of 105 healthcare workers were enlisted in the study with 35 participants in each group (scrub A, polyester fabric with an unknown antimicrobial; scrub B, polyester/cotton fabric finished with two unknown antimicrobials and silver; control scrub, polyester/cotton blend with no antimicrobial finish). The authors found no significant differences in the contamination of uniforms amongst all three types of scrubs [74]. In another study, Boutin et al. [75] conducted a blinded, randomized crossover study design with 90 healthcare workers who were assigned an antimicrobial-treated scrub and a control scrub to wear during a hospital shift. Sampling of bacteria and frequency of pathogenic bacteria (i.e. *Staphylococcus aureus*, *Enterococcus* or gram-negative rods) was taken between 8 and 12 h after the beginning of the shift. No difference in aerobic bacterial counts was found between the control scrub and the antimicrobial-treated scrub. The authors stated the antimicrobial was proprietary but that chitosan was one of the active ingredients [75].

Evidence of Antimicrobial-Treated Textile Effect on HAIs

One of the few clinical trials evaluating the effect of antimicrobial-treated textiles involved copper oxide-impregnated linens on patient HAIs in a long-term care ward [76]. The protocol involved comparing the number of HAIs, fever days and administration of antibiotics over two parallel 6-month periods (i.e. in the first 6-month period December 2010–June 2011, regular hospital linens were used; in the second 6-month period December 2011–June 2012, copper oxide-treated sheets, pillowcases and patients' clothing were used). Data was collected from patient medical records, and healthcare workers directly caring for patients were not involved in the data collection, although treated linens did look noticeably different from regular hospital linens. The authors stated that 108 patients were involved in the study (57 in the first period and 51 in the second period), but it was not clear whether any of these patients were present in both periods. A significant reduction in HAIs associated with the eyes and gastrointestinal tract, as well as significantly less numbers of fever days and days of antibiotic use, was observed. The study has been reviewed as having "very low quality of evidence" under the GRADE (Grading of Recommendations Assessment, Development and Evaluation) system for critiquing clinical trials [78]. More recently two more clinical trials have been published on the use of copper-oxide impregnated textiles in hospital facilities, with one showing a significant reduction in HAIs due to multidrug resistant organisms or *Clostridium difficile* [79] and the other significant reductions in the use of antibiotics and fever days [80]. Despite the poor evaluation using the GRADE system for the Lazary et al. [76] study, these studies do suggest that there is the potential for copper oxide-treated textiles to lead to a reduction in HAIs.

Conclusions

As part of the inanimate environment, clothing and textiles used in hospitals can harbour potentially pathogenic micro-organisms. As a result they may be implicated in the trans-mission of HAIs. Many of the published cases where textiles have been recognized as the source of an infectious outbreak, or an isolated case of infection, inadequate hygiene practices while handling dirty laundry or contamination occurring during or following laundering has been identified as the issue. These studies highlight how important it is to follow recommended procedures for laundering hospital textiles. Antimicrobial efficacy can be highly variable even with some commercially acquired antimicrobial textiles not exhibiting any efficacy at all, despite being labelled as anti-microbial. The conditions under which an antimicrobial tex-tile may be used in can vary considerably from the conditions under which most in vitro standard tests for antimicrobial efficacy occur. Unfortunately, the research evaluating how antimicrobial-treated textiles perform in reducing microbial load within a healthcare setting is minimal, and limited stud-ies have been found that examine their impact on HAIs. Therefore, the evidence showing that antimicrobial-treated textiles are beneficial in reducing HAIs is negligible.

Nonetheless, in theory, antimicrobial-treated textiles have considerable potential to contribute to reducing HAIs, but must be used in conjunction with well-established, thorough hygiene practices (e.g. hand washing, hospital cleaning and laundering), and certainly not in replacement of such prac-tices. Two antimicrobials showing good potential are copper oxide and N-halamine, both of which have rapid kill times. Many copper products already have EPA approval to allow public health claims to be made, and in situ studies of treated textiles have shown reduction in microbial loads, with one clinical trial finding when sheets and clothing were replaced with copper oxide-treated textiles, a reduction in some types of HAIs occurred [76]. N-Halamine-impregnated textiles have shown astoundingly rapid and effective broad-spectrum antimicrobial activity in the laboratory [62], although there is limited availability of the textiles commercially. The abil-ity of N-halamine treated textiles to be recharged through

chlorine bleaching compatible with hospital laundering pro-cesses may not be suitable for all types of textiles. Nonetheless, it is clear that considerably more research examining antimicrobial-treated textiles within a clinical set-ting is still required.

References

1. Borkow G, Gabbay J. Biocidal textiles can help fight nosocomial infections. Med Hypotheses. 2008;70(5):990–4. doi:10.1016/j. mehy.2007.08.025.
2. Wiener-Well Y, Galuty M, Rudensky B, Schlesinger Y, Attias D, Yinnon AM. Nursing and physician attire as possible source of nosocomial infections. Am J Infect Control. 2011;39(7):555–9. doi:10.1016/j.ajic.2010.12.016.
3. Fijan S, Turk SS. Hospital textiles, are they a possible vehicle for healthcare-associated infections? Int J Environ Res Public Health. 2012;9(9):3330–43. doi:10.3390/ijerph9093330.
4. Burden M, Cervantes L, Weed D, Keniston A, Price CS, Albert RK. Newly cleaned physician uniforms and infrequently washed white coats have similar rates of bacterial contamination after an 8-hour workday: a randomized controlled trial. J Hosp Med. 2011;6(4):177–82. doi:10.1002/jhm.864.
5. Bureau-Chalot F, Piednoir E, Camus J, Bajolet O. Microbiologic quality of linen and linen rooms in short-term care units. J Hosp Infect. 2004;56(4):328–9. doi:10.1016/j.jhin.2003.12.016.
6. Dancer SJ. How do we assess hospital cleaning? A proposal for microbiological standards for surface hygiene in hospitals. J Hosp Infect. 2004;56(1):10–5. doi:10.1016/j.jhin.2003.09.017.
7. Perry C, Marshall R, Jones E. Bacterial contamination of uniforms. J Hosp Infect. 2001;48(3):238–41. doi:10.1053/jhin.2001.0962.
8. Treakle AM, Thom KA, Furuno JP, Strauss SM, Harris AD, Perencevich EN. Bacterial contamination of health care workers' white coats. Am J Infect Control. 2009;37(2):101–5. doi:10.1016/j. ajic.2008.03.009.
9. Wong D, Nye K, Hollis P. Microbial flora on doctors' white coats. BMJ. 1991;303:1602–4.
10. Albrich WC, Harbarth S. Health-care workers: source, vec-tor, or victim of MRSA? Lancet Infect Dis. 2008;8(5):289–301. doi:10.1016/S1473-3099(08)70097-5.
11. Ohl M, Schweizer M, Graham M, Heilmann K, Boyken L, Diekema D. Hospital privacy curtains are frequently and rapidly contami-nated with potentially pathogenic bacteria. Am J Infect Control. 2012;40(10):904–6. doi:10.1016/j.ajic.2011.12.017.
12. Dohmae S, Okubo T, Higuchi W, et al. Bacillus cereus noso-comial infection from reused towels in Japan. J Hosp Infect. 2008;69(4):361–7. doi:10.1016/j.jhin.2008.04.014.
13. Weernink A, Severin WPJ, Tjernberg I, Dijkshoorn L. Pillows, an unexpected source of Acinetobacter. J Hosp Infect. 1995;29(3):189–99.
14. Trillis F, Eckstein EC, Budavich R, Pultz MJ, Donskey CJ. Contamination of hospital curtains with health care-associated pathogens. Infect Control Hosp Epidemiol. 2008;29(11):48–50. doi:10.1086/591863.
15. Dancer SJ. Importance of the environment in methicillin-resistant *Staphylococcus aureus* acquisition: the case for hospi-tal cleaning. Lancet Infect Dis. 2008;8(2):101–13. doi:10.1016/ S1473-3099(07)70241-4.
16. Neely AN, Maley MP. Survival of enterococci and staphylococci on hospital fabrics and plastic. J Clin Microbiol. 2000;38(2):724–6. doi:10.1016/S0001-2092(06)61994-7.
17. Shiomori T, Miyamoto H, Makishima K, et al. Evaluation of bedmaking-related airborne and surface methicillin-resistant

Staphylococcus aureus contamination. J Hosp Infect. 2002;50(1): 30–5. doi:10.1053/jhin.2001.1136.

18. Brunton WAT. Infection and hospital laundry. Lancet. 1995;345(8964):1574–5.

19. Sasahara T, Hayashi S, Morisawa Y, Sakihama T, Yoshimura A, Hirai Y. Bacillus cereus bacteremia outbreak due to contaminated hospital linens. Eur J Clin Microbiol Infect Dis. 2011;30(2):219–26. doi:10.1007/s10096-010-1072-2.

20. Wright SN, Gerry JS, Busowski MT, et al. Gordonia bronchialis sternal wound infection in 3 patients following open heart surgery: intraoperative transmission from a healthcare worker. Infect Control Hosp Epidemiol. 2012;33(12):1238–41. doi:10.1086/668441.

21. Duffy J, Harris J, Gade L, et al. Mucormycosis outbreak associated with hospital linens. Pediatr Infect Dis J. 2014;33(5):472–6. doi:10.1097/INF.0000000000000261.

22. Thomas MC, Giedinghagen DH, Hoff GL. An outbreak of scabies among employees in a hospital-associated commercial laundry. Infect Control. 1987;8(10):427–9. doi:10.1017/S0195941700066613.

23. Shah PC, Krajden S, Kane J, Summerbell RC. Tinea corporis caused by Microsporum canis: report of a nosocomial outbreak. Eur J Epidemiol. 1988;4(1):33–8.

24. Standaert SM, Hutcheson RH, Schaffner W. Nosocomial transmission of Salmonella gastroenteritis to laundry workers in a nursing home. Infect Control Hosp Epidemiol. 1994;15(1):22–6. Available at: http://www.ncbi.nlm.nih.gov/pubmed/8133005

25. Munoz-Price LS, Arheart KL, Lubarsky DA, Birnbach DJ. Differential laundering practices of white coats and scrubs among health care professionals. Am J Infect Control. 2013;41(6):565–7. doi:10.1016/j.ajic.2012.06.012.

26. Loh W, Ng VV, Holton J. Bacterial flora on the white coats of medical students. J Hosp Infect. 2000;45(1):65–8. doi:10.1053/jhin.1999.0702.

27. Pilonetto M, Rosa EAR, Brofman PRS, et al. Hospital gowns as a vehicle for bacterial dissemination in an intensive care unit. Braz J Infect Dis. 2004;8(3):206–10. doi:/S1413-86702004000300003

28. Boyce JM, Potter-Bynoe G, Chenevert C, King T. Environmental contamination due to methicillin-resistant *Staphylococcus aureus*: possible infection control implications. Infect Control Hosp Epidemiol. 1997;18(9):622–7. Available at: http://www.ncbi.nlm.nih.gov/pubmed/9309433

29. Braswell ML, Spruce L. Implementing AORN recommended practices for surgical attire. AORN J. 2012;95(1):122–40. doi:10.1016/j.aorn.2011.10.017.

30. Wilson JA, Loveday HP, Hoffman PN, Pratt RJ. Uniform: an evidence review of the microbiological significance of uniforms and uniform policy in the prevention and control of healthcare-associated infections. Report to the Department of Health (England). J Hosp Infect. 2007;66(4):301–7. doi:10.1016/j.jhin.2007.03.026.

31. Wilkoff LJ, Westbrook L, Dixon GJ. Factors affecting the persistence of *Staphylococcus aureus* on fabrics. Appl Microbiol. 1969;17(2):268–74.

32. Borkow G, Monk A. Fighting nosocomial infections with biocidal non-intrusive hard and soft surfaces. World J Clin Infect Dis. 2012;2(4):77–90. doi:10.5527/wjn.v4.i3.379.

33. McMurry LM, Oethinger M, Levy SB. Triclosan targets lipid synthesis. Nature. 1998;394(6693):531–2. doi:10.1038/28970.

34. Levy SB. Antibiotic and antiseptic resistance: impact on public health. Pediatr Infect Dis J. 2000;19(10):S120–2. Available at: http://www.ncbi.nlm.nih.gov/pubmed/11052402

35. Braoudaki M, Hilton AC. Adaptive resistance to biocides in Salmonella enterica and *Escherichia coli* O157 and cross-resistance to Antimicrobial agents. J Clin Microbiol. 2004;42(1):73–8. doi:10.1128/JCM.42.1.73.

36. Mcmurry LM, Mcdermott PF, Levy SB, Murry LMMC, Dermott PFMC. Genetic evidence that InhA of Mycobacterium

smegmatis is a target triclosan. Antimicrob Agents Chemother. 1999;43(3):711–3.

37. Windler L, Height M, Nowack B. Comparative evaluation of antimicrobials for textile applications. Environ Int. 2013;53:62–73. doi:10.1016/j.envint.2012.12.010.

38. Schettler T. Antimicrobials in hospital furnishings: do they help reduce healthcare-associated infections? 2016. Available at: http://sehn.org/wp-content/uploads/2016/03/Antimicrobials-Report-2016.pdf.

39. Thorpe B. Chemicals in consumer products are draining trouble into the Great Lakes ecosystem. Canadian Environmental Law Association Toronto; 2014.

40. Borkow G, Gabbay J. Copper as a biocidal tool. Curr Med Chem. 2005;12(18):2163–75. doi:10.2174/0929867054637617.

41. Monteiro DR, Gorup LF, Takamiya AS, Ruvollo-Filho AC, de Camargo ER, Barbosa DB. The growing importance of materials that prevent microbial adhesion: antimicrobial effect of medical devices containing silver. Int J Antimicrob Agents. 2009;34(2):103–10. doi:10.1016/j.ijantimicag.2009.01.017.

42. Gao Y, Cranston R. Recent advances in antimicrobial treatments of textiles. Text Res J. 2008;78(1):60–72. doi:10.1177/0040517507082332.

43. Textiles Intelligence Ltd. Antimicrobial fibres, fabrics and apparel: innovative weapons against infection. Perform Appar Mark. 2013;47:25–57.

44. Lorenz C, Windler L, Von Goetz N, et al. Characterization of silver release from commercially available functional (nano) textiles. Chemosphere. 2012;89(7):817–24. doi:10.1016/j.chemosphere.2012.04.063.

45. Gabbay J, Borkow G, Mishal J, Magen E, Zatcoff R, Shemer-Avni Y. Copper oxide impregnated textiles with potent biocidal activities. J Ind Text. 2006;35(4):323–35. doi:10.1177/1528083706060785.

46. International Copper Association. Protection is about the person, not the product. 2015. Available at: http://www.antimicrobialcopper.org/uk/public-health-claims. Accessed 27 May 2016.

47. Humphreys H. Self-disinfecting and microbiocide-impregnated surfaces and fabrics: what potential in interrupting the spread of healthcare-associated infection? Clin Infect Dis. 2014;58(6):848–53. doi:10.1093/cid/cit765.

48. Li Y, Leung P, Yao L, Song QW, Newton E. Antimicrobial effect of surgical masks coated with nanoparticles. J Hosp Infect. 2006;62(1):58–63. doi:10.1016/j.jhin.2005.04.015.

49. Messaoud M, Chadeau E, Chaudouët P, Oulahal N, Langlet M. Quaternary ammonium-based composite particles for antibacterial finishing of cotton-based textiles. J Mater Sci Technol. 2014;30(1):19–29. doi:10.1016/j.jmst.2013.09.012.

50. McDonnell G, Russell AD. Antiseptics and disinfectants: activity, action, and resistance. Clin Microbiol Rev. 1999;12(1):147–79.

51. Schneider PM. New technologies in sterilization and disinfection. Am J Infect Control. 2013;41(5):S81–6. doi:10.1016/j.ajic.2012.12.003.

52. Chen-Yu JH, Eberhardt DM, Kincade DH. Antibacterial and laundering properties of AMS and PHMB as finishing agents on fabric for health care workers' uniforms. Cloth Text Res J. 2007;25(3):258–72. doi:10.1177/0887302X07303625.

53. Simoncic B, Tomsic B. Structures of novel antimicrobial agents for textiles – a review. Text Res J. 2010;80(16):1721–37. doi:10.1177/0040517510363193.

54. Moore K, Gray D. Using PHMB antimicrobial to p0revent wound infection. Wound UK. 2007;3(2):96–102.

55. Butcher M. PHMB: an effective antimicrobial in wound bioburden management. Br J Nurs. 2012;21(12):S16–21.

56. Kawabata A, Taylor JA. The effect of reactive dyes upon the uptake and antibacterial efficacy of poly(hexamethylene biguanide) on cotton. Part 3: reduction in the antibacterial efficacy of poly(hexamethylene biguanide) on cotton, dyed with

bis(monochlorotriazinyl) reactive dyes. Carbohydr Polym. 2007;67(3):375–89. doi:10.1016/j.carbpol.2006.06.022.

57. Sun Y, Sun G. Durable and regenerable antimicrobial textile materials prepared by a continuous grafting process. J Appl Polym Sci. 2002;84(8):1592–9. doi:10.1002/app.10456.

58. Kenawy ER, Worley SD, Broughton R. The chemistry and applications of antimicrobial polymers: a state-of-the-art review. Biomacromolecules. 2007;8(5):1359–84. doi:10.1021/bm061150q.

59. Liu S, Sun G. Durable and regenerable biocidal polymers: acyclic N-halamine cotton cellulose. Ind Eng Chem Res. 2006;45(19):6477–82. doi:10.1021/ie060253m.

60. He WD, Pan CY, Lu T. Novel regenerable N-halamine polymeric biocides. I. Synthesis, characterization, and antibacterial activity of hydantoin-containing polymers. J Appl Polym Sci. 2001;80(13):2460–7. doi:10.1002/app.1353.

61. Sun Y, Sun G. Grafting hydantoin-containing monomers onto cotton cellulose. J Appl Polym Sci. 2001;81:617–24.

62. Sun G, Worley SD. Chemistry of durable and regenerable biocidal textiles. J Chem Educ. 2005;82(1):60. doi:10.1021/ed082p60.

63. Tanner BD. Antimicrobial fabrics – issues and opportunities in the era of antibiotic resistance. AATCC Rev. 2009;9(11):30–3.

64. International Organization for Standardization. ISO 20743: textiles – determination of antibacterial activity of textile products. Geneva; 2013.

65. Tomsic B, Simoncic B, Orel B, et al. Sol-gel coating of cellulose fibres with antimicrobial and repellent properties. J Sol-Gel Sci Technol. 2008;47(1):44–57. doi:10.1007/s10971-008-1732-1.

66. Risti T, Fras L, Novak M, et al. Antimicrobial efficiency of functionalized cellulose fibres as potential medical textiles. In: Méndez-Vilas A, editor. Science against microbial pathogens: communicating current research and technological advances. Badajoz: Formatex; 2011. p. 36–51.

67. McQueen R, Keelan M, Kannayiram S. Determination of antimicrobial efficacy for textile products against odor-causing bacteria. AATCC Rev. 2010;10(4):58–63.

68. Kulthong K, Srisung S, Boonpavanitchakul K, Kangwansupamonkon W, Maniratanachote R. Determination of silver nanoparticle release from antibacterial fabrics into artificial sweat. Part Fibre Toxicol. 2010;7(1):8. doi:10.1186/1743-8977-7-8.

69. McQueen RH, Keelan M, Xu Y, Mah T. In vivo assessment of odour retention in an antimicrobial silver chloride-treated polyester textile. J Text Inst. 2013;104(1):108–17. doi:10.1080/00405000.2012.697623.

70. Alvarez E, Uslan DZ, Malloy T, Sinsheimer P, Godwin H. It is time to revise our approach to registering antimicrobial agents for health care settings. Am J Infect Control. 2015;44:228–32. doi:10.1016/j.ajic.2015.09.015.

71. Bearman GML, Rosato A, Elam K, et al. A crossover trial of antimicrobial scrubs to reduce methicillin-resistant *Staphylococcus aureus* burden on healthcare worker apparel. Infect Control Hosp Epidemiol. 2012;33(3):268–75. doi:10.1086/664045.

72. Schweizer M, Graham M, Ohl M, Heilmann K, Boyken L, Diekema D. Novel hospital curtains with antimicrobial properties: a randomized, controlled trial. Infect Control Hosp Epidemiol. 2012;33(11):1081–5. doi:10.1086/668022.

73. Taylor L, Phillips P, Hastings R. Reduction of bacterial contamination in a healthcare environment by silver antimicrobial technology. J Infect Prev. 2009;10(1):6–12. doi:10.1177/1757177408099083.

74. Burden M, Keniston A, Frank MG, et al. Bacterial contamination of healthcare workers' uniforms: a randomized controlled trial of antimicrobial scrubs. J Hosp Med. 2013;8(7):380–5. doi:10.1002/jhm.2051.

75. Boutin MA, Thom KA, Zhan M, Johnson JK. A randomized crossover trial to decrease bacterial contamination on hospital scrubs. Infect Control Hosp Epidemiol. 2014;35(11):1411–3. doi:10.1086/678426.

76. Lazary A, Weinberg I, Vatine JJ, et al. Reduction of healthcare-associated infections in a long-term care brain injury ward by replacing regular linens with biocidal copper oxide impregnated linens. Int J Infect Dis. 2014;24:23–9. doi:10.1016/j.ijid.2014.01.022.

77. Renaud FNR, Dore J, Freney HJ, Coronel B, Dusseau JY. Evaluation of antibacterial properties of a textile product with antimicrobial finish in a hospital environment. J Ind Text. 2006;36(1):89–94. doi:10.1177/1528083706066438.

78. Muller MP, MacDougall C, Lim M, et al. Antimicrobial surfaces to prevent healthcare-associated infections: a systematic review. J Hosp Infect. 2016;92(1):7–13. doi:10.1016/j.jhin.2015.09.008.

79. Sifri CD, Burke GH, Enfield KB. Reduced health care-associated infections in an acute care community hospital using a combination of self-disinfecting copper-impregnated composite hard surfaces and linens. Am J Infect Control. 2016;44(12):1565–1571. doi: 10.1016/j.ajic.2016.07.007.

80. Marcus EL, Yosef H, Borkow G, Caine Y, Sasson A, Moses AE. Reduction of health care-associated infection indicators by copper oxide-impregnated textiles: Crossover, double-blind controlled study in chronic ventilator-dependent patients. Am J Infect Control. 2017;45(4):401–403. doi:10.1016/j.ajic.2016.11.022.

Multidrug-Resistant Gram-Negative Bacilli: Infection Prevention Considerations

14

Oryan Henig, David E. Katz, and Dror Marchaim

Introduction

Gram-negative bacilli (GNB) pathogens cause a variety of serious infections. Their role as causative offending pathogens increased in the past years, and in many regions, they are considered the most common human pathogens [1, 2]. Emergence of resistance to antimicrobials among GNB has become a worldwide threat in both healthcare settings and the community, including among previously healthy and young individuals [3–5].

In 2008, Rice LB established a definition that was later embraced by the Infectious Diseases Society of America (IDSA) called "ESKAPE," in order to designate the pathogens that cause the majority of US hospital infections, while effectively "escaping" the activities of the commonly used antimicrobials (*Enterococcus faecium, Staphylococcus aureus, Klebsiella pneumoniae, Acinetobacter baumannii, Pseudomonas aeruginosa,* and *Enterobacter* species) [6, 7]. "ESKAPE" was changed later on into "ESCAPE," in order to include the "C" for *Clostridium difficile* and "E" for *Enterobacteriaceae* as a group (as opposed to the "K" of *Klebsiella* and "E" of *Enterobacter*) [8]. Among the ESCAPE group, GNBs are the pathogens that pose the highest epidemiological threat, due to extreme shortage of effective therapeutics [9]. In a large point-prevalence analysis conducted among 13,796 intensive care unit (ICU) patients from all over the world, GNB accounted for 62% of ICU infections [1].

The epidemiology of GNB has evolved dramatically during past years in several aspects: the incidence of infections increased, the distribution of resistances changed (in terms of geographic locations, facilities involved, unit composition, and populations affected), new mechanisms of resistance emerged, and, moreover, the definitions and detection rates changed, enabling more efficient monitoring and analysis of multidrug-resistant (MDR) GNBs [9]. Although the extent and diversity of antimicrobial resistance among GNB is very broad, non-susceptibility to beta-lactam agents, particularly to carbapenems and to extended-spectrum cephalosporins, frequently defines the epidemiological significance of the GNB pathogen [10]. Therefore, control of beta-lactam-resistant pathogens is commonly central to most infection control programs [10–12]. The use of beta-lactams as the backbone of treatment for serious GNB-related infections (being the oldest, safest, and frequently the least expensive with established efficacy per post-marketing controlled trials) [5, 13] contributed to the development and spread of resistance mechanisms. This chapter will focus primarily on infection control measures aimed at curbing the emergence and spread of four phenotypic resistance traits among the ESCAPE GNBs: (1) carbapenem-resistant *Enterobacteriaceae* (CRE), (2) carbapenem-resistant *Pseudomonas aeruginosa* (CRPA), (3) *Acinetobacter baumannii* (including but not solely limited to carbapenem-resistant *A. baumannii* [CRAB]), (4) *Enterobacteriaceae* resistant to extended-spectrum cephalosporins. This latter group will include pathogens expressing various types of beta-lactamases, including the Ambler A extended-spectrum beta-lactamases (ESBLs) and the Ambler C bla_{AmpC} (AmpC).

In general, there are two major approaches for limiting the emergence and spread of MDR organisms (MDRO). One is to address the spread of resistant organisms from one patient to the next (e.g., via healthcare staff, patient environment, and shared equipment). Alternatively, one may try to attenuate the emergence of resistance among susceptible strains the patient is already harboring. The possible infection control measures and interventions that address patient-to-patient transmission include (1) hand hygiene (HH), (2) contact isolation precautions (CIP), (3) cohorting with or without dedicated staff, (4) environmental cleaning, (5) surveillance programs to identify asymptomatic carriers, and (6) decolonization protocols [14–19]. In contrast, attenuating emergence of resistance requires enforcing adherence to antimicrobial stewardship policies [20]. In this chapter, we

O. Henig • D.E. Katz • D. Marchaim (✉)
Department of Infectious Diseases, Assaf Harofeh Medical Center, Zerifin 7030001, Israel
e-mail: oryan.henig@gmail.com; dekatz1@gmail.com; drormarchaim@gmail.com

© Springer International Publishing AG 2018
G. Bearman et al. (eds.), *Infection Prevention*, DOI 10.1007/978-3-319-60980-5_14

will review the role and available scientific data for each one of those measures, for each one of the aforementioned four groups of pathogens. When no conclusive controlled data is available, we will state our recommendations based on expert opinion.

Carbapenem-Resistant *Enterobacteriaceae* (CRE)

Epidemiology and Microbiology

The first carbapenem-resistant case of *Klebsiella pneumoniae*, through bla_{KPC} production, was reported from North Carolina in 2001 [21]. A few years later, it was identified in New York and spread to the south and west parts of the USA, eventually involving almost every US state [22–24]. Data from the Center for Disease Control and Prevention's (CDC) National Healthcare Safety Network (NHSN) indicated that by 2014, 2.8–12% of the *Enterobacteriaceae* healthcare-associated infections (HAIs) were CRE [25]. There was also an increase of CRE in Europe. The European Antimicrobial Resistance Surveillance Network (EARS-Net) reported in 2014 a mean of 7.3% CRE among *K. pneumoniae* (with rates over 60% in Greece) and 1.2% among *Escherichia coli* [26].

CRE were once considered exclusively nosocomial pathogens [27]; however, over the last decade, the boundaries between hospitals and long-term care facilities (LTCF) including skilled nursing facilities and long-term acute-care hospitals (LTACH) changed, due to the modern continuity of healthcare [28]. In a 2011 point-prevalence survey in an LTACH in Chicago, CRE was detected among 30% of residents [29, 30]. Today, every infection control program in an acute-care hospital must involve its surrounding LTCFs, in order to be successful [28].

The main resistant mechanism of CRE is by hydrolyzing the carbapenem by carbapenemase enzymes often carried on mobile genetic elements (i.e., CRE-CP) [21, 31]. The current major carbapenemase in the USA and worldwide is the Ambler- A bla_{KPC} [32], but Ambler- B (bla_{NDM}, bla_{VIM}, bla_{IMP}) and Ambler- D (bla_{OXA-48}) are additional carbapenemases reported in various frequencies from various parts of the world [33]. Non-carbapenemase-producing CRE (CRE-non-CP) is becoming more and more prevalent worldwide [31], particularly since the Clinical and Laboratory Standards Institute (CLSI) and the European Committee on Antimicrobial Susceptibility Testing (EUCAST) lowered the breakpoints defining non-susceptibility to carbapenems among *Enterobacteriaceae* [34, 35]. Not much is known about the epidemiology of CRE-non-CP. It is speculated that this group of pathogens is heterogenic, consisting of various mechanisms of resistance, including unidentified (or misdiagnosed) carbapenemases and non-carbapenemase beta-lactamases coupled with loss of expression of outer-membrane proteins and/or expression of efflux pumps [36]. The epidemiological implications of CRE-CP versus CRE-non CP are controversial [37], and tests for resistance mechanisms are utilized differently in various geographic areas [38]. For instance, while the Israeli ministry of health advocates to test every CRE for carbapenemase production, preferably through molecular methods, and to implement different infection control measures guided by carbapenemase production results, the US CDC does not require mandatory testing for carbapenemase production for the definition of CRE. Infection control measures for CRE-CP and CRE-non-CP carriers could be similar in some states and institutions [24, 39]. CRE are extensively drug-resistant organisms (XDRO) [40], with very few therapeutic options available [41]. Recently, colistin resistance, one of the very few therapeutic options, was found in 43% of 191 isolates of CRE-*K. pneumoniae* (CRKP) strains [42]. Moreover, a plasmid-mediated colistin resistance gene (mcr-1) was reported in *E. coli*, which, if disseminated, might lead to a truly pan-resistant pathogen [43].

Measures to Decrease CRE Patient-to-Patient Transmission

Hand Hygiene

Hand hygiene (HH) is considered one of the important interventions and measures to prevent patient-to-patient transmission of CRE. HH is a vital part of standard precautions and of contact isolation precautions (CIP); however, data demonstrating the impact of HH as a stand-alone intervention are lacking. Nevertheless, it is simple and considered the most efficacious intervention [24, 44]. Unfortunately, compliance with this simple and basic practice is inadequate [45]. A mathematical model estimated the impact of HH on CRKP transmission in a surgical unit with low HH compliance (21%). The authors demonstrated that an increase in HH compliance to a rate of 60% succeeded in containing CRKP transmission and was the most important and effective intervention in curbing CRKP spread [46]. HH adherence should be monitored, adherence rates distributed to staff and managers, feedback obtained, and education systematically provided. HH must serve as the backbone for every CRE prevention plan, and resources should be allocated accordingly.

Contact Isolation Precautions (CIP)

CIP include three components: HH before donning a gown and gloves, donning a gown and gloves before entering the patient's room, and removing gown and gloves and performing HH before leaving the patient's room [24, 47]. CRE carriers should be subjected to CIP [24].

Several studies demonstrated that CIP may limit the spread of CRE [48, 49]. A national intervention program in Israel reduced the incidence of CRE detected in clinical cultures from 55.5 to 11.7 per 100,000 patient-days [49]. In an ICU in a New York City hospital, the incidence of CRE detected in clinical cultures decreased from 9.7 to 3.7 per 1000 patient-days following implementation of CIP as part of a prevention bundle [49, 50]. Other examples for bundles implemented to reduce CRE spread were described worldwide, all including CIP as the pivotal measure. For example, in an outbreak in an ICU in Italy, several interventions were implemented in several stages. CIP were implemented as the first stage, whereas cohorting was implemented later. Implementing CIP as well as cohorting and enforcing other measures (including improvements in environmental cleaning), helped avoid the closure of the ICU [51].

There is no consensus as for the duration of CIP for CRE carriers. In one study, the duration of carriage was found to be prolonged; specifically, the mean duration of carriage was 387 days (95% CI 312–463 days), and 39% of the patients were positive for at least 12 months [52, 53]. Predictors of CRE persistence or recrudesce include antimicrobial use, subsequent admission to an institution or another hospital, and a time interval less than or equal to 3 months since the first positive CRE culture. It was shown that having one predictor was associated with a 50% chance of having a positive result [54]. In an Israeli study, risk factors for recurrent carriage in patients who were predefined as "CRE-free" (i.e., two negative cultures collected on different days) included short time between last positive culture, readmission to a healthcare facility, and the presence of foreign bodies [55]. We believe that the duration of CIP should be for at least 12 months. Moreover, as long as the patient is incontinent, we advocate not to remove the patient from CIP, due to high rate of recrudesce, though this recommendation is not scientifically supported. CIP, just like HH, depends on healthcare worker (HCW) compliance; therefore, adherence to correct CIP should be monitored closely, followed by adequate education and feedback.

Patient Cohorting and Dedicated Staff

Cohorting refers to placing patients with the same pathogen or mechanism of resistance together, preferably cared by dedicating staff who do not care for other patients during the same shift. In a detailed review of studies that evaluated bundles with different combinations of interventions, the interventions that were common to all studies were HH and CIP [22, 50]. In the Israeli national CRE-CP epidemic, the outbreak was further curbed and contained only following the institution of a set of regulations that mandated every institution to designate a specified cohort unit for CRE-CP carriers, treated by dedicated nursing staff [49, 56].

"United cohort units" containing several types of carriers (i.e., CRE and CRAB) are strongly discouraged given the risk of transferring mobile genetic elements containing resistance traits that could cross the interspecies barriers [57], resulting to pan-resistant isolates. In a multicenter trial, co-carriage of CRE-CP along with *A. baumannii* or *P. aeruginosa* was associated with increased overall mortality and with emergence of CRE-CP resistant to colistin. This was evident in the center where a united cohort unit (for all carbapenem-resistant GNBs) was present in one of the ICUs [57, 58]. Currently, the CDC recommends cohorting of patients with CRE in both hospitals and LTCFs [24].

Environmental Cleaning and Disinfection

Surface level cleanliness in healthcare environments has been shown to be important for controlling infections caused by Gram-positive microorganisms such as MRSA, VRE, and *C. difficile* [59]. Controlled studies demonstrating the impact of cleaning alone for controlling *Enterobacteriaceae* infections, however, are lacking. Regardless, studies demonstrate that a colonized patient's immediate environment becomes colonized with the same MDR-GNB relatively fast [60]. It has been observed that GNBs tend to survive longer than Gram-positives [61]. While *Enterobacteriaceae* were thought to survive less than non-fermenters GNB (*A. baumannii*, *P. aeruginosa*), recent data have demonstrated longer survival periods; for example, isolation of *E. coli* on metal surfaces lasted for 16 months following the initial exposure [62, 63].

The evidence supporting CRE environmental contamination is controversial. In a report that studied the rate of CRE contamination in bedrooms of seven patients colonized or infected with CRE, only 8.4% of the samples from different surfaces grew CRE. The majority of pathogens survived less than 72 h [64]. Alternatively, an Israeli study showed higher rates of environmental contamination [60]. In this study, two environmental sampling methods were used, i.e., direct CHROM-agar KPC contact plates and eSWAB. Direct CHROM-agar contact plates were more sensitive than eSWAB for detecting environmental CRE on flat surfaces (e.g., bedside table/tray), and the eSWAB was superior on non-flat surfaces (e.g., pillows) [60, 65]. The areas closest to the patient had the highest pathogen recovery. In other studies, the areas with the highest contamination rate were the toilet and the floor near the toilet [64]. In other ICU outbreaks, sinks were shown to be an important reservoir [66].

Evidence from controlled CRE outbreak investigations demonstrated that cleaning the patient environment, specifically high-touch surfaces, can assist in reducing potential transmission [22, 60, 67, 68]. Even though evidence evaluating the sole impact of cleaning on CRE acquisitions is lacking, maintaining a clean environment must be perceived as fundamental for all hygienic measures in preventing CRE infections [59]. Rooms occupied by patients with CRE should be cleaned and disinfected thoroughly at least once per day. Moreover, we advocate cleaning the high-touch surfaces (e.g., bedrails, bedside tables or trays, infusion pumps, monitors [including its wires], charts hung on beds, nurse call buttons, light switches of night lights, door handles, and toilet, sinks) every shift, i.e., multiple times a day. Following patient discharge, any facility should establish an internal "terminal cleaning" protocol, which details the measures that should be applied specifically for this indication. Training is important, and the process of terminal cleaning should be monitored, and results should be distributed to all involved personnel. CDC further encourages institutions to optimize their policies and procedures related to environmental disinfection in both CRE endemic and epidemic settings [69].

New methods for disinfection of the patient's environment after discharge were evaluated in recent years, including ultraviolet (UV) C-emitted light and hydrogen peroxide vapor systems. These methods were not tested specifically for CRE, but they were tested for *P. aeruginosa* and *A. baumannii* and are undergoing further testing and evaluation [70, 71].

Monitoring of Cleaning

Given the potential role of cleaning in the control of CRE outbreaks, monitoring the adherence to cleaning policies as well as the efficacy of cleaning is now considered fundamental additives for prevention [69]. A visual inspection does not suffice, and culturing methods on routine basis (i.e., in non-outbreak settings) yield unsatisfactory recovery rates [60]. Monitoring cleanliness may be accomplished using invisible fluorescent markers or adenosine triphosphate (ATP) bioluminescence measurements. Utilizing ATP bioluminometers has provided quantitative evidence of improved cleanliness in terms of Gram-positive pathogens from high-touch surfaces [72, 73]. In a study that used fluorescent markers to objectively evaluate the thoroughness of terminal cleaning before and after implementing an educational intervention for environmental services personnel, cleaning improved from 49.5 to 82% (of surfaces cleaned) and helped to increase compliance with proper procedures [74]. However, the impact of evaluating the quality and compliance of cleaning practices on clinical outcomes, including acquisitions of CRE, is lacking.

Shared Equipment

Shared equipment refers to objects used by more than one patient or physician, which can potentially be contaminated with MDRO (including CRE) and provide a vector for transmission. CRE was isolated from ambu bags, phones, toys, pens, keyboards, and stethoscopes [75]. Protocols for cleaning, disinfection, and sterilizing shared equipment should be

established and followed closely. The importance of equipment disinfection with regard to CRE was recently highlighted following an outbreak of CRE infection associated with use of duodenoscopes (2012–2015) [76–78]. About 65% of sites reported positive cultures of the duodenoscopes even after proper reprocessing per manufacturer's instructions. The complex design of the duodenoscopes limited access to parts of the scopes, which were found to be contaminated with CRE [76, 79].

Active Surveillance

Active surveillance has become one of the central measures used in infection control programs. Active screening cultures (ASC) reflect colonization pressure better than clinical specimens [56, 80] and identify patients who serve as a reservoir for potential MDRO transmission. When accompanied by preemptive CIP [22, 81], ASC was shown to reduce colonization pressure [82] and limit the spread of MDROs, including CRE [56]. In addition, since CRE colonization is a risk factor for CRE infection [83], ASC may lead to improve outcomes for patients infected with CRE, by reducing the delay in instituting appropriate antimicrobial therapy, which is the strongest independent predictor for mortality in severe sepsis [84, 85].

ASC is now recommended by both national and international societies for CRE prevention [11, 24, 86]. Cultures for screening should be taken from the rectum (samples should contain stool), and the perirectal area should be sampled only in specified populations (e.g., neutropenic patients) [84]. The methods used for processing surveillance samples are various and include cultures and fast molecular techniques to identify CRE and relevant carbapenemases [39]. Local policies for CRE screening should be developed to target certain populations based of risk stratification in any given facility. Major risks to be considered include patients who were recently hospitalized (i.e., within the past 6–12 months), LTCF residents, elderly incontinent individuals with reduced cognition, and foreign patients from endemic countries (i.e., "medial tourism") [24, 87, 88]. Both the CDC and ESCMID recommend that patients being treated at cancer centers, in an ICU, and/or in endemic units/floors should be periodically (i.e., weekly) screened to further reduce the colonization pressure [11, 24]. In addition, in the case of new acquisition, contacts should be rescreened.

Clinical laboratories should have an established protocol for timely notification of clinical and/or infection prevention personnel when CRE are identified by clinical or surveillance culture. Facilities should also establish a flagging system to point to staff of CRE carriage status upon future admissions or whenever the patient is transferred between locations inside the institution [11, 24, 81]. In Israel, a national registry governed by the ministry of health assists in improving inter-facilities communications on national level and may have contributed to the containment of a huge outbreak in 2006–2009 [49, 56].

Decolonization for CRE

As a concept, selective digestive decontamination (SDD) and selective oropharyngeal decontamination (SOD) involves administration of antibiotics (mainly oral nonabsorbable agents), to eradicate gastrointestinal (GI) carriage of MDR-GNB, in order to reduce the risk of progressing from colonization to infection. This measure was mainly studied in preventing hospital-acquired pneumonia (HAP) and ventilator-associated pneumonia (VAP) [89, 90]. Several randomized controlled trials evaluated the impact of anti-CRE decolonization on CRE carriage eradication and CRE infection prevention, with conflicting results. Saidel Odes et al. demonstrated a decrease in *K. pneumoniae* CRE (CRKP) carriage following 7 days of SDD and SOD using polymyxin and gentamicin (compared to a placebo-controlled group), but colonization rate later increased after 6 weeks [91]. In another study, the use of colistin and/or gentamicin for SDD was associated with significant eradication of CRE as well as decreased mortality [92]. However, in the same study, 26% of the patients treated with gentamicin were later colonized with gentamicin-resistant CRE. Lubbert C et al. used colistin and gentamicin as SDD and SOD and did not observe a significant difference in the eradication rate compared to control group. Moreover, at the 48-day stool culture follow-up, there was a 19% increase in colistin resistance and a 45% increase in gentamicin resistance among CRKP isolates, whereas no emergence of resistance was detected among the control group [93]. Since CRE is a XDRO with very limited therapeutic options [40], we do not recommend using a potentially therapeutic agent (e.g., colistin) for CRE prevention or for decolonization of asymptomatic carriers. SDD could be considered for unique indications only (e.g., candidates for transplant or for intensive chemotherapy) [81, 94].

One potential intervention to eradicate CRE colonization in the GI tract is by fecal microbiota transplantation (FMT). FMT is now used for recurrent *C. difficile* infection and was recently reported to have success in eradication of GI ESBL-producing *K. pneumoniae* in immunocompromised patients. Trials of FMT for decolonization of CRE are currently underway with initial promising results [95]. Efficacy and safety data from larger cohorts of carriers are needed in order to advocate specific and clear recommendations.

Antimicrobial Stewardship

Antibiotic stewardship has an important role in curbing the emergence of antimicrobial resistance and should be incorporated into every infection control program [24, 96]. There is no antibiotic found consistently to be associated with CRE acquisition, not even carbapenems [20]. However, exposure to antibiotics in general was the strongest independent predictor associated with CRE acquisition in many trials [41]. An ecological study conducted in India has shown that an antimicrobial stewardship program that included routine shortening of the duration of antibiotics administration was associated with reduction of CRE isolation [97, 98]. In an Israeli study, restricting the use of carbapenems showed remarkable success in lowering CRE rates, but that was part of a bundle that included among others, ASC and cohorting [99].

Carbapenem-Resistant *Pseudomonas aeruginosa*

Epidemiology and Microbiology

P. aeruginosa is the most prevalent GNB causing HAP and VAP in the USA [100]. Data from the National Healthcare Safety Network (NHSN) from 2006 to 2007 reported that 25.3% of *P. aeruginosa* causing HAI were carbapenem resistant [101]. CRPA infections have been associated with increased mortality, length of hospitalization, and costs [102].

P. aeruginosa possesses numerous resistance mechanisms to carbapenems. Efflux pumps, encoded both chromosomally and on numerous plasmids, confer resistance to multiple classes of drugs (except polymyxins) and are the predominant mechanism of multidrug resistance among *P. aeruginosa*, along with beta-lactamases (including carbapenemases) [103]. Therapeutic failure due to resistance that emerges during treatment is frequently reported [104]. Apart from resistance, *P. aeruginosa* is known for its ability to produce biofilm, which contributes to its resistance and survival on environmental surfaces, medical devices, and the airways of patients with chronic lung diseases [105]. These features of CRPA necessitate collaborations with infection control and antibiotic stewardship teams to control its spread and limit emergence of resistance.

Patient-to-Patient Transmission

Outbreaks associated with CRPA are typically described in ICU settings, immunocompromised patients, and neonates. Important reservoirs are contaminated sinks, scopes, water taps, and mechanical ventilators [106]. Other risk factors include ICU stays, use of invasive devices, being bedridden, and exposure to antimicrobials [107]. The mechanisms of transmission vary, and the contribution of patient-to-patient or environment-to-patient transmission is in debate. Though several studies demonstrated low cross transmission rate during ICU outbreaks [56, 80, 82], other studies estimated that the proportion of patient-to-patient transmission varied between 18% in hospital wards, 36–64% in ICUs [108], and above 70% in LTCFs [14]. A recent study showed that colonization pressure was a significant factor in new CRPA acquisition [109]. Another important population are patients with cystic fibrosis (CF), shown to be a source of patient-to-patient transmission. Samples of air within 3 ft of patients with CF were shown to be contaminated with *P. aeruginosa* during 8.2% of visits [110].

Hand Hygiene and Contact Isolation Precautions (CIP)

In a point-prevalence analysis of stool cultures, it was found that 13% of healthcare workers (HCW) carry *P. aeruginosa*. In addition, hand colonization was detected among 15% of ICU personnel and was demonstrated to persist on hands for up to 4 weeks [108]. An outbreak investigation in a neonatal ICU (NICU) found the same strain of *P. aeruginosa* among patients and the long artificial nails of one of the staff. Improving HH and restriction of nail length reduced the rate of infection [111]. In a study that focused on CRPA infection rate before and after increasing hand sanitizer use among HCWs, the rate of CRPA infections was negatively correlated to the volume of alcohol being consumed by hand sanitizers [112]. Other studies, however, demonstrated failure of HH and CIP to limit the rate of CRPA infections [50, 109]. Since the pathways of transmissions vary and the contributions of patient-to-patient transmission in endemic settings are controversial, the rationale behind recommending CIP to limit the spread of CRPA is based primarily on extrapolations from other better-designed studies pertaining to other MDRO acquisitions [18].

Whereas the ESCMID guidelines recommend the use of CIP in cases of MDR-PA in both epidemic and endemic settings, CDC recommendations defer, as with other MDROs, to the clinical and epidemiological judgment of the attending personnel at any given site [11]. Most facilities subject only patients with CRPA to CIP, since resistance to carbapenems is the epidemiological marker for the isolate becoming an XDRO [9]. In this context, it is important to note that CIP in general has been associated with less attention and personal contact from HCW because of the additional effort required in adhering to CIP [113]. CIP may be stressful for patients and their families, and isolated patients are prone to higher rates of dissatisfaction with care, anxiety, depression, preventable adverse events, and medical errors [114]. However, CIP is one of our only tools to reduce the colonization pressure that contributes to the risk of patients becoming colonized and of colonized patients becoming infected with the offending pathogen [115–117]. Our recommendation is to implement CIP for CRPA carriers.

Patient Cohorting and Dedicated Staff

There are no solid evidence-based studies that measured the impact of cohorting and instituting dedicated staff on the rate of CRPA infections. In one ICU outbreak, cohorting ended the outbreak [118]. However, united cohorting (i.e., cohorting patients with CRPA with carriers of other carbapenem-resistant GNB), as discussed above, was associated with co-colonization of CRE, *A. baumannii*, and *P. aeruginosa* and increased antimicrobial resistance to carbapenems and to colistin [58]. Therefore, we recommend against united cohorting as an infection control measure for such settings, in order to avoid emergence of pan-resistant GNBs [58].

Environmental Cleaning and Disinfection

P. aeruginosa is capable of colonizing a wide range of healthcare environments, mainly moistened sites, but it was isolated after prolonged periods from dry surfaces as well [61]. Several properties of *P. aeruginosa* favor its persistence in the hospital environment, as discussed above. In addition, *P. aeruginosa* is inherently resistant to some disinfectants such as biguanides and quaternary ammonium compounds through the action of efflux pumps [119]. The significance of tap water and other moistened sites (e.g., connection pieces and basins) as a reservoir for patients' colonization was demonstrated in both outbreak and endemic settings [120]. In several outbreaks, only manipulation of the water tap and water-associated sites, such as pasteurizing the water or replacement of the water source, was effective in abating the outbreaks [121–123]. Following one outbreak in an ICU, a combination of measures were applied: increasing the water temperature, using copper silver ionization, replacement of drinking water with *P. aeruginosa*-free bottle water, reinforcement of standard precaution, and hand disinfection with alcohol solutions instead of soap. These measures significantly reduced the rate of exogenous acquisition of *P. aeruginosa* (i.e., patient-to-patient transmission or faucet-to-patient transmission), whereas the endogenous acquisition remained without change [124]. There were, however, several methodological controversies associated with case allocation in this study. In a different ICU, the presence of *P. aeruginosa* in tap water was associated with patients' colonization of the same strain [125]. In another study that evaluated colonization in intubated patients, tap water in the patients' rooms was colonized in 63% of samples [126]. While clinical data evaluating the impact of cleaning methods on CRPA associated with HAI are lacking, maintaining a clean environment provides the fundamental basis for all hygienic measures in preventing infection [59].

Active Surveillance

Since patients colonized with CRPA exert colonization pressure, and patient-to-patient transmission is important in CRPA spread, it would be reasonable to screen patients.

However, current data to support the practice of ASC on CRPA spread are scarce. Several studies demonstrated prior colonization in 56.5–100% of ICU patients who had *P. aeruginosa* infection [108, 127, 128]. A study that screened ICU patients demonstrated increased risk for infection in patients who were colonized on admission compared to non-colonized patients (14.65-fold) [129]. Rectal colonization was consistently reported to have the highest yield of screening cultures, followed by pharyngeal or other respiratory cultures [108, 129, 130]. In mechanically ventilated patients or patients with chronic lung diseases (e.g., CF), deep respiratory surveillances are preferable [84]. Overall, colonization rates are high in the ICU setting and range between 26% and 43% [128, 129], but currently there is no evidence supporting routine screening (in endemic settings) as a measure for reducing CRPA acquisition rates [50]. We recommend implementing ASC only in ICUs during outbreaks or if significant increases in basal endemic rates are observed.

Decolonization for *P. aeruginosa*

Most decolonization regimens studied were for the prevention of HAP and VAP. Not many of the regimens had established antipseudomonal activity, and they did not evaluate the impact on *P. aeruginosa* colonization exclusively. However, *P. aeruginosa* is the most common GNB causing VAP. Since emergence of resistance was demonstrated with these regimens [91], and the clinical efficacy was not evaluated, this practice is discouraged, particularly in areas with higher burden of resistance.

Antimicrobial Stewardship

Various methodologies were used in different studies to evaluate the impact of carbapenem exposure and the emergence of CRPA [131]. Though studies conducted at the ecological level (i.e., correlating hospital antimicrobial usage and incidence of diagnosing resistance strains) showed no impact [102], studies conducted at the individual level (case-control analyses) demonstrated an association between previous exposure to imipenem and CRPA infection [132, 133]. Antibiotic stewardship interventions that were implemented to curb the emergence of new CRPA demonstrated a favorable impact of restricting carbapenems on CRPA rates. In a 22-university hospital study, eight hospitals restricted the use of carbapenems between 2002 and 2006 and showed a significant reduction in the CRPA rates [134]. In a quasi-experimental study conducted at a rehabilitation center, the impact of an antibiotic stewardship program on patterns of resistance before (between 2011 and 2012) and after (between 2012 and 2014) the intervention was evaluated. Reduced consumption of carbapenems and fluoroquinolones was associated with a decrease in emergence of the XDR phenotype among offending *P. aeruginosa* strains (from 55% in 2011 to 12% in 2014, $p < 0.001$). Of note, reduction of resistance rate was demonstrated among other pathogens as well [135].

Numerous studies in the past years were conducted to assess the impact of ertapenem use instead of group 2 carbapenems (i.e., imipenem, meropenem, and doripenem) on CRPA rate isolation. Most of these studies were sponsored by the pharmaceutical industry and showed that the substitution of ertapenem (group 1 carbapenem) with other broad-spectrum, non-carbapenem agents was not associated with an increase in CRPA rates [136–138]. In summary, antibiotic stewardship has a major role in curbing antimicrobial resistance among *P. aeruginosa*.

Acinetobacter Baumannii

Epidemiology and Microbiology

A. baumannii has become a major cause of nosocomial infections in the last two decades. The ability to resist environmental stresses and cleaning materials, as well as the rapid emergence of antimicrobial resistance, has made *A. baumannii* one of the most prevalent causes of outbreaks in ICUs [139]. The prevalence of MDR and mainly carbapenem-resistant *A. baumannii* (CRAB) has increased dramatically in most of the world. Rates of CRAB increased from 1% in the 1990s to 70% in certain areas in Europe and the USA [140, 141]. *A. baumannii* outbreaks were initially restricted to ICUs. Over time, *A. baumannii* became a pathogen found in other departments (i.e., internal medicine wards), as well as in patients from LTCF and LTACH, who serves as reservoir for transmission [25, 142–144]. CRAB identified in the community usually reflects previous exposure to health system, to procedures, or to broad-spectrum antibiotics [142].

It is yet to be determined whether CRAB deserves a greater focus in terms of infection control measures than carbapenem-susceptible *A. baumannii* (CSAB). Since certain mechanisms of resistance to carbapenem are chromosomally encoded, CSAB may become CRAB in the same patient under certain stressors [145]. A recent controlled study has shown similar outcomes between patients with CRAB and CSAB bloodstream infections after controlling for confounders, including the delay in initiating appropriate therapy (DAAT) [10]. Based on this analysis and available data, we propose that infection control measures should focus on reducing patient-to-patient transmission of all *A. baumannii*, not only CRAB. *A. baumannii* resistant to colistin has recently been reported in outbreaks in Italy and Greece [146]. Some patients in this study came from the "community," which highlights the importance of limiting transmission in acute-care hospitals of pan-resistant isolates from patients admitted from LTCFs [28].

Measures to Decrease *A. baumannii* Patient-to-Patient Transmission

Patient-to-Patient Transmission Role and Hand Hygiene

In detailed and robustly conducted analyses, which aimed to quantify all transmission opportunities between *A. baumannii* carriers, it was shown repeatedly that patient-to-patient transmission is the major mode for *A. baumannii* acquisition in acute-care hospitals, compared to emergence of resistance [147, 148]. Colonized patients may serve as reservoirs, and HCW hands, shared equipment, and/or contaminated close environment can all serve as vectors for transmission. A study that evaluated the transmission of MDR organisms in the ICU showed that HCW hands were contaminated (before entry into patient rooms) twice as more often with *A. baumannii* (5.1%) compared to other MDROs (0.6–3.6%) [149]. This same study also demonstrated that after glove removal and before HH was performed, hands and gloves were contaminated with MDR *A. baumannii* in 4.2% and 29.3%, respectively. Gowns were also significantly contaminated after patient care. In a Spanish ICU, the contamination rate by MDR *A. baumannii* was 12–20% among HCWs [150]. As with CRE, the isolated impact of HH on the rate of *A. baumannii* transmission is hard to quantify. However, HH should be implemented as part of every infection control intervention to reduce transmission of *A. baumannii*. Data from experimentally contaminated hands show that alcohol-based hand rub could reduce *A. baumannii* counts by 98% [151].

Contact Isolation Precautions (CIP)

The efficacy of CIP in controlling *A. baumannii* outbreaks (irrespective of resistance pattern) was repeatedly demonstrated to be effective [152]. In one study, the incidence rates of *A. baumannii* colonization and infections decreased during CIP and increased again when CIP was discontinued [152]. Another study demonstrated the efficacy of CIP as part of a bundle in an endemic setting [150]. In this study, a marked and sustained decrease in MDR *A. baumannii* infections was demonstrated as well, including BSI episodes. The success of containing outbreaks by implementing CIP depends on adherence to HH recommendations [151], proper environmental cleaning (e.g., appropriate disposal of contaminated equipment) [150], and preemptive isolation while cultures of suspected carriers are being processed [152]. Although the APIC recommends CIP for patients with MDR *A. baumannii* in acute-care hospitals [153], we believe that all patients with *A. baumannii* strains should be subjected to

CIP (not related to *Acinetobacter* of non-*A. baumannii* complex). In LTCFs, APIC recommends that the individual patient's clinical condition, as well as the incidence of MDR *A. baumannii* in the facility, and the type of LTCF should determine whether CIP should be implemented [153].

Patient Cohorting and Dedicated Staff

Patient cohorting and dedicating staff has not been evaluated independently for *A. baumannii* prevention. In a trial that instituted cohorting along with CIP, the prevention bundle was effective [152]. Cohorting patients (preferably with dedicated staff and always accompanied with CIP) should be implemented whenever patient isolation in a private room is not feasible. APIC recommends cohorting of patients with MDR *A. baumannii* only [153]; we think that any intervention should apply to all patients with *A. baumannii*, regardless of the phenotypic resistance profile [10, 84].

Environmental Cleaning and Disinfection

Environmental contamination of dry and moist areas is an established mechanism for *A. baumannii* dissemination. Colonized and infected patients shed *A. baumannii* for prolonged periods, which can contaminate hospital surfaces and medical devices [139, 154–156]. In some studies, *A. baumannii* was cultured from various surfaces and devices (e.g., ventilators, suctioning equipment, resuscitation equipment, bed rails, bedside tables, sinks, pillows, and radiology machines) for up to 5 months [61]. In an ICU that evaluated transmission of various MDROs between HCWs, patients, and the environment, *A. baumannii* was present in 78% of rooms hosting known carriers. The authors estimated that one third of occurrences where HCW enters a room of a patient with *A. baumannii* results in contamination of their gowns and gloves [149]. Most of the data pertaining to the efficacy of environmental cleaning in controlling outbreaks of GNBs are derived from *A. baumannii* outbreak investigations [157–159]. Several outbreak reports from general ICU, neurosurgery, and pediatric burn units were controlled only after initiating and implementing environmental screening and cleaning interventions [11].

A. baumannii is more resistant to some products commonly used for cleaning and disinfecting the environment [160]. Persistent contamination by *A. baumannii* was demonstrated even after four routine cleaning and disinfecting sessions [161]. In that study, the addition of hydrogen peroxide vapor (HPV) improved the reduction of site contamination. Novel methods, such as HPV and UV light, have been shown to be significantly more effective in reducing contamination rates [162]. However, clinical efficacies on actual infectious clinical outcomes studied in controlled design are lacking. In addition, current high turnaround time in many acute-care hospitals, and the need to empty the room prior the use of one of these novel methodologies, may hinder their implementation in hospitals [29, 71]. As discussed in other sections, infection control programs for curbing *A. baumannii* spread should always include specified policies that address cleaning techniques, products, and responsibilities at all levels. Both cleaning procedures while the patient is in the room and after the patient is discharged should be established. Audits and monitoring of cleanliness, as well as feedback and education back to the teams, are part of implementing environmental cleaning as an infection control measure.

Active Surveillance

The role of *A. baumannii* screening is still under debate. In general, *A. baumannii* asymptomatic carriers increase the colonization pressure, and early identification accompanied by preemptive CIP has the potential to limit patient-to-patient transmission [163]. This is important since patient-to-patient transmission has a pivotal role in *A. baumannii* spread [147, 148]. In addition, patients colonized with *A. baumannii* are at higher risk for *A. baumannii* infection than patients without colonization [164], and appropriate antimicrobial therapy in *A. baumannii* infections is frequently delayed [165]. All these factors theoretically support the use of active surveillance cultures (ASC) in order to prevent *A. baumannii* acquisitions.

There are, however, limitations to ASC in the field of *A. baumannii*. First, the sensitivity of surveillance cultures using traditional methods was found to be low and varied between studies, ranging between 55 and 85% [166, 167], even when multiple body sites were concurrently sampled. Second, the optimal body site to screen has not been determined, as opposed to the rectum for CRE and VRE screening or the nares for MRSA. Studies that evaluated screening sensitivity for different body sites using different sampling techniques (e.g., swab versus sponge), and different microbiological processing methodologies, have yielded various results. The only clear recommendation is to obtain respiratory specimens for ASC obtained through deep suction in mechanically ventilated patients [166].

In a Monte-Carlo simulation analysis with three possible carriage prevalences of *A. baumannii* (2%, 4%, and 6%) in a theoretical acute-care hospital settings, significant decreases in transmission, infection, and mortality rates were associated with *A. baumannii* ASC intervention, even when the sensitivity rate of the test was as low as 55% [168]. This study also demonstrated cost-effectiveness for *A. baumannii* ASC, with cost reductions of 19–53%, unless the prevalence of *A. baumannii* was lower than 2% and the sensitivity of the test was lower than 55% [168]. In a study conducted in Thailand, a bundle that included ASC, along with CIP, cohorting, and enhanced environmental cleaning, the acquisition rate was reduced by 76% [169]. The ESCMID guide-

lines recommend ASC for *A. baumannii* during outbreaks, coupled with CIP and cohorting.

Decolonization for *A. baumannii*

Though polymyxins have been evaluated in decolonization protocols for CRE (as discussed above), and typically these agents are active against *A. baumannii* (including CRAB) [47], there are no clinical data to support this practice. When weighing the potential for the emergence of resistance to colistin [170], decolonization is strongly discouraged.

Antimicrobial Stewardship

Numerous controlled studies investigated the independent predictors for colonization and infection with *A. baumannii* [171, 172]. In a case-control study that evaluated predictors for CRAB versus CSAB, carbapenem use was found to be associated with CRAB colonization and infection [173]. In a systematic review of risk factors for MDR *A. baumannii*, antimicrobial exposures, including to carbapenems, were reported as independent predictors for MDR *A. baumannii* in 11/20 of the studies [174]. These studies highlight the importance of both mechanisms of CRAB spread, i.e., patient-to-patient transmission and the emergence of resistance among susceptible strains.

Few studies evaluated the impact of antibiotic stewardship intervention on the emergence of carbapenem resistance among susceptible species of *A. baumannii* and on the emergence of *A. baumannii* in general (regardless of resistance profile), with conflicting results [132, 175]. The relation between colistin exposure and pan-resistant colistin-resistant *A. baumannii* acquisition is clearly evident [57, 170]. Despite the lack of controlled trials, the association between *A. baumannii* emergence and antimicrobial exposure mandates implementing a strong stewardship program. The rate of *A. baumannii* acquisitions should be one of the measurable elements for the program. As In CRE cases, restricting and monitoring antimicrobial use in general, and not only carbapenems, may impact the rates of *A. baumannii* and CRAB, as well as other MDROs [20, 132].

ESBL- and/or AmpC-Producing *Enterobacteriaceae*

Epidemiology and Microbiology

The first plasmid-mediated beta-lactamase in Gram-negative bacteria was discovered in Greece in the 1960s and had a narrow spectrum of activity against penicillin [176]. With greater use of broad-spectrum cephalosporins, beta-lactamases with broader spectrum of activity were discovered, and in 1983, the first extended-spectrum beta-lactamase (ESBL) bacterial strain was reported from Germany and later on spread exponentially throughout the globe [176]. Data from the Study of Monitoring Antimicrobial Resistance Trends (SMART), which evaluate trends of antimicrobial susceptibilities in different geographic regions among patients with urinary tract infections (UTI) between 2002 and 2010, revealed an increase in ESBL-producing *Enterobacteriaceae* strains (e.g., *E. coli*, *K. pneumoniae*, *K. oxytoca*, and *Proteus mirabilis*) from less than 20% in 2002 to more than 40% in 2010 in Asia [177]. A similar increase was demonstrated in the Middle East [178]. In 2015, the prevalence of ESBLs among pathogens associated with HAIs in the USA was 17.8% [25].

ESBLs are classified as Ambler A beta-lactamases and consist of various families of enzymes (TEM, SHV, and CTX-M). These enzymes can hydrolyze broad-spectrum penicillins and cephalosporins as well as monobactams and are typically inhibited by beta-lactamase inhibitors (e.g., clavulanate, tazobactam) [179]. Carbapenems are relatively active against these isolates and are considered the treatment of choice for severe ESBL infections [180]. There are other prevalent resistance mechanisms to broad-spectrum cephalosporins, most notably AmpC (bla_{AmpC}), which are Ambler C beta-lactamases. AmpC are not inhibited by beta-lactamase inhibitors and are usually chromosomally encoded among typical *Enterobacteriaceae* (e.g., *Enterobacter*, *Citrobacter*, *Morganella*, *Serratia*, and *Providencia*), though it could reside on mobile genetic elements as well (e.g., bla_{CMY-2}-producing *E. coli*) [181]. Despite the different type of enzymes in ESBL and AmpC outbreaks, the two modes of resistance acquisitions (i.e., patient-to-patient transmission and the emergence of resistance) play a role [84]. Therefore, infection control measures addressing both modes should be rigorously implemented in order to effectively control an outbreak [16].

In the past, ESBLs were considered as nosocomial infections, particularly in the intensive care unit (ICU) setting. Over the last two decades, the boundaries between inpatient and certain outpatient services were nearly abolished, with ESBL dissemination to LTCFs and back to acute-care hospitals [182]. This resulted in conflicting recommendations pertaining to infection control prevention measures [16]. Later on, ESBL strains were isolated also among young and previously healthy individuals with no established exposures to healthcare settings [183, 184]. The misuse of antimicrobials among patients in the community (e.g., fluoroquinolones and broad-spectrum beta-lactams [185, 186]), coupled with the dissemination through contaminated food and agriculture products (probably resulting from the large quantities of antimicrobials that are administered to food-producing animals for growth promotion) might have also played a pivotal role in the spread of ESBL strains in the community [187, 188].

In many regions around the world, ESBLs are now considered common offending strains among patients with community-acquired or community-onset infections [84]. An outbreak of an ESBL (bla_{CTX-M})-producing *E. coli* strain associated with dozens of deaths in 2011 among previously young and healthy individuals, mainly from Western Europe, was traced to a contaminated food product [189]. A meta-analysis also demonstrated strong association between traveling to endemic areas and ESBL carriage upon return (a risk ratio of 2.4, 95% CI 1.26, 4.58) [190].

Since ESBLs became endemic in so many regions worldwide, the exact role of patient-to-patient transmission versus emergence of resistance is not well defined. Various studies reported a patient-to-patient transmission rate ranging from 1.5 to 52% [14, 191, 192]. There is also variability among ESBL species: patient-to-patient transmission as well as patient-to-environment contamination rates were shown to be higher for *K. pneumoniae* compared to *E. coli* [15, 193, 194].

Measures to Decrease Patient-to-Patient Transmission of ESBLs and AmpCs

Hand Hygiene

Even though the rate of patient-to-patient transmission is variable, hand hygiene as part of standard precautions should be implemented and audited before and after every contact with ESBL carriers. Several studies have demonstrated that HCW hands are contaminated with GNB, including resistant GNB (e.g., ESBL and AmpC) [195, 196]. There is significant reduction in hand GNB inoculums by performing hand hygiene [44, 45, 197]. A recent study in the ICU setting demonstrated HH as the most efficient infection control measure to control ESBL. Their model showed that improving hand hygiene compliance from 55 to 80% before patient contact, and from 60 to 80% after patient contact, reduced the proportion of patients who acquired ESBL within 90 days by 91% [198].

Contact Isolation Precautions (CIP)

Studies that evaluated CIP impact on the spread of ESBLs were conducted mainly in a setting of an outbreak and as part of an entire bundle. In certain regions, where ESBL became so common in community settings, implementing CIP for all ESBL carriers upon admission to an acute-care hospital may not be worthwhile. When too many patients in a given department are subjected to CIP (not in an ICU), the compliance with CIP measures are known to decrease considerably, specifically HH [199]. This recommendation should not apply of course to regions with low endemic ESBL rates, or to special circumstances or events (i.e., an outbreak in certain units, e.g., neonatal ICUs) [16, 84]. One retrospective study that included two hospitals in France with similar rates of ESBL *E. coli* carriage, but with CIP applied in only one of the hospitals, demonstrated similar rates of ESBL *E. coli* transmission in both institutions [200].

The European guidelines for infection prevention of MDR-GNB recommend implementing CIP in both epidemic and endemic settings of ESBL prevalence [11]. In Switzerland, national guidelines recommend CIP for all patients colonized or infected with ESBL in acute-care facilities [191, 201]. Considering the lack of evidence to support CIP as a common practice for every ESBL carrier, we propose that CIP should be implemented during outbreaks or in specified units with prone populations, where the benefit may outweigh the disadvantages associated with CIP (as discussed above).

Patient Cohorting and Dedicated Staff

Evidence pertaining to the benefit of cohorting patients with ESBLs is lacking. An analysis from France modeled an ESBL outbreak in an ICU and evaluated the contribution of several strategies on ESBL acquisition. Cohorting was the second most effective intervention in reducing ESBL acquisitions, following HH [198]. As discussed in the section of CIP above, cohorting patients colonized with ESBL in endemic settings might be perceived as a futile intervention that might not always be effective [16, 84].

Environmental Cleaning and Disinfection

The role of environmental contamination for curbing ESBL transmission is similar to that discussed above, in detail, in the CRE section. In brief, there are controlled data suggesting that a colonized patient's immediate environment becomes colonized with the same MDR-*Enterobacteriaceae* genotype relatively fast and for prolonged periods of time [60, 62, 63]. Evidence from controlled ESBL outbreak investigations demonstrated that cleaning the patient environment, specifically high-touch surfaces, can assist in reducing potential transmission [22, 60, 67, 68]. Even though evidence evaluating the sole impact of cleaning on ESBL acquisitions is lacking, maintaining a clean environment must be perceived as fundamental for all hygienic measures in preventing ESBL transmission and infections [59].

Active Surveillance

Asymptomatic colonization with ESBL is associated with future ESBL infection [202, 203]. Therefore, screening for colonization was considered as one of the measures to reduce ESBL infections. However, of 287 patients who were screened in one endemic hospital, 69 (24%) were colonized during the study period (very high proportion), while only five developed ESBL infection. Moreover, only in three infected patients the same genotype as the colonizing organism was isolated [204]. Therefore, quantifying the exact ben-efit of ASC in endemic settings is problematic. Moreover, the sensitivity and negative predictive value of screening the perirectal area and groin vary from 42 to 95% [11]. The resources associated with a comprehensive ESBL ASC program could be overwhelming in endemic settings, and as with CIP, we recommend, based on the current data, to implement ASC for ESBLs only during outbreaks or for specified prone populations.

Decolonization for ESBLs and AmpCs

Data from a large meta-analysis that included 28,909 healthy individuals revealed fecal colonization rate of 2% in North America and 22% in Southeast Asia and Africa. Carriage of ESBL and AmpC could be prolonged (i.e., 18% of returned travelers remained colonized even after 6 months) [190, 205]. Several studies reported persistent colonization of ESBL among 25–43% of colonized patients after 12 months, particularly if they had recurrent healthcare exposure during that time [206, 207].

Data pertaining to the impact of SDD regimens on clinical outcomes of ESBL or AmpC carriers are scarce. A randomized controlled trial from Switzerland showed no significant decrease in the ESBL carriage, and in patients who did respond, the effect lasted only 4 weeks [208]. Other non-randomized studies that evaluated SDD for eradication of ESBL have shown inconsistent results pertaining to the success rate of decolonization, as well as to the impact on clinical outcomes [209]. Considering the risk of resistance spread and the lack of data to support SDD for ESBL (or AmpC) carriers, we recommend not implementing such a practice, except for individual specified scenarios.

Antimicrobial Stewardship

Emergence of resistance has an important role in the spread of ESBL and AmpC. Misuse and overuse of broad-spectrum antibiotics across healthcare systems (i.e., hospitals and LTCFs) and in the community are correlated with the prevalence of resistance [5, 41]. A study conducted in Greece demonstrated the importance of an antimicrobial stewardship team and policy: total antibiotic consumption decreased by 3.3%, restricted antibiotics decreased by 42% (primarily cefepime), and the resistance rate of *K. pneumoniae* resistant to third- and fourth-generation cephalosporins (representing both ESBL- and AmpC-producing strains) decreased from 29–37% to 12–15% [210]. In a prospective study conducted in Vanderbilt, TN, between 2002 and 2005, implementing stewardship program was associated with significant reduction in the use of anti-GNB antibiotics, coupled with a decrease in HAIs due to MDR *Enterobacteriaceae* [132]. In Denmark, the restricted use of cephalosporins, fluoroquinolones, and carbapenems as part of an infection control bundle resulted in a sustained reduction in the incidence of both colonization and infections caused by ESBLs [211].

References

1. Vincent JL, et al. International study of the prevalence and outcomes of infection in intensive care units. JAMA. 2009;302(21):2323–9.
2. Marchaim D, et al. Epidemiology of bacteremia episodes in a single center: increase in Gram-negative isolates, antibiotics resistance, and patient age. Eur J Clin Microbiol Infect Dis. 2008;27(11):1045–51.
3. Antibiotic resistance threats in the United States, 2013. https://www.cdc.gov/drugresistance/pdf/ar-threats-2013-508.pdf, 2013.
4. Marchaim D, et al. National multicenter study of predictors and outcomes of bacteremia upon hospital admission caused by Enterobacteriaceae producing extended-spectrum beta-lactamases. Antimicrob Agents Chemother. 2010;54(12):5099–104.
5. Adler A, Katz DE, Marchaim D. The continuing plague of extended-spectrum beta-lactamase-producing Enterobacteriaceae infections. Infect Dis Clin N Am. 2016;30(2):347–75.
6. Boucher HW, et al. Bad bugs, no drugs: no ESKAPE! An update from the Infectious Diseases Society of America. Clin Infect Dis. 2009;48(1):1–12.
7. Rice LB. Federal funding for the study of antimicrobial resistance in nosocomial pathogens: no ESKAPE. J Infect Dis. 2008;197(8):1079–81.
8. Peterson LR. Bad bugs, no drugs: no ESCAPE revisited. Clin Infect Dis. 2009;49(6):992–3.
9. Peleg AY, Hooper DC. Hospital-acquired infections due to gram-negative bacteria. N Engl J Med. 2010;362(19):1804–13.
10. Tal-Jasper R, et al. Clinical and epidemiological significance of Carbapenem resistance in Acinetobacter baumannii infections. Antimicrob Agents Chemother. 2016;60(5):3127–31.
11. Tacconelli E, et al. ESCMID guidelines for the management of the infection control measures to reduce transmission of multidrug-resistant Gram-negative bacteria in hospitalized patients. Clin Microbiol Infect. 2014;20(Suppl 1):1–55.
12. Richter SS, Brown SA, Mott MA. The impact of social support and self-esteem on adolescent substance abuse treatment outcome. J Subst Abus. 1991;3(4):371–85.
13. Tal Jasper R, et al. The complex epidemiology of extended-spectrum beta-lactamase-producing Enterobacteriaceae. Future Microbiol. 2015;10(5):819–39.
14. Harris AD, McGregor JC, Furuno JP. What infection control interventions should be undertaken to control multidrug-resistant gram-negative bacteria? Clin Infect Dis. 2006;43(Suppl 2):S57–61.
15. Harris AD, et al. Patient-to-patient transmission is important in extended-spectrum beta-lactamase-producing *Klebsiella pneumoniae* acquisition. Clin Infect Dis. 2007;45(10):1347–50.
16. Harris AD, et al. How important is patient-to-patient transmission in extended-spectrum beta-lactamase *Escherichia coli* acquisition. Am J Infect Control. 2007;35(2):97–101.
17. Harris AD. How important is the environment in the emergence of nosocomial antimicrobial-resistant bacteria? Clin Infect Dis. 2008;46(5):686–8.
18. Barnes SL, et al. Preventing the transmission of multidrug-resistant organisms: modeling the relative importance of hand hygiene and environmental cleaning interventions. Infect Control Hosp Epidemiol. 2014;35(9):1156–62.
19. Ajao AO, et al. Risk of acquiring extended-spectrum beta-lactamase-producing Klebsiella species and *Escherichia coli* from prior room occupants in the intensive care unit. Infect Control Hosp Epidemiol. 2013;34(5):453–8.
20. Bogan C, Marchaim D. The role of antimicrobial stewardship in curbing carbapenem resistance. Future Microbiol. 2013;8(8):979–91.
21. Yigit H, et al. Novel carbapenem-hydrolyzing beta-lactamase, KPC-1, from a carbapenem-resistant strain of *Klebsiella pneumoniae*. Antimicrob Agents Chemother. 2001;45(4):1151–61.
22. Munoz-Price LS, Quinn JP. Deconstructing the infection control bundles for the containment of carbapenem-resistant Enterobacteriaceae. Curr Opin Infect Dis. 2013;26(4):378–87.
23. Patients with KPC-producing Carbapenem-resistant Enterobacteriaceae (CRE) reported to the Centers for Disease Control and Prevention (CDC) as of January 2017, by state. https://www.cdc.gov/hai/organisms/cre/trackingcre.html, 2017.
24. CDC, Facility Guidance for Control of Carbapenem-resistant Enterobacteriaceae (CRE). https://www.cdc.gov/hai/pdfs/cre/CRE-guidance-508.pdf, 2015.
25. Weiner LM, et al. Vital signs: preventing antibiotic-resistant infections in hospitals – United States, 2014. Am J Transplant. 2016;16(7):2224–30.
26. Antimicrobial resistance interactive database (EARS-Net). http://atlas.ecdc.europa.eu/public/index.aspx?Instance=GeneralAtlas, 2014.
27. Hussein K, et al. Carbapenem resistance among *Klebsiella pneumoniae* isolates: risk factors, molecular characteristics, and susceptibility patterns. Infect Control Hosp Epidemiol. 2009;30(7):666–71.
28. Marchaim D, et al. The burden of multidrug-resistant organisms on tertiary hospitals posed by patients with recent stays in long-term acute care facilities. Am J Infect Control. 2012;40(8):760–5.
29. Otter JA. What's trending in the infection prevention and control literature? From HIS 2012 to HIS 2014, and beyond. J Hosp Infect. 2015;89(4):229–36.
30. Lin MY, et al. The importance of long-term acute care hospitals in the regional epidemiology of *Klebsiella pneumoniae* carbapenemase-producing Enterobacteriaceae. Clin Infect Dis. 2013;57(9):1246–52.
31. Perez F, Van Duin D. Carbapenem-resistant Enterobacteriaceae: a menace to our most vulnerable patients. Cleve Clin J Med. 2013;80(4):225–33.
32. Munoz-Price LS, et al. Clinical epidemiology of the global expansion of *Klebsiella pneumoniae* carbapenemases. Lancet Infect Dis. 2013;13(9):785–96.
33. Perez F, et al. Treatment options for infections caused by carbapenem-resistant Enterobacteriaceae: can we apply "precision medicine" to antimicrobial chemotherapy? Expert Opin Pharmacother. 2016;17(6):761–81.
34. EUCAST. European Committee on Antimicrobial Susceptibility Testing. Clinical breakpoints. 2010; Available from: ≤http://www.srga.org/eucastwt/MICTAB/index.html>.
35. CLSI. Performance standards for antimicrobial susceptibility testing. Twenty-sixth informational supplement. Approved standard M100-S20. Wayne: Clinical and Laboratory Standards Institute; 2010.
36. Adler A, et al. A swordless knight: epidemiology and molecular characteristics of the blaKPC-negative sequence type 258 *Klebsiella pneumoniae* clone. J Clin Microbiol. 2012;50(10):3180–5.
37. Tamma PD, et al. Comparing the outcomes of patients with Carbapenemase-producing and non-Carbapenemase-producing Carbapenem-resistant Enterobacteriaceae bacteremia. Clin Infect Dis. 2017;64(3):257–64.

38. Miller S, Humphries RM. Clinical laboratory detection of carbapenem-resistant and carbapenemase-producing Enterobacteriaceae. Expert Rev Anti-Infect Ther. 2016;14(8):705–17.

39. Richter SS, Marchaim D. Screening for carbapenem-resistant Enterobacteriaceae: who, when, and how? Virulence. 2016; 8(4): 417–426.

40. Magiorakos AP, et al. Multidrug-resistant, extensively drug-resistant and pandrug-resistant bacteria: an international expert proposal for interim standard definitions for acquired resistance. Clin Microbiol Infect. 2012;18(3):268–81.

41. Marchaim D, et al. Recent exposure to antimicrobials and carbapenem-resistant Enterobacteriaceae: the role of antimicrobial stewardship. Infect Control Hosp Epidemiol. 2012;33(8):817–30.

42. Monaco M, et al. Colistin resistance superimposed to endemic carbapenem-resistant Klebsiella pneumoniae: a rapidly evolving problem in Italy, November 2013 to April 2014. Euro Surveill. 2014;19(42):14–18.

43. McGann P, et al. Escherichia coli Harboring mcr-1 and blaCTX-M on a novel IncF plasmid: first report of mcr-1 in the United States. Antimicrob Agents Chemother. 2016;60(7):4420–1.

44. Maragakis LL. Recognition and prevention of multidrug-resistant Gram-negative bacteria in the intensive care unit. Crit Care Med. 2010;38(8 Suppl):S345–51.

45. Erasmus V, et al. Systematic review of studies on compliance with hand hygiene guidelines in hospital care. Infect Control Hosp Epidemiol. 2010;31(3):283–94.

46. Sypsa V, et al. Transmission dynamics of carbapenemase-producing Klebsiella pneumoniae and anticipated impact of infection control strategies in a surgical unit. PLoS One. 2012;7(7):e41068.

47. Siegel JD, et al. 2007 guideline for isolation precautions: preventing transmission of infectious agents in health care settings. Am J Infect Control. 2007;35(10 Suppl 2):S65–164.

48. Lledo W et al. Guidance for control of infections with carbapenem-resistant or carbapenemase-producing Enterobacteriaceae in acute care facilities. MMWR Morb Mortal Wkly Rep. 2009;58(10):256–60.

49. Schwaber MJ, et al. Containment of a country-wide outbreak of carbapenem-resistant Klebsiella pneumoniae in Israeli hospitals via a nationally implemented intervention. Clin Infect Dis. 2011;52(7):848–55.

50. Kochar S, et al. Success of an infection control program to reduce the spread of carbapenem-resistant Klebsiella pneumoniae. Infect Control Hosp Epidemiol. 2009;30(5):447–52.

51. Agodi A, et al. Containment of an outbreak of KPC-3-producing Klebsiella pneumoniae in Italy. J Clin Microbiol. 2011;49(11):3986–9.

52. Zimmerman FS, et al. Duration of carriage of carbapenem-resistant Enterobacteriaceae following hospital discharge. Am J Infect Control. 2013;41(3):190–4.

53. Poirel L, et al. Long-term carriage of NDM-1-producing Escherichia coli. J Antimicrob Chemother. 2011;66(9):2185–6.

54. Schechner V, et al. Predictors of rectal carriage of carbapenem-resistant Enterobacteriaceae (CRE) among patients with known CRE carriage at their next hospital encounter. Infect Control Hosp Epidemiol. 2011;32(5):497–503.

55. Bart Y, et al. Risk factors for recurrence of Carbapenem-resistant Enterobacteriaceae carriage: case-control study. Infect Control Hosp Epidemiol. 2015;36(8):936–41.

56. Schwaber MJ, Carmeli Y. An ongoing national intervention to contain the spread of carbapenem-resistant enterobacteriaceae. Clin Infect Dis. 2014;58(5):697–703.

57. Marchaim D, et al. Outbreak of colistin-resistant, carbapenem-resistant Klebsiella pneumoniae in metropolitan Detroit, Michigan. Antimicrob Agents Chemother. 2011;55(2):593–9.

58. Marchaim D, et al. "Swimming in resistance": co-colonization with carbapenem-resistant Enterobacteriaceae and Acinetobacter baumannii or Pseudomonas aeruginosa. Am J Infect Control. 2012;40(9):830–5.

59. Dancer SJ. Hospital cleaning in the 21st century. Eur J Clin Microbiol Infect Dis. 2011;30(12):1473–81.

60. Lerner A, et al. Environmental contamination by carbapenem-resistant Enterobacteriaceae. J Clin Microbiol. 2013; 51(1):177–81.

61. Kramer A, Schwebke I, Kampf G. How long do nosocomial pathogens persist on inanimate surfaces? A systematic review. BMC Infect Dis. 2006;6:130.

62. Wilks SA, Michels H, Keevil CW. The survival of Escherichia coli O157 on a range of metal surfaces. Int J Food Microbiol. 2005;105(3):445–54.

63. Williams AP, et al. Persistence of Escherichia coli O157 on farm surfaces under different environmental conditions. J Appl Microbiol. 2005;98(5):1075–83.

64. Weber DJ, Anderson D, Rutala WA. The role of the surface environment in healthcare-associated infections. Curr Opin Infect Dis. 2013;26(4):338–44.

65. Obee P, et al. An evaluation of different methods for the recovery of meticillin-resistant Staphylococcus aureus from environmental surfaces. J Hosp Infect. 2007;65(1):35–41.

66. Wolf I, et al. The sink as a correctable source of extended-spectrum beta-lactamase contamination for patients in the intensive care unit. J Hosp Infect. 2014;87(2):126–30.

67. Ciobotaro P, et al. An effective intervention to limit the spread of an epidemic carbapenem-resistant Klebsiella pneumoniae strain in an acute care setting: from theory to practice. Am J Infect Control. 2011;39(8):671–7.

68. Munoz-Price LS, et al. Successful control of an outbreak of Klebsiella pneumoniae carbapenemase-producing K. pneumoniae at a long-term acute care hospital. Infect Control Hosp Epidemiol. 2010;31(4):341–7.

69. Carling PC, Huang SS. Improving healthcare environmental cleaning and disinfection: current and evolving issues. Infect Control Hosp Epidemiol. 2013;34(5):507–13.

70. Weber DJ, Kanamori H, Rutala WA. 'No touch' technologies for environmental decontamination: focus on ultraviolet devices and hydrogen peroxide systems. Curr Opin Infect Dis. 2016;29(4):424–31.

71. Anderson DJ, et al. Decontamination of targeted pathogens from patient rooms using an automated ultraviolet-C-emitting device. Infect Control Hosp Epidemiol. 2013;34(5):466–71.

72. Boyce JM, et al. Monitoring the effectiveness of hospital cleaning practices by use of an adenosine triphosphate bioluminescence assay. Infect Control Hosp Epidemiol. 2009;30(7):678–84.

73. Chow A, et al. Alcohol handrubbing and chlorhexidine handwashing protocols for routine hospital practice: a randomized clinical trial of protocol efficacy and time effectiveness. Am J Infect Control. 2012;40(9):800–5.

74. Carling PC, et al. Improving environmental hygiene in 27 intensive care units to decrease multidrug-resistant bacterial transmission. Crit Care Med. 2010;38(4):1054–9.

75. Tschopp C, et al. Predictors of heavy stethoscope contamination following a physical examination. Infect Control Hosp Epidemiol. 2016;37(6):673–9.

76. Ha J, Son BK. Current issues in Duodenoscope-associated infections: now is the time to take action. Clin Endosc. 2015;48(5):361–3.

77. Rutala WA, Weber DJ. Outbreaks of carbapenem-resistant Enterobacteriaceae infections associated with duodenoscopes: what can we do to prevent infections? Am J Infect Control. 2016;44(5 Suppl):e47–51.

78. O'Horo JC, et al. Carbapenem-resistant Enterobacteriaceae and endoscopy: an evolving threat. Am J Infect Control. 2016;44:1032–6.

79. Rubin ZA, Murthy RK. Outbreaks associated with duodenoscopes: new challenges and controversies. Curr Opin Infect Dis. 2016;29(4):407–14.

80. Harris AD, et al. Co-carriage rates of vancomycin-resistant enterococcus and extended-spectrum beta-lactamase-producing bacteria among a cohort of intensive care unit patients: implications for an active surveillance program. Infect Control Hosp Epidemiol. 2004;25(2):105–8.

81. Temkin E, et al. Carbapenem-resistant Enterobacteriaceae: biology, epidemiology, and management. Ann N Y Acad Sci. 2014;1323:22–42.

82. Bonten MJ. Colonization pressure: a critical parameter in the epidemiology of antibiotic-resistant bacteria. Crit Care. 2012;16(4):142.

83. Dickstein Y, et al. Carbapenem-resistant Enterobacteriaceae colonization and infection in critically ill patients: a retrospective matched cohort comparison with non-carriers. J Hosp Infect. 2016;94(1):54–9.

84. Adler A, Friedman ND, Marchaim D. Multidrug-resistant gram-negative bacilli: infection control implications. Infect Dis Clin N Am. 2016;30(4):967–97.

85. Leibman V, et al. Simple bedside score to optimize the time and the decision to initiate appropriate therapy for carbapenem-resistant Enterobacteriaceae. Ann Clin Microbiol Antimicrob. 2015;14:31.

86. Palmore TN, Henderson DK. Managing transmission of carbapenem-resistant enterobacteriaceae in healthcare settings: a view from the trenches. Clin Infect Dis. 2013;57(11):1593–9.

87. Schwaber MJ, Carmeli Y. Carbapenem-resistant Enterobacteriaceae: a potential threat. JAMA. 2008;300(24):2911–3.

88. Bhargava A, et al. Risk factors for colonization due to carbapenem-resistant Enterobacteriaceae among patients exposed to long-term acute care and acute care facilities. Infect Control Hosp Epidemiol. 2014;35(4):398–405.

89. Pugin J, et al. Oropharyngeal decontamination decreases incidence of ventilator-associated pneumonia. A randomized, placebo-controlled, double-blind clinical trial. JAMA. 1991;265(20):2704–10.

90. Bergmans DC, et al. Prevention of ventilator-associated pneumonia by oral decontamination: a prospective, randomized, double-blind, placebo-controlled study. Am J Respir Crit Care Med. 2001;164(3):382–8.

91. Saidel-Odes L, et al. A randomized, double-blind, placebo-controlled trial of selective digestive decontamination using oral gentamicin and oral polymyxin E for eradication of carbapenem-resistant Klebsiella pneumoniae carriage. Infect Control Hosp Epidemiol. 2012;33(1):14–9.

92. Oren I, et al. Eradication of carbapenem-resistant Enterobacteriaceae gastrointestinal colonization with nonabsorbable oral antibiotic treatment: a prospective controlled trial. Am J Infect Control. 2013;41(12):1167–72.

93. Lubbert C, et al. Rapid emergence of secondary resistance to gentamicin and colistin following selective digestive decontamination in patients with KPC-2-producing Klebsiella pneumoniae: a single-centre experience. Int J Antimicrob Agents. 2013;42(6):565–70.

94. Septimus EJ, Schweizer ML. Decolonization in prevention of health care-associated infections. Clin Microbiol Rev. 2016;29(2):201–22.

95. Bilinski J, et al. Fecal microbiota transplantation inhibits multidrug-resistant gut pathogens: preliminary report performed in an immunocompromised host. Arch Immunol Ther Exp. 2016;64(3):255–8.

96. Barlam TF, et al. Implementing an antibiotic stewardship program: guidelines by the Infectious Diseases Society of America and the Society for Healthcare Epidemiology of America. Clin Infect Dis. 2016;62(10):e51–77.

97. Ghafur A, et al. "Save Antibiotics, Save lives": an Indian success story of infection control through persuasive diplomacy. Antimicrob Resist Infect Control. 2012;1(1):29.

98. Kritsotakis EI, et al. Antibiotic use and the risk of carbapenem-resistant extended-spectrum-{beta}-lactamase-producing Klebsiella pneumoniae infection in hospitalized patients: results of a double case-control study. J Antimicrob Chemother. 2011;66(6):1383–91.

99. Borer A, et al. Risk factors for developing clinical infection with carbapenem-resistant Klebsiella pneumoniae in hospital patients initially only colonized with carbapenem-resistant K pneumoniae. Am J Infect Control. 2012;40(5):421–5.

100. Sader HS, et al. Antimicrobial susceptibility of Gram-negative organisms isolated from patients hospitalised with pneumonia in US and European hospitals: results from the SENTRY Antimicrobial Surveillance Program, 2009-2012. Int J Antimicrob Agents. 2014;43(4):328–34.

101. Hidron AI, et al. NHSN annual update: antimicrobial-resistant pathogens associated with healthcare-associated infections: annual summary of data reported to the National Healthcare Safety Network at the Centers for Disease Control and Prevention, 2006–2007. Infect Control Hosp Epidemiol. 2008;29(11):996–1011.

102. Lautenbach E, et al. Imipenem resistance in Pseudomonas aeruginosa: emergence, epidemiology, and impact on clinical and economic outcomes. Infect Control Hosp Epidemiol. 2010;31(1):47–53.

103. Santajit S, Indrawattana N. Mechanisms of antimicrobial resistance in ESKAPE pathogens. Biomed Res Int. 2016;2016:2475067.

104. Mayhall CG. Hospital epidemiology and infection control. 4th ed. Lippincott Williams & Wilkins Philadelphia.

105. Breidenstein EB, de la Fuente-Nunez C, Hancock RE. Pseudomonas aeruginosa: all roads lead to resistance. Trends Microbiol. 2011;19(8):419–26.

106. Corona-Nakamura AL, et al. Epidemiologic study of Pseudomonas aeruginosa in critical patients and reservoirs. Arch Med Res. 2001;32(3):238–42.

107. Aloush V, et al. Multidrug-resistant Pseudomonas aeruginosa: risk factors and clinical impact. Antimicrob Agents Chemother. 2006;50(1):43–8.

108. Olson B, et al. Epidemiology of endemic Pseudomonas aeruginosa: why infection control efforts have failed. J Infect Dis. 1984;150(6):808–16.

109. DalBen MF, et al. Colonization pressure as a risk factor for colonization by multiresistant Acinetobacter spp and carbapenem-resistant Pseudomonas aeruginosa in an intensive care unit. Clinics (Sao Paulo). 2013;68(8):1128–33.

110. Clifton IJ, Peckham DG. Defining routes of airborne transmission of Pseudomonas aeruginosa in people with cystic fibrosis. Expert Rev Respir Med. 2010;4(4):519–29.

111. Moolenaar RL, et al. A prolonged outbreak of Pseudomonas aeruginosa in a neonatal intensive care unit: did staff fingernails play a role in disease transmission? Infect Control Hosp Epidemiol. 2000;21(2):80–5.

112. Pires dos Santos R, et al. Hand hygiene, and not ertapenem use, contributed to reduction of carbapenem-resistant Pseudomonas aeruginosa rates. Infect Control Hosp Epidemiol. 2011;32(6):584–90.

113. Kirkland KB, Weinstein JM. Adverse effects of contact isolation. Lancet. 1999;354(9185):1177–8.

114. Stelfox HT, Bates DW, Redelmeier DA. Safety of patients isolated for infection control. JAMA. 2003;290(14):1899–905.

115. Muto CA, et al. SHEA guideline for preventing nosocomial transmission of multidrug-resistant strains of Staphylococcus

aureus and enterococcus. Infect Control Hosp Epidemiol. 2003;24(5):362–86.

116. Levin PF. Improving compliance with universal precautions: effectiveness of interventions. AAOHN J. 1995;43(7):362–70.

117. Lai KK, et al. Failure to eradicate vancomycin-resistant enterococci in a university hospital and the cost of barrier precautions. Infect Control Hosp Epidemiol. 1998;19(9):647–52.

118. Rosenberger LH, et al. Effective cohorting and "superisolation" in a single intensive care unit in response to an outbreak of diverse multi-drug-resistant organisms. Surg Infect. 2011;12(5):345–50.

119. Kerr KG, Snelling AM. Pseudomonas aeruginosa: a formidable and ever-present adversary. J Hosp Infect. 2009;73(4):338–44.

120. Marchaim D, et al. Hospital bath basins are frequently contaminated with multidrug-resistant human pathogens. Am J Infect Control. 2012;40(6):562–4.

121. Bert F, et al. Multi-resistant Pseudomonas aeruginosa outbreak associated with contaminated tap water in a neurosurgery intensive care unit. J Hosp Infect. 1998;39(1):53–62.

122. Hota S, et al. Outbreak of multidrug-resistant Pseudomonas aeruginosa colonization and infection secondary to imperfect intensive care unit room design. Infect Control Hosp Epidemiol. 2009;30(1):25–33.

123. Bukholm G, et al. An outbreak of multidrug-resistant Pseudomonas aeruginosa associated with increased risk of patient death in an intensive care unit. Infect Control Hosp Epidemiol. 2002;23(8):441–6.

124. Petignat C, et al. Exogenous sources of pseudomonas aeruginosa in intensive care unit patients: implementation of infection control measures and follow-up with molecular typing. Infect Control Hosp Epidemiol. 2006;27(9):953–7.

125. Rogues AM, et al. Contribution of tap water to patient colonisation with Pseudomonas aeruginosa in a medical intensive care unit. J Hosp Infect. 2007;67(1):72–8.

126. Valles J, et al. Patterns of colonization by Pseudomonas aeruginosa in intubated patients: a 3-year prospective study of 1,607 isolates using pulsed-field gel electrophoresis with implications for prevention of ventilator-associated pneumonia. Intensive Care Med. 2004;30(9):1768–75.

127. Bertrand X, et al. Endemicity, molecular diversity and colonisation routes of Pseudomonas aeruginosa in intensive care units. Intensive Care Med. 2001;27(8):1263–8.

128. Gomez-Zorrilla S, et al. Prospective observational study of prior rectal colonization status as a predictor for subsequent development of Pseudomonas aeruginosa clinical infections. Antimicrob Agents Chemother. 2015;59(9):5213–9.

129. Cohen R, et al. A prospective survey of Pseudomonas aeruginosa colonization and infection in the intensive care unit. Antimicrob Resist Infect Control. 2017;6:7.

130. Bonten MJ, et al. Characteristics of polyclonal endemicity of Pseudomonas aeruginosa colonization in intensive care units. Implications for infection control. Am J Respir Crit Care Med. 1999;160(4):1212–9.

131. Voor In't Holt AF, et al. A systematic review and meta-analyses show that carbapenem use and medical devices are the leading risk factors for carbapenem-resistant Pseudomonas aeruginosa. Antimicrob Agents Chemother. 2014;58(5):2626–37.

132. Dortch MJ, et al. Infection reduction strategies including antibiotic stewardship protocols in surgical and trauma intensive care units are associated with reduced resistant gram-negative healthcare-associated infections. Surg Infect. 2011;12(1):15–25.

133. Carmeli Y, et al. Emergence of antibiotic-resistant Pseudomonas aeruginosa: comparison of risks associated with different antipseudomonal agents. Antimicrob Agents Chemother. 1999;43(6):1379–82.

134. Pakyz AL, Oinonen M, Polk RE. Relationship of carbapenem restriction in 22 university teaching hospitals to carbapenem use

and carbapenem-resistant Pseudomonas aeruginosa. Antimicrob Agents Chemother. 2009;53(5):1983–6.

135. Tedeschi S, et al. An Antimicrobial Stewardship Program Based on Systematic Infectious Disease Consultation in a Rehabilitation Facility. Infect Control Hosp Epidemiol. 2017;38(1):76–82.

136. Carmeli Y, et al. The effects of group 1 versus group 2 carbapenems on imipenem-resistant Pseudomonas aeruginosa: an ecological study. Diagn Microbiol Infect Dis. 2011;70(3):367–72.

137. Goldstein EJ, et al. Introduction of ertapenem into a hospital formulary: effect on antimicrobial usage and improved in vitro susceptibility of Pseudomonas aeruginosa. Antimicrob Agents Chemother. 2009;53(12):5122–6.

138. Nicolau DP, et al. Carbapenem stewardship: does ertapenem affect Pseudomonas susceptibility to other carbapenems? A review of the evidence. Int J Antimicrob Agents. 2012;39(1):11–5.

139. Munoz-Price LS, Weinstein RA. Acinetobacter infection. N Engl J Med. 2008;358(12):1271–81.

140. CDC's antibiotic resistance patient safety atlas https://www.cdc.gov/hai/surveillance/ar-patient-safety-atlas.html, 2015.

141. Reddy T, et al. Trends in antimicrobial resistance of Acinetobacter baumannii isolates from a metropolitan Detroit health system. Antimicrob Agents Chemother. 2010;54(5):2235–8.

142. Sengstock DM, et al. Multidrug-resistant Acinetobacter baumannii: an emerging pathogen among older adults in community hospitals and nursing homes. Clin Infect Dis. 2010;50(12):1611–6.

143. de Medina T, Carmeli Y. The pivotal role of long-term care facilities in the epidemiology of Acinetobacter baumannii: another brick in the wall. Clin Infect Dis. 2010;50(12):1617–8.

144. Eveillard M, et al. Reservoirs of Acinetobacter baumannii outside the hospital and potential involvement in emerging human community-acquired infections. Int J Infect Dis. 2013;17(10):e802–5.

145. Bonomo RA, Szabo D. Mechanisms of multidrug resistance in Acinetobacter species and Pseudomonas aeruginosa. Clin Infect Dis. 2006;43(Suppl 2):S49–56.

146. Agodi A, et al. Spread of a carbapenem- and colistin-resistant Acinetobacter baumannii ST2 clonal strain causing outbreaks in two Sicilian hospitals. J Hosp Infect. 2014;86(4):260–6.

147. Marchaim D, et al. Molecular and epidemiologic study of polyclonal outbreaks of multidrug-resistant Acinetobacter baumannii infection in an Israeli hospital. Infect Control Hosp Epidemiol. 2007;28(8):945–50.

148. Marchaim D, et al. Clinical and molecular epidemiology of Acinetobacter baumannii bloodstream infections in an endemic setting. Future Microbiol. 2017;12:271–83.

149. Morgan DJ, et al. Transfer of multidrug-resistant bacteria to healthcare workers' gloves and gowns after patient contact increases with environmental contamination. Crit Care Med. 2012;40(4):1045–51.

150. Rodriguez-Bano J, et al. Long-term control of hospital-wide, endemic multidrug-resistant Acinetobacter baumannii through a comprehensive "bundle" approach. Am J Infect Control. 2009;37(9):715–22.

151. Cardoso CL, et al. Effectiveness of hand-cleansing agents for removing Acinetobacter baumannii strain from contaminated hands. Am J Infect Control. 1999;27(4):327–31.

152. Gbaguidi-Haore H, et al. Ecological study of the effectiveness of isolation precautions in the management of hospitalized patients colonized or infected with Acinetobacter baumannii. Infect Control Hosp Epidemiol. 2008;29(12):1118–23.

153. Rebmann T, Rosenbaum PA. Preventing the transmission of multidrug-resistant Acinetobacter baumannii: an executive summary of the Association for Professionals in infection control and epidemiology's elimination guide. Am J Infect Control. 2011;39(5):439–41.

154. Peleg AY, et al. The success of acinetobacter species; genetic, metabolic and virulence attributes. PLoS One. 2012;7(10):e46984.

155. Doi Y, et al. Extensively drug-resistant Acinetobacter baumannii. Emerg Infect Dis. 2009;15(6):980–2.

156. Peleg AY, Seifert H, Paterson DL. Acinetobacter baumannii: emergence of a successful pathogen. Clin Microbiol Rev. 2008;21(3):538–82.

157. Doidge M, et al. Control of an outbreak of carbapenem-resistant Acinetobacter baumannii in Australia after introduction of environmental cleaning with a commercial oxidizing disinfectant. Infect Control Hosp Epidemiol. 2010;31(4):418–20.

158. Landman D, et al. Transmission of carbapenem-resistant pathogens in New York City hospitals: progress and frustration. J Antimicrob Chemother. 2012;67(6):1427–31.

159. Simor AE, et al. An outbreak due to multiresistant Acinetobacter baumannii in a burn unit: risk factors for acquisition and management. Infect Control Hosp Epidemiol. 2002;23(5):261–7.

160. Nseir S, et al. Risk of acquiring multidrug-resistant Gram-negative bacilli from prior room occupants in the intensive care unit. Clin Microbiol Infect. 2011;17(8):1201–8.

161. Manian FA, et al. Isolation of Acinetobacter baumannii complex and methicillin-resistant *Staphylococcus aureus* from hospital rooms following terminal cleaning and disinfection: can we do better? Infect Control Hosp Epidemiol. 2011;32(7):667–72.

162. Boyce JM. Modern technologies for improving cleaning and disinfection of environmental surfaces in hospitals. Antimicrob Resist Infect Control. 2016;5:10.

163. Maragakis LL, et al. Incidence and prevalence of multidrug-resistant acinetobacter using targeted active surveillance cultures. JAMA. 2008;299(21):2513–4.

164. Corbella X, et al. Relevance of digestive tract colonization in the epidemiology of nosocomial infections due to multiresistant Acinetobacter baumannii. Clin Infect Dis. 1996;23(2):329–34.

165. Ku K, et al. Retrospective evaluation of colistin versus tigecycline for the treatment of Acinetobacter baumannii and/or carbapenem-resistant Enterobacteriaceae infections. Am J Infect Control. 2012;40(10):983–7.

166. Marchaim D, et al. Surveillance cultures and duration of carriage of multidrug-resistant Acinetobacter baumannii. J Clin Microbiol. 2007;45(5):1551–5.

167. Doi Y, et al. Screening for Acinetobacter baumannii colonization by use of sponges. J Clin Microbiol. 2011;49(1):154–8.

168. Coyle JR, et al. Effectiveness and cost of implementing an active surveillance screening policy for Acinetobacter baumannii: a Monte Carlo simulation model. Am J Infect Control. 2014;42(3):283–7.

169. Apisarnthanarak A, et al. A multifaceted intervention to reduce pandrug-resistant Acinetobacter baumannii colonization and infection in 3 intensive care units in a Thai tertiary care center: a 3-year study. Clin Infect Dis. 2008;47(6):760–7.

170. Qureshi ZA, et al. Colistin-resistant Acinetobacter baumannii: beyond carbapenem resistance. Clin Infect Dis. 2015;60(9):1295–303.

171. Abbo A, et al. Multidrug-resistant Acinetobacter baumannii. Emerg Infect Dis. 2005;11(1):22–9.

172. Chopra T, et al. Risk factors and outcomes for patients with bloodstream infection due to Acinetobacter baumannii-calcoaceticus complex. Antimicrob Agents Chemother. 2014;58(8):4630–5.

173. Lee SO, et al. Risk factors for acquisition of imipenem-resistant Acinetobacter baumannii: a case-control study. Antimicrob Agents Chemother. 2004;48(1):224–8.

174. Falagas ME, Kopterides P. Risk factors for the isolation of multi-drug-resistant Acinetobacter baumannii and Pseudomonas aeruginosa: a systematic review of the literature. J Hosp Infect. 2006;64(1):7–15.

175. Jaggi N, Sissodia P, Sharma L. Control of multidrug resistant bacteria in a tertiary care hospital in India. Antimicrob Resist Infect Control. 2012;1(1):23.

176. Sievert DM, et al. Antimicrobial-resistant pathogens associated with healthcare-associated infections: summary of data reported to the National Healthcare Safety Network at the Centers for Disease Control and Prevention, 2009-2010. Infect Control Hosp Epidemiol. 2013;34(1):1–14.

177. Morrissey I, et al. A review of ten years of the study for monitoring antimicrobial resistance trends (SMART) from 2002 to 2011. Pharmaceuticals (Basel). 2013;6(11):1335–46.

178. Bertrand X, Dowzicky MJ. Antimicrobial susceptibility among gram-negative isolates collected from intensive care units in North America, Europe, the Asia-Pacific rim, Latin America, the Middle East, and Africa between 2004 and 2009 as part of the Tigecycline Evaluation and Surveillance Trial. Clin Ther. 2012;34(1):124–37.

179. Bush K. Extended-spectrum beta-lactamases in North America, 1987–2006. Clin Microbiol Infect. 2008;14(Suppl 1):134–43.

180. Ofer-Friedman H, et al. Carbapenems versus piperacillin-Tazobactam for bloodstream infections of Nonurinary source caused by extended-Spectrum Beta-lactamase-producing Enterobacteriaceae. Infect Control Hosp Epidemiol. 2015;36(8):981–5.

181. Jacoby GA, Munoz-Price LS. The new beta-lactamases. N Engl J Med. 2005;352(4):380–91.

182. Ben-Ami R, et al. Influx of extended-spectrum beta-lactamase-producing enterobacteriaceae into the hospital. Clin Infect Dis. 2006;42(7):925–34.

183. Hayakawa K, et al. Epidemiology and risk factors for isolation of *Escherichia coli* producing CTX-M-type extended-spectrum beta-lactamase in a large U.S. Medical Center. Antimicrob Agents Chemother. 2013;57(8):4010–8.

184. Ben-Ami R, et al. A multinational survey of risk factors for infection with extended-spectrum beta-lactamase-producing enterobacteriaceae in nonhospitalized patients. Clin Infect Dis. 2009;49(5):682–90.

185. Bonkat G, et al. Increasing prevalence of ciprofloxacin resistance in extended-spectrum-beta-lactamase-producing *Escherichia coli* urinary isolates. World J Urol. 2013;31(6):1427–32.

186. Tukenmez Tigen E, et al. Outcomes of fecal carriage of extended-spectrum beta-lactamase after transrectal ultrasound-guided biopsy of the prostate. Urology. 2014;84(5):1008–15.

187. Guo Y, et al. Frequency, antimicrobial resistance and genetic diversity of *Klebsiella pneumoniae* in food samples. PLoS One. 2016;11(4):e0153561.

188. Nakane K, et al. Long-term colonization by bla(CTX-M)-harboring *Escherichia coli* in healthy Japanese people engaged in food handling. Appl Environ Microbiol. 2016;82(6):1818–27.

189. King LA, et al. Outbreak of Shiga toxin-producing *Escherichia coli* O104:H4 associated with organic fenugreek sprouts, France, June 2011. Clin Infect Dis. 2012;54(11):1588–94.

190. Karanika S, et al. Fecal colonization with extended-spectrum beta-lactamase-producing Enterobacteriaceae and risk factors among healthy individuals: a systematic review and metaanalysis. Clin Infect Dis. 2016;63:310–8.

191. Tschudin-Sutter S, et al. Rate of transmission of extended-spectrum beta-lactamase-producing enterobacteriaceae without contact isolation. Clin Infect Dis. 2012;55(11):1505–11.

192. Alves M, et al. Extended-spectrum beta-lactamase – producing enterobacteriaceae in the intensive care unit: acquisition does not mean cross-transmission. BMC Infect Dis. 2016;16:147.

193. Hilty M, et al. Transmission dynamics of extended-spectrum beta-lactamase-producing Enterobacteriaceae in the tertiary care hospital and the household setting. Clin Infect Dis. 2012;55(7):967–75.

194. Freeman JT, et al. Predictors of hospital surface contamination with extended-spectrum beta-lactamase-producing *Escherichia*

coli and *Klebsiella pneumoniae*: patient and organism factors. Antimicrob Resist Infect Control. 2014;3(1):5.

195. Pittet D, et al. Bacterial contamination of the hands of hospital staff during routine patient care. Arch Intern Med. 1999;159(8):821–6.

196. Guenthner SH, Hendley JO, Wenzel RP. Gram-negative bacilli as nontransient flora on the hands of hospital personnel. J Clin Microbiol. 1987;25(3):488–90.

197. Weintrob AC, et al. Natural history of colonization with gram-negative multidrug-resistant organisms among hospitalized patients. Infect Control Hosp Epidemiol. 2010;31(4):330–7.

198. Pelat C, et al. Hand hygiene, cohorting, or antibiotic restriction to control outbreaks of multidrug-resistant Enterobacteriaceae. Infect Control Hosp Epidemiol. 2016;37(3):272–80.

199. Dhar S, et al. Contact precautions: more is not necessarily better. Infect Control Hosp Epidemiol. 2014;35(3):213–21.

200. Zahar JR, et al. About the usefulness of contact precautions for carriers of extended-spectrum beta-lactamase-producing *Escherichia coli*. BMC Infect Dis. 2015;15:512.

201. Tietz A, Francioli P, Widmer AF. Extended -spectrum beta-lactamase (ESBL): spitalhygienische Implikationen. Swiss Noso. 2004;11:29–32.

202. Reddy P, et al. Screening for extended-spectrum beta-lactamase-producing Enterobacteriaceae among high-risk patients and rates of subsequent bacteremia. Clin Infect Dis. 2007;45(7):846–52.

203. Cornejo-Juarez P, et al. Fecal ESBL *Escherichia coli* carriage as a risk factor for bacteremia in patients with hematological malignancies. Support Care Cancer. 2016;24(1):253–9.

204. Gardam MA, et al. Is surveillance for multidrug-resistant enterobacteriaceae an effective infection control strategy in the absence of an outbreak? J Infect Dis. 2002;186(12):1754–60.

205. Kennedy K, Collignon P. Colonisation with *Escherichia coli* resistant to "critically important" antibiotics: a high risk for international travellers. Eur J Clin Microbiol Infect Dis. 2010;29(12):1501–6.

206. Birgand G, et al. Duration of colonization by extended-spectrum beta-lactamase-producing Enterobacteriaceae after hospital discharge. Am J Infect Control. 2013;41(5):443–7.

207. Titelman E, et al. Faecal carriage of extended-spectrum beta-lactamase-producing Enterobacteriaceae is common 12 months after infection and is related to strain factors. Clin Microbiol Infect. 2014;20(8):O508–15.

208. Huttner B, et al. Decolonization of intestinal carriage of extended-spectrum beta-lactamase-producing Enterobacteriaceae with oral colistin and neomycin: a randomized, double-blind, placebo-controlled trial. J Antimicrob Chemother. 2013;68(10):2375–82.

209. Rieg S, et al. Intestinal decolonization of Enterobacteriaceae producing extended-spectrum beta-lactamases (ESBL): a retrospective observational study in patients at risk for infection and a brief review of the literature. BMC Infect Dis. 2015;15:475.

210. Ntagiopoulos PG, et al. Impact of an antibiotic restriction policy on the antibiotic resistance patterns of Gram-negative microorganisms in an intensive care unit in Greece. Int J Antimicrob Agents. 2007;30(4):360–5.

211. Knudsen JD, Andersen SE. A multidisciplinary intervention to reduce infections of ESBL- and AmpC-producing, gram-negative bacteria at a university hospital. PLoS One. 2014;9(1):e86457.

Active Surveillance Cultures for MRSA, VRE, Multidrug-Resistant Gram-Negatives

15

Amar Krishna and Teena Chopra

Introduction and Definition

Infections due to multidrug-resistant (MDR) bacteria including Gram-positive and Gram-negative bacteria are responsible for a significant proportion of healthcare-associated infections [1]. Infections caused by MDR pathogens are associated with worse patient outcomes including increased morbidity, mortality, healthcare costs, and increased hospital lengths of stay when compared to infections by more drug-sensitive pathogens [2, 3]. Methicillin-resistant *Staphylococcus aureus* [MRSA], vancomycin-resistant *Enterococcus* [VRE], and multidrug-resistant Gram-negative bacteria [MDR-GN] including extended spectrum beta-lactamase producing *Enterobacteriaceae* [ESBL], carbapenem-resistant *Enterobacteriaceae* [CRE], MDR *Pseudomonas*, and MDR *Acinetobacter* have been mainly responsible for most drug-resistant infections that occur in healthcare settings [1]. Patients can be also colonized with these pathogens without developing infection, and studies have shown that most often colonization by these bacteria precedes development of infection [4–6]. Patients who are colonized or infected by MRSA, VRE, and MDR-GN can be a source of spread to other patients in a healthcare facility usually through hands of healthcare workers, contaminated environment, or contaminated fomites [7]. There is also frequent movement of patients colonized or infected with MRSA, VRE, and MDR-GN between healthcare facilities including acute care hospitals, nursing homes, and long-term acute care facilities leading to organism spread [8–10].

Various infection control measures are used to prevent spread of these pathogens among patients and between healthcare facilities especially in the setting of an outbreak. Active surveillance [AS] is one such infection control measure which involves detection of patients who are colonized

with the targeted MDR pathogen by the use of culture or molecular methods. This approach is based on the observation that patients colonized with MDR pathogens might go undetected if a healthcare facility relies on detection of these pathogens based on clinical cultures only [passive surveillance].

Once colonization by MDR pathogens is detected by the use of active surveillance, further spread to other patients can be prevented with the use of infection control measures including contact precautions, isolation, and environmental cleaning. Active surveillance is also used to estimate the incidence and prevalence of MDR pathogens in patients of a healthcare facility or during investigation of an outbreak due to MDR pathogen [11–13]. Other instance where active surveillance is used includes preoperative detection of nasal MRSA carriers to provide decolonization and appropriate antibiotic prophylaxis during surgery [14].

Evidence to Support or Refute Active Surveillance

Despite the use of active surveillance as part of routine infection control, studies have been conflicting on the effectiveness of surveillance to control or decrease MDR organism spread in a healthcare facility. This is especially true in studies where the MDR pathogen is known to be endemic or sporadically detected in a facility [14–18]. Since AS by itself will not lead to control of MDR pathogen spread, studies evaluating the effectiveness of active surveillance are usually combined with other infection control measures including barrier precautions and cohorting in private rooms or separate units of patients known or suspected to be colonized by the MDR pathogen. Most of these studies have targeted a single MDR pathogen, pathogens having similar resistance mechanisms or pathogens resistant to same class of antibiotics and generally targeted patients admitted in wards or intensive care units where the likelihood of patients to be colonized with the MDR pathogen is high [18–20].

A. Krishna (✉) • T. Chopra
Division of Infectious Diseases, Harper University Hospital,
Detroit Medical Center/Wayne State University,
3990 John R, Detroit, MI 48201, USA
e-mail: akrishn@med.wayne.edu; tchopra@med.wayne.edu

© Springer International Publishing AG 2018
G. Bearman et al. (eds.), *Infection Prevention*, DOI 10.1007/978-3-319-60980-5_15

There are several factors which can influence the outcome of studies determining the efficacy of AS, and these factors must be closely considered when such studies are evaluated. Since studies use multiple infection control interventions concomitantly or sequentially, each of these interventions can influence the outcome. For example, if patients are receiving decolonization therapy or other infection control interventions are concomitantly started to reduce other healthcare-associated infections, then this can influence the outcome unless controlled during the study analysis. In studies with before/after study design which fail to control for secular trends, then it will be unclear if changes in outcomes are due to the intervention or due to persistence of secular trends itself [21]. Outcomes will also depend on compliance with AS, hand hygiene, and contact precautions which are frequently not measured in studies. Lastly it is also important to consider the sensitivity and specificity of microbiologic methods used to identify the pathogen and the turnaround time of the test. Since this will accurately identify the population targeted for the infection control interventions and help implement them in a timely manner to derive the maximum benefit.

MRSA

With regard to MRSA, there are a handful of studies that are usually mentioned to support or refute the effectiveness of AS in controlling spread. The Veterans Affairs [VA] study which was implemented in VA hospitals nationwide was able to show a decrease in MRSA transmission and healthcare-associated MRSA infections in both ICUs and non-ICUs when compared to baseline with the use of universal AS and contact precautions in patients who tested positive for MRSA [22]. Hand hygiene and a change in the institutional culture whereby infection control became responsibility of everyone who had contact with patients were also promoted during the intervention period. Routine decolonization was not recommended and use of mupirocin for nasal decolonization of MRSA did not increase during the intervention period.

In another retrospective study with an interrupted time series design done in eight ICUs where a series of infection control interventions were implemented one at a time, only AS for nasal MRSA carriage with use of contact precautions for patients who tested positive showed a decrease in MRSA bacteremia in intensive care units [ICUs] and hospital wide [20]. Other interventions such as use of sterile barrier precautions during central venous catheter placement, alcohol-based hand rub use, or hand hygiene promotion were not associated with a decrease in MRSA bacteremia. This is despite a compliance with hand hygiene increasing to 80% in the campaign year. Although AS and isolation was imple-

mented in only ICUs, the authors hypothesized that reduction in opportunities for MRSA transmission in non-ICUs was because of fewer MRSA carriers being discharged from ICUs likely leading to hospital wide decrease in MRSA bacteremia. In addition, there are multiple studies where AS and contact isolation have proved successful in controlling outbreaks due MRSA in different type of healthcare settings [7].

However, results from randomized trials on AS have been less encouraging. STAR ICU study was a cluster randomized trial in eight ICUs where patients in intervention ICUs were assigned to contact precautions if clinical or surveillance cultures were positive for MRSA or VRE; all other patients in the intervention group were assigned to care with universal gloving until discharge or until surveillance cultures obtained at admission came back negative [23]. Patients in control group were maintained on standard precautions, and contact precautions were only assigned if MRSA or VRE were identified on clinical cultures. Despite surveillance cultures identifying a large proportion of colonized patients, this study did note a difference in ICU level incidence of MRSA or VRE infection or colonization in intervention and control groups. Prolonged turnaround time of 5 days for reporting culture results which increased the proportion of time MRSA or VRE-positive patients was assigned to universal gloving instead of contact precautions; less compliance with contact precautions than required especially during contact with environment only and the short duration of the intervention period were some of the reasons that were noted for lack of effectiveness of AS.

Similarly, in the REDUCE MRSA cluster randomized trial in 74 ICUs, authors noted a decrease in MRSA-positive clinical cultures and a decrease in ICU-attributable blood stream infection due to any pathogen in the universal decolonization group when compared to targeted decolonization or screening and isolation groups [24]. However, it has to be noted that screening and isolation for MRSA was already a standard of care in all ICUs with 90% of admitted patients undergoing screening; therefore, the effectiveness or otherwise of AS cannot be evaluated, but this study did provide evidence that universal decolonization might provide added benefit to control MRSA.

In another three-phase ICU study, baseline period was followed by interrupted time series study of universal chlorhexidine bathing combined with hand hygiene improvement for 5 months [phase 2] [25]. This was then followed by a cluster randomized where conventional AS for MRSA and VRE was compared with rapid-based screening for MRSA, VRE, and highly resistant *Enterobacteriaceae* [phase 3]. The study reported decrease in MDR acquisition in phase 2 mainly due to decreased acquisition of MRSA and no further decrease in acquisition noted in phase 3 regardless of whether screening was done with conventional or rapid testing. [25].

Another study that has been extensively quoted to recommend against use of AS is a prospective interventional cohort study with crossover design conducted in Switzerland involving surgical patients [14]. This study found that the use of AS surveillance with contact isolation, decolonization with chlorhexidine and nasal mupirocin, and adjustment of preoperative antibiotics in nasal MRSA carriers did not decrease nosocomial MRSA infections when compared to control group. However, only 31% of MRSA carriers were identified prior to surgery, and in the intervention group, only 66% of MRSA-positive patients received appropriate preoperative antibiotics, and only 41% of MRSA carriers received decolonization prior to surgery. In addition, none of the 26 patients who were identified as MRSA positive as outpatients and received appropriate decolonization and preoperative antibiotics developed MRSA infection.

In addition, a systematic review in 2008 concluded that although the existing evidence may favor the use of active surveillance for MRSA in ICUs, evidence is of poor quality, and definitive recommendations cannot be made [15]. In another systematic review and meta-analysis in 2009, there was no reduction in MRSA acquisition with rapid screening when compared to conventional screening [26]. There was however reduction in MRSA blood stream infection with rapid screening when compared to no screening. Both these reviews noted that there were other interventions such as decolonization with nasal mupirocin and chlorhexidine baths and hand hygiene promotion used concomitantly at time of AS making efficacy of each intervention difficult to assess [15, 26].

VRE

As noted above, randomized trials on VRE failed to show decrease in VRE infection or colonization with AS and contact isolation [23, 25]. However, in an outbreak setting, VRE have been successfully controlled with the use of AS, contact precautions, and isolation/cohorting [27–29]. VRE outbreak has also been successfully controlled in an entire region involving many different healthcare facilities with the use of AS of high-risk patients, contact precautions, and communication between healthcare facilities about VRE status of patients at time of transfer [13]. Most of these studies have concurrently used other interventions including hand hygiene promotion, use of alcohol-based hand rubs, decolonization, staff cohorting, ward closure, environmental cleaning, and antibiotic restriction to contain a VRE outbreak making the efficacy of individual interventions difficult to assess [13, 27–29].

Control is particularly successful if molecular techniques identified a single or few VRE strains as responsible for an outbreak indicating that cases of VRE colonization and infection are acquired mainly from cross transmission which can be controlled by AS and contact isolation [13, 27, 29]. A study conducted in the Netherlands differentiated outbreak from non-outbreak VRE strains with the help of pulsed-field gel electrophoresis [PFGE] and used contact precautions and cohorting on patients infected or colonized with outbreak strain only, and this leads to successful control of the outbreak [30].

In a study comparing two hospitals, there was twofold more cases of VRE bacteremia in the hospital which did not routinely screen patients for VRE colonization compared to the hospital which conducted weekly AS and used contact precautions in VRE-colonized patients in high-risk wards including ICUs [17]. In the hospital not conducting AS, VRE bacteremia was mainly identified in ICUs further indicating increased patient to patient cross transmission of VRE with subsequent development of bacteremia occurred in the absence of screening and contact isolation [other hospital was using AS in ICUs]. Furthermore, PFGE indicated that bacteremic VRE strains in hospital not using AS were more clonally related indicating that cross transmission was occurring. However, it is to be noted that the hospital not using AS performed mainly liver transplants and more abdominal surgeries which might have increased risk of VRE bacteremia in patients [17].

MDR-GN Studies demonstrating successful control of MDR-GN outbreaks have showed that only one or few closely related strains were responsible for the outbreaks indicating infection control measures prevented patient to patient cross transmission [31–34]. Outbreaks of CRE, ESBL *Enterobacteriaceae*, other MDR *Enterobacteriaceae*, MDR *Pseudomonas*, and MDR *Acinetobacter* have been successfully controlled with IC measures either implemented concomitantly or sequentially [31–35]. In a review which evaluated efficacy of stepwise implementation of infection control bundles in control of CRE concluded that combination of AS and patient/staff cohorting is the most effective strategy [36]. With regard to some Gram negatives such as *Acinetobacter* and *Pseudomonas*, hospital environment can play an important role in organism persistence, and surveillance cultures have been used to identify possible sources [32, 37].

In an endemic setting, efficacy of AS and other infection control measures might depend on whether endemicity is due to efficient cross transmission of the organism or due to denevo acquisition of organism from antibiotic selection pressure [11, 16, 38, 39]. In the slatter scenario, which is seen with Amp-C producers and ESBL *E. coli*, studies have shown infection control measures are unlikely to be effective in decreasing endemicity [16, 38]. Molecular analysis has also confirmed that such strains isolated from different patients are polyclonal and unrelated [38]. Such strains arising from patients own flora might not be efficiently cross transmitted among patients. In a retrospective study, no outbreaks of ESBL *E. coli* were noted despite one hospital stopped isolating patients colonized with this organism [39]. In another observational study, there were only two instances of cross transmission among roommates despite many other patients cared for in the same room as patients found to be colonized with ESBL *Enterobacteriaceae* who were not on contact precautions [16]. These studies also noted increased compliance with hand hygiene and contact precautions might also have decreased opportunities for cross transmission [16, 39].

CRE acquisition in endemic setting likely depends on colonization pressure in a hospital or unit indicating patient to patient transmission playing an important role in CRE spread [40]. Therefore, infection control measures have proved effective in decreasing CRE rates in an endemic setting including when such measures have been implemented nationwide [41]. However, this might only apply to CRE where carbapenem resistance is due to production of beta-lactamases capable of hydrolyzing carbapenems rather than resistance to carbapenems due to other mechanisms [41]. In the latter case, organism acquisition is likely from patients own flora. Although various infection control measures have been implemented to control CRE making efficacy of each intervention difficult to assess, one study indicated that AS was likely responsible for decrease in carbapenem-resistant *Klebsiella pneumoniae* in their ICU [11]. With regard to other Gram-negative pathogens including MDR *Acinetobacter* and *Pseudomonas*, only few studies on efficacy of infection control measures have been done in an endemic setting [11, 42].

Sites and Method of Surveillance

MRSA Studies have consistently shown that specimens from nares have high negative predictive value for ruling out MRSA colonization [43, 44]. In addition cultures from site of skin breakdown are also recommended [43]. Screening for MRSA has traditionally relied on conventional culture methods which usually have a turnaround time of few days leading to delay in implementation of contact precautions for MRSA-positive patients, and if preemptive contact isolation is being used, and then it will lead to unnecessary use of isolation in patients who would eventually found to be negative for MRSA colonization [23]. To circumvent these drawbacks, various rapid screening methods have been used for earlier detection. Rapid screening methods for MRSA can be broadly classified into two categories: those using chromogenic media and those relying on molecular methods. Real-time PCR have the shortest test time of less than 1 h, and results of chromogenic media can be obtained as early as 22 h [45, 46]. In addition, both categories of rapid screening

have been shown to have high sensitivity [45, 46]. Despite the short turnaround time and decrease in isolation days with rapid screening, it is unclear whether they reduce MRSA transmission compared to conventional cultures as previously noted in the meta-analysis and a cluster randomized trial [25, 26].

VRE

Stool, rectal, and perirectal swabs are all sensitive methods to detect VRE colonization [47, 48]. Studies have also used stool specimens sent for *Clostridium difficile* testing to screen for VRE [49]. However, using this method as the only surveillance strategy can miss significant proportion of VRE-colonized patients [49]. Similar to MRSA, both rapid methods and conventional culture have been used to detect VRE colonization [47, 50]. Among the rapid methods, chromogenic agars have high sensitivity and specificity when compared to culture-based methods for VRE detection [47, 50]. They also reduce turnaround time of screening [47]. Sensitivity of culture and chromogenic agar is lowered by low vancomycin MIC of the tested VRE isolates, low fecal VRE density of the tested sample, and high vancomycin concentration in the culture media [51].

Real-time PCR methods are also increasing used for VRE screening which detect VanA and VanB genes directly from stool or rectal samples [47]. PCR has high sensitivity and NPV but generally has low positive predictive value especially for VanB-containing Enterococci [47, 50]. Therefore, a positive result would require culture confirmation since this could be due to detection on VanB genes in non-enterococcal species including Gram-positive anaerobic bacteria. [47] Poor PPV of PCR-based screening could also be due to low prevalence of VRE in the tested specimens or the gold standard culture method used for comparison with PCR [47, 50].

MDR-GN

Rectal or stool samples are usually used for detection of CRE, ESBL *Enterobacteriaceae*, and other multidrug-resistant *Enterobacteriaceae* [52–54]. With regard to surveillance samples for *Pseudomonas* and *Acinetobacter* species, it is unclear which sites are associated with highest sensitivity. Usually studies have used culture from multiple sites to increase sensitivity. These sites have included rectum, skin, pharynx, nose, wounds, urine, and tracheal aspirate if patient is on mechanical ventilation [32, 35, 55]. Despite taking surveillance samples from multiple sites, one study found sensitivity of detecting patients colonized with *A. baumannii* was only 55%. [55].

The most commonly used culture methods to screen for ESBL *Enterobacteriaceae* are MacConkey agar and Drigalski agar with or without enrichment, and they are usually supplemented with third-generation cephalosporin to select growth of resistant bacteria [38, 56]. Chromogenic agars are also used for screening purposes due to their short turnaround time and increased sensitivity [57]. Confirmation of ESBL phenotype is by double disk synergy test [38].

Screening for CRE can also be done with conventional culture-based methods or use of chromogenic agars [11, 52, 53]. Among the chromogenic agars, SUPERCARBA has the highest sensitivity for CRE detection [53]. If screening is positive, then confirmation of carbapenemase production is required. This can be done by phenotypic methods or confirmation with PCR [52]. Carba-NP test which is based on in vitro hydrolysis of imipenem resulting in change of pH value of the indicator is a very sensitive and specific method to confirm carbapenemase production [53]. Currently PCR can be used directly on rectal surveillance samples to detect CRE and have a test time of <1 h [58]. However main drawback with PCR-based screening is the increased cost and inability to detect previously unidentified resistance genes [53].

Patient Populations to Screen, Frequency of Screening, and Duration of Colonization

Studies on VRE and MDR-GN have mainly targeted patients admitted in high-risk units such as ICUs and units housing immunocompromised patients [17, 19, 38, 41]. Some studies have also targeted patients known to be at high risk of colonization such as patients with prolonged hospitalization, history of recent antibiotic use, patients coming from nursing home, or known contacts of colonized patients [6, 41]. In addition to the above population, studies on AS for MRSA have used universal screening as a surveillance strategy [22]. Studies have also been conducted to define populations at increased risk for colonization who need to be targeted for AS [5, 28, 59]. Decision on which populations to target for AS should depend on the epidemiology of the MDR pathogen in that facility as well as in surrounding facilities who frequently transfer their patients.

With regard to frequency of screening, studies have either screened patients at admission or discharge, weekly and at time of discharge [18, 23, 24]. Screening is continued in patients who test negative at time of admission to determine new acquisition during that hospitalization. Since frequent screening requires considerable resource and increases laboratory workload and workload of staff responsible for taking surveillance samples, healthcare facilities who plan to implement AS should determine the frequency of AS after considering these factors. Another strategy which can be utilized in areas with low MDR prevalence is conducting point prevalence surveys in units or populations where the MDR pathogen is initially detected [31].

Another issue that needs to be considered by facilities employing AS is to determine when to repeat surveillance to document clearance of the MDR pathogen to avoid unnecessary contact isolation in patients with history of previous colonization. Colonization with MRSA, VRE, and MDR-GNs can persist for many months to years [44, 55, 60]. A study on duration of colonization by MRSA and VRE in patients with prolonged hospital stay found that 11% of MRSA carriers and 18% of VRE carriers cleared their colonization a median of 23 and 26.5 days, respectively, and hence repeat surveillance after this period should be considered [61]. With regard to CRE, 50–70% of colonized patients had cleared the organism at least 90 days after their last positive culture, so repeat surveillance cultures to document clearance should be considered after this time frame [41, 60]. Similarly in patients colonized with *A. baumannii*, only 17% patients were still colonized after a median duration of last isolation of 16 months [55].

Conclusions

AS has been used as an infection control strategy for control of MDR pathogen spread in healthcare facilities during the past few decades. Outbreaks due to many MDR pathogens including MRSA, VRE, and MDR-GN have been successfully controlled with this strategy when combined with other infection control measures. More recent studies however have questioned the effectiveness of AS especially in studies done in setting where the MDR pathogen is known to be endemic. In addition, AS is unlikely to be effective when the prevalence of the MDR pathogen is low in a facility. A comparative effectiveness review conducted by Agency of Healthcare Research and Quality in 2013 on MRSA screening concluded that there is low strength of evidence that universal screening of hospitalized patients decreases MRSA infections [21]. There was also insufficient evidence on other outcomes of universal MRSA screening and to support or refute MRSA screening on any outcomes in other settings [21]. Following this review, there has been one major randomized trial which did not show benefit of screening and isolation for MRSA and VRE when added to a policy of universal chlorhexidine and hand hygiene improvement [25]. To further complicate matters, MRSA has been successfully controlled in several European countries with prevalence as low as <0.5% by using a search and destroy strategy which involves active surveillance and strict application of contact precautions and isolation in colonized and infected patients [7]. Similarly, studies on use of AS to control endemic VRE have come to varied conclusions. With regard to MDR-GN, effectiveness of AS might depend on mechanism of endemicity of the particular pathogen with AS combined with other infection control measures more likely to be effective where the mechanism is more likely due to cross transmission such as in case of CRE especially those that produce beta-lactamases which hydrolyze carbapenems. Some of this heterogenicity could also be due to studies not controlling for important confounders such as secular trends, compliance with infection control measures, and concomitant use of other infection control measures which can influence outcomes of interest [21].

Future studies should use design features and analytical strategies to control for these important confounders to arrive at definite conclusions to support causal inference. Until then, a two-tiered approach to implementation of AS and other infection control measures as recommended by CDC should be considered [62]. This approach should be tailored to each healthcare facility based on the local circumstances, feasibility, and the specific MDR pathogen which is being transmitted with frequent reassessment to determine the efficacy of the implemented measures [62].

References

1. Weiner LM, Webb AK, Limbago B, et al. Antimicrobial-resistant pathogens associated with healthcare-associated infections: summary of data reported to the national healthcare safety network at the centers for disease control and prevention, 2011–2014. Infect Control Hosp Epidemiol. 2016;37(11):1288–301.
2. Cosgrove SE. The relationship between antimicrobial resistance and patient outcomes: mortality, length of hospital stay, and health care costs. Clin Infect Dis. 2006;42(Suppl 2):S82–9.
3. DiazGranados CA, Zimmer SM, Klein M, Jernigan JA. Comparison of mortality associated with vancomycin-resistant and vancomycin-susceptible enterococcal bloodstream infections: a meta-analysis. Clin Infect Dis. 2005;41(3):327–33.
4. Huang SS, Rifas-Shiman SL, Pottinger JM, et al. Improving the assessment of vancomycin-resistant enterococci by routine screening. J Infect Dis. 2007;195(3):339–46.
5. Ben-Ami R, Schwaber MJ, Navon-Venezia S, et al. Influx of extended-spectrum beta-lactamase-producing enterobacteriaceae into the hospital. Clin Infect Dis. 2006;42(7):925–34.
6. Calfee DP, Giannetta ET, Durbin LJ, Germanson TP, Farr BM. Control of endemic vancomycin-resistant enterococcus among inpatients at a university hospital. Clin Infect Dis. 2003;37(3):326–32.
7. Muto CA, Jernigan JA, Ostrowsky BE, et al. SHEA guideline for preventing nosocomial transmission of multidrug-resistant strains of Staphylococcus aureus and enterococcus. Infect Control Hosp Epidemiol. 2003;24(5):362–86.
8. Elizaga ML, Weinstein RA, Hayden MK. Patients in long-term care facilities: a reservoir for vancomycin-resistant enterococci. Clin Infect Dis. 2002;34(4):441–6.
9. Polgreen PM, Beekmann SE, Chen YY, et al. Epidemiology of methicillin-resistant Staphylococcus aureus and vancomycin-resistant enterococcus in a rural state. Infect Control Hosp Epidemiol. 2006;27(3):252–6.
10. Marquez P, Terashita D, Dassey D, Mascola L. Population-based incidence of carbapenem-resistant Klebsiella pneumoniae along the continuum of care, Los Angeles County. Infect Control Hosp Epidemiol. 2013;34(2):144–50.
11. Kochar S, Sheard T, Sharma R, et al. Success of an infection control program to reduce the spread of carbapenem-resistant Klebsiella pneumoniae. Infect Control Hosp Epidemiol. 2009;30(5):447–52.
12. Thiebaut AC, Arlet G, Andremont A, et al. Variability of intestinal colonization with third-generation cephalosporin-resistant Enterobacteriaceae and antibiotic use in intensive care units. J Antimicrob Chemother. 2012;67(6):1525–36.
13. Ostrowsky BE, Trick WE, Sohn AH, et al. Control of vancomycin-resistant enterococcus in health care facilities in a region. N Engl J Med. 2001;344(19):1427–33.
14. Harbarth S, Fankhauser C, Schrenzel J, et al. Universal screening for methicillin-resistant Staphylococcus aureus at hospital admission and nosocomial infection in surgical patients. JAMA. 2008;299(10):1149–57.
15. McGinigle KL, Gourlay ML, Buchanan IB. The use of active surveillance cultures in adult intensive care units to reduce methicillin-resistant Staphylococcus aureus-related morbidity, mortality, and costs: a systematic review. Clin Infect Dis. 2008;46(11):1717–25.
16. Tschudin-Sutter S, Frei R, Dangel M, Stranden A, Widmer AF. Rate of transmission of extended-spectrum beta-lactamase-producing enterobacteriaceae without contact isolation. Clin Infect Dis. 2012;55(11):1505–11.
17. Price CS, Paule S, Noskin GA, Peterson LR. Active surveillance reduces the incidence of vancomycin-resistant enterococcal bacteremia. Clin Infect Dis. 2003;37(7):921–8.
18. Souweine B, Traore O, Aublet-Cuvelier B, et al. Role of infection control measures in limiting morbidity associated with multi-resistant organisms in critically ill patients. J Hosp Infect. 2000;45(2):107–16.
19. Almyroudis NG, Osawa R, Samonis G, et al. Discontinuation of systematic surveillance and contact precautions for Vancomycin-Resistant Enterococcus (VRE) and its impact on the incidence of VRE faecium bacteremia in patients with hematologic malignancies. Infect Control Hosp Epidemiol. 2016;37(4):398–403.
20. Huang SS, Yokoe DS, Hinrichsen VL, et al. Impact of routine intensive care unit surveillance cultures and resultant barrier precautions on hospital-wide methicillin-resistant Staphylococcus aureus bacteremia. Clin Infect Dis. 2006;43(8):971–8.
21. Noorani HZ, Adams E, Glick S, Weber S, Belinson S, Aronson N. Screening for Methicillin-Resistant Staphylococcus aureus (MRSA): future research needs: identification of future research needs from comparative effectiveness review no. 102. Rockville: Agency for Healthcare Research and Quality (US); 2013.
22. Jain R, Kralovic SM, Evans ME, et al. Veterans affairs initiative to prevent methicillin-resistant Staphylococcus aureus infections. N Engl J Med. 2011;364(15):1419–30.
23. Huskins WC, Huckabee CM, O'Grady NP, et al. Intervention to reduce transmission of resistant bacteria in intensive care. N Engl J Med. 2011;364(15):1407–18.
24. Huang SS, Septimus E, Kleinman K, et al. Targeted versus universal decolonization to prevent ICU infection. N Engl J Med. 2013;368(24):2255–65.
25. Derde LP, Cooper BS, Goossens H, et al. Interventions to reduce colonisation and transmission of antimicrobial-resistant bacteria in intensive care units: an interrupted time series study and cluster randomised trial. Lancet Infect Dis. 2014;14(1):31–9.
26. Tacconelli E, De Angelis G, de Waure C, Cataldo MA, La Torre G, Cauda R. Rapid screening tests for meticillin-resistant Staphylococcus aureus at hospital admission: systematic review and meta-analysis. Lancet Infect Dis. 2009;9(9):546–54.
27. Rupp ME, Marion N, Fey PD, et al. Outbreak of vancomycin-resistant enterococcus faecium in a neonatal intensive care unit. Infect Control Hosp Epidemiol. 2001;22(5):301–3.

28. Byers KE, Anglim AM, Anneski CJ, et al. A hospital epidemic of vancomycin-resistant enterococcus: risk factors and control. Infect Control Hosp Epidemiol. 2001;22(3):140–7.

29. Hanna H, Umphrey J, Tarrand J, Mendoza M, Raad I. Management of an outbreak of vancomycin-resistant enterococci in the medical intensive care unit of a cancer center. Infect Control Hosp Epidemiol. 2001;22(4):217–9.

30. Mascini EM, Troelstra A, Beitsma M, et al. Genotyping and pre-emptive isolation to control an outbreak of vancomycin-resistant enterococcus faecium. Clin Infect Dis. 2006;42(6):739–46.

31. Munoz-Price LS, Hayden MK, Lolans K, et al. Successful control of an outbreak of Klebsiella pneumoniae carbapenemase-producing K. pneumoniae at a long-term acute care hospital. Infect Control Hosp Epidemiol. 2010;31(4):341–7.

32. Simor AE, Lee M, Vearncombe M, et al. An outbreak due to multiresistant Acinetobacter baumannii in a burn unit: risk factors for acquisition and management. Infect Control Hosp Epidemiol. 2002;23(5):261–7.

33. Piagnerelli M, Kennes B, Brogniez Y, Deplano A, Govaerts D. Outbreak of nosocomial multidrug-resistant Enterobacter aerogenes in a geriatric unit: failure of isolation contact, analysis of risk factors, and use of pulsed-field gel electrophoresis. Infect Control Hosp Epidemiol. 2000;21(10):651–3.

34. Giuffre M, Cipolla D, Bonura C, et al. Outbreak of colonizations by extended-spectrum beta-lactamase-producing Escherichia coli sequence type 131 in a neonatal intensive care unit, Italy. Antimicrob Resist Infect Control. 2013;2(1):8.

35. Ciofi Degli Atti M, Bernaschi P, Carletti M, et al. An outbreak of extremely drug-resistant Pseudomonas aeruginosa in a tertiary care pediatric hospital in Italy. BMC Infect Dis. 2014:14–494.

36. Munoz-Price LS, Quinn JP. Deconstructing the infection control bundles for the containment of carbapenem-resistant Enterobacteriaceae. Curr Opin Infect Dis. 2013;26(4):378–87.

37. Yakupogullari Y, Otlu B, Dogukan M, et al. Investigation of a nosocomial outbreak by alginate-producing pan-antibiotic-resistant Pseudomonas aeruginosa. Am J Infect Control. 2008;36(10):e13–8.

38. Gardam MA, Burrows LL, Kus JV, et al. Is surveillance for multidrug-resistant enterobacteriaceae an effective infection control strategy in the absence of an outbreak? J Infect Dis. 2002;186(12):1754–60.

39. Zahar JR, Poirel L, Dupont C, Fortineau N, Nassif X, Nordmann P. About the usefulness of contact precautions for carriers of extended-spectrum beta-lactamase-producing Escherichia coli. BMC Infect Dis. 2015;15:512.

40. Swaminathan M, Sharma S, Poliansky Blash S, et al. Prevalence and risk factors for acquisition of carbapenem-resistant Enterobacteriaceae in the setting of endemicity. Infect Control Hosp Epidemiol. 2013;34(8):809–17.

41. Schwaber MJ, Carmeli Y. An ongoing national intervention to contain the spread of carbapenem-resistant enterobacteriaceae. Clin Infect Dis. 2014;58(5):697–703.

42. Apisarnthanarak A, Pinitchai U, Thongphubeth K, et al. A multifaceted intervention to reduce pandrug-resistant Acinetobacter baumannii colonization and infection in 3 intensive care units in a Thai tertiary care center: a 3-year study. Clin Infect Dis. 2008;47(6):760–7.

43. Manian FA, Senkel D, Zack J, Meyer L. Routine screening for methicillin-resistant Staphylococcus aureus among patients newly admitted to an acute rehabilitation unit. Infect Control Hosp Epidemiol. 2002;23(9):516–9.

44. Sanford MD, Widmer AF, Bale MJ, Jones RN, Wenzel RP. Efficient detection and long-term persistence of the carriage of methicillin-resistant Staphylococcus aureus. Clin Infect Dis. 1994;19(6):1123–8.

45. Perry JD, Davies A, Butterworth LA, Hopley AL, Nicholson A, Gould FK. Development and evaluation of a chromogenic agar medium for methicillin-resistant Staphylococcus aureus. J Clin Microbiol. 2004;42(10):4519–23.

46. Huletsky A, Lebel P, Picard FJ, et al. Identification of methicillin-resistant Staphylococcus aureus carriage in less than 1 hour during a hospital surveillance program. Clin Infect Dis. 2005;40(7):976–81.

47. Faron ML, Ledeboer NA, Buchan BW. Resistance mechanisms, epidemiology, and approaches to screening for vancomycin-resistant enterococcus in the health care setting. J Clin Microbiol. 2016;54(10):2436–47.

48. Usacheva EA, Ginocchio CC, Morgan M, et al. Prospective, multicenter evaluation of the BD GeneOhm VanR assay for direct, rapid detection of vancomycin-resistant enterococcus species in perianal and rectal specimens. Am J Clin Pathol. 2010;134(2):219–26.

49. Shadel BN, Puzniak LA, Gillespie KN, Lawrence SJ, Kollef M, Mundy LM. Surveillance for vancomycin-resistant enterococci: type, rates, costs, and implications. Infect Control Hosp Epidemiol. 2006;27(10):1068–75.

50. Humphreys H. Controlling the spread of vancomycin-resistant enterococci. Is active screening worthwhile? J Hosp Infect. 2014;88(4):191–8.

51. Wijesuriya TM, Perry P, Pryce T, et al. Low vancomycin MICs and fecal densities reduce the sensitivity of screening methods for vancomycin resistance in enterococci. J Clin Microbiol. 2014;52(8):2829–33.

52. Nordmann P, Gniadkowski M, Giske CG, et al. Identification and screening of carbapenemase-producing Enterobacteriaceae. Clin Microbiol Infect. 2012;18(5):432–8.

53. Nordmann P, Poirel L. Strategies for identification of carbapenemase-producing Enterobacteriaceae. J Antimicrob Chemother. 2013;68(3):487–9.

54. Hacek DM, Bednarz P, Noskin GA, Zembower T, Peterson LR. Yield of vancomycin-resistant enterococci and multidrug-resistant Enterobacteriaceae from stools submitted for Clostridium difficile testing compared to results from a focused surveillance program. J Clin Microbiol. 2001;39(3):1152–4.

55. Marchaim D, Navon-Venezia S, Schwartz D, et al. Surveillance cultures and duration of carriage of multidrug-resistant Acinetobacter baumannii. J Clin Microbiol. 2007;45(5):1551–5.

56. Grohs P, Podglajen I, Guerot E, et al. Assessment of five screening strategies for optimal detection of carriers of third-generation cephalosporin-resistant Enterobacteriaceae in intensive care units using daily sampling. Clin Microbiol Infect. 2014;20(11):O879–86.

57. Abbott IJ, Jenney AW, Spelman DW, et al. Active surveillance for multidrug-resistant gram-negative bacteria in the intensive care unit. Pathology. 2015;47(6):575–9.

58. Tato M, Ruiz-Garbajosa P, Traczewski M, et al. Multisite evaluation of Cepheid Xpert Carba-R assay for detection of Carbapenemase-producing organisms in rectal swabs. J Clin Microbiol. 2016;54(7):1814–9.

59. Harbarth S, Sax H, Fankhauser-Rodriguez C, Schrenzel J, Agostinho A, Pittet D. Evaluating the probability of previously unknown carriage of MRSA at hospital admission. Am J Med. 2006;119(3):275 e215–23.

60. Zimmerman FS, Assous MV, Bdolah-Abram T, Lachish T, Yinnon AM, Wiener-Well Y. Duration of carriage of carbapenem-resistant Enterobacteriaceae following hospital discharge. Am J Infect Control. 2013;41(3):190–4.

61. Ghosh A, Jiao L, Al-Mutawa F, et al. Value of an active surveillance policy to document clearance of meticillin-resistant Staphylococcus aureus and vancomycin-resistant enterococci amongst inpatients with prolonged admissions. J Hosp Infect. 2014;88(4):230–3.

62. Siegel JD, Rhinehart E, Jackson M, Chiarello L. Healthcare infection control practices advisory C. Management of multidrug-resistant organisms in health care settings, 2006. Am J Infect Control. 2007;35(10 Suppl 2):S165–93.

C. difficile Microbiome Manipulation

16

Jenna Wick, Tinzar Basein, and Shira Doron

Introduction

The burden of *Clostridium difficile* infection (CDI) has been increasing in the past decade in terms of incidence, mortality, morbidity, recurrence, and healthcare cost [1–4]. Rates of CDI in US hospitals have increased steadily since 1993. In 2009, there were more than 336000 CDI-related hospital stays, comprising 0.9% of all hospital stays. Almost half a million infections among patients in the United States in a single year are caused by *C. difficile* [3]. Approximately 29000 patients died within 30 days of the initial diagnosis of *C. difficile*. Of those, about 15000 deaths were estimated to be directly attributable to *C. difficile* infections, making *C. difficile* a very important cause of infectious disease death in the United States. Recurrent CDI occurs after 20–30% of initial episodes and after as many as 40–60% of first recurrences [5]. In a 2011 prevalence survey, *C. difficile* was the most commonly reported pathogen causing 12.1% of the healthcare-associated infections identified [4]. The economic burden of CDI is substantial, with up to $4.8 billion each year in excess costs for acute care facilities alone [3].

With increasing incidence and recurrence rates of CDI, prevention and control measures are critical. *C. difficile* transmission occurs not only via the contaminated hands of healthcare workers but also from the environment, where the spores can persist for a long period of time [6]. Skin contamination and environmental shedding of *C. difficile* often persist after resolution of diarrhea and for 1–4 weeks after therapy [7]. Moreover, *C. difficile* spores can remain viable on hard surfaces for up to 5 months, providing a reservoir for infection transmission. Current guidelines for control of CDI recommend contact precautions, meticulous hand hygiene, proper environmental decontamination, and antimicrobial

J. Wick • T. Basein • S. Doron (✉)
Division of Geographic Medicine and Infectious Diseases, Tufts Medical Center, 800 Washington Street, Box 238, Boston, MA 02111, USA
e-mail: JWick@tuftsmedicalcenter.org; TBasein@ tuftsmedicalcenter.org; sdoron@tuftsmedicalcenter.org

stewardship [8]. Despite efforts by hospitals to adhere to these guidelines, however, the incidence of CDI is increasing [9]. Since one of the risk factors for developing CDI is alteration of the ecological environment of the gut by antimicrobial use, manipulation of the human gut microbiome holds promise as a strategy to prevent and control CDI.

Clostridium difficile

CDI manifests as a range of symptoms from mild diarrhea to, in the severe complicated cases, pseudomembranous colitis, toxic megacolon, sepsis, or death [10]. The symptoms are a result of *C. difficile* enterotoxin TcdA and cytotoxin TcdB, which act together to deplete intestinal cytoskeleton integrity and tight junctions, reducing transepithelial resistance and causing fluid accumulation. Further degradation of intestinal epithelium occurs from inflammatory cytokines mediated by TcdA and TcdB causing neutrophil chemotaxis and damage to the mucosa [10]. This drastic disturbance to the intestine is both a result and cause of profound destruction of resident gut bacteria.

Intestinal Microbiome

The human intestine contains an estimated 1000 microbial species with a genome 100-fold greater than the human host [11]. This gut microbiome contributes to vital functions for host homeostasis including nutrient metabolism, vitamin production, immunity, gastrointestinal motility, and preservation of the intestinal epithelial barrier [12]. In 2012, the Human Microbiome Project Consortium performed a study with 242 participants analyzing the healthy Western microbiome [13]. The study found considerable variation in microbial composition, particularly in abundance of the genus *Bacteroides* [13]. However, the metagenomic carriage of metabolic pathways was constant among the participants, suggesting that a healthy microbiome may be better defined

G. Bearman et al. (eds.), *Infection Prevention*, DOI 10.1007/978-3-319-60980-5_16

by its ability to maintain normal metabolic functions rather than by its proportions of particular species [13]. The study found that an average of 86% of genes in the gut were found to encode an unknown function [13]; thus, our microbial inhabitants remain largely illusive.

Microbiome and *C. difficile*

While significant interpersonal variation in gut microbes is the rule, there are also clear differences between cohorts that differ by age, environment, and diet [11]. Furthermore, alterations of the microbiota—dysbiosis—have been consistently correlated with disease, including CDI [14]. Antibiotic therapy leads to gut dysbiosis characterized by low diversity, enabling growth of pathogens, which no longer need to compete for resources, and can utilize carbon produced from bacterial lysis [15].

These altered conditions enable *C. difficile* proliferation and infection, which in turn further drive dysbiosis [16]. Murine models have demonstrated that susceptibility to CDI after antibiotic therapy is associated with an overall decrease in bacterial diversity, with a relative increase in the abundance of the phylum Proteobacteria, and relative decreases in *Bacteroidetes* and *Firmicutes* [17]. Schubert et al. used a murine model to study the effect of seven antibiotics from six classes at different doses and subsequent challenge with *C. difficile* spores. Different antibiotics caused distinct alterations of bacterial compositions, which resulted in significant differences in *C. difficile* colonization susceptibility [18]. Skraban et al. studied the human gut microbiome associated with *C. difficile* by comparing fecal samples from patients who tested positive for *C. difficile* with those of healthy controls. Healthy participants had a larger number of bacterial groups and significantly greater diversity than participants positive for *C. difficile*. Within the participants positive for *C. difficile*, there were considerable differences in microbial composition among different *C. difficile* ribotypes. Stools positive for the particularly virulent ribotype 027 had the smallest number of bacterial groups and least diversity [19]. Thus, it appears that *C. difficile* colonization may be associated less with changes in abundance of specific groups of bacteria and more with the composition of microbes working in a consortium [18, 19].

Studies of Microbiome Manipulation and *C. difficile*

Existing prospective studies of microbiome manipulation and *C. difficile* are limited by small sample sizes. Yet combining or comparing studies is difficult because of their heterogeneity in methodology, patient populations, severity of disease, and microbial preparations.

Probiotics

In the United States, probiotics are marketed as dietary supplements, and thus data to support claims of their health benefits are not reviewed by the FDA [20]. The World Health Organization (WHO) and Food and Agriculture Organization (FAO) of the United Nations define probiotics as "live microorganisms that confer a health benefit on the host when administered in adequate amounts" [20]. *Lactobacillus* and *Bifidobacterium* are common probiotic genera and largely considered safe by the FAO. They may even be safe for high-risk populations; systematic reviews of studies testing *Lactobacillus* and *Bifidobacterium* in medium-risk and critically ill patients observed no adverse events associated with the probiotics [21]. However, reports of infection in patients who were immunocompromised or had artificial heart valves do suggest a need for caution when recommending or administering probiotics to vulnerable patients until clinical trials have definitively determined their safety [21].

Probiotics for Primary Prevention of *C. difficile*

Studies of probiotics to prevent primary infection (the first episode of CDI) have found conflicting results. In 2007, Hickson et al. performed a randomized double-blind, placebo-controlled study with 135 hospitalized patients receiving antibiotics [22]. The probiotic studied was a mixture of *Lactobacillus casei*, *Lactobacillus bulgaricus*, and *Streptococcus thermophilus* administered in a yogurt drink twice a day during antibiotic administration and for one additional week after completion of the antibiotic course. In the ensuing 4 weeks, 9 out of 53 in the placebo group developed diarrhea caused by *C. difficile*, whereas none of the 56 participants in the probiotic group had positive *C. difficile* tests, a statistically significant difference. Additionally, there were no reported adverse events attributable to the probiotic. Of note, over 80% of patients screened were excluded, which limits the applicability of the results to the general population [22].

In contrast to the significant results found by Hickson et al. and others [23, 24], the largest single published study of probiotics for *C. difficile* prevention did not find a significant effect. The study was carried out at five hospitals in England and Wales and included 2941 patients aged 65 and older who were exposed to at least one antibiotic [25]. Participants consumed a probiotic with a combination of *Lactobacillus* and *Bifidobacterium* for 21 days. Within 12 weeks, 0.8% of patients in the probiotic group and 1.2% of patients taking the placebo experienced diarrhea due to *C. difficile*. Measures of diarrhea severity, abdominal symptoms, length of hospital stay, and quality of life also showed no statistical difference [25]. This study adds to others studying

Lactobacillus, *Bifidobacterium*, and the yeast *Saccharomyces boulardii* that have failed to detect a difference between probiotics and placebo in prevention of CDI [26, 27].

In 2013, Goldenberg et al. performed a systematic review including randomized controlled trials of adults and children co-administered probiotics with antibiotics, which separately considered studies for prevention of CDAD (*C. difficile*-associated diarrhea) and CDI (which includes manifestations other than diarrhea, ranging from asymptomatic colonization to toxic megacolon) [28]. Although the 23 studies for CDAD prevention, which included 4213 patients, concluded a 64% reduction, the 13 trials for CDI including 961 participants found no statistical difference in outcomes [28]. A systematic review and meta-analysis published in 2016 by Lau et al. included 26 randomized controlled trials with 7957 patients and found a 60.5% lower risk of CDAD in the probiotic group as well [29]. Subgroup analyses found the evidence for efficacy to be strongest for *Lactobacillus*, *Saccharomyces*, and mixed probiotic formulations [29].

Conflicting results from trials likely result from their heterogeneity and may depend on different patient populations. Probiotics may also have greater utility in higher-risk groups, such as patients taking proton pump inhibitors, and studies could be targeted to the these populations [30].

Guidelines for Use of Probiotics for Primary *C. difficile* Prevention

Currently, national guidelines do not recommend probiotics to prevent initial episodes of *C. difficile*. The 2010 SHEA/IDSA guidelines advise against prescribing probiotics for primary *C. difficile* prevention [31], and the 2013 American College of Gastroenterology guidelines state there is insufficient evidence to recommend probiotics for primary prevention [32].

Probiotics for Secondary Prevention of *C. difficile*

Probiotics may be more effective for secondary prevention of recurrent CDI, once *C. difficile*-associated dysbiosis has occurred, than for primary prevention. Approximately one third of patients who develop CDI will later suffer from recurrent CDI [31], and these infections are not only more challenging to treat but can be drastically more expensive. The estimated cost per case for primary CDI is $5243, in comparison to $13655 per case for recurrent CDI [33].

In 1994, McFarland et al. studied the effect of *S. boulardii* for prevention of recurrent CDI in a randomized double-blind, placebo-controlled multicenter trial and found a significant reduction in later recurrent episodes when given in combination with standard antibiotics to treat *C. difficile*. However, antibiotic therapy, dosage, and duration were not controlled [34]. In 2000, Surawicz et al. expanded upon this research by performing a randomized double-blind, placebo-controlled trial with *S. boulardii* for prevention of recurrent CDI while controlling antibiotic therapy. Participants, who were randomized to high- or low-dose vancomycin or metronidazole, received *S. boulardii* or placebo starting on day 7 of antibiotic therapy and continuing for 28 days. *S. boulardii* effectively decreased both the frequency and number of CDI recurrences at 8 weeks in the patients who received high-dose vancomycin but not in those who received low-dose vancomycin or metronidazole [35].

Guidelines for Use of Probiotics for Secondary *C. difficile* Prevention

There are slightly more confident recommendations for the use of probiotics as secondary prevention for *C. difficile* as compared with the recommendations for primary prevention. The 2010 Society for Hospital Epidemiology of America/Infectious Diseases Society of America guidelines state *S. boulardii* may decrease the number of *C. difficile* recurrences but should be avoided in critically ill and immunosuppressed patients [33]. The 2013 American College of Gastroenterology guidelines state that "although there is moderate evidence that two probiotics (*L. rhamnosus GG* and *S. boulardii*) decrease the incidence of antibiotic associated diarrhea, there is insufficient evidence that probiotics prevent Clostridium difficile infection" [32].

Probiotics as Adjunctive Therapy for *C. difficile*

In 2006, McFarland conducted a meta-analysis including randomized controlled trials of probiotics for the treatment of *C. difficile* [36]. Six studies including 354 subjects were analyzed. Of these, five were for treatment of *C. difficile* and one was for prevention. Two (33%) reported significant reduction of *C. difficile* by probiotics. All of the studies enrolled adults only, and half included only patients with recurrent disease. Antibiotics for *C. difficile* were administered concurrently, and the type and dose of antibiotic were not randomized or standardized. Doses, strains, and duration of probiotics varied among the studies. When combined for meta-analysis, data revealed a relative risk of 0.59 (95% CI 0.41–0.85) indicating a significant benefit associated with the use of probiotics for *C. difficile*. Dendukuri et al. [37] criticized the McFarland meta-analysis [36] for combining results from studies that could not have been drawn from the same population, resulting in, in their estimation, an artificial narrowing of the overall confidence interval for the efficacy of probiotics. They cited other reasons why they deemed the use of meta-analysis in this case inappropriate, such as the different types and doses of probiotic, different lengths of follow-up, and different definitions of diarrhea and response to therapy. These authors contended that the point estimate of the pooled odds ratio for effectiveness in *C. difficile* was almost entirely determined by the one study that showed a statistically significant benefit, while the confidence interval became narrower due to the increased sample size achieved by combining the studies. They pointed out that a systematic review would have been more appropriate. Indeed, these authors had published just such a review on the use of probiotics for prevention and treatment of CDAD in adults in 2005 [37]. Four randomized controlled studies (all included in the McFarland meta-analysis) were identified, with CDAD as the primary outcome. Four additional randomized controlled studies identified CDAD as a secondary outcome. Only two studies showed a benefit for probiotics in treatment of *C. difficile*, particularly in patients with more severe disease; however, the variability in the use of concomitant antibiotics against *C. difficile* makes interpretation of the results difficult.

In 2008, Pillai and Nelson performed a systematic review on the use of probiotics for the treatment of *C. difficile* infections in adults [38]. The review, which included some of the same studies that had been included in the McFarland meta-analysis [36] and the Dendukuri systematic review [37], included four randomized controlled studies. They concluded that probiotics did not show a significant consistent beneficial effect when used in the treatment of *C. difficile*. Only one study found a benefit in the treatment of recurrent CDI, but not in the initial episode. Data were not pooled for analysis because of the variations in recruitment criteria, the type of probiotics used, and the type of concomitant antibiotic therapy and high dropout rates.

Due to the limited information and variable results of studies on the efficacy of probiotics for the treatment of *C. difficile*, Schoster et al. performed in vitro analysis of 17 probiotic strains [39]. Five of the 17 tested probiotic strains inhibited the growth of *C. difficile*. Those five strains included *L. plantarum* (BG112), *L. rhamnosus* (LRH19), *L. plantarum* (LPAL), *L. rhamnosus* (SP1), and *B. animalis* ssp. *lactis* (BLC1).

More recently, given the promising results of FMT trials for treatment of *C. difficile*, attention has turned to the use of multi-strain probiotic combinations, which perhaps more closely approximate stool (or perhaps not), for treatment of CDI. The ongoing phase 2 probiotics for *Clostridium difficile* infection in adults (PICO) study is a randomized, double-blind, placebo-controlled trial by Barker et al. studying the efficacy of a combination of four strains of probiotics in adult patients with CDI [40].

Probiotic Mechanisms

The potential mechanism by which probiotics might treat or prevent CDI has been debated, but likely involves multiple components. Probiotics are thought to provide enhanced colonization resistance, improve integrity of the intestinal barrier, secrete antimicrobial peptides, and cause downregulation of gene expression through quorum sensing [21]. *Lactobacillus* has a direct inhibitory effect against many pathogens, believed to be due to secretion of organic acids, hydrogen peroxide, and bacteriocins [41]. The probiotic formulation Bio-K+ (*Lactobacillus acidophilus* CL1285, *Lactobacillus casei* LBC80R, and *Lactobacillus rhamnosus* CLR2) has been found to effectively neutralize *C. difficile* toxins in addition to having cytotoxic effects [41]. All *Lactobacillus* species do not appear to have equal activity against *C. difficile*. Lactobacillus mixed cultures have strong inhibitory effects against *C. difficile*, while *L. casei* and *L. rhamnosus* pure cultures have demonstrated less pronounced inhibition compared to the mixed cultures, and *L. acidophilus* has no effect [41]. *S. boulardii*, not a normal inhabitant of the intestine, has been shown to increase host concentrations of immunoglobulin A and antitoxin A and to produce a protease that hydrolyzes *C. difficile* toxins A and B [20].

A better understanding of the mechanisms of action of probiotics could in the future allow for intervention at several different stages of the disease process. An emerging concept is the use of prebiotics for infection prevention. A prebiotic is defined as "a selectively fermented ingredient that allows specific changes, both in the composition and/or activity in the gastrointestinal microflora that confers benefits upon host well-being and health" [42]. Prebiotics can also be combined with probiotics as synbiotics [43]. Prebiotics are thought to alleviate diarrheal disease by increasing short-chain fatty acids, or reducing the pH of the intestine [44], but research has yet to ascertain whether prebiotics would be effective for *C. difficile*.

Fecal Microbiota Transplantation for *C. difficile*

Permanent alteration of the gut microbiota is challenging because of immune tolerance to the resident microbes, which inhibits colonization of new organisms [45], requiring a drastic event to significantly change the composition. FMT may be a more effective method of *C. difficile* treatment and/or prevention because the procedure provides three times the order of magnitude of bacteria compared to that from probiotics [46]. FMT has been shown to considerably alter the recipients' microbiota for at least 24 weeks, whereas probiotics are associated with short-term microbiota modifications of 10–14 days [47].

Although the research on FMT is still limited, the early results are promising. In 2013, Van Nood et al. conducted a single center open-label trial for recurrent CDI with three arms: vancomycin alone, vancomycin with bowel lavage, and vancomycin with bowel lavage and donor feces infusion via naso-duodenal tube [48]. The study terminated early after an interim analysis because of its striking success. Out of the 16 patients receiving the infusion of donor feces, 13 had no further evidence of infection after one infusion and two others experienced resolution of their relapsing CDI after a second infusion. Resolution occurred in only 3 out of 13 patients in the bowel lavage group and 4 of 13 in the vancomycin alone group. Analysis of stool samples from participants in the infusion group demonstrated increased fecal microbiota diversity following the procedure, with a greater proportion of *Bacteroidetes* and *Clostridium* clusters IV and XIVa and a reduction in Proteobacteria. Except for mild diarrhea and abdominal cramping on the day of infusion, there were no significant differences in adverse events among patients in the three arms [48].

A study by Shankar et al. in 2014 treated three recurrent CDI patients with FMT from one stool donor. Within 2 days, all patients had reduced diarrheal symptoms, and at 2 months, *C. difficile* toxin B could not be detected in their stool samples by qPCR. Two of the patients had developed formed stools by day three and did not have reinfection at least 2 years later. The third patient suffered from ulcerative colitis, complicating the treatment course, and relapsed a year and a half after FMT during a course of antibiotic therapy for UTI. The researchers utilized a phylogenetic microbiota array to analyze distal gut microbiota of the donor and the recipients prior to transplantation and throughout the follow-up period. Prior to FMT, the stool samples of all CDI patients had high proportions of species belonging to the classes *Gammaproteobacteria* and *Bacilli*, while in the healthy donors' samples, the classes *Clostridia*, *Actinobacteria*, *Erysipelotrichi*, and *Bacteroidia* predominated. Following FMT, the patient samples had a composition that matched that of the donors in both taxonomy of organisms present and relative abundances, and this composition remained stable during the 4-month follow-up [49].

The high rate of resolution of recurrent CDI following FMT remains when all studies are combined in systematic reviews. A meta-analysis by Kassam et al. in 2013 included 11 observational studies comprised of 273 patients, and the weighted pooled rate of clinical resolution was 89% [50]. FMT was associated with minor adverse effects of cramping, belching, and abdominal discomfort, but no serious adverse events [50]. A systematic review in 2014 of case series, case reports, and a randomized controlled study testing FMT for recurrent CDI found a resolution rate of 87% [46].

Stool transplants can be delivered through many different routes: nasogastric or nasojejunal tube, oral capsules, upper endoscopy, retention enema, as well as colonoscopy [51], and it is unknown whether the routes differ in efficacy. Youngster et al. studied 20 patients with refractory or recurrent CDI who received frozen stool suspension from an unrelated donor via colonoscopic or nasogastric administration. At 8 weeks, 14 patients (70%) experienced resolution of diarrhea and no recurrences. Five patients received a second infusion and four were cured bringing overall resolution rate to 90%. The study did not find a significant difference between the colonoscopic or nasogastric routes [52]; however, systematic reviews and meta-analysis have found some differences between the lower and upper GI routes of donor stool administration. Kassam et al. detected a trend toward an improved response for delivery via a lower GI route [50], and Cammarota et al. observed lower GI administration resulted in a slightly higher rate of resolution than upper GI routes, 81–86% compared to 84–93%, respectively [46]. Costs of each method may be an important factor in the decision, as well as patient characteristics. The optimal route of administration may even depend on the most desired species to be delivered. Some spore-forming *Firmicutes* species need to pass through the upper GI tract for efficacy [53], whereas *Bacteroidetes* may need administration via a lower route to prevent destruction by gastric acids [54].

Another debated question is whether there is an increase in efficacy when the recipient is related to the donor. A systematic review in 2011 of 27 case series and reports, comprising 317 patients, observed a slight increase in resolution with stool from a related donor (93% vs. 84%) [55]. However, the meta-analysis by Kassam et al. found no significant differences in resolution whether or not the donor was related [50].

Little is known about FMT for *C. difficile* in children. *C. difficile* colonizes the intestine of 60–70% of infants in their first month, but by 1 year of age carriage decreases to 10%, and at adulthood drops to 0–3% [56]. CDI is more commonly viewed as a disease of older adults, but there has been a concerning rise of CDI incidence in children, with a tenfold increase between 1991 and 2009 [57]. In 2014, both Pierog et al. and Walia et al. reported case series of FMT performed on children with recurrent CDI. Pierog et al. described cases of stool donation from parents to six children, with the youngest age 21 months, who all recovered post FMT [58]. Walia et al. reported two children under 3 years old with recurrent CDI who received the donation from a mother and grandmother [59]. Both children experienced resolution of CDI and remained without symptoms over 6 months after the procedure. This adds to the limited literature on pediatric FMT for CDI and suggests the procedure is safe and effective for infants and children, but more robust trials are needed.

FMT for Immunocompromised Patients

Like probiotic research, in which nearly all studies for probiotics exclude immunocompromised patients [29], FMT trials also exclude these patients due to safety concerns, yet immunocompromised individuals are at a particularly high risk of developing CDI and of having complications such as recurrences.

There are 15 published case reports and case series of FMT in immunosuppressed patients, with 132 total recipients. Combined analysis shows efficacy is comparable to non-immunocompromised patients: over 80% resolution after first FMT procedure and over 90% after the second [60]. However, one study found a higher relapse rate in cancer patients [61], and there have been severe adverse events in patients with IBD, although infectious complications are uncommon [60]. The evidence of FMT for immunocompromised patients is extremely limited and heterogeneous, but encouraging, and indicates trials with safety precautions are warranted.

FMT Mechanisms

Antibiotic therapy has been shown to cause many metabolic alterations. These enhance the capacity of C. difficile to proliferate; thus, some of the proposed mechanisms of FMT involve restoration of traditional metabolic, rather than microbial, composition.

Antibiotics deplete normally occurring gut bacteria that convert primary bile acids to secondary bile acids [17]. Weingarden et al. analyzed the fecal microbiota of 12 recurrent CDI patients prior to and post FMT and found substantial differences in bile acids. Prior to FMT, primary bile acids were elevated compared to their concentration post procedure, and three types of secondary bile acids were present post FMT that were absent prior [62]. Taurocholate (the conjugated bile acid of cholic acid with the amino acid taurine) and glycine have been shown to bind to C. difficile spores and activate germination [63]. CamSA is a meta-benzene sulfonic acid derivative of taurocholate and competitively inhibits taurocholate-mediated germination of C. difficile spores. In mice inoculated with a high concentration of C. difficile spores, those treated with a high dose of CamSA did not develop CDI, and the mice given a lower dose experienced delayed onset and decreased severity of disease [63]. The results of these studies indicate that FMT restores primary and secondary bile acid proportions that may prevent the conditions for C. difficile proliferation. In an analysis of the metabolome of the C. difficile susceptibility state, researchers compared the cecal content of healthy and CDI mice. In the CDI susceptible state, there was a marked increase in primary bile acids, taurocholate, and other tauroconjugated bile acids and a decrease in the secondary bile acid deoxycholate [64].

In the same study there were also considerable differences in metabolites other than bile acids. The researchers found an increase in carbohydrates and decrease in short-chain fatty acids, indicating a decrease in carbohydrate fermentation [64]. In a murine model it was found that antibiotic treatment transiently increases succinate and C. difficile upregulates a metabolic pathway to convert succinate to butyrate [65]. In a study with 75 CDI participants and 40 healthy controls, the CDI microbiome displayed a significant reduction in butyrate-producing C2–C4 anaerobic fermenters [66]. Additional metabolites, including butyrate and succinate, appear to be associated with CDI, and FMT may reestablish normal proportions for resolution.

In vitro experiments with primary bile acids and specific carbohydrates directly indicated that C. difficile utilizes metabolites of the antibiotic-altered microbiome for germination and proliferation [64].

The next direction in FMT research is to determine the specific beneficial groups of organisms and isolate these protective strains for transplantation. One study found both human and mouse fecal matter transplanted into mice with recurrent CDI increased Bacteroidetes groups, which include Bacteroides and Porphyromonadaceae, and Firmicutes groups, which include Clostridiales and Lachnospiraceae [67]. Another study also found key Bacteroidetes species conferred CDI protection through FMT when stool from CDI-resistant mice was transplanted to CDI susceptible mice. Further analysis showed that these species induce the antimicrobial peptide Reg3γ which prevented C. difficile from accessing colonic crypts and the resulting intestinal inflammation and stem cell injury [68]. A compound in development by Seres Therapeutics, SER-262, is a second-generation composition of purified bacterial spores which has been shown to be highly effective for prevention of CDI in mice [69]. The company's first product, SER-109, failed to show a difference in subsequent CDI recurrence when given to patients with recurrent CDI in a phase 2 study [70]. Unlike SER-109, SER-262 is completely synthetic.

Guidelines for Use of FMT in CDI

The only US FMT guidelines available are from the Fecal Microbiota Transplantation Workgroup [71]. Without stating the basis for their recommendations, the authors suggest consideration of FMT for patients with refractory or recurrent CDI, moderate CDI that did not respond to treatment after 1 week, and severe CDI that didn't respond to treatment after 48 h. The workgroup cautions performing FMT in immunocompromised patients and does not recommend specific criteria for stool donors other than exclusions (see Table 16.1), citing a lack of data [71]. European guidelines strongly recommend FMT only for multiple recurrences [72].

The lack of standard protocol for screening of FMT donors raises the concern of uncontrolled transmission of known infections and unknown ramifications from an altered microbiota. The Fecal Microbiota Transplantation Workgroup has put forth proposed donor qualifications shown in Table 16.1. The workgroup recommends a questionnaire and then serum and stool testing. Serum tests should screen for HIV, hepatitis A virus, hepatitis B virus, hepatitis C virus, and syphilis, and stool should be screen for typical enteric pathogens, *C. difficile* toxin, Giardia antigens, *Cryptosporidium* antigens, *Helicobacter pylori* antigens, helminths, ova, and parasites [71].

Purified Culture as Treatment for or for Prevention of *C. difficile*

FMT may shift into administration of purified intestinal stool cultures, also known as "human probiotic" or "synthetic stool" which could prevent the "ick factor" of traditional stool infusions and reduce concerns of disease transmission. In 1989, Tvede and Rask-Madsen reported that a cocktail of ten facultative aerobes and anaerobes was effective against recurrent CDI in five patients [73]. Petrof et al. tested the effect of purified intestinal bacterial cultures, which they called "RePOOPulate," containing 33 strains from a healthy

Table 16.1 Fecal microbiota transplantation workgroup proposed FMT donor for CDI characteristics

Absolute contraindications	Human immunodeficiency virus (HIV); hepatitis B or C infections; exposure to HIV or viral hepatitis within the previous 12 months; high-risk sexual behaviors; use of illicit drugs; tattoos or body piercing performed within 6 months; incarceration or history of incarceration; current communicable disease (e.g., upper respiratory tract infection); risk factors for variant Creutzfeldt–Jakob disease; travel within the last 6 months to areas high risk of traveler's diarrhea; history of inflammatory bowel disease, irritable bowel syndrome, and other functional diseases; history of gastrointestinal malignancy or known polyposis; use of antibiotics within the preceding 3 months, immunosuppressant, chemotherapeutic drugs; and recent consumption of a potential allergen for the recipient
Relative contraindications	History of major gastrointestinal surgery; metabolic syndrome, autoimmune diseases, atopic diseases, and chronic pain syndromes

stool donor for recurrent CDI. Two patients with CDI who failed at least three antibiotic courses received the stool substitute via colonoscopy. Both patients experienced resolution of diarrhea in 2–3 days and remained without symptoms for 6 months. Additionally, the patients' microbiota compositions following the procedure resembled the stool substitute, as is seen in traditional FMT [74].

Although it has been established that a healthy intestinal microbiome provides resistance to CDI that is disrupted by antibiotic use, the specific elements of the microbiome responsible for this protection remain unknown. Buffie et al. sought to determine the specific bacterial changes within the intestine that provide resistance to CDI [75]. Mice were administered different antibiotics, which created varied disturbances in the microbial communities and in turn varied vulnerability to CDI. The researchers then correlated the microbial changes to the acquisition of CDI. They found that individual species were responsible for CDI prevention rather than a community structure and identified 11 bacterial operation taxonomic units (OTUs) associated with CDI prevention, the greatest association being with *Clostridium scindens*. The study continued with a human population of 24 allo-HSCT patients, 12 of whom were diagnosed with CDI, and the remaining 12 were *C. difficile* carriers without infection. The bacteria that exhibited protection against CDI in the human cohort were then compared to those in the murine cohort, and two OTU associated with resistance to CDI were shared in both groups, with the strongest again being *C. scindens*. To determine whether this correlation was causal, the researchers adoptively transferred a four-bacteria consortium associated with *C. difficile* inhibition, *C. scindens* alone, or vehicle (PBS). Adoptive transfer of the consortium or of *C. scindens* alone ameliorated CDI, associated weight loss and mortality, while adoptive transfer of the other three bacterial isolates individually did not have a substantial impact on resistance to CDI. Using a bile-acid sequestrant, the researchers determined that the bile-acid production was the mechanism of *C. scindens* CDI protection [75].

Reeves et al. had determined that after a cocktail of five antibiotics and *C. difficile* challenge, mice with mild CDI were primarily colonized with bacteria from the family *Lachnospitacea*, whereas moribund mice had a predominance of *E. coli* [76]. Reeves et al. then analyzed the effect of *Lachnospitacea* and CDI in germ-free mice [76] by precolonizing a cohort with *Lachnospitacea* before *C. difficile* challenge. These precolonized mice had significantly decreased *C. difficile* colonization, toxin levels, and disease, compared to mice that were not precolonized or that were precolonized with *E. coli*, and only 20% mortality compared to 100% in the *E. coli* precolonized mice. Further study of the *Lachnospitacea* family may result in greater knowledge of the mechanisms of CDI resistance as well as mechanisms for prevention and treatment [76].

Conclusions

Research on treatment and prevention of *C. difficile* infection through the manipulation of the microbiome likely has a promising future that could take many different paths.

Further study is required, with larger trials to elucidate the many contradictions and questions that remain. Studies testing specific probiotic strains under controlled conditions should resolve conflicting results regarding which probiotic strains are protective against primary and secondary CDI in which patients and which strains might be useful as adjunctive therapy for treatment of disease. Data are needed to determine if different modes of delivery of probiotics, FMT, or purified culture have greater efficacy, in all or certain patient types. Research on safety should be conducted in probiotic, FMT, and purified culture studies to determine if benefits outweigh the risks in vulnerable patients. Lastly, clear protocols will be needed to ensure standardized, safe treatment for patients undergoing microbiome manipulation for *C. difficile*.

References

1. Lucado J, Gould C, Elixhauser A. Clostridium difficile infections (CDI) in hospital stays, 2009. HCUP. 2012.
2. Gerding DN, LF. The epidemiology of Clostridium difficile infection inside and outside health care institutions. Infect Dis Clin N Am. 2015;29(1):37–50.
3. CDC Press Releases. CDC. n.d.. http://www.cdc.gov/media/releases/2015/p0225-clostridium-difficile.html. Published January 1, 2016. Accessed 4 Mar 2016.
4. Magill SS, Edwards JR, Bamberg W, et al. Multistate point-prevalence survey of health care–associated infections. N Engl J Med. 2014;370:1198–208.
5. Johnson S. Recurrent Clostridium difficile infection: causality and therapeutic approaches. Int J Antimicrob Agents. 2009;33:S33–6.
6. Barbut F. How to eradicate Clostridium difficile from the environment. J Hosp Infect. 2015;89(4):287–96.
7. Sethi AK, Al-Nassir WN, Nerandzic MM, Bobulsky GS, Donskey CJ. Persistence of skin contamination and environmental shedding of Clostridium difficile during and after treatment of *C. difficile* infection. Infect Control Hosp Epidemiol. 2010;31(1):21–7.
8. Rebmann T, Carrico RM, Association for Professionals in Infection Control and Epidemiology. Preventing Clostridium difficile infections: an executive summary of the association for professionals in infection control and epidemiology's elimination guide. Am J Infect Control. 2011;39(3):239–42.
9. Roberts K, Smith CF, Snelling AM, et al. Aerial dissemination of Clostridium difficile spores. BMC Infect Dis. 2008;8:7.
10. Rupnik M, Wilcox MH, Gerding DN. Clostridium difficile infection: new developments in epidemiology and pathogenesis. Nat Rev Microbiol. 2009;29(1):37–50.
11. Guinane CM, Cotter PD. Role of the gut microbiota in health and chronic gastrointestinal disease: understanding a hidden metabolic organ. Therap Adv Gastroenterol. 2013;6(4):295–308.
12. Sekirov I, Russell SL, Antunes LC, Finlay BB. Gut microbiota in health and disease. Physiol Rev. 2010;90(3):859–904.
13. Human Microbiome Project Consortium. Structure, function and diversity of the healthy human microbiome. Nature. 2012;486(7402):207–14.
14. Bäckhed F, Fraser CM, Ringel Y, et al. Defining a healthy human gut microbiome: current concepts, future directions, and clinical applications. Cell Host Microbe. 2014;12(5):611–22.
15. Britton RA, Young VB. Role of the intestinal microbiota in resistance to colonization by Clostridium difficile. Gastroenterology. 2014;146(6):1547–53.
16. Brandt LJ. Fecal transplantation for the treatment of Clostridium difficile infection. Gastroenterol Hepatol. 2012;8(3):191–4.
17. Theriot CM, Young VB. Interactions between the gastrointestinal microbiome and Clostridium difficile. Annu Rev Microbiol. 2015;69:445–61.
18. Schubert AM, Sinani H, Schloss PD. Antibiotic-induced alterations of the murine gut microbiota and subsequent effects on colonization resistance against Clostridium difficile. MBio. 2015;6:4.
19. Skraban J, Dzeroski S, Zenko B, et al. Gut microbiota patterns associated with colonization of different Clostridium difficile ribotypes. PLoS One. 2013;8(2):e58005.
20. Crow JR, Davis SL, Chaykosky DM, Smith TT, Smith JM. Probiotics and fecal microbiota transplant for primary and secondary prevention of Clostridium difficile infection. Pharmacotherapy. 2015;35(11):1016–25.
21. Allen SJ. The potential of probiotics to prevent Clostridium difficile infection. Infect Dis Clin N Am. 2015;29(1):135–44.
22. Hickson M, D'Souza AL, Muthu N, et al. Use of probiotic lactobacillus preparation to prevent diarrhoea associated with antibiotics: randomised double blind placebo controlled trial. BMJ. 2007;335:80–3.
23. Gao XW, Mubasher M, Fang CY, Reifer C, Miller LE. Dose-response efficacy of a proprietary probiotic formula of lactobacillus acidophilus CL1285 and lactobacillus casei LBC80R for antibiotic-associated diarrhea and Clostridium difficile-associated diarrhea prophylaxis in adult patients. Am J Gastroenterol. 2010;105(7):1636–41.
24. Rafiq R. Prevention of Clostridium difficile (*C. difficile*) diarrhea with probiotic in hospitalized patients treated with antibiotics. Gastroenterology. 2007;132:A187.
25. Allen SJ, Wareham K, Wang D, et al. Lactobacilli and bifidobacteria in the prevention of antibiotic-associated diarrhoea and *Clostridium difficile* diarrhoea in older inpatients (PLACIDE): a randomised, double-blind, placebo-controlled, multicentre trial. Lancet. 2013;382(9900):1249–57.
26. McFarland LV. Probiotics for the primary and secondary prevention of *C. difficile* infections: a meta-analysis and systematic review. Antibiotics. 2015;4:160–78.
27. Beausoleil M, Fortier N, Guénette S, et al. Effect of a fermented milk combining *lactobacillus acidophilus* CL1285 and *lactobacillus casei* in the prevention of antibiotic-associated diarrhea: a randomized, double-blind, placebo-controlled trial. Can J Gastroenterol. 2007;21(11):732–6.
28. Goldenberg JZ, Ma SS, Saxton JD, et al. Probiotics for the prevention of Clostridium difficile associated diarrhea in adults and children. Cochrane Database Syst Rev. 2013;5:1–150.
29. Lau CSM, CR. Probiotics are effective at preventing Clostridium difficile-associated diarrhea: a systematic review and meta-analysis. Int J Gen Med. 2016;9:27–37.
30. Kwok CS, Arthur AK, Anibueze CI, Singh S, Cavallazzi R, Loke YK. Risk of Clostridium difficile infection with acid suppressing drugs and antibiotics: meta-analysis. Am J Gastroenterol. 2012;107(7):1011–9.
31. Cohen SH, Gerding DN, Johnson S, et al. Clinical practice guidelines for Clostridium difficile infection in adults: 2010 update by the Society for Healthcare Epidemiology of America (SHEA) and the Infectious Diseases Society of America (IDSA). Infect Control Hosp Epidemiol. 2010;31(5):431–55.
32. Surawicz CM, Brandt LJ, Binion DG, et al. Guidelines for diagnosis, treatment, and prevention of Clostridium difficile infections. Am J Gastroenterol. 2013;108(4):478–4.

33. Ghantoji SS, Sail K, Lairson DR, DuPont HL, Garey KW. Economic healthcare costs of Clostridium difficile infection: a systematic review. J Hosp Infect. 2010;74(4):309–18.

34. McFarland LV, Surawicz CM, Greenberg RN, et al. A randomized placebo-controlled trial of saccharomyces boulardii in combination with standard antibiotics for Clostridium difficile disease. JAMA. 1994;271(24):1913–8.

35. Surawicz CM, McFarland LV, Greenberg RN, et al. The search for a better treatment for recurrent Clostridium difficile disease: use of high-dose vancomycin combined with saccharomyces boulardii. Clin Infect Dis 2000. 2000;31(4):1012–7.

36. McFarland LV. Meta-analysis of probiotics for the prevention of antibiotic associated diarrhea and the treatment of Clostridium difficile disease. Am J Gastroenterol. 2006;101(4):812–22.

37. Dendukuri N, Costa V, McGregor M, Brophy JM. Probiotic therapy for the prevention and treatment of Clostridium difficile-associated diarrhea: a systematic review. CMAJ. 2005;173(2):167–70.

38. Pillai A, Nelson R. Probiotics for treatment of Clostridium difficile-associated colitis in adults. Cochrane Database Syst Rev. 2008;23(1):CD004611.

39. Schoster A, Kokotovic B, Permin A, Pedersen PD, Dal Bello F, Guardabassi L. In vitro inhibition of Clostridium difficile and clostridium perfringens by commercial probiotic strains. Anaerobe. 2013;20:36.

40. Barker A, Duster M, Valentine S, Archbald-Pannone L, Guerrant R, Safdar N. Probiotics for Clostridium difficile infection in adults (PICO): study protocol for a double-blind, randomized controlled trial. Contemp Clin Trials. 2015;44:26–32.

41. Auclair J, Frappier M, Millette M. Lactobacillus acidophilus CL1285, lactobacillus casei LBC80R, and lactobacillus rhamnosus CLR2 (bio-K+): characterization, manufacture, mechanisms of action, and quality control of a specific probiotic combination for primary prevention of Clostridium difficile infection. CID. 2015:S135–43.

42. Roberfroid M. Prebiotics: the concept revisited. J Nutr. 2007;137(3):830S–7S.

43. Vyas U, Ranganathan N. Probiotics, prebiotics, and synbiotics: Gut and beyond. Gastroenterol Res Prac. 2012.

44. de Vrese M, Schrezenmeir J. Probiotics, prebiotics, and synbiotics. Adv Biochem Eng Biotechnol. 2008;111:1–66.

45. Rineh A, Kelso MJ, Vatansever F, Tegos GP, Hamblin MR. Clostridium difficile infection: molecular pathogenesis and novel therapeutics. Expert Rev Anti-Infect Ther. 2014;12(1):131–50.

46. Cammarota G, Ianiro G, Gasbarrini A. Fecal microbiota transplantation for the treatment of Clostridium difficile infection: a systematic review. J Clin Gastroenterol. 2014;48(8):693–702.

47. Grehan MJ, Borody TJ, Leis SM, Campbell J, Mitchell H, Wettstein A. Durable alteration of the colonic microbiota by the administration of donor fecal flora. J Clin Gastroenterol. 2010;44(8):551–61.

48. Van Nood E, Vrieze A, Nieuwdorp M, et al. Duodenal infusion of donor feces for recurrent Clostridium difficile. N Engl J Med. 2013;368:407–15.

49. Shankar V, Hamilton MJ, Khoruts A, et al. Species and genus level resolution analysis of gut microbiota in Clostridium difficile patients following fecal microbiota transplantation. Microbiome. 2014;13(2).

50. Kassam Z, Lee CH, Yuan Y, Hunt RH. Fecal microbiota transplantation for Clostridium difficile infection: systematic review and meta-analysis. Am J Gastroenterol. 2013;108(4):500–8.

51. Bakken JS, Polgreen PM, Beekmann SE, Susan E, Riedo FX, Streit JA. Treatment approaches including fecal microbiota transplantation for recurrent Clostridium difficile infection (RCDI) among infectious disease physicians. Anaerobe 2013; 24:20–4.

52. Youngster I, Russell GH, Pindar C, Ziv-Baran T, Sauk J, Hohmann EL. Oral, capsulized, frozen fecal microbiota trans-

plantation for relapsing Clostridium difficile infection. JAMA. 2014;312(17):1772–8.

53. Burns DA, Heap JT, Minton NP. Clostridium difficile spore germination: an update. Res Microbiol. 2010;161(9):730–4.

54. Damman CJ, Miller SI, Surawicz CZ, Zisman TL. The microbiome and inflammatory bowel disease: is there a therapeutic role for fecal microbiota transplantation? Am J Gastroenterol. 2012;107(10):1452–9.

55. Gough E, Shaikh H, Manges AR. Systematic review of intestinal microbiota transplantation (fecal bacteriotherapy) for recurrent Clostridium difficile infection. Clin Infect Dis. 2011;53(10):994–1002.

56. Jangi S, Lamont JT. Asymptomatic colonization by Clostridium difficile in infants: implications for disease in later life. J Pediatr Gastroenterol Nutr. 2010;51(1):2–7.

57. Khanna S, Pardi DS, Kelly CR, et al. A novel microbiome therapeutic increases gut microbial diversity and prevents recurrent Clostridium difficile infection. JID. 2016;214:173–81.

58. Pierog A, Mencin A, Reilly NR. Fecal microbiota transplantation in children with recurrent Clostridium difficile infection. Pediatr Infect Dis J. 2014;33(11):1198–200.

59. Walia R, Garg S, Song Y, et al. Efficacy of fecal microbiota transplantation in 2 children with recurrent Clostridium difficile infection and its impact on their growth and gut microbiome. J Pediatr Gastroenterol Nutr. 2014;59(5):565–70.

60. Di Bella S, Gouliouris T, Petrosillo N. Fecal microbiota transplantation (FMT) for Clostridium difficile infection: focus on immunocompromised patients. J Infect Chemother. 2015;21(4):230–7.

61. Rubin MR, Bilezikian JP, Birken S, et al. Human chorionic gonadotropin measurements in parathyroid carcinoma. Eur J Endocrinol. 2008;159(4):469–74.

62. Weingarden AR, Dosa PI, DeWinter E, et al. Changes in colonic bile acid composition following fecal microbiota transplantation are sufficient to control Clostridium difficile germination and growth. PLoS One. 2016;11(1).

63. Howerton A, Patra M, Abel-Santos E. A new strategy for the prevention of Clostridium difficile infection. J Infect Dis. 2013;207(10):1498–504.

64. Theriot CM, Koenigsknecht MJ, Carlson PE Jr, et al. Antibiotic-induced shifts in the mouse gut microbiome and metabolome increase susceptibility to Clostridium difficile infection. Nat Commun. 2014;5:3114.

65. Ferreyra JA, Wu KJ, Hryckowian AJ, Bouley DM, Weimer BC, Sonnenburg JL. Gut microbiota-produced succinate promotes *C. difficile* infection after antibiotic treatment or motility disturbance. Cell Host Microbe. 2014;16(6):770–7.

66. Antharam VC, Li EC, Ishmael A, et al. Intestinal dysbiosis and depletion of butyrogenic bacteria in Clostridium difficile infection and nosocomial diarrhea. J Clin Microbiol. 2013;51(9):2884–92.

67. Seekatz AM, Young VB. *Clostridium difficile* and the microbiota. J Clin Invest. 2014;124(10):4182–48.

68. Bangar H. Intestinal stem cell injury caused by Clostridium difficile is averted by Bacteroidales-induced crypt defenses. 2015.

69. Wortman JR, Lachey J, Lombardo M-J, et al. Design and evaluation of SER-262: a fermentation-derived microbiome therapeutic for the prevention of recurrence in patients with primary Clostridium difficile infection. Cambridge, MA: Seres Therapeutics; 2016.

70. Mullard A. Leading microbiome-based therapeutic falters in phase II trial. Nat Rev Drug Discov. 2016;15(595).

71. Bakken JS, Borody T, Brandt LJ, et al. Perspective: treating Clostridium difficile infection with fecal microbiota. Clin Gastroenterol Hepatol. 2011;9:1044–9. doi:10.1016/j.cgh.2011.08.014.

72. Debast SB, Bauer MP, Kuijper EJ. European society of clinical microbiology and infectious diseases: update of the treatment

guidance document for Clostridium difficile infection. Clin Microbiol Infect. 2014;20:1–26.

73. Tvede M, Rask-Madsen J. Bacteriotherapy for chronic relapsing Clostridium difficile diarrhoea in six patients. Lancet. 1989;8648(1):1156–60.

74. Petrof EO, Gloor GB, Vanner SJ, et al. Stool substitute transplant therapy for the eradication of Clostridium difficile infection: 'RePOOPulating' the gut. Microbiome. 2013;1(1).

75. Buffie CG, Bucci V, Stein RR, et al. Precision microbiome restoration of bile acid-mediated resistance to Clostridium difficile. Nature. 2015;517(7533):205–8.

76. Reeves AE, Koenigsknecht MJ, Bergin IL, Young VB. Suppression of Clostridium difficile in the gastrointestinal tracts of germfree mice inoculated with a murine isolate from the family lachnospiraceae. Infect Immun. 2012;80(11):3786–94.

Air Contamination in the Hospital Environment

Luis A. Shimose, Eriko Masuda, Ana Berbel Caban,
and Luisa Silvia Munoz-Price

Introduction

Air is postulated to be a mode of transmission for multiple infectious organisms. The importance of air in the transmission of infectious processes has always interested the medical community; this is well exemplified by the use of the terms "miasma" or "malaria" in which "bad air" was thought to be responsible for the origin of many diseases [1]. This phenomenon has been extensively studied in diseases caused by organisms such as *Mycobacterium tuberculosis*, *Aspergillus* species, and respiratory viruses, among others [2].

Nowadays, in the era of multidrug-resistant organisms, there is a clear relationship between environmental contamination and nosocomial infections; nonetheless, there is still an unanswered question of whether or not air plays a role in the horizontal transmission of such infections, contributing to the development of outbreaks in this setting [3, 4]. Air has also been implicated as a possible vector in the spread of different mechanisms of resistance between organisms [1, 4].

Furthermore, in recent years, there has been an increase interest to better understand the close relationship between the different components of hospital environment, including indoor air [4]. This phenomenon is owe to a dramatic increase in infections caused by multidrug-resistant organisms that are acquired during hospital admissions, and also due to the increasing number of potentially susceptible population such as transplant or oncological patients, resulting in increased morbidity and mortality [5].

So far, there is no standardization regarding the indications for air sampling in the hospital setting, what method should be used, and how to interpret the results in order to put them into practice from an infection control point of view [5]. This review aims to summarize the existing data on and controversies related to air contamination within the healthcare system.

General Principles

Biological aerosol is defined as a collection, either naturally or artificially created, of biological particles that are diffused in the air or in another gaseous phase [2, 6–8]. Based on this principle, microorganisms can be found in the air in two forms. The first one is a conglomeration that includes microorganisms, small dust particles, and water or body fluid droplets, forming the so-called nuclei droplets [2, 6, 7, 9]. This corresponds to the mode of transmission of airborne pathogens such as *M. tuberculosis* [10, 11]. The second form is an aggregate of microorganisms associated with dry particles, either from body sources (e.g., skin, fecal patina) or fomites [2, 9]. This is the suspected mechanism implicated in the spread of healthcare-associated pathogens, such as methicillin-resistant *Staphylococcus aureus* (MRSA) and carbapenem-resistant gram-negative bacteria [2, 9, 11].

The size of airborne microbial particles contained within biological aerosols varies greatly from 2 μm up to 100 μm [2, 12]. The larger particles will settle very fast, being deposited over the floor or other horizontal surfaces, and will not travel more than couple of meters from their site of origin [12]. In

L.A. Shimose
Critical Care Medicine, Cleveland Clinic, Cleveland, OH, USA
e-mail: lshimose@gmail.com

E. Masuda
Internal Medicine, LAC+USC Medical Center,
Los Angeles, CA, USA
e-mail: emasuda10@gmail.com

A.B. Caban
Department of Internal Medicine, University of Miami Hospital/
Jackson Memorial Hospital, Miami, FL, USA
e-mail: aberbe01@gmail.com

L.S. Munoz-Price (✉)
Department of Medicine-Division of Infectious Diseases, Froedtert
and the Medical College of Wisconsin, Froedtert Hospital,
9200 W Wisconsin Ave, Milwaukee, WI 53226, USA
e-mail: smunozprice@mcw.edu

© Springer International Publishing AG 2018
G. Bearman et al. (eds.), *Infection Prevention*, DOI 10.1007/978-3-319-60980-5_17

contrast, smaller particles could evaporate to form droplet nuclei, which could contain pathogenic organisms [2]. These small particles will settle very slowly. It has been described that a 2 um droplet nucleus could take up to 4 h to fall a distance of 2 m [12]. Given this long suspension time, these particles can be carried long distances by air currents and thus be distributed widely throughout a hospital [2]. For this reason, the behavior of some forms of biological aerosol is influenced greatly by the ventilation conditions within each room [12].

Another important factor contributing to the ability of biological aerosols to cause environmental contamination, and later on development of nosocomial infections, is the intrinsic characteristics of the organisms themselves. Some bacteria are not designed to be aerosolized, finding the air to be a hostile environment where they are subject to desiccation, nutrient deprivation, and damaged by radiation, oxygen, and free radicals [3]. Other bacteria will form spores when aerosolized, allowing them to survive for extended period of times; such is the case for the *Clostridium* and *Bacillus* species [3, 6]. Some gram-positive bacteria have also been described to survive desiccation for prolong periods of times, such is the case of *S. aureus* [13]. On the other hand, gram-negative bacteria are thought to survive for shorter periods when aerosolized [14]. There are few exceptions to this, as in the case of *Acinetobacter* spp. and *Pseudomonas* species [15, 16].

Thus, the effect of biological aerosols will depend greatly on the characteristic of the environment where they were formed and released and its biological composition including the ability of the organisms to survive free in the environment.

Indications for Sampling Air in the Hospital Setting

There are several potential indications for air sampling in the hospital setting [2, 5, 7]. Epidemiological investigation of nosocomial infections and outbreaks is one of such indications. While the acquisition of most nosocomial infections is associated with direct person-to-person contact leading to cross-contamination of the hospital surfaces, and hence the use of contact precautions with gowns and gloves implemented around patients colonized or infected with multidrug-resistant organism such as MRSA, the possible role of airborne transmission of nosocomial infections is also under consideration [17]. This observation arises in cases in which the degree of contamination of the hospital environment is much heavier and more extensive than expected, implying the presence of a different mechanism [18]. Airborne transmission is thought to be responsible for as much as 10% of nosocomial infections including MRSA, *Acinetobacter*, and *Aspergillus* spp. [12]. In fact, orthopedic prosthetic joint infection rates correlate with the number of airborne bacteria within 30 cm of the surgical wounds [19]. Furthermore, air filtration through HEPA filters

has been shown to reduce the rate of invasive pulmonary aspergillosis in immune-compromised patients [20]. When evaluating air contamination in the setting of clinical infections, it is imperative that the aerosolized isolate is identical to the patient's isolate and that the degree of air contamination is clinically significant [5].

Even in the absence of outbreaks, air sampling can be used for research purposes. When patients are colonized with MRSA, it is standard practice to implement contact precaution with gowns and gloves [21]. However, recent studies demonstrated aerial dispersal of MRSA from patients infected or colonized with this organism, proposing the use of masks around such patients [22]. Further research is necessary to determine its clinical significance [13]. Consequently, studying the aerial dissemination patterns of microorganisms can help elucidate the appropriate level of infection precautions (contact, droplet, airborne) that should be exercised, which in turn will lead to containment of such infections.

Culturing air samples can be used to identify hazardous procedures and confirm resolution of the problem after necessary changes are implemented. Certain healthcare equipments like the ultrasonic cleaners used for disinfection of surgical equipment release bioaerosols into the environment [23]. Air sampling can be used to assess the quantity of released microbes and determine the efficacy of repair [9]. Similarly, in the setting of bioterrorism, air sampling can be used to detect presence of hazardous agents and confirm successful removal after appropriate cleansing [24].

Finally, air sampling can act as quality measures in infection control to ensure proper system function. Maintaining properly installed HVAC filters by preventing air leakages and dust overloads is fundamental to controlling infections [25, 26]. One can inspect air samples around the filters during periodic filter inspections and also after filter manipulation (i.e., repair, cleaning) to ensure proper operation. What is more, hospital renovations and construction projects are very common in the world of ever-expanding healthcare. Surveillance of airborne environmental disease during these times is imperative for patient safety [25].

Blindly obtaining air samples without an objective is discouraged due to the ambiguous clinical significance of the result [11]. For instance, in order to investigate the continued *Aspergillus* contamination of tissue culture in a research laboratory, air samples were used to determine that a contaminated filter of the incubator was the culprit [9]. Such as this, there should always be a purpose and an intention to act on the results obtained.

Air Sampling Methods

The method chosen to sample air will depend on various factors, including the purpose for which air sampling is being performed, the type of organism being studied, the expertise or preferences of the investigator, and the resources available for such task. Ideally, all of the points mentioned above should be fulfilled when selecting a method.

Methods used for sampling air can be classified into two categories: passive and active methods [27]. The passive methods are based on sedimentation, whereas the active ones use more complex devices such as air impactors, centrifugal air machines, or filtration systems [9].

Passive Methods for Sampling Air

Passive air sampling is performed using settle plates, relying on gravity to deposit biological particles containing bacteria, into a culture plate [9, 27]. The average particle size encountered in the hospital setting is of approximately 13 μm [9]. It has been described that an agar plate of 100 mm in diameter could potentially collect particles from 1 ft³ of air in approximately 15 min at a sedimentation speed of 0.46 cm/s [9, 27, 28].

The main advantages of settle plates include being an easy method to use, affordable (especially important in poor-resources settings), and readily available [27]. Also the results obtained with this method are considered reproducible and reliable, in contrast to active sampling methods, mainly because settle plates directly measure bacterial sedimentation on horizontal surfaces, rather than suspended biological particles in the air, where it would be difficult to predict where and when they would sediment [29, 30].

The main limitation of the passive method is that it provides a qualitative result of air contamination, which might weakly correlate with the real degree of contamination of the environment being tested [1, 27]. Also this method is easily influenced by airflow present in the vicinity of the plate, making the results vary depending on the location of the plate [9]. It can be insensitive in cases in which the bacterial load is low [27, 31, 32]. Passive methods also require longer periods of sampling compared to the active methods, of at least 1 h [27]. There have been reports in which settle plates have been left open for periods equal or longer than 24 h, making the plates dry upon collection [31, 32]. In this instance, it has been described that swabbing the plates with a premoistened Q-tip and later transfer into liquid media could increase chances of recovering organisms [31–33].

Active Methods for Sampling Air

These devices forces airflow directly onto the surface of culture media [6]. The standard measurement of air contamination with these methods is based on the number of CFU per cubic meter of air suctioned (CFU/m³) [27]. This is based on the principle that each particle that impacts the culture media

will form a colony [6, 7]. There are several different types of devices that belong to this category (Table 17.1).

Several studies have been done comparing the different devices for active air sampling. The majority of these studies showed that there is a great variability of the results when using them, even at the same place and same time, making it difficult to determine a superior device among the others [7, 27, 34–38].

The main benefit of active air sampling is the proposed higher sensitivity to detect air contamination [7, 27, 38]. As mentioned earlier, this method provides more detailed and specific results including the volume of air suctioned during their use and the numbers of colonies in each plate, expressed as CFU/m³ of air sampled [7, 27, 34–37]. Some specific air impactors could also provide an exact time in which air contamination occurred, allowing the investigator to correlate those findings with activities happening inside the patients rooms [18, 39].

There are many drawbacks with the use of these devices. They are expensive and its use is time-consuming. Machines are noisy, thus making it difficult to use for prolong periods of time in occupied rooms [38]. They are also difficult to sterilize, fact that could give false-positive results due to prior contamination of the device [27]. There is one major limitation with these methods, that is, the limited sample size of air being tested, probably requiring multiple cycles of sampling to obtain a representative indoor air sample [27]. Also, it is believed that the growth of some of the organisms could be inhibited by the impact into the culture media [6, 33, 38, 40]. It has also been reported that the sampling time also affects greatly the successful recovery of bacteria from air, finding that prolong periods of sampling could potentially inhibit growth of susceptible bacteria or could cause bacteria to bounce out of the culture media into the environment [6, 41].

Active or Passive Air Sampling?

Comparisons between active and passive methods for air sampling have shown mixed results. There are some reports that conclude that there is correlation between both methods for detecting air contamination [7, 28]. One study concluded that in instances in which the level of air contamination was low, there was a discrepancy between both methods, probably due to the relative low sensitivity of settle plates when compared with air impactors [7].

Given the differences between active sampling methods with each other, the mixed results obtained when comparing active versus passive methods, and the lack of standardization, it is difficult to determine which type of method is superior among the others. Factors that can affect the results when comparing methods for sampling air include the levels of contamination in the environment, the type of airflow in the room being tested, and the different activities happening inside the room [7].

Table 17.1 Different types of the most common commercially available air samplers

Impactors:	*Slit type*
These are the most commonly used active sampling methods. Air is drawn into a sampling head by a pump or fan into a solid media, via narrow slit (slit samplers) or perforated plate (sieve samplers). The velocity of the air is determined by the width of the slit in slit samplers and the diameter of the holes in sieve samplers. When air hits the surface of the media plate, it makes a tangential change of direction, and any suspended particles are thrown out by inertia, impacting onto the agar plate. After incubating the plate, counting the number of visible colonies gives a direct quantitative estimate of the number of colony-forming units in the sampled air	Casella single slit and four slit sampler
	Mattson-Garvin air sampler
	New Brunswick STA air sampler
	Bourdillon sampler
	BIAP slit sampler
	Reyniers slit sampler
	Sieve type
	Andersen 2-, 6-, and 8-stage sampler
	Ross-Microban sieve air sampler
	Personal particulate aerosol collector
	Surface Air System (SAS) system
	Joubert 3-stage biocollector
Impingers:	All-glass impinger 30 and pre-impinger
Impingers use a liquid media for particle collection. Sampled air is drawn by a suction pump through a narrow inlet tube into a small flask containing the collection media. When the air hits the surface of the liquid, it changes direction abruptly, and any suspended particles are impinged into the collection liquid. Once the sampling is complete, the collected liquid can be cultured to enumerate viable microorganisms. Since the sample volume can be calculated using the flow rate and sampling time, the result is quantitative	Midget impinger with personal air sampler
	May 3-stage glass impinger
	Folin bubbler
	Cyclone sampler
Filtration samplers:	Millipore membrane filtered monitor
In this method, air is drawn by a pump or vacuum through a membrane filter. The filter medium may be a polycarbonate or cellulose acetate, which can be incubated directly by transferring onto the surface of an agar medium, or gelatine, which can be dissolved and analyzed by regular culture methods	Gelman membrane filter air sampler
	MSF 37 monitor
	Sartorius MD8 air sampler
Centrifugal samplers:	Rotary centrifugal air sampler (RCS)
In this method, air is forced by an impeller drum concentrically into the surface of a culture media. After collecting the sample, the agar media is incubated and the colonies counted. Because this method draws a precise amount of air per minute, the detected number of colonies can be calculated per unit volume of air	Well sampler

The ideal method for sampling air should be easy to use, should not be expensive in order to be widely available, should be able to detect all aerosolized biological particles present, should provide a quantitative result that strongly correlates with the real degree of contamination of the environment, should minimize the amount of nonviable organisms in the culture media, and should provide an specific time in which air contamination occurred [9].

Gram-Positive Organisms

Classically, it has been thought that gram-positive bacteria, such as *Staphylococcus aureus*, are the dominant type of bacteria contaminating the indoor air of hospitals as described in several reports [42, 43].

Methicillin-Resistant *Staphylococcus aureus*

MRSA was first reported in 1962 in the British Medical Journal, which at that time was named "Celbenin"-resistant staphylococci [13, 44]. Currently, it is recognized as a major hospital-acquired pathogen in community hospitals, long-term care facilities, and tertiary care hospitals [45]. This pathogen has become endemic in hospitals worldwide, presenting a major concern in hospital hygiene [46], especially, since studies have shown that *S. aureus* has the potential to survive for long periods and is resistant to desiccation [47]. It has been documented that the primary route of transmission is via the hands of healthcare workers and that colonized or infected patients are the primary reservoirs [47]. That being said, handwashing is widely recognized as the single most important factor for preventing subsequent colonization and infection [48]. Conversely, MRSA has been recovered from many sites, including floors, linen, medical equipment, and furniture; therefore, transmission via inanimate environments that may also play an important role, however, remains uncertain [45].

The role of environmental contamination and transmission of MRSA has been studied for many years now. As early as in 1960, Colbeck described one human experiment, which was made with a woolen threat and dried for 10 days. In this experiment, a superficial scratch was made on the skin and the woolen thread was rubbed on the linear scratch. After 3 days, there was definite abscess formation, as well as edema and axillary adenitis [49]. Although there is no evidence demonstrating the direct transmission through MRSA from the environment to patients, there is evidence that contamination of the environment with MRSA is sufficient to contaminate the gloves of HCW's and, thus, leading to transmission to patients [47].

More recently, Hardy et al. from the University of Birmingham in the UK conducted a study aimed to examine the presence of MRSA in the environment and its relationship to the patients' acquisition of MRSA [47]. This prospective study was conducted in a 9-bed ICU for 14 months, and at every environmental screening, samples were obtained from the four sites in each bed space, these being underneath the bed, workstation, control buttons on the monitors, and a ledge positioned behind the bed. Results demonstrated that MRSA was isolated from the environment at every environmental screening, when both small and large numbers of patients were colonized. In only 20 (37.5%) of 56 occasions were the strains isolated from the patient and the strains isolated from their immediate environment indistinguishable. However, there was a strong evidence to suggest that 3 of 26 patients who acquired MRSA while in the intensive care unit acquired MRSA from the environment [47]. These observations show the magnitude of the spread of the organism within the hospital environment and provide evidence that there is another mechanism, such as air, involved in the spread of MRSA besides direct person-to-person contact.

Another study performed by Huang et al. examined the duration of survival of two strains of MRSA on three types of hospital fomites. Results demonstrated MRSA survived for 11 days on plastic patient chart, more than 12 days on a laminated tabletop, and 9 days on a cloth curtain [50]. The fact that MRSA can survive in dry conditions at room temperatures for the periods demonstrated by this study suggests air and environmental contamination may be an important and an overlooked reservoir of the MRSA through which noncolonized patients can acquire the organism.

Airborne transmission of MRSA is generally considered to occur at lower frequency than transmission via direct contact, but MRSA in the form of bioaerosol can contaminate air and cause airborne infection [45]. In a study conducted in Japan by Shiomori et al., the number of airborne MRSA before, during, and after bed making was investigated with an Andersen air samples in the rooms of 13 inpatients with either MRSA infection or colonization. MRSA-containing particles isolated were 2–3 μm in diameter before bed making and >5 μm during bed making. The number was significantly higher 15 min after bed making suggesting that MRSA was recirculated in the air, especially after movement [45]. Another study conducted by Wilson et al. at the Nepean Hospital ICU in New South Wales studied air sampling at six locations three times weekly over a period of 32 weeks in a new, initially MRSA-free ICU to examine if this organism

was found in air samples and whether its presence was affected by the number of MRSA-colonized patients present. A significant correlation was found between the daily numbers of MRSA-colonized or MRSA-infected patients in the unit and the daily number of MRSA positive air sample cultures obtained [51]. However, airborne transmission from patients colonized with MRSA warrants further investigation, not only in terms of improving infection control recommendations for patients but also for the indication and use of personal protective devices by healthcare workers [13].

Vancomycin-Resistant Enterococci

The two most common human pathogens within the *Enterococcus* family are *E. faecalis* and *E. faecium*. They are well known to cause different infections including wound infections, urinary tract infections, and bacteremias, most commonly in the healthcare setting [52, 53]. It is estimated that 30% of the enterococci infections caused by these organisms are due to vancomycin-resistant strains [52].

The role of environmental contamination with VRE has been studied and described in the literature as an important contributor to the spread of these organisms within hospitals [54]. The importance of air contamination and its implications from the infection control point of view have not been established, and the evidence is scant or almost not existing. A study performed in a hospital in London looked into the spread of enterococci into the environment from patients that were either colonized or infected with these organisms [53]. They incorporated air sampling as part of the investigation, using a MAS Eco air sampler for 10-min periods [53]. Air and environmental samples were taken twice per week for a total length of 17 weeks and were obtained from a combined medical and surgical ward that consisted of single occupancy rooms and also common bays with four beds each. Air samples were positive during this surveillance, and more than 80% of the positive air samples belongedVancomycin-resistant enterococci (VRE) to a single unrecognized carrier that was taking laxatives during the surveillance period when increased rates of air contamination were observed. Molecular typing was performed by PFGE and confirmed clonality between the patient and air isolates [53].

It is thought that aerosolization of enterococci poses little direct risk for patients, but contributes greatly to environmental contamination, which has been shown to increase the risk of inpatients to acquire these pathogens [55].

Clostridium difficile

Clostridium difficile is a spore-forming gram-positive bacterium. In recent years, the emergence of an epidemic strain of

C. difficile known as North American pulsed-field gel electrophoresis type NAP1 – polymerase chain reaction type 027 – has been associated with large outbreaks mainly in the USA, Canada, and Europe [56, 57]. As mentioned before, given its ability to form spores, *C. difficile* can survive for several months or even years in hospital surfaces when shedded in the stools, not only from infected patients but also from asymptomatic carriers [58–60]. It has been reported that up 15% of patients that are asymptomatic could be carriers of toxigenic strains of *C. difficile*, fact that poses an enormous challenge from the infection control point of view in order to control outbreaks due to this organism [60].

The role of environmental contamination in the spread of spores contributing to outbreaks has been studied [58]. The possibility of aerosolization of *C. difficile* spores has been studied in the past decades with no apparent success. In 1981, a study conducted by Fekety and colleagues looked into possible air contamination with spores of this organism [59]. Air samples were obtained with a slit impactor, but the sampling time was not reported. In this study, all of the air samples were negative for *C. difficile* [59]. One strong reason to believe why air could contribute to the spread of this organism is the extensive contamination of surfaces seen not only inside the rooms of infected patients but also in other common areas in the hospital [56, 57].

It has not been until recent years that the possible implication of the aerial route in the spread of *C. difficile* was demonstrated [58]. The first report of aerosolization of *C. difficile* into the environment is from 2008 when Roberts and colleagues used a portable cyclone air sampler in a geriatric ward housing patients with confirmed *C. difficile* infection (CDI) [61]. The air sampler was used for 15-min periods at 30-min intervals for two consecutive days. Air was blown into an enriched liquid media specially designed by the investigators to isolate the organism of interest [61]. In this surveillance, 23 out of 32 air samples were positive with the bacterium, and molecular typing showed isolates were indistinguishable from each other [61].

Best et al. looked into concomitant contamination of air and environmental surfaces with *C. difficile* [18]. Here, air samples were obtained using an AirTrace Environmental sampler that rotates the plate constantly over 360° allowing to determine the exact time in which air contamination happened during the surveillance period [18]. The air sampling was separated into three different periods [18]. The first one was performed for 1-h sampling time, which yielded only 12% of positive air samples. The second one was performed in patients with suspected CDI but not yet confirmed diagnosis, for 10-h period each time. One air sample was positive in a patient prior to confirming the diagnosis of *C. difficile*, which could suggest that the shedding of the spores happens on patients before being placed on contact precautions [18]. The final air sampling period was performed also for 10 h,

but this phase was done on patients with confirmed *C. difficile* colitis. Among the latter, air samples were positive in seven out of the ten patients studied. Molecular typing was performed showing that the air, environmental, and clinical isolates were related to each other [18]. Increased rates of air contamination were associated with activities happening inside the rooms such as bed changing or medical rounds [18].

Subsequently, the same investigators evaluated the influence of toilets after flushing in the degree of air contamination with *C. difficile* [62]. For this experiment, both settle plates and an AirTrace Environmental sampler were used. Experiments were performed using preparation with fecal suspension from patients with confirmed CDI [62]. Spores were found in the air after flushing the toilets and remained in the air for up to 90 min. Positive settle plates were obtained when toilets were flushed only with the lid open, but no air contamination was found on settle plates when the lids were closed [62].

Gram-Negative Organisms

Acinetobacter baumannii

Carbapenem-resistant *A. baumannii* has become an important nosocomial pathogen in recent years given the limited therapeutic options available to treat this organism [52, 63]. In 2013, the Center for Disease Control and Prevention estimated that multidrug-resistant *A. baumannii* causes more than 7,000 infections and leads to more than 500 deaths per year solely in the USA [52]. These numbers have increased in the following years. Certainly, this pathogen has become endemic in several hospitals around the globe [64–67]. An important characteristic of *A. baumannii* is its ability to survive desiccation for prolonged periods of time, making the hospital environment a major reservoir for this organism [63, 66, 68, 69]. For this reason, air has been postulated to be a possible vector contributing to environmental contamination.

There have been several reports in the literature describing outbreak investigations due to *Acinetobacter* species in which air samples were obtained. The first one is from 1987, when Gerner-Smidt and colleagues found positive air samples with *A. calcoaceticus* serovar *anitratus* during a 2-year outbreak in a Danish ICU [68]. Here, air samples were obtained using a slit sampler and settle plates that were left open for 3–6-h periods [68]. In the same year, an outbreak investigation caused by *A. anitratus* in two hospitals in the UK reported positive *Acinetobacter* samples from air. Air sampling was performed using settle plates placed 3 m from the patients, obtaining 16 positive samples with *Acinetobacter* spp. from a total of 82 settle plates used [69]. The time for which plates were left open was not reported [69]. A study from 1989 conducted in the Netherlands found *Acinetobacter* in the air using slit samplers in 12 out of 104 (11%) samples, but these isolates did not match with the epidemic strain when molecular testing was performed [70]. A report from a hospital in Turkey from 2006 described an epidemiological investigation of all *A. baumannii* isolates found at that institution [67]. Molecular testing was performed and found that there were various genotypes that were endemic during the surveillance period. Some of the isolates analyzed were obtained from the air using an air impactor [67]. One study from Argentina published in 2008 aimed to evaluate the prevalence of multidrug-resistant *A. baumannii* [71]. Air samples were obtained as part of their surveillance project using three different methods that included settle plates, an air impactor, and a liquid impinge [71]. In this study, *A. baumannii* was found only on 4 samples out of 54 total air samples; all of them were obtained by the air impactor [71].

More recently, a group from the University of Miami looked into aerosolization of carbapenem-resistant *A. baumannii* in a single ICU in a teaching hospital in Florida where this organism is endemic and where patient-to-patient transmission was observed [72]. Air samples were obtained in three different days in rooms occupied by *A. baumannii*-positive patients. Air was sampled using open blood agar plates left open for 24 h. It was found that 23% of air samples were positive with *A. baumannii* [72]. PFGE was performed to the clinical and air isolates, proving clonality [72]. Later on, the same group evaluated presence of *A. baumannii* in consecutive days among inpatients colonized with this organism in either the rectum or respiratory tract [31]. Samples were collected daily for up to 10 days using settle plates. Air samples were positive for *A. baumannii* in 21% of the instances [31]. Interestingly on this study, patients with rectal colonization contaminated more their ambient air compared to patients colonized in the respiratory tract (26% and 11%, respectively; *p* = 0.01). Rep-PCR demonstrated clonality of the isolates [31]. In another study from the same institution, air and environmental samples were obtained concomitantly among inpatients admitted in adult ICUs [32]. This study confirmed the prior results, showing higher degree of air contamination in patients with rectal colonization with *A. baumannii* compared to patients with respiratory colonization (38% and 13% respectively; *p* = 0.0001). In this study, it was also evaluated if the type of ICU (single occupancy rooms versus open layout ICU) where patients were admitted to played a role in the results. There was no difference between the two types of ICU with regard to the degree of air contamination, but there was a higher degree of clonality by PFGE between air and patient's isolates in the single occupancy ICUs [32].

Contradictory data exists in regard to the presence of *A. baumannii* in the air. In a study published by a group from the University of Maryland, only 1 out of 12 air samples belonging to rooms occupied by *A. baumannii*-positive patients was positive for this organism [73]. This study used an air impactor as the sampling method, for a testing period of 1 h [73]. Another study from Thailand also evaluated the presence of air contamination in ICUs housing closed-circuit mechanical ventilated *A. baumannii*-positive patients. Their air sampling technique consisted of placing two settle plates next to each patient twice per week. None of the air samples were positive for *A. baumannii* [73].

There are several hypotheses regarding the presence or not of *A. baumannii* in the air that we can take from the aforementioned studies. We could imply that closed-circuit ventilation could prevent the bacteria to aerosolized in the air or maybe that the rectum is a more prolific spreader of *A. baumannii* and other bacteria in general into the air and the environment. The difference in the ventilation systems among different hospitals could also explain the difference in findings [74]. The overall body of evidence favors the fact that air plays an important role in the horizontal transmission among inpatients with this organism.

Pseudomonas aeruginosa

P. aeruginosa is a common pathogen associated with hospital-acquired infections including pneumonias, bloodstream infections, urinary tract infections, and surgical site infections, among others [52]. Nearly 8% of all healthcare-associated infections are caused by *P. aeruginosa* and that 13% of these infections are caused by multidrug-resistant strains leading to increased morbidity and mortality among inpatients [52].

Patients with cystic fibrosis (CF) comprise a special population since they tend to have chronic and recurrent respiratory infections with multiple organisms, most commonly due to *P. aeruginosa* [75–77]. These patients are exposed frequently to multiple classes of antibiotics, being more prone to acquired resistant strains [75–77]. Once patients with CF acquired this organism, it is almost impossible to eradicate it from their airways, making them of special interest from the infection control point of view [76, 77]. Given this phenomenon, they can contribute to aerosolization of such organisms into the environment [75]. It has been described that *Pseudomonas* can survive desiccation for up to 5 days when released in sputum, making this an important characteristic that could contribute to contamination of the environment and potentially leading to horizontal transmission among inpatients [75].

The presence of *P. aeruginosa* in the air has been described in the literature. The main body of evidence is based on studies among patients with CF. In 1983, a study performed in Denmark in a CF clinic aimed to determine the prevalence of environmental contamination with this organism [75]. Here, environmental and air samples were taken as part of the investigation from both the CF clinic and from other areas of the hospital that served as the control group. Air was cultured using both settle plates and a centrifugal air sampler. Settle plates were left open for 2-h periods. The air samples obtained from the clinic were all positive for *P. aeruginosa*, compared to none in the control group [75]. In another study from 2005 in a CF center in the UK, it also evaluated the presence of an endemic strain of *P. aeruginosa* in the air as part of a surveillance study [78]. Air samples were collected using a slit sampler for 15-min sampling time. The endemic strain was detected in 80% of the air samples taken from inside the patient's rooms and in 60% from samples taken in the corridors of the ward [78]. Interestingly, the presence of the organism was not detected after terminal cleaning, highlighting the importance of cleaning in the prevention of environmental contamination [78].

The use of air humidifiers for respiratory therapy among inpatients has also been shown to produce high degree of air contamination with *P. aeruginosa* [79]. In a study from 1970 performed by Grieble et al., it showed that the presence of this organism in the air correlated with the use of these instruments [79]. Air sampling was performed by using settle plates that were placed randomly inside the rooms. The degree of air contamination decreased after thorough disinfection with phenolic acid, but it did not halted the presence of *Pseudomonas* in the air in the following days [79].

Klebsiella-Producing Carbapenemase (KPC)-Producing Gram-Negative Rods

KPCs are plasmid-mediated enzymes belonging to the Ambler class A of beta-lactamases [80, 81]. They were first described in a *Klebsiella pneumoniae* isolate in 1996 [82]. In recent years, it has spread to many other gram-negative bacteria, thus making them of special concern from the infection control point of view due to high morbidity and mortality associated with these pathogens when infection develops given the limited therapeutic options available [83–87].

Certainly, KPC-producing organisms have become endemic in multiple hospitals around the world [83]. The implementation of bundles to decrease the incidence of infections due to these organisms has served as a proof that hospital environment serves as a reservoir for them [88]. It has also been proposed that air contamination – leading to later environmental contamination – is involved in the horizontal transmission of these organisms.

There is scant data regarding air contamination with KPC organisms. Munoz-Price et al. evaluated concomitant air and surface contamination in patients that were either colonized or infected with KPC-producing organisms [89]. Most of the

isolates studied in this project were *K. pneumoniae* as the organism harboring this enzyme, but also *E. coli*, *Enterobacter aerogenes*, and *Citrobacter freundii* were present [89]. Patients were either colonized in the rectum or respiratory tract or had positive clinical cultures. Air was sampled using settle plates located close to the head of the bed of the patients [89]. KPC organisms were detected in the air, but there was no difference in the degree of air contamination between the three groups [89].

Conclusions

The role of air in the spread of healthcare-associated organisms has been revised here with different degrees of evidence. Sampling the air in patient care areas is still controversial, even during outbreaks.

Air sampling is not routinely done in the hospital setting, and the results obtained will depend mainly on the indication for performing such task, the resources available in each hospital, the circumstances in which it will be performed, and the intrinsic characteristics of the pathogen being studied. Less importance should be given to the method used, whether it is a passive or an active method, since there is no clear evidence demonstrating which method is superior among others, and results obtained can be similar with either of them, especially if the points mentioned above are taken into consideration.

There is no doubt that contamination of the hospital environment with nosocomial pathogens is a crucial step for the development of horizontal transmission with such organisms among inpatients. In instances where the degree of contamination is much greater than expected, it might be logical to think of air as a possible "vector" as demonstrated by the evidence displayed in this chapter.

References

1. Humphreys H. Microbes in the air – when to count! The role of air sampling in hospitals. J Med Microbiol. 1992;37(2):81–2.
2. Beggs CB. The airborne transmission of infection in hospital buildings: fact or fiction? Indoor Built Environ. 2003;12(1):9–18.
3. Greene VW, et al. Microbiological contamination of hospital air. I. Qualitative studies. Appl Microbiol. 1962;10(6):567–71.
4. Bernard MC, et al. Air contamination around patients colonized with multidrug-resistant organisms. Infect Control Hosp Epidemiol. 2012;33(9):949–51.
5. Li CS, et al. Bioaerosol characteristics in hospital clean rooms. Sci Total Environ. 2003;305(1–3):169–76.
6. Lacey J, et al. Bioaerosols and occupational lung disease. J Aerosol Sci. 1994;25(8):1371–404.
7. Griffiths WD, et al. The assessment of bioaerosols: a critical review. J Aerosol Sci. 1994;25(8):1425–58.
8. Douwes J, et al. Bioaerosol health effects and exposure assessment: progress and prospects. Ann Occup Hyg. 2003;47(3):187–200.

9. Gröschel DH. Air sampling in hospitals. Ann N Y Acad Sci. 1980;353:230–40.

10. Escombe AR, et al. The detection of airborne transmission of tuberculosis from HIV-infected patients, using an in vivo air sampling model. Clin Infect Dis. 2007;44(10):1349–57.

11. Eickhoff TC. Airborne nosocomial infection: a contemporary perspective. Infect Control Hosp Epidemiol. 2016;11(4):849–67.

12. Beggs C. The use of engineering measures to control airborne pathogens in hospital buildings. J Chem Inf Model. 2013;53(9):1689–99.

13. Gehanno J, et al. Aerial dispersal of methicillin-resistant Staphylococcus aureus in hospital rooms by infected or colonised patients. J Hosp Infect. 2009;71(3):256–62.

14. Heidelberg JF, et al. Effect of aerosolization on culturability and viability of gram-negative bacteria. Appl Environ Microbiol. 1997;63(9):3585–8.

15. Blessing-Moore J, et al. Mucosal droplet spread of Pseudomonas aeruginosa from cough of patients with cystic fibrosis. Proc Br Thorac Soc. 1982;8:778–92.

16. Jawad A, et al. Influence of relative humidity and suspending menstrua on survival of Acinetobacter spp. on dry surfaces. Influence of relative humidity and suspending menstrua on survival of Acinetobacter spp. on dry surfaces. J Clin Microbiol. 1996;34(12):2881.

17. Napoli C, et al. Air sampling procedures to evaluate microbial contamination: a comparison between active and passive methods in operating theatres. BMC Public Health. 2012;12:594.

18. Best EL, et al. The potential for airborne dispersal of Clostridium difficile from symptomatic patients. Clin Infect Dis. 2010;50(11):1450–7.

19. Gosden PE, et al. Importance of air quality and related factors in the prevention of infection in orthopaedic implant surgery. J Hosp Infect. 1998;39(3):173–80.

20. Oren I, et al. Invasive pulmonary aspergillosis in neutropenic patients during hospital construction: before and after chemoprophylaxis and institution of HEPA filters. Am J Hematol. 2001;66(4):257–62.

21. Centers for Disease Control and Prevention. Precautions to prevent the spread of MRSA in healthcare settings 2007. Atlanta: Centers for Disease Control and Prevention; 2007. http://www.cdc.gov/hicpac/pdf/isolation/Isolation2007.pdf

22. Sherertz RJ, et al. A cloud adult: the Staphylococcus aureus-virus interaction revisited. Ann Intern Med. 1996;124(6):539–47.

23. Singh S, et al. Hospital infection control guidelines: principles and practice. Jaypee Brothers Medical Publishers (P) Ltd.; 2012.

24. McDermott HJ. Air monitoring for toxic exposures. John Wiley & Sons; 2004.

25. Sehulster L, et al. Guidelines for environmental infection control in health-care facilities. Recommendations of CDC and the healthcare infection control practices advisory committee (HICPAC). MMWR Recomm Rep. 2003;52(RR-10):1–42.

26. Ohsaki Y, et al. Undetected bacillus pseudo-outbreak after renovation work in a teaching hospital. J Inf Secur. 2007;54(6):617–22.

27. Pasquarella C, et al. The index of microbial air contamination. J Hosp Infect. 2000;46(4):241–56.

28. Whyte W. Sterility assurance and models for assessing airborne bacterial contamination. J Parenter Sci Technol. 1986;40(5):188–97.

29. Friberg B, et al. Inconsistent correlation between aerobic bacterial surface and air counts in operating rooms with ultra clean laminar air flows: proposal of a new bacteriological standard for surface contamination. J Hosp Infect. 1999;42(4):287–93.

30. Friberg B, et al. Correlation between surface and air counts of particles carrying aerobic bacteria in operating rooms with turbulent ventilation: an experimental study. J Hosp Infect. 1999;42(1):61–8.

31. Shimose LA, et al. Contamination of ambient air with Acinetobacter baumannii on consecutive inpatient days. J Clin Microbiol. 2015;53(7):2346–8.

32. Shimose LA, et al. Carbapenem-resistant Acinetobacter baumannii: concomitant contamination of air and environmental surfaces. Infect Control Hosp Epidemiol. 2016;37(07):777–81.

33. Kingston D. Selective media in air sampling: a review. J Appl Microbiol. 1971;34(1):221–32.

34. Pasquarella C, et al. Air microbial sampling: the state of the art. Ig Sanità Pubblica. 2008;64(1):79–120.

35. Jensen PA, et al. Evaluation of eight bioaerosol samplers challenged with aerosols of free bacteria. Am Ind Hyg Assoc J. 1992;53(10):660–7.

36. Casewell MW, et al. Bacterial air counts obtained with a centrifugal (RCS) sampler and a slit sampler-the influence of aerosols. J Hosp Infect. 1984;5(1):76–82.

37. Nakhla LS, et al. A comparative evaluation of a new centrifugal air sampler (RCS) with a slit air sampler (SAS) in a hospital environment. J Hosp Infect. 1981;2(C):261–6.

38. Mehta SK, et al. Evaluation of portable air samplers for monitoring airborne culturable bacteria. Aihaj. 2000;61(6):850–4.

39. Shimose LA, et al. A comparison of two methods for sampling air: settle plates versus impactor. ID Week 2015 Abstract # 1774. San Diego.

40. Stewart SL, et al. Effect of impact stress on microbial recovery on an agar surface. Appl Environ Microbiol. 1995;61(4):1232–9.

41. Macher JM, et al. Performance criteria for bioaerosol samplers. J Aerosol Sci. 1992;23(SUPPL. 1):647–50.

42. Messi P, et al. Prevalence of multi-drug-resistant (MDR) bacteria in air samples from indoor and outdoor environments. Aerobiologia (Bologna). 2015;31(3):381–7.

43. Huang PY, et al. Airborne and surface-bound microbial contamination in two intensive care units of a medical center in central Taiwan. Aerosol Air Qual Res. 2013;13(3):1060–9.

44. Coia JE, et al. Guidelines for the control and prevention of methicillin-resistant Staphylococcus aureus (MRSA) in healthcare facilities. J Hosp Infect. 2006;63(SUPPL. 1):1–44.

45. Shiomori T, et al. Evaluation of bedmaking-related airborne and surface methicillin-resistant Staphylococcus aureus contamination. J Hosp Infect. 2002;50(1):30–5.

46. Rohr U, et al. Colonization of patients and contamination of the patients' environment by MRSA under conditions of single-room isolation. Int J Hyg Environ Health. 2009;212(2):209–15.

47. Hardy KJ, et al. A study of the relationship between environmental contamination with methicillin-resistant Staphylococcus aureus (MRSA) and patients' acquisition of MRSA. Infect Control Hosp Epidemiol. 2006;27(2):127–32.

48. French GL, et al. Tackling contamination of the hospital environment by methicillin-resistant Staphylococcus aureus (MRSA): a comparison between conventional terminal cleaning and hydrogen peroxide vapour decontamination. J Hosp Infect. 2004;57(1):31–7.

49. Cimolai N. MRSA and the environment: implications for comprehensive control measures. Eur J Clin Microbiol Infect Dis. 2008;27(7):481–93.

50. Huang R, et al. Methicillin-resistant Staphylococcus aureus survival on hospital fomites. Infect Control Hosp Epidemiol. 2012;27(11):1267–9.

51. Wilson RD, et al. The correlation between airborne methicillin-resistant Staphylococcus aureus with the presence of MRSA colonized patients in a general intensive care unit. Anaesth Intensive Care. 2004;32(2):202–9.

52. Centers for Disease Control and Prevention. Antibiotic resistance threats in the United States, 2013. Atlanta: Centers for Disease Control and Prevention; 2013. http://www.cdc.gov/drugresistance/pdf/ar-threats-2013-508.pdf

53. Muzslay M, et al. Dissemination of antibiotic-resistant enterococci within the ward environment: the role of airborne bacteria and the risk posed by unrecognized carriers. Am J Infect Control. 2013;41(1):57–60.

54. Mayer RA, et al. Role of fecal incontinence in contamination of the environment with vancomycin-resistant enterococci. Am J Infect Control. 2003;31(4):221–5.

55. Drees M, et al. Prior environmental contamination increases the risk of acquisition of vancomycin-resistant enterococci. Clin Infect Dis 2008;46(5):678–685.

56. Leffler DA, et al. Clostridium difficile infection. N Engl J Med. 2015;372(16):1539–48.

57. Kelly CP, et al. Clostridium difficile. More difficult than ever. N Engl J Med. 2015;372(16):1539–48.

58. Donskey CJ. Preventing transmission of Clostridium difficile: is the answer blowing in the wind? Clin Infect Dis. 2010;50(11): 1458–61.

59. Fekety R, et al. Epidemiology of antibiotic-associated colitis. Isolation of clostridium difficile from the hospital environment. Am J Med. 1981;70(4):906–8.

60. Alasmari F, et al. Prevalence and risk factors for asymptomatic clostridium difficile carriage. Clin Infect Dis. 2014;59(2):216–22.

61. Roberts K, et al. Aerial dissemination of Clostridium difficile spores. BMC Infect Dis. 2008;8.(February 2006:7.

62. Best EL, et al. Potential for aerosolization of Clostridium difficile after flushing toilets: the role of toilet lids in reducing environmental contamination risk. J Hosp Infect. 2012;80(1):1–5.

63. Munoz-Price LS, et al. Acinetobacter infection. N Engl J Med. 2008;358(12):1271–81.

64. Munoz-Price LS, et al. Control of a two-decade endemic situation with carbapenem-resistant Acinetobacter baumannii: electronic dissemination of a bundle of interventions. Am J Infect Control. 2014;42(5):466–71.

65. Munoz-Price LS, et al. Eighteen years of experience with Acinetobacter baumannii in a tertiary care hospital. Crit Care Med. 2013;41(12):2733–42.

66. Catalano M, et al. Survival of Acinetobacter baumannii on bed rails during an outbreak and during sporadic cases. J Hosp Infect. 1999;42(1):27–35.

67. Akalin H, et al. Epidemiology of Acinetobacter baumannii in a university hospital in Turkey. Infect Control Hosp Epidemiol. 2006;27(4):404–8.

68. Gerner-Smidt P. Endemic occurrence of Acinetobacter calcoaceticus biovar anitratus in an intensive care unit. J Hosp Infect. 1987;10(3):265–72.

69. Allen KD, et al. Hospital outbreak of multi-resistant Acinetobacter anitratus: an airborne mode of spread? J Hosp Infect. 1987;9(2):110–9.

70. Crombach WH, et al. Control of an epidemic spread of a multi-resistant strain of Acinetobacter calcoaceticus in a hospital. Intensive Care Med. 1989;15(3):166–70.

71. Barbolla RE, et al. Molecular epidemiology of Acinetobacter baumannii spread in an adult intensive care unit under an endemic setting. Am J Infect Control. 2008;36(6):444–52.

72. Munoz-Price LS, et al. Aerosolization of Acinetobacter baumannii in a trauma ICU*. Crit Care Med. 2013;41(8):1915–8.

73. Rock C, et al. Infrequent air contamination with Acinetobacter baumannii of air surrounding known colonized or infected patients. Infect Control Hosp Epidemiol. 2015;36(7):830–2.

74. Munoz-Price LS. Acinetobacter in the air: did Maryland get it wrong? Infect Control Hosp Epidemiol. 2015;36(7):833–4.

75. Zimakoff J, et al. Epidemiology of Pseudomonas aeruginosa infection and the role of contamination of the environment in a cystic fibrosis clinic. J Hosp Infect. 1983;4(1):31–40.

76. Hart CA, et al. Persistent and aggressive bacteria in the lungs of cystic fibrosis children. Br Med Bull. 2002;61:81–96.

77. Govan JR, et al. Microbial pathogenesis in cystic fibrosis: mucoid Pseudomonas aeruginosa and Burkholderia cepacia. Microbiol Rev. 1996;60(3):539–74.

78. Panagea S, et al. Environmental contamination with an epidemic strain of Pseudomonas aeruginosa in a Liverpool cystic fibrosis centre, and study of its survival on dry surfaces. J Hosp Infect. 2005;59(2):102–7.

79. Brooks AM, et al. Fine-particle humidifier* source of Pseudomonas aeruginosa infections in a respiratory-disease unit. N Engl J Med. 1970;282(10):531–5.

80. Munoz-Price LS, et al. Clinical epidemiology of the global expansion of Klebsiella pneumoniae carbapenemases. Lancet Infect Dis. 2013;

81. Vasoo S, et al. Emerging issues in gram-negative bacterial resistance: an update for the practicing clinician. Mayo Clin Proc. 2015;

82. Nordmann P, et al. The real threat of Klebsiella pneumoniae carbapenemase-producing bacteria. Lancet Infect Dis. 2009;

83. Munoz-Price LS, et al. Clinical epidemiology of the global expansion of Klebsiella pneumoniae carbapenemases. Lancet Infect Dis. 2015;13(9):785–96.

84. Kim YA, et al. Features of infections due to Klebsiella pneumoniae carbapenemase-producing Escherichia coli: emergence of sequence type 131. Clin Infect Dis. 2012;

85. Ahn C, et al. Microbiological features of KPC-producing Enterobacter isolates identified in a U.S. hospital system. Diagn Microbiol Infect Dis. 2014;80(2):154–8.

86. Falagas ME, et al. Deaths attributable to carbapenem-resistant enterobacteriaceae infections. Emerg Infect Dis. 2014;

87. Fraenkel-Wandel Y, et al. Mortality due to bla KPC Klebsiella pneumoniae bacteraemia. J Antimicrob Chemother. 2015;

88. Munoz-Price LS, et al. Successful eradication of a monoclonal strain of Klebsiella pneumoniae during a K. pneumoniae carbapenemase– producing K. pneumoniae outbreak in a surgical intensive care unit in Miami, Florida. Infect Control Hosp Epidemiol. 2010;31(3110):1074–7.

89. Shimose LA, et al. Air and environmental contamination with KPC-producing gram-negative rods. ID Week 2015 Abstract # 1790. San Diego.

Vertical Versus Horizontal Infection Control Interventions

Salma Muhammad Abbas, Michelle Doll, and Michael P. Stevens

Vertical Versus Horizontal Infection Control Interventions

Healthcare-associated infections (HAIs) are often preventable diseases that are not only a major concern for patient safety but also represent a major economic burden on a nation's healthcare system [1, 2]. These include, but are not limited to, surgical site infections (SSIs), central line-associated bloodstream infections (CLABSIs), catheter-associated urinary tract infections (CAUTIs), ventilator-associated pneumonias (VAPs), and bloodstream infections (BSIs) caused by multidrug-resistant organisms (MDROs) such as methicillin-resistant *Staphylococcus aureus* (MRSA), vancomycin-resistant *Enterococcus* (VRE), carbapenem-resistant *Enterobacteriaceae* (CRE), and carbapenem-resistant *Acinetobacter baumannii* (CRAB) [3, 4]. Reducing the spread of these organisms has been an area of major focus in the realm of infection control, and numerous strategies such as implementation of hand hygiene, contact precautions, and chlorhexidine bathing have been implemented to achieve this. Some of these target specific microorganisms and are called "vertical" strategies, while others aim to reduce infections caused by multiple pathogens simultaneously and are known as "horizontal" strategies (see Fig. 18.1) [5].

S.M. Abbas (✉) • M. Doll
Department of Internal Medicine, Virginia Commonwealth University, 1000 E Marshall Street, Suite 205, Richmond, VA 23298, USA
e-mail: salma.abbas@vcuhealth.org; michelle.doll@vcuhealth.org

M.P. Stevens
Department of Internal Medicine, Division of Infectious Diseases, Virginia Commonwealth University Medical Center, 1300 East Marshall Street, North Hospital, 2nd Floor, Room 2-100, P.O. Box 980019, Richmond, VA 23298, USA

Infectious Diseases/Epidemiology, Virginia Commonwealth University Health System, Richmond, VA, USA
e-mail: michael.stevens@vcuhealth.org

Compare and Contrast Vertical and Horizontal Strategies

Patients are at risk for being exposed to organisms such as MRSA, VRE, and CRE during hospital admissions and can become colonized with them. They may go on to develop infections with these organisms or transmit them to other patients. A vertical strategy targets patients colonized or infected with a specific microorganism and aims to decrease the number of infections caused by this single pathogen. On the contrary, the horizontal approach is a more holistic strategy adopted to reduce infections caused by all microorganisms sharing a common means of transmission. As a result, the horizontal approach is generally a utilitarian strategy, while the vertical strategy supports exceptionalism by prioritizing the eradication of some pathogens [5]. Resource utilization for vertical strategies typically surpasses horizontal strategies. Horizontal strategies are more patient-centric, in so much that patients benefit from prevention of all infections simultaneously, not just those caused by specific microorganisms. In addition, vertical strategies are short term as efforts are made to prevent the spread of infections caused by a specific pathogen at a given point in time, while horizontal strategies, by virtue of their larger scale, are not only relevant to a hospital's current situation but may play a greater role in the long-term prevention of infections as well. Finally, both types differ in the types of infection-prevention approaches used: examples of vertical programs include active surveillance for MRSA and vaccination against specific pathogens, whereas those for horizontal strategies encompass measures such as implementation of hand hygiene, bathing patients with antiseptics such a chlorhexidine gluconate (CHG), antimicrobial stewardship, and environmental disinfection to name a few [5]. Both strategies have been used to prevent infections, and many studies have been conducted to determine their effectiveness (see Table 18.1).

© Springer International Publishing AG 2018
G. Bearman et al. (eds.), *Infection Prevention*, DOI 10.1007/978-3-319-60980-5_18

Fig. 18.1 Vertical vs.
horizontal infection
prevention strategies [5]

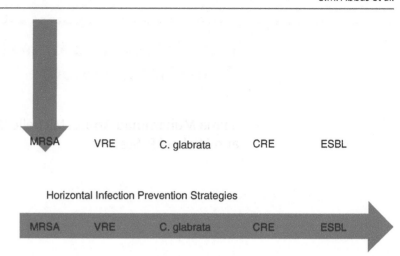

Table 18.1 Vertical vs. horizontal infection control strategies [5]

	Horizontal	Vertical
Focus	Population based	Pathogen based
Population	Universal	Selective or universal
Resource costs	Relatively low	Usually high
Philosophy	Utilitarian	Exceptionalism
Values favored	Patient	Hospital, infection prevention experts
Temporal focus	Present, future	Present

Evidence for Vertical Infection Control Strategies

Vertical strategies are mostly based on the results of active surveillance and testing (AST), a strategy aimed at reducing colonization of various anatomic sites by pathogens and thereby reducing infection and transmission of these by identifying carriers. This approach has been most widely implemented for the eradication of MRSA, VRE, and CRE, and numerous studies have been conducted to elucidate the effects of AST with or without additional decolonization measures [6, 7].

Methicillin-Resistant *Staphylococcus aureus*

Overall, the incidence of MRSA infections has increased significantly since its emergence in the 1960s. Additionally, due to the virulence of community-acquired MRSA strains and their growing contribution to HAIs, MRSA identification and eradication has been identified as an important infection control strategy [8]. Intensive care units (ICUs) are considered high-risk settings for the transmission of MDROs such as MRSA, and multiple studies have been conducted to determine the impact of infection prevention strategies on the incidence of HAIs in these units. Huskins and colleagues conducted a cluster-randomized trial in adult ICUs to evalu-

ate the effect of active surveillance and isolation for MRSA and VRE compared with standard practice. During a 6-month study period, 5,434 admissions to ten ICUs were assigned to the intervention arm, and 3705 admissions to eight ICUs were assigned to the control arm. The results of this study did not demonstrate any benefit of AST and isolation for infection prevention as the difference in the mean incidence of MRSA and VRE colonization and infection-related events per 1000-patient days between the two groups was not statistically significant (40.4 ± 3.3 and 35.6 ± 3.7 in the intervention and control groups, respectively, $P = 0.35$) [9]. Similarly, a comparative effectiveness review performed by Glick and colleagues found insufficient evidence for the use of targeted MRSA screening as a sole infection prevention strategy [10]. Zafar and colleagues conducted a prospective observational study to assess the prevalence of nasal colonization among patients with community-associated MRSA infection admitted to a 600-bed urban academic center between 2004 and 2006. A total of 51 patients underwent nasal swab cultures, and only 41% were found to have nasal colonization with MRSA. The results of this study demonstrate that MRSA infections may occur in a high percentage of patients without nasal MRSA carriage which argues against the utility of vertical infection prevention strategies given their narrow focus [11]. Moreover, MRSA screening does not have an impact on other organisms such as VRE and CRE (as opposed to many horizontal infection control strategies that impact multiple organisms simultaneously) [8].

Given the widespread use of mupirocin for MRSA decolonization, emerging resistance is an area of major concern. Mupirocin is a protein synthesis inhibitor which acts by inhibiting bacterial isoleucyl-tRNA synthetase. *S. aureus* strains may harbor alterations in the isoleucyl-tRNA synthetase *ileS* gene which confers low-level resistance (MIC = 8–256 μ(micro)g/ml) or *mupA* gene which is associated with high-level resistance (MIC ≥ 512 μ(micro)g/ml) [12]. Fritz and colleagues conducted a study to determine the prevalence of high-level mupirocin resistance among 1089 pediatric patients admitted with skin and soft tissue infections. Cultures were obtained from the axillae, anterior nares, and inguinal folds, and 483 patients were found to be colonized with *S. aureus*. Of these, 23 isolates (2.1%) carried the *mupA* gene. A total of 408 patients, including four patients colonized with *S. aureus* harboring a *mupA* gene, underwent nasal decolonization with twice-daily application of mupirocin for 5 days (with or without antimicrobial baths), and 258 underwent daily CHG bathing for 5 days. Patients were followed with colonization cultures for up to 12 months. Among the patients carrying mupirocin-resistant *S. aureus*, 100% remained colonized at 1 month compared to 44% of the patients who were carriers of mupirocin-sensitive *S. aureus* ($P = 0.041$) [12].

Carbapenem-Resistant Enterobacteriaceae and *Acinetobacter baumannii*

Carbapenems are an important antimicrobial class given their activity against gram-negative organisms with Amp-C-mediated β(beta)-lactamases or extended-spectrum β(beta)-lactamases (ESBLs) [13]. Selection of carbapenem-tolerant *Enterobacteriaceae* was uncommon in the United States in the 1990s, prior to the recognition of novel β(beta)-lactamases with carbapenem-hydrolyzing activity. *Klebsiella pneumoniae* carbapenemase (KPC) is the most commonly identified carbapenemase in the United States. Others such as the metallo-β(beta)-lactamases are more common in other parts of the world. The Centers for Disease Control and Prevention (CDC) currently recommends point-prevalence surveys to identify CRE carriers in units where infections caused by these organisms have been identified over the past 6–12 months. The recommendations to prevent their transmission include implementation of hand hygiene, contact precautions, and testing contacts of CRE patients. Infection prevention personnel should be promptly notified regarding the detection of CRE, and additional measures such as skin decolonization may be employed if felt necessary [14].

CRE is a major challenge given the frequency of infections caused by these organisms as well as the associated mortality which may be as high as 50% among ICU patients [15]. Patel and colleagues conducted two matched case-control studies to determine the epidemiology of CRE infections and determine risk factors and clinical outcomes associated with infections secondary to carbapenem-resistant isolates among 99 patients when compared with a similar number of patients with infections caused by carbapenem-susceptible organisms. It was concluded that infections caused by KPC producers were associated with a longer duration of mechanical ventilation ($P = 0.04$), exposure to antimicrobials (cephalosporins, $P = 0.02$; carbapenems, $P < 0.001$), and higher mortality due to infection (38% vs. 12%, $P < 0.001$) [15]. Measures such as chlorhexidine

gluconate (CHG) bathing for skin antisepsis have also been studied in addition to standard precautions to prevent the spread of resistant gram-negative organisms. Chung and colleagues carried out an interrupted time series study to determine the effect of daily CHG bathing on carbapenem-resistant *Acinetobacter baumannii* acquisition in a medical ICU. A 12-month CHG bathing period was compared with a 14-month control period. A reduction of 51.8% was observed in CRAB acquisition rates following the introduction of CHG bathing (44.0 vs. 21.2 cases/1000 at-risk patient-days, $P < 0.001$) [16].

In addition to the inpatient setting, CRE infections are an emerging threat in long-term acute-care hospitals (LTACHs) where patients are at high risk for acquisition and transmission of these organisms. Moreover, the residents of these facilities can also introduce CRE into hospitals during admissions. In a study conducted in four LTACHs, a stepped-wedge design was used to assess the effect of a bundled intervention (screening patients for KPC rectal colonization, contact isolation, daily CHG bathing for all patients, and healthcare worker education and compliance monitoring). A total of 3894 patients from the preintervention period were compared to 2951 patients admitted after the introduction of the intervention bundle. With this strategy, the incidence rate of KPC colonization demonstrated a significant decline in the intervention arm (4 vs. 2 acquisitions per 100 patient-weeks; $P = 0.004$) [17].

Vancomycin-Resistant Enterococcus

VRE have been recognized as a cause of HAIs since the 1980s and are implicated in about 20,000 infections in the United States annually [18]. Guidelines for VRE prevention have been in place for over two decades. Recommendations include surveillance testing, contact precautions, hand hygiene, and limiting the use of vancomycin, without a consensus on the best approach [19]. A recent meta-analysis identified hand hygiene as a more effective strategy to prevent VRE infections when compared to contact precautions [20]. Of note, the small number of studies focusing primarily on VRE precluded meta-analysis for surveillance screening and environment decontamination.

Evidence for Horizontal Infection Control Strategies

This approach encompasses the implementation of measures such as hand hygiene, universal decolonization, selective digestive tract decolonization (SDD), antimicrobial stewardship, and environmental decontamination to prevent infections and emergence of MDROs regardless of the colonization status of patients [6].

Hand Hygiene

Hand hygiene has been the cornerstone of infection prevention for over a century and is often considered the most important infection prevention strategy [21]. Transmission of healthcare-associated organisms through contamination of healthcare workers' (HCWs) hands has been well studied and established as an area of major focus. To be transmissible, the organisms must be present on a patient's skin or have contaminated the environment; come in contact with and be transferred to hands of HCWs; survive on their skin for several minutes, with failure to be eradicated due to inadequate hand hygiene; and spread to another patient as a result of direct skin contact. The adherence of HCWs to hand hygiene varies across centers and ranges from 5 to 89% [22]. Hand hygiene is effective at preventing spread of organisms such as MRSA, VRE, and resistant gram-negative organisms. The CDC currently recommends the following five moments for hand hygiene: before patient contact, before performing aseptic procedures, following exposure to body fluids, after contact with patients, and following contact with their surroundings [23]. Strict compliance with hand hygiene may reduce the rates of HAIs by up to 40% [24].

Universal Decolonization

While conventional methods, such as hand hygiene, have been in place for a long time, there has been a recent surge in the use of CHG for universal decolonization with its use being more widespread in ICUs. Multiple studies have been carried out to examine the effect of CHG bathing on the acquisition of MDROs and the incidence of HAIs. Several studies evaluating CHG bathing were published in 2013. Climo and colleagues carried out a multicenter cluster-randomized, nonblinded crossover trial to evaluate the effect of daily CHG bathing for 6 months compared to bathing with nonantimicrobial washcloths in nine intensive care units and bone marrow transplant units. A total of 7727 patients were included in the study. The results showed a significant reduction in overall bloodstream infections (4.78 cases per 1000 patient-days with CHG bathing vs. 6.60 cases per 1000 patient-days with nonantimicrobial cloth; $P = 0.007$) as well as the acquisition of MDROs (5.10 cases per 1000 patient-days with CHG bathing vs. 6.60 cases per 1000 patient-days with nonantimicrobial washcloths; $P = 0.03$) [25]. Huang and colleagues conducted a pragmatic cluster-randomized trial among 74,256 ICU patients randomized to three different strategies: screening and isolation for MRSA, targeted MRSA decolonization, and universal decolonization. The hazard ratios for bloodstream infection with any pathogen

were 0.99, 0.78, and 0.56 among the three groups, respectively ($P < 0.001$), demonstrating a significant reduction in the universal decolonization group [26]. Similarly, a cluster-randomized crossover trial including 4947 pediatric ICU admissions investigated the impact of daily bathing either with CHG or standard practice on infection acquisition during two 6-month study periods. Per-protocol analysis demonstrated a lower incidence of bacteremia among the CHG bathing group when compared with standard practice (3.28 per 1000 days vs. 4.93 per 1000 days; $P = 0.044$) [27]. While the results of these studies were promising, a recent pragmatic cluster-randomized crossover trial did not support daily CHG bathing. A total of 9340 patients admitted to five adult ICUs were included in the study and bathed daily with either CHG or nonantimicrobial cloths for 10 weeks, with a 2-week washout period prior to switching to the alternate bathing treatment for 10 weeks. Intervention with CHG bathing did not lead to a significant reduction in the incidence of HAIs [28]. It is important to note that the overall low rates of HAIs and single-center design of this study may have impacted its results.

With the heightened interest in the use of CHG as a disinfectant in the healthcare setting, emerging resistance has been a concern. CHG resistance is attributed to qacA/B genes among MRSA and qacE genes among Klebsiella species which encode multidrug efflux systems [29, 30]. CHG susceptibility testing is not routinely performed; no breakpoints have been established by the Clinical and Laboratory Standards Institute (CLSI) [30]. In the pediatric study conducted by Fritz and colleagues mentioned above, 10/10891 (0.9%) patients harbored CHG-resistant S. aureus at baseline and two of these underwent daily CHG bathing for 5 days. At 1 month, there was no difference in colonization status among these patients when compared to patients carrying no CHG-resistant microorganisms ($P = 1.0$) [12]. The lack of an appreciable association may be attributed to the low overall prevalence of CHG resistance in the study, however. Continued vigilance for emerging CHG resistance seems warranted.

Selective Digestive Tract Decolonization

SDD is a prophylactic measure to reduce infections caused by Candida, Staphylococcus aureus, and gram-negative organisms among patients with gastrointestinal carriage of these organisms. Protocols vary across centers but can include the following: a short course of parenteral antibiotics such as a third- or fourth-generation cephalosporin, nonabsorbable enteral agents (e.g. polymyxin E, amphotericin B and vancomycin), and oral and rectal surveillance cultures on admission and at 2-week intervals thereafter to monitor the effectiveness of SDD. Although multiple trials have demonstrated its effectiveness in reducing pneumonias and bloodstream infections among critically ill patients, its use remains controversial due to concerns such as the selection of resistant organisms [31]. Reig and colleagues conducted a retrospective observational study to evaluate the efficacy of intestinal decolonization among 45 patients with a history of at least two ESBL *E. coli* infections and persistent intestinal carriage (determined by positive rectal and/or stool cultures). Patients were treated with either low- or high-dose oral colistin or oral rifaximin for 4 weeks. ESBL *E. coli* eradication occurred in 19/45 (42%) patients. The use of single-drug oral regimens for intestinal decolonization is not well established, and additional studies are required to further explore this [32].

Antimicrobial Stewardship

Antimicrobial stewardship programs (ASPs) are considered crucial for combatting the emergence of antimicrobial resistance and can be linked with infection prevention programs. According to the CDC, 20–50% of all antibiotics used in the United States are unnecessary. Antibiotic use is associated with drug reactions, *Clostridium difficile* infections, as well as antibiotic resistance [33]. A bundle approach consisting of staff education, early identification, expanded infection control measures including hand hygiene, and judicious use of antibiotics was introduced at a tertiary care center in the United States to manage high *C. difficile* infection rates (7.2 per 1000 hospital discharges). The rate of *C. difficile* infections fell to 3.0 per 1000 hospital discharges within 6 years (71% reduction, $P < 0.001$) [34].

Environmental Cleaning

Contaminated surfaces such as bedrails, bed surfaces, nurse call buttons, television remotes, and medical equipment have been identified as reservoirs for organisms such as MRSA, VRE, *C. difficile*, *Acinetobacter* species, *Pseudomonas aeruginosa*, and norovirus. Persistence of these organisms in the environment and ineffective environmental cleaning strategies result in transmission of these organisms to other patients [35]. The current CDC recommendations for effective environmental decontamination include assignment of dedicated staff members to clean different units, thorough decontamination of surfaces such as bedrails, charts, and doorknobs along with frequent monitoring of units to assess for adherence to outlined protocols [19].

Financial Considerations

According to a decision tree analysis to compare costs of various MRSA surveillance strategies, universal MRSA screening was deemed more cost intensive compared to targeted surveillance, but interestingly, the latter was more cost-effective than no screening [36]. However, when MRSA surveillance strategies with and without decolonization were compared to other approaches such as universal contact precautions and universal decolonization in a recent cost-effectiveness model using a hypothetical cohort of 10,000 adult ICU patients, universal decolonization was deemed the most cost-effective infection prevention strategy for MRSA colonization prevalence of up to 12%; as this drops from 12 to 5%, AST with selective decolonization may be the more optimal approach, emphasizing the consideration of local factors prior to making decisions regarding the best infection prevention strategy [37]. According to an estimate focusing mainly on infection prevention in the ICU setting and surgical units, interventions such as hand hygiene, contact isolation in the setting of known MDRO infections, or colonization and environmental cleaning led to a net global saving of US $13,179 per month between 2009 and 2014 by reducing HAIs such as central line-associated bloodstream infections, ventilator-associated pneumonias, and surgical site infections [38].

Conclusion

MDROs are a major healthcare concern and along with HAIs have become a major infection prevention focus. Vertical and horizontal infection control strategies have been used to combat HAIs. These strategies include measures such as active surveillance testing, hand hygiene programs, universal skin decolonization with antiseptics such as CHG, and antimicrobial stewardship. Many studies have shown beneficial results with lower rates of HAIs resulting from both vertical and horizontal strategies. However, there is still controversy over which strategies are most optimal in different settings. In terms of HAI prevention, generally horizontal strategies are more likely to have a broader impact and are more cost-effective. For a pathogen such as *Clostridium difficile*, for which direct surveillance is not a current practice, horizontal measures such as compliance with hand hygiene measures, empiric contact precautions for presumptive infectious diarrhea, and antimicrobial stewardship are the only strategies available. While a horizontal approach seems optimal for many situations, adverse effects of horizontal strategies must also be considered. For instance, a theoretical concern is the development of CHG resistance with the wide deployment of CHG bathing. Although vertical strategies have a role in the management of outbreaks of specific pathogens, in general, horizontal strategies have a greater impact at a lower cost.

References

1. Scott DR. 2009. Center for Disease Control and Prevention. The direct medical costs of healthcare-associated infections in US hospitals and the benefits of prevention. Available at: http://www.cdc.gov/HAI/pdfs/hai/Scott_CostPaper.pdf

2. Zimlichman E, Henderson D, Tamir O. Health care–associated infections: a meta-analysis of costs and financial impact on the US Health Care System. JAMA Intern Med. 2013;173(22):2039–46.

3. Centers for Disease Control and Prevention. 2013. National and State Healthcare-Associated Infections Progress Report. Published January 14, 2015. Available at: www.cdc.gov/hai/progress-report/index.html

4. Magill SS, Jonathan RE. Multistate point-prevalence survey of health care–associated infections. N Engl J Med. 2014;370:1198–208.

5. Edmond MB, Wenzel RP. Screening inpatients for MRSA – case closed. N Engl J Med. 2013;368:2314–5.

6. Septimus E, Weinstein RA, Perl TM, Goldmann DA, Yokoe DS. Approaches for preventing healthcare-associated infections: go long or go wide? Infect Control Hosp Epidemiol. 2014;35(7):797–801.

7. Wenzel RP, Edmond MB. Infection control: the case for horizontal rather than vertical interventional programs. Int J Infect Dis. 2010;14(Suppl 4):S3–5.

8. Wenzel RP, Bearman G, Edmond MB. Screening for MRSA: a flawed hospital infection control intervention. Infect Control Hosp Epidemiol. 2008;29(11):1012–8.

9. Huskins WC, Huckabee CM, O'Grady NP, et al. Intervention to reduce transmission of resistant bacteria in intensive care. N Engl J Med. 2011;364:1407–18.

10. Glick SB, Samson DJ, Huang ES, Vats V, Aronson N, Weber SG. Screening for methicillin-resistant *Staphylococcus aureus*: a comparative effectiveness review. Am J Infect Control. 2014;42(2):148–55.

11. Zafar U, Johnson LB, Hanna M, Riederer K, Sharma M, Fakih MG, Thirumoorthi MC, Farjo R, Khatib R. Prevalence of nasal colonization among patients with community-associated methicillin-resistant *Staphylococcus aureus* infection and their household contacts. Infect Control Hosp Epedemiol. 2007;28(8):966–9.

12. Fritz SA, Hogan PG, Camins BC, Ainsworth AJ, Patrick C, Martin MS, Krauss MJ, Rodriguez M, Burnham CD. Mupirocin and chlorhexidine resistance in *Staphylococcus aureus* in patients with community-onset skin and soft tissue infections. Antimicrob Agents Chemother. 2013;57(1):559–68.

13. Gupta N, Limbago BM, Patel JB, Kallen AJ. Carbapenem-resistant Enterobacteriaceae: epidemiology and prevention. Clin Infect Dis. 2011;53(1):60–7.

14. Centers for Disease Control and Prevention. n.d. Available at: http://www.cdc.gov/hai/pdfs/cre/CRE-guidance-508.pdf

15. Patel G, Huprikar S, Factor SH, Jenkins SG, Calfee DP. Outcomes of carbapenem-resistant *Klebsiella pneumoniae* infection and the impact of antimicrobial and adjunctive therapies. Infect Control Hosp Epidemiol. 2008;29:1099–106.

16. Chung YK, Kim JS, Lee SS, Lee JA, Kim HS, Shin KS, Park EY, Kang BS, Lee HJ, Kang HJ. Effect of daily chlorhexidine bathing

17. Hayden MK, Lin MY, Lolans K, Weiner S, Blom D, Moore NM, Fogg L, Henry D, Lyles R, Thurlow C, Sikka M, Hines D, Weinstein RA. Prevention of colonization and infection by *Klebsiella pneumoniae* carbapenemase-producing Enterobacteriaceae in long-term acute-care hospitals. Clin Infect Dis. 2015;60(8):1153–61.

18. Centers for Disease Control and Prevention. n.d. Available at: http://www.cdc.gov/drugresistance/pdf/ar-threats-2013-508.pdf

19. Centers for Disease Control and Prevention. n.d. Available at: http://www.cdc.gov/hicpac/pdf/MDRO/MDROGuideline2006.pdf

20. De Angelis G, Cataldo MA, De Waure C, Venturiello S, La Torre G, Cauda R, Carmeli Y, Tacconelli E. Infection control and prevention measures to reduce the spread of vancomycin-resistant enterococci in hospitalized patients: a systematic review and meta-analysis. De Angelis G1, Cataldo MA, de Waure C, Venturiello S, La Torre G, cauda R, Carmeli Y, Tacconelli E. Author information abstract OBJECTIVES: Vancomycin. J Antimicrob Chemother. 2014;69(5):1185–92.

21. Lankford MG, Zembower TR, Trick WE, Hacek DM, Noskin GA, Lance RP. Influence of role models and hospital design on the hand hygiene of health-care workers. Emerg Infect Dis. 2003;9(2):217–23.

22. The World Health Organization. n.d. Available at: http://www.who.int/gpsc/5may/tools/who_guidelines-handhygiene_summary.pdf

23. Centers for Disease Control and Prevention. n.d. Available at: http://www.cdc.gov/handhygiene/training.html

24. Kampf G, Löffler H, Gastmeier P. Hand hygiene for the prevention of nosocomial infections. Dtsch Arztebl Int. 2009;106(40):649–55.

25. Climo MW, Yokoe DS, Warren DK. Effect of daily chlorhexidine bathing on hospital-acquired infection. N Engl J Med. 2013;368(6):533–42.

26. Huang SS, Septimus E, Kleinman K, et al. For the CDC prevention epicenters program and the AHRQ DECIDE network and healthcare-associated infections program. Targeted versus universal decolonization to prevent ICU infection. N Engl J Med. 2013;368:2255–65.

27. Milstone AM, Elward A, Song X, et al. Daily chlorhexidine bathing to reduce bacteremia in critically ill children: a multi-center, cluster-randomized, two-period crossover trial. Lancet. 2013;381(9872):1099–106.

28. Noto MJ, Domenico HJ, Byrne DW, et al. Chlorhexidine bathing and healthcare-associated infections: a randomized clinical trial. JAMA. 2015;313(4):369–78.

29. Warren DK, Prager M, Munigala S, Wallace MA, Kennedy CR, Bommarito KM, Mazuski JE, Burnham CD. Prevalence of qacA/B genes and mupirocin resistance among methicillin-resistant *Staphylococcus aureus* (MRSA) isolates in the setting of chlorhexidine bathing without mupirocin. Infect Control Hosp Epidemiol. 2016;2:1–8.

30. Vali L, Dashti AA, El-Shazly S, Jadaon MM. *Klebsiella oxytoca* with reduced sensitivity to chlorhexidine isolated from a diabetic foot ulcer. Int J Infect Dis. 2015;34:112–6.

31. Silvestri L, van Saene HKF. Selective decontamination of the digestive tract: an update of the evidence. HSR Proc Intensive Care Cardiovasc Anesth. 2012;4(1):21–9.

32. Rieg S, Küpper MF, Kd W, Serr A, Bohnert JA, Kern VW. Intestinal decolonization of Enterobacteriaceae producing extended-spectrum β-lactamases (ESBL): a retrospective observational study in patients at risk for infection and a brief review of the literature. BMC Infect Dis. 2015;15:475.

33. Centers for Disease Control and Prevention. n.d. Available at: http://www.cdc.gov/getsmart/healthcare/implementation/core-elements.html

34. Muto CA, Blank MK, Marsh JW, Vergis EN, O'Leary MM, Shutt KA, Pasculle AW, Pokrywka M, Garcia JG, Posey K, Roberts TL, Potoski BA, Blank GE, Simmons RL, Veldkamp P, Harrison LH, Paterson DL. Control of an outbreak of infection with the hypervirulent Clostridium difficile BI strain in a university hospital using a comprehensive "bundle" approach. Clin Infect Dis. 2007;45(10):1266–73.

35. Gandra S, Ellison RT. Modern trends in infection control practices in intensive care units. J Intensive Care Med. 2014;29(6):311–26.

36. Tübbicke A, Hübner C, Hübner NO, Wegner C, Kramer A, Fleßa S. Cost comparison of MRSA screening and management – a decision tree analysis. BMC Health Serv Res. 2012;12:438.

37. Gidengil CA, Gay C, Huang SS, Platt R, Yokoe D, Lee GM. Cost-effectiveness of strategies to prevent methicillin-resistant *Staphylococcus aureus* transmission and infection in an intensive care unit. Infect Control Hosp Epidemiol. 2015;36(1):17–27.

38. Arefian H, Vogel M, Kwetkat A, Hartmann M. Economic evaluation of interventions for prevention of hospital acquired infections: a systematic review. PLoS One. 2016;11:e0146381, 10.1371.

The Role of the Hospital Epidemiologist

Kristina A. Bryant

Background

Ignaz Semmelweis has been described as the original hospital epidemiologist, and his work is not dissimilar to that of modern practitioners [1]. In the mid-nineteenth century, he identified an outbreak of puerperal fever and conducted a stepwise investigation that implicated a lack of handwashing between autopsy and the operating room as the likely cause. He designed and implemented a hand hygiene intervention and measured the effect on infection rates. Despite objective evidence, his colleagues dismissed the importance of his work [2]. Semmelweis left the practice of medicine, and it would take another century for the value of the epidemiologist in preventing healthcare-acquired infections to be realized.

New York physician Joseph Felsen is credited with being the first to use the term "hospital epidemiologist" to describe an expert in the "investigation of infectious disease outbreaks arising or spreading within an institution" [3]. In a 1939 presentation before the epidemiology section of the American Public Health Association, Felsen called for the appointment of an epidemiologist to the staff of every hospital as part of a comprehensive program to prevent infectious diarrhea [4].

Unfortunately, his ideas were slow to catch on despite a growing recognition of the problem of healthcare-acquired infections. More than a decade later, Felsen made the same argument in a letter to JAMA [5]. "…we are stressing the importance of the hospital epidemiologist," he wrote. "As you know, intramural outbreaks of various types occur frequently in our hospitals but are poorly managed or inadequately studied." Fellow physician Leopold Brahdy likewise noted the occurrence of preventable diseases among doctors, nurses, other hospital personnel, and patients in medical institutions [6]. "A hospital epidemiologist is a major step

toward ending unnecessary illness and unnecessary death from disease acquired right in our own territory," he wrote.

In 1962, public health authorities in New York City ordered the creation of a local hospital epidemiology program, in part to foster collaboration between the health department and medical facilities and "enhance preventive medical activities [7]." As part of a pilot project, 16 hospitals in the borough of Brooklyn each designated a medical staff member to serve in the position of epidemiologist. These physicians participated in a standardized training program (ten weekly lecture-seminars organized by the Columbia University School of Public Health) and were paid as part-time employees of the health department in recognition of the incremental increase in their work responsibilities. Their duties mirrored those of many healthcare epidemiologists today: they identified and investigated outbreaks; developed a system for reporting select diseases to the health department, including HAIs; and provided education to their peers as well as nonprofessional staff. They chaired infection control committees, worked with employee health services, and coordinated immunization programs. Citing improvements in the timely investigation of syphilis cases as well as more efficient use of public health and hospital laboratories for the diagnosis of viral and rickettsial diseases, organizers declared the program and success and proposed expansion to every hospital in the city.

The Study on the Efficacy of Nosocomial Infection Control [SENIC], conducted by the Centers for Disease Control and Prevention (CDC) in 1976–1977, provided additional objective evidence about the value of the healthcare epidemiologist. SCENIC demonstrated that hospital infection prevention programs led by a physician with expertise in healthcare epidemiology had lower rates of HAIs [8, 9]. More than half of study hospitals had a physician or microbiologist serving in a leadership role, with higher rates among larger hospitals and those affiliated with academic medical centers [10]. Most physician leaders were pathologists (40 %), surgeons (11.7 %), internists (9.2 %), or infection disease specialists (8.7 %). Just over a quarter had

K.A. Bryant (✉)
University of Louisville, Healthcare Epidemiologist,
Norton Children's Hospital, 571 South Floyd Street, Suite 321,
Louisville, KY 40202, USA
e-mail: k0brya01@louisville.edu

© Springer International Publishing AG 2018
G. Bearman et al. (eds.), *Infection Prevention*, DOI 10.1007/978-3-319-60980-5_19

completed formal training in healthcare epidemiology and most (62 %) devoted only between 1 and 4 h weekly to infection surveillance and control activities.

When hospitals were resurveyed in 1983, the overall percentage with a physician hospital epidemiologist was slightly better (57 % vs. 51 %), but few individuals appeared to be pursuing hospital epidemiology as a career. Only 15 % had received specific training in the field and there was a high rate of turnover in the position.

In 1997, the CDC partnered with the Association for Professionals in Infection Control and Epidemiology (APIC) to reassess the state of infection prevention programs in the United States [11]. In the prior year, 47.6 % of 187 participating healthcare facilities had at least one part-time or full-time epidemiologist, but only 66 % provided financial compensation for epidemiology services. Most epidemiologists were individuals with an MD or PhD with training in infectious diseases, and they spent a small fraction of their work assignment (median 15 % or less) on infection control activities. In 2011, in a similar sample of acute care facilities, half still lacked an epidemiologist [12]. While more recent data are not available, it seems likely that the vision articulated in the 1960s—a trained, adequately compensated epidemiologist in every hospital—has not yet been realized.

Training

In the twenty-first century, healthcare epidemiologists are most often physicians with subspecialty training in infectious diseases and a background in internal medicine or pediatrics. Although the ranks of epidemiologists occasionally include professionals from fields other than medicine (e.g., nursing or clinical microbiology specialists with graduate degrees in public health), guidance from the Society for Healthcare Epidemiology of America (SHEA) suggests that the clinical insight of a physician is invaluable in this role [13]. In particular, the physician epidemiologist brings an understanding of the nuances of clinical care that affect the development and implementation of infection prevention practices.

While the Accreditation Council for Graduate Medical Education program requirements stipulate that trainees in infectious diseases (adult and pediatric) "demonstrate knowledge of infection control and hospital epidemiology," not every fellowship graduate will have the necessary skills and training required of the healthcare epidemiologist [14, 15]. A 2012 survey of pediatric infectious disease training programs in the United States found that little time was devoted to formal instruction or experiential learning in healthcare epidemiology [16]. Only a third of programs had a dedicated "infection control" rotation, and didactic sessions were limited, typically only 1–2 h.

SHEA has published a comprehensive review of the skills and competencies required of the healthcare epidemiologist, many of which are beyond the scope of most infectious disease training programs. Additional education is available through online courses offered by professional societies. A training certificate course in healthcare epidemiology is offered by SHEA in partnership with the CDC.

At present, there is no national certification process for healthcare epidemiologists analogous to the certification for infection preventionists nor is a single, recommended training pathway. One state, California, has established mandatory minimum requirements for physicians who have authority over the infection prevention and control program [17].

Duties of the Healthcare Epidemiologist

In the twenty-first century, HAIs are increasingly occurring outside acute care hospitals [18]. The burden in long-term care facilities is well recognized, with as many as two million infections occurring in US nursing homes annually [19]. Formal systematic surveillance in ambulatory settings is lacking but outbreak reports document healthcare-associated infections in doctors' and dentists' offices, outpatient surgery centers, pain clinics, and imaging facilities [20]. Although ambulatory and community settings are even less likely than acute care settings to have adequate epidemiology support, the term "healthcare epidemiologist" has largely replaced the term "hospital epidemiologist" in recognition of the need for this specialized expertise across the healthcare continuum. Alternately, the title "medical director for infection prevention" is used in some organizations.

Healthcare epidemiologists provide oversight of a facility's infection prevention program, often in collaboration with an infection preventionist. They serve as subject matter experts on topics ranging from pathogen transmission to diagnosis and treatment of infectious diseases. While specific responsibilities may vary according to institutional needs and priorities, common duties are listed below.

Administration

In some facilities, the healthcare epidemiologist functions as a manager: he or she is involved in day-to-day operations, supervising other professionals, overseeing budgets, and directing projects. In every facility, the healthcare epidemiologist has the opportunity to serve as a leader, broadly defined as person of influence within an organization and one who has the opportunity to effect change in the behavior of others [21]. Outlining the functions of a leader, Richard Wenzel wrote that healthcare epidemiologist leader must "articulate the mission, convince others to follow, create the high standards and the philosophy for success, and help design the culture of an organization" [22]. This may happen in both formal and informal settings. For example, the epidemiologist is often called upon to chair interdisciplinary committees, including the infection control committee. Leadership also happens in the doctors' lounge or the cafeteria. As a respected expert on infectious diseases and infection prevention, the epidemiologist is in a position to recruit support from peers and others for initiatives to reduce HAIs, even when these require changes in personal practice.

In some organizations, epidemiologists are involved in formal or informal review of physician practice. As such, their duties could include communication with surgeons about their surgical site infection rates, with hospitalists about hand hygiene compliance or intensivists about adherence to central venous catheter insertion bundles. The inherent tension associated with giving negative feedback to colleagues can create particular challenges for the epidemiologist who also maintains an infectious disease practice that is dependent on referrals [23].

Surveillance

Surveillance—the process of gathering, managing, analyzing, and reporting data—has been a core function of the healthcare epidemiologist since the days of Semmelweis. The modern epidemiologist participates in the development of a risk assessment, which is used in combination with regulatory mandates to drive the data that is collected. He or she must have a working knowledge of the National Healthcare Safety Network surveillance definitions for healthcare-associated infections and be able to articulate the difference between these and clinical definitions of infection to both frontline providers and administrators. In mature programs, data collection and preliminary data analysis are done by another member of the infection prevention team, while the healthcare epidemiologist is focused on interpretation of data and using it to develop interventions and improve patient outcomes. As noted by Robert Haley in an address at Columbia University in 1986, it is the job of the epidemiologist to report surveillance data in a way that is clinically relevant to other physicians [23].

Outbreak Investigation

Outbreak investigation is no less important now than in the 1960s, when hospital outbreaks of dysentery fueled the demand for physician epidemiologists. In the 2010 survey of a representative sample of US hospitals, one third had investigated an outbreak in the preceding 24 months [24]. The health epidemiologist participates in all phases of an outbreak investigation, including recognition, case finding, conduct of a case control, and implementation of control measures. He or she may be responsible for communication with internal stakeholders (facility administrators, healthcare providers, risk management) and external stakeholders (public health authorities, regulatory agencies, and the media).

Public Health/Emergency Preparedness

Healthcare epidemiologists may be involved with public health at the international and national level, working with the World Health Organization, the Centers for Disease Control and Prevention, or a nonprofit organization focused on health outcomes. They also serve in leaderships positions in state and local health departments. Those employed in community healthcare facilities still have the opportunity to shape national policies and practices related to infection prevention by serving on the Healthcare Infection Control Practices Advisory Committee (HICPAC), a federal advisory committee assembled to provide advice and guidance to CDC and the Secretary of the Department of Health and Human Services (HHS), or as members of guidelines committee of professional organizations. At the local level, healthcare epidemiologists collaborate with public health authorities on a number of issues, including recognition and investigation of infectious disease outbreaks.

They are often at the forefront of emergency preparedness activities ranging from pandemic influenza to bioterrorism to new and emerging infections such as Ebola virus disease (EVD). This was illustrated in late 2014 as US hospitals ramped up to identify and care for patients with EVD. A subset of SHEA members who were largely epidemiologists reported spending a median of 40 h per week on EVD preparedness activities, sometimes at the expense of other infection prevention duties [25].

Education

Education of personnel, patients, and families is a core activity of IP/HE programs. Healthcare epidemiologists must utilize adult learning principles to develop and implement educational activities for peers, other professional and non-professional staff, and the public. "Education" may take a number of forms, including formal lecture presentations, workshops, hands-on simulations, computer-based modules, small group discussions, and printed materials.

Employee Health

The healthcare epidemiologists may serve as the medical director for employee health services. Potential duties include policy development, evaluation and treatment of personnel after blood and body fluid exposure or other infectious disease exposure, oversight of immunization programs, and clearance of employees to return to work after an illness [26].

Quality Improvement and Patient Safety

The tools used by the healthcare epidemiologist to reduce HAI are also key to reducing noninfectious adverse outcomes. Many healthcare epidemiologists have developed expertise in the use of performance improvement methodologies and can serve as resource for design and implementation of projects not specifically related to infection prevention. The healthcare epidemiologist works collaboratively with the patient safety officer to reduce patient harm.

Antimicrobial Stewardship

The goals of antimicrobial stewardship include the optimization of drug selection, dosing, route of administration, and duration of therapy in order to improve patient outcomes and reduce adverse events. The Infectious Diseases Society of America and SHEA have recommended that antimicrobial stewardship programs (ASP) be led by infectious disease physicians with additional stewardship training [27]. Critical skills and competencies for required antimicrobial stewardship leaders have been defined and are distinct from those required of the healthcare epidemiologist, because effective antimicrobial stewardship is considered essential to efforts to eliminate healthcare-associated infections, including those caused by multidrug-resistant organisms and *Clostridium difficile*. Collaboration between the HE and ASP program is essential, and in some facilities, the healthcare epidemiologist also leads the ASP.

Research

Most HE are involved in work that advances the science of infection prevention. Research is a broad term that encompasses investigator initiated, randomized-controlled trials involving interventions, products or devices, retrospective observational studies, and outbreak investigations. Those without significant protected time devoted to research can still contribute data to research networks and multicenter collaboratives.

Resources and Compensation

The SCENIC study suggested that optimal staffing for infection control programs in the United States included one infection control professional for every 250 occupied beds in acute care facilities [8]. As the scope and complexity of infection prevention have increased, the concept of staffing based on occupied beds has been challenged [28]. In 2015, APIC conducted a workforce survey of its members that is expected to reshape recommendations for IP staffing in various healthcare settings.

Guidance for epidemiology staffing has also evolved. While noting the value of a part-time physician "with expertise in healthcare epidemiology," SCENIC investigators shopped short of making formal staffing recommendations. Guidance on epidemiology staffing remained limited for the next 30 years, although in 2007, members of the Dutch Society of Infection Prevention and Control in the healthcare setting (VHIG) and the Dutch Society of Medical Microbiology, the Netherlands, recommended one full-time equivalent epidemiologist or medical microbiologist per 25,000 admissions [29]. In 2016, SHEA published recommendations describing minimum staffing requirements for healthcare epidemiology based on the size of a facility and anticipated complexity of the patient population served (Table 19.1) [30].

Models for remuneration of hospital epidemiology services include hourly rate payments, a global fee for defined services, and a salaried position within an organization [31]. Among SCENIC participants, only 5 % of physicians received compensation specifically for their infection surveillance and control work, although in a minority some received at least a part-time salary for other services. A 2006 survey of SHEA members indicated gains, but on the whole, hospital epidemiologists remained undercompensated based on the time dedicated [32]. Only 65 % of the 526 survey respondents reported any compensation for they HE/IC services provided; the median percentage of total income provided by HE/IC services was 25 % [32]. Hourly compensation was reported by 102 individuals, at a median range of $101–150/h.

Table 19.1 Compensation for healthcare epidemiologists

	Recommended compensation	
	>300 beds and/or over 50 ICU beds	<300 beds and/or <50 ICU beds
Academic institutions	≥1.5 FTE of full professor salary[a]	≥1 FTE of full professor salary[a]
Community-based hospitals	≥1.0 FTE salary of regional market value	≥0.5 FTE regional market value

[a]Based on Association of American Medical Colleges norms (Adapted from [32])

Centers for Medicare and Medicaid Services pay-for-performance initiatives that impose financial penalties on hospitals for HAIs have created an unintended benefit for the healthcare epidemiologist: it has never been easier to demonstrate the financial value of the epidemiologist to an organization. Frameworks for negotiating appropriate compensation for managing infection prevention and control activities have been published [26, 31]. In addition to salary or consulting fees, contracts should clearly delineate scope of duties, the anticipated time commitment, available administrative support, physical resources necessary to perform the requested duties (including but not limited to computer hardware, software, access to administrative databases, availability of molecular typing, etc.), as well as protected time and reimbursement for professional development/continuing medical education.

Conclusions

Healthcare epidemiologists improve the quality of care for patients and are instrumental in reducing HAIs across the healthcare spectrum. Effective epidemiologists have mastered a unique set of skills and competencies through specialized training. They should be compensated adequately and appropriately for their work by the healthcare facility or entity utilizing their services.

References

1. Smith PW, Watkins K, Hewlett A. Infection control through the ages. Am J Infect Control. 2012;40:35–42.
2. Noakes TD, Borresen J, Hew-Butler T, Lambert MI, Jordaan E. Semmelweis and the aetiology of puerperal sepsis 160 years on: an historical review. Epidemiol Infect. 2008;136:1–9.
3. Felsen J, Wolarshy W. The hospital epidemiologist. Hospitals. 1940.
4. Auster LS. Applied epidemiology in a general hospital. JAMA. 1941:158.
5. Felsen J. Epidemiologists in hospitals. JAMA. 1950;144:65.
6. Brahdy L. Hospitals and epidemiologists. JAMA. 1950;144:783.
7. Fuerst HT, Lichtman HS, James G. Hospital epidemiology: its development and potential. JAMA. 1965;194:329–32.
8. Haley RW, Culver DH, White JW, et al. The efficacy of infection surveillance and control programs in preventing nosocomial infections in US hospitals. Am J Epidemiol. 1985;121:182–20.
9. Haley RW, Morgan WM, Culver DH, et al. Update from the SENIC project. Hospital infection control: recent progress and opportunities under prospective payment. Am J Infect Control. 1985;13:97–108.
10. Haley RW. The "hospital epidemiologist" in U.S. hospitals, 1976–1977: a description of the head of the infection surveillance and control program. Report of the SCENIC project. Infect Control. 1980;1:21–32.
11. Nguyen GT, Proctor SE, Sinkowitz-Cochran RL, Garret DO, Jarvis WR, Association for Professionals in Infection Control and Epidemiology, Inc. Status of infection surveillance and control programs in the United States, 1992–1996. Am J Infect Control. 2000;28:392–400.
12. Stone PW, Pogorzelska-Maziarz M, Herzig CT, et al. State of infection prevention in US hospitals enrolled in the National Health and Safety Network. Am J Infect Control. 2014;42(2):94–9.
13. Kaye KS, Anderson DL, Cook E, Huang SS, Siegel J, Zuckerman JL, Talbot TR. Guidance for infection prevention and healthcare epidemiology program: healthcare epidemiology skills and competencies. Infect Control Hosp Epidemiol. 2015;36:369–80.
14. Accreditation Council for Graduate Medical Education. ACGME Program Requirements for Graduate Medical Education in Pediatric Infectious Diseases. http://www.acgme.org/Portals/0/PFAssets/ProgramRequirements/335_infectious_disease_peds_2016.pdf?ver=2016-03-23-113832-480
15. Accreditation Council for Graduate Medical Education. ACGME Program Requirements for Graduate Medical Education in Infectious Disease (Internal Medicine). http://www.acgme.org/Portals/0/PFAssets/ProgramRequirements/146_infectious_disease_int_med_2016.pdf?ver=2016-03-23-113050-250
16. Sandora TJ1, Esbenshade JC, Bryant KA, Pediatric Leadership Council of SHEA. Pediatric infectious diseases fellowship training in healthcare epidemiology: a national needs assessment. Infect Control Hosp Epidemiol. 2013;34(2):195–9.
17. California Senate bill no. 158. 2008. California Legislative website. http://www.leginfo.ca.gov/pub/07-08/bill/sen/sb_0151-0200/sb_158_bill_20080925_chaptered.pdf. Published 2008. Accessed 5 Sept 2014.
18. Centers for Disease Control and Prevention. Guide to infection prevention in outpatient settings: minimum expectations for safe care. Available at http://www.cdc.gov/hai/pdfs/guidelines/Ambulatory-Care+Checklist_508_11_2015.pdf. Accessed 9 Sept 2016.
19. Strausbaugh L, Joseph C. The burden of infection in long-term care. Infect Control Hosp Epidemiol. 2000;21:674–9.
20. Centers for Disease Control and Prevention. Outbreaks and patient notifications in outpatient settings, selected examples, 2010–2014. Available at http://www.cdc.gov/HAI/settings/outpatient/outbreaks-patient-notifications.html. Accessed 1 Oct 2016.
21. Saint S, Kowalski CP, Banaszak-Holl, Forman J, Damschroder L, Krein SL. The importance of leadership in preventing healthcare-associated infection: results of a multisite qualitative study. Infect Control Hosp Epidemiol. 2010;31:901–7.
22. Wenzel RP. Leadership and management for healthcare epidemiology. In: Wenzel RP, editor. Prevention and control of noscomial infections. 4th ed. Philadelphia: Lippincott, Williams and Wilkins; 2003. p. 609–16.
23. Haley RW. The role of infectious disease physicians in hospital infection control. Bull NY Acad Med. 1987;63:597–604.
24. Rhinehart E, Walker S, Murphy D, O'Reilly K, Leeman P. Frequency of outbreak investigations in US hospitals: results of a national survey of infection preventionists. Am J Infect Control. 2012;40:2–8.
25. Morgan DJ, Braun B, Milstone AM, et al. Lessons learned from hospital Ebola preparation. Infect Control Hosp Epidemiol. 2015;36:627–31.
26. Simmons BP, Parry MF, Williams M, Weinstein RA. The new era of hospital epidemiology: what you need to succeed. Clin Infect Dis. 1996;22:550–3.
27. Barlam TF, Cosgrove SE, Abbo LM, et al. Implementing an antibiotic stewardship program: guidelines by the Infectious Diseases Society of America and the Society for Healthcare Epidemiology of America. Clin Infect Dis. 2016;62(10):e51–77.
28. O'Boyle C, Jackson M, Henly SJ. Staffing requirements for infection control programs in US health care facilities: Delphi project. Am J Infect Control. 2002. 2002;30:321–33.

29. van den Broek PJ, Kluytmans JA, Ummels LC, Voss A, Vandenbroucke-Grauls CM. How many infection control staff do we need in hospitals? J Hosp Infect. 2007;65:108–11.

30. Bryant KA, Harris AD, Gould CV, Humphreys E, Lundstrom T, Murphy DM, Olmsted R, Oriola S, Zerr D. Necessary infrastructure of infection prevention and healthcare epidemiology programs: a review. Infect Control Hosp Epidemiol 2016;37:371–80.

31. McQuillen DP, Petrak RM, Wasserman RB, Nahass RG, Scull JA, Martinelli LP. The value of infectious disease specialists: non-patient care activities. Clin Infect Dis. 2008;47:1051–63.

32. Wright SB, Ostrowsky B, Fishman N, Deloney VM, Mermel L, Perl TM. Expanding roles of healthcare epidemiology and infection control in spite of limited resources. Infect Control Hosp Epidemiol. 2010;31:127–32.

Whole Genome Sequencing for Outbreak Investigation

20

Tara N. Palmore

Introduction

Whole genome microbial sequencing provides information at a level of detail previously unattainable with the molecular biology techniques that have long served as tools for public health and epidemiology. Instead of making educated guesses based on epidemiologic data and helpful but imprecise estimates of microbial relatedness, epidemiologists can use the unambiguous results of sequencing to understand an outbreak.

Whole genome sequencing enables tracking of antimicrobial-resistant bacterial strains at a resolution that could not be achieved with older methods, such as pulsed-field gel electrophoresis, repetitive extragenic palindromic (Rep-) PCR, and multilocus sequence typing, which compare isolates using a small fraction of the organism's nucleic acids.

Overview of Whole Genome Sequencing and Older Typing Methods

Genome sequencing has advanced over the past 15 years from the Sanger method to next-generation sequencing. The original Sanger method enabled sequencing of a single DNA fragment at a time up to 1000 bp in length, using radiolabeled or fluorescently labeled nucleotides. Whether sequencing was performed manually, using a glass plate, or by automated capillary devices, Sanger sequencing was an extremely laborious and time-consuming method of sequencing the entire genome of a microbe, much less a multicellular organism. Despite its limitations, Sanger sequencing was used to complete the Human Genome Project [1].

T.N. Palmore (✉)
Hospital Epidemiology Service, National Institutes of Health Clinical Center, 10 Center Drive, Room 12C103A, MSC 1899, Bethesda, MD 20892, USA
e-mail: tpalmore@mail.nih.gov

Next-Generation Sequencing

Next-generation sequencing refers to high-throughput sequencing by large instruments in which thousands of DNA fragments are amplified and sequenced in parallel ("massively parallel") and the fluorescently labeled nucleotides are detected as they are incorporated. The highest-throughput devices typically are large and reserved for shared use in core facilities. In the past five years, tabletop sequencers have become increasingly available and popular. These sequencers are medium throughput, thus capable of sequencing a microbial genome but not an entire human genome. They are, however, far more accessible than high-throughput sequencers since they can be dedicated for use by individual labs. A number of high-throughput and tabletop sequencing devices are available on the market; their various sequencing platforms use similar workflow but different chemistry and methods of imaging to capture sequences as they are built [2].

Before sequencing begins, a library of DNA fragments is prepared from the genome of interest. The fragments are amplified and attached to complementary adapters or sequences that are recognized by the device. Sequencing proceeds as described, with parallel sequencing and detection of the thousands of fragments. After sequencing is completed (usually hours to days, depending on the quantity of genomic data and the depth, or duplication, of sequencing), the multiple copies of short, overlapping sequence reads (approximately 50–300 bp) are assembled de novo by computer programs [3]. The assembly is error-prone and thus relies on the depth of sequencing, or the generation of many fragments covering each area of the genome, and, ideally, the presence of a high-quality reference genome for comparison [4]. Assembled sequences are laboriously calibrated and corrected by expert "finishers" for misalignments and gaps [3]. The finished sequences can then be compared to other sequences. Genome sequences are deposited in public databases that enable researchers to access reference genomes and compare strains.

© Springer International Publishing AG 2018

G. Bearman et al. (eds.), *Infection Prevention*, DOI 10.1007/978-3-319-60980-5_20

"Third-Generation" Sequencing

Single-molecule real-time (SMRT) sequencing devices, sometimes called "third-generation sequencers," read the sequences of hundreds of thousands of individual long fragments of DNA ("single molecules"). The long reads – up to 1000 base pairs – are easier to assemble than short-read sequences and therefore allow better assessment of variation in repeat regions of the genome [5]. Short-read sequences from next-generation platforms can then be aligned to the long reads for error correction [6]. SMRT sequencing can be used for chromosomal DNA as well as plasmid DNA. Plasmids contain repeat regions and mobile genetic elements that make their contiguous assembly from short-read sequences challenging. Long-read SMRT sequencing can be used to recreate the framework of plasmids, where shorter sequences may not have sufficient overlap with unique sequences to differentiate a plasmid's structure [6]. Plasmid sequencing can be used to determine whether isolates of the same or different species may share the same plasmid – i.e., whether horizontal plasmid transmission between the isolates has occurred [6].

Older Bacterial Typing Methods

Many methods of typing have been used over the decades since public health and healthcare epidemiology experts began trying to determine relatedness of isolates. Pulsed-field gel electrophoresis (PFGE), Rep-PCR, and multilocus sequence typing are just few of the most common methods employed at various times since the 1970s. Of these, PFGE has been used to analyze the broadest range of bacterial species. In PFGE, bacterial DNA undergoes cleavage by restriction enzymes, and the resulting large DNA fragments are separated by size due to multidirectional electrical pulses. The resulting bands for each isolate are compared, and established criteria are used to label the isolates as related or unrelated [7]. This technique is useful if isolates have sufficiently different band patterns that they are deemed unrelated, but similar or identical band patterns may give only a gross, qualitative estimate of relatedness. An example is the community-acquired USA300 pulsotype of methicillin-resistant Staphylococcus aureus, whose isolates will all, by definition, have similar band patterns despite significant sequence variation [9]. The technique is laborious, time-consuming (at least three days), and low throughput.

Rep-PCR utilizes the arrangement of numerous repetitive DNA sequences interspersed between coding regions of genomes to distinguish between strains of bacteria [8]. The process can be automated, with repetitive sequences amplified to produce amplicons of varying length and separated by electrophoresis, giving band patterns that can be read and compared by software. As with PFGE, this technique is most helpful if it shows that isolates belong to different strains, whereas those deemed similar can still vary significantly.

Multilocus sequence typing (MLST) compares 400–500 bp sequences around seven loci that are selected in housekeeping genes. The sequences are amplified using primers specific for those loci, followed by Sanger sequencing of the amplified fragment of DNA from each locus. Each unique combination of sequences, or alleles, defines the sequence type of the organism, a classification that is standardized worldwide [10]. With the plummeting price of whole genome sequencing [11], MLST performed by this traditional method costs more than whole genome sequencing [10].

With the availability of whole genome sequences, MLST is implemented using the same loci and alleles that are identified using the whole genome sequences of the relevant bacterial isolates. The combination of alleles detected in the whole genome sequence is then labeled with the predicted sequence type. MLST using loci in core genes, the genome sequences that are common to all members of the set of bacteria being studied, has expanded the resolution of whole genome sequence-based MLST [12, 13]. This technique can miss sequence variation at loci that are not used for the comparison, but requires less computational labor and expertise than whole genome comparison of single nucleotide polymorphisms (SNPs).

Comparison of Whole Genome Sequencing with Older Methods

Numerous published studies have compared whole genome sequencing with older techniques in the course of investigating microbial relatedness during outbreaks. For example, in a report on the use of whole genome sequencing to elucidate an outbreak of blaKPC+ *Klebsiella pneumoniae*, Snitkin et al. noted that both Rep-PCR and PFGE were performed on outbreak isolates and that neither technique had the resolution to demonstrate differences. When microbial sequencing was performed, isolate sequences varied only within a range of 41 base pairs [14]. The differences, though minute, were sufficient to elucidate the chain of transmission within the outbreak. Even some more recent investigations have utilized PFGE as the first-line typing method, followed by whole genome sequencing to achieve higher resolution [15, 16].

Sequence Analysis

When the goal of sequencing is to detect minor variations or relatedness among isolates, assembled sequences may be aligned and compared for the presence of SNPs. Such analysis is labor intensive and, more importantly, requires a high level of expertise to handle the variations that occur in repetitive sequences, gene rearrangements, and inserted mobile genetic elements. Another approach, which does not require de novo assembly of the sequenced genome, is to compare shared genomic sections with reference strains; this approach would not examine large-scale genomic variation, such as insertions and deletions of genes. When analysis at that level is not possible, investigators have used core genome SNP analysis or multilocus sequence typing as described above. There is no standard algorithm or threshold for determining what magnitude of allelic or single nucleotide differences is considered closely related or clonal.

Once the sequence variants of a clonal outbreak strain are fully characterized by whole genome sequencing, researchers can develop a clone-specific set of PCR primers as a rapid diagnostic tool to identify isolates belonging to the outbreak strain [17–19]. Another technique, pan-PCR, is enabled by analyzing known sequences of a given bacterial species and generating a set of primers that can differentiate among strains of that species, providing species-specific strain typing [20].

Use of Whole Genome Sequencing for Outbreak Investigation

The power of whole genome sequencing for outbreak investigation lies in uniting its output with the relevant epidemiologic data. Epidemiological and genomic data can be joined to develop putative models of transmission for healthcare or public health epidemiology. Genomic data lend precision to intrinsically inexact epidemiologic data, and epidemiologic observations provide essential real-world context for the abstract results of genome sequencing. Examples from outbreaks on various scales demonstrate the remarkable insights that can be gleaned from this combination.

International Outbreak Investigation

Whole genome sequencing has been used to track the evolution and transmission of bacteria over great temporal and geographic distances. A now-infamous example is the use of sequencing to trace the origin of the Haitian cholera epidemic that began in 2010 in the wake of a devastating earthquake, and is still ongoing, leaving thousands dead. Haiti had no previous evidence of cholera in the historical record [21], and when infections first appeared in October 2010, officials speculated that the strain could have been introduced from the Americas or further afield.

Scientists were already conducting whole genome sequencing on historical and contemporaneous *Vibrio chol-*

erae isolates from around the world for an ongoing study to better understand the transmission dynamics of the seventh known cholera pandemic (in progress since the 1960s) [22]. The researchers included isolates from the Haitian outbreak and, through analysis of SNPs, determined that they were indeed part of the pandemic and in fact were closely related to recent South Asian strains [22]. Comparison of the SMRT sequences from the Haitian outbreak strain to sequences from around the world further confirmed clonality of the Haitian outbreak and supported recent importation of cholera from South Asia via "human activity" [23]. The indisputable genomic evidence from multiple studies [21–24] that the epidemic was introduced by a United Nations peacekeeper from Nepal has had enormous, unresolved legal and policy implications [25].

In addition to identifying the origins and international context of the Haitian cholera outbreak, whole genome sequencing has been used to study the outbreak's further spread in the years since the organism was introduced to the nation's cholera-naive population [24]. Eppinger and colleagues analyzed optical maps and SNPs from 116 whole genome sequences, including 45 from Haitian isolates, together with epidemiological data, to define "phylogeographic" patterns as isolates were carried across the country by people and by water. The authors noted that investigation of future cholera epidemics will be assisted greatly by hundreds of genomes that are accessible in public databases [24].

Although the focus of this review is bacterial sequencing, *Candida auris* is an important, emerging pathogen that has recently materialized in healthcare settings on multiple continents. The organism, which has caused serious healthcare-associated outbreaks, provides another example of sequencing used to trace the relatedness of isolates from around the globe. *C. auris* was first appreciated as a distinct species when it appeared in a clinical culture in Japan in 2009 [26]. Database searches have identified very few isolates from before 2009 [27]. In the past two years, nosocomial outbreaks of *C. auris* have occurred in India, Pakistan, South Africa, and Venezuela, with high rates of resistance to antifungal drugs and high associated mortality. Scientists from the US Centers for Disease Control and Prevention (CDC) conducted whole genome sequencing of isolates from each of the affected countries, as well as the initial isolate from Japan. Sequencing showed distinct clades in each region (South Asia, East Asia, South America, South Africa), suggesting that *C. auris* emerged simultaneously in each area rather than being transmitted by recent travelers or other vectors [27].

In a CDC report of the first seven patients identified with *C. auris* in the United States, whole genome sequencing demonstrated that isolates from patients who had been inpatients in the same hospitals were closely related, and that each of the isolates could be traced to one of the international clades [28]. Investigators further showed that environmental isolates found in the investigation of two cases from the same hospital in Illinois closely matched the relevant patient isolates (<10 SNPs). In contrast, isolates from each of the international clades differed by tens of thousands of SNPs [28]. Since the report of the first seven cases, the CDC has identified dozens more US cases of *C. auris* [29], and the growing database of sequences is used to trace their origins.

Hospital Outbreak Investigation

A first retrospective use of whole genome sequencing to investigate a hospital outbreak was published in 2012 by Koser et al. [30]. The investigators sequenced 14 isolates of methicillin-resistant *Staphylococcus aureus* (MRSA), including those from neonates involved in a suspected nosocomial outbreak in 2009 and, for comparison, contemporaneous MRSA-infected patients in other hospital wards. Analysis of SNPs in the isolates' core genome sequences confirmed that seven babies were indeed part of a clonal outbreak, but surprisingly revealed that two of the intended control MRSA patients had isolates that differed by only one SNP, likely representing unrecognized transmission. Of note, the authors reported that the isolates were sequenced within 1.5 days of extracting DNA from cultures. Although the sequencing and analysis were performed after the resolution of the outbreak, the researchers demonstrated the rapidity and feasibility of utilizing whole genome sequencing as a nosocomial outbreak investigative tool, in combination with a classical epidemiological inquiry [30].

Real-Time Whole Genome Sequencing During a Nosocomial Outbreak

The first real-time use of whole genome sequencing to investigate a hospital outbreak took place in 2011, when the US National Institutes of Health (NIH) Clinical Center, the clinical research hospital at the NIH, experienced a nosocomial outbreak of bla_{KPC}-carrying *K. pneumoniae* that had reduced susceptibility to colistin [14]. The outbreak began with an index patient who was known to be colonized in multiple sites with bla_{KPC}+ *K. pneumoniae* and was placed in contact isolation on admission. Five weeks elapsed between the index patient's presence in the ICU and detection of a second case of bla_{KPC}+ *K. pneumoniae* colonization, which led the infection control team to question whether there might have been two separate introductions of the organism into the ICU. Further screening cultures identified additional cases.

In the second month of the outbreak, Snitkin and Segre sequenced the first five isolates from patients who were colonized or infected with bla_{KPC}+ *K. pneumoniae*.

The genomics experts used SNP analysis to confirm the clonality of the outbreak and the likely chain of transmission among the first few cases. Their results prompted a shift in infection-control efforts toward conducting increasingly broad and ultimately hospital-wide microbial screening for the outbreak organism. These efforts ended the outbreak in December 2011; among 17 patients who had developed infection or colonization with the outbreak strain, six had died of bacteremia by the time the outbreak ended. Snitkin and Segre sequenced the remaining outbreak isolates, and the rapid mutation rate of the organism made it possible to elucidate the chain of transmission throughout the entire outbreak. They constructed a putative model of transmission using an innovative algorithm to combine genomic relatedness with epidemiological data such as the timing of patient locations in the various hospital wards. The sequencing of three slightly different isolates from different sites of colonization on the index patient demonstrated the disquieting finding that three distinct transmission events had occurred from the index patient, who had been isolated with barrier precautions for staff [14].

Six months later, in July 2012, an instance of nosocomial transmission from a chronically colonized patient to an immunocompromised patient resulted in a 17th case and, ultimately, a seventh death; whole genome sequencing was used rapidly to confirm the transmission and identify the source patient [6].

Numerous research teams throughout the world have since used whole genome sequencing as a tool to investigate suspected nosocomial outbreaks with a range of organisms, in combination with classical epidemiological techniques [31–35]. Whole genome sequencing has not only replaced older bacterial typing methods but has also become a tool for understanding the sequence of events in an outbreak setting [36].

Plasmid Sequencing to Identify Horizontal Transmission of Resistance Genes

While infection control precautions for resistant bacteria are designed around their most likely modes of transmission – the hands of healthcare personnel, contaminated surfaces, or contaminated equipment – the dynamics of plasmid dissemination may be far more complex. In addition, mobile genetic elements such as plasmids and transposons may spread undetected, and there are no infection control measures that specifically address this problem.

Conlan retrospectively studied the NIH outbreak isolates and a number of other environmental and patient isolates, identified through screening cultures, using SMRT sequencing to identify instances of horizontal transmission of carbapenemase genes and their plasmids. Horizontal transmission was ruled out in several cases and confirmed in others. Environmental cultures done to investigate one patient's unexpected colonization with a non-outbreak strain of bla_{KPC}+ K. pneumoniae led to isolation of bla_{KPC}+ Citrobacter freundii and bla_{KPC}+Enterobacter cloacae from a faucet aerator and a sink drain, respectively, in the patient's room. Conlan demonstrated horizontal transfer of the patient's bla_{KPC}+ plasmid to the two sink isolates. In addition, the E. cloacae isolate contained two other bla_{KPC}+ plasmids – including one containing a different bla_{KPC} subtype – that did not match those from any patient or environmental isolates. Thus SMRT long-read sequencing and plasmid assembly enabled determinations of plasmid transmission involving three different bacterial species and the simultaneous presence of multiple bla_{KPC}+ plasmids [6].

Investigators at the University of Pittsburgh used long-read sequencing with analysis of chromosomal and plasmid sequences to delineate an outbreak of resistant K. pneumoniae associated with duodenoscopes [37]. They found not only that there had been transmission of bla_{KPC}+ K. pneumoniae ST258 but that person-to-person spread of bla_{KPC}+ plasmids may have occurred via contaminated scopes [37].

Other investigators have described the horizontal transfer of plasmids carrying resistance genes in a variety of settings, using short-read sequencing platforms. Skalova et al. sequenced isolates from 20 patients who harbored Enterobacteriaceae with $bla_{OXA-48-like}$ carbapenemases (the first known cases in the Czech Republic). Several of the isolates came from nosocomial clusters, some were associated with travel, and some appeared to be community acquired. The researchers identified a plasmid-mediated outbreak, with polyclonal bla_{OXA-48}+ isolates sharing a common plasmid, whereas OXA48-like carbapenemases were carried on distinct plasmids [38].

Mathers and colleagues described a plasmid-mediated outbreak involving 16 isolates belonging to six species of Enterobacteriaceae; 12 isolates contained a distinct, promiscuous plasmid. The plasmid sequencing analysis was combined with epidemiologic data to develop hypothesized routes of spread within the hospital [18]. From plasmid sequence analysis, Mathers developed PCR primers specific for the outbreak plasmid and was able to deploy the PCR as a rapid diagnostic test to identify outbreak isolates [18]. In a later paper, the team demonstrated that plasmid sequencing combined with epidemiologic data could discriminate between multiple independent importations of bla_{KPC}+ K. pneumoniae and transmission of the previously identified bla_{KPC}-carrying endemic plasmid [39].

The ability to sequence and track mobile genetic elements adds an important dimension to our understanding of the spread of antimicrobial resistance. Much research is needed to translate these observations into measures that can reign in the dispersion of mobile genetic elements within the healthcare setting.

Sequencing of Endemic-Multidrug-Resistant Organisms

In addition to its use for elucidating outbreaks, whole genome sequencing can be used to describe the epidemiology of endemic multidrug-resistant organisms in order to better understand the dynamics of spread within communities and social networks. For example, Popovich et al. conducted SNP analysis of whole genome sequences of the USA300 pulsotype of MRSA from surveillance swabs collected from individuals seeking care within an urban community. They identified four pairs of people with closely related isolates, some of whom had in common illicit drug use and homelessness or residence in shelters. They also identified distinct transmission clusters among individuals who were African-American and infected with HIV, and a tendency for these clusters to be located in neighborhoods with high rates of past incarceration. The authors posited that transmission may have occurred in prisons or through activity associated with imprisonment [40].

Hospitals that have the ability to conduct whole genome sequencing can develop their own institutional databases of genome sequences from endemic multidrug-resistant bacteria (or other organisms of interest). Pecora et al. reported their experience in building such a database, which included plasmid sequences, that informs their epidemiological observations and provides comparators for determining whether subsequent isolates represent nosocomial transmission [41].

Interinstitutional Outbreak Investigation

Several studies have used whole genome sequencing to elucidate the transmission of highly resistant organisms between healthcare facilities or even among healthcare facilities in a region.

Zhou reported the use of whole genome sequencing in combination with epidemiologic data to track the spread of a high-risk clone of bla_{CTX-M}+ K. pneumoniae from a single source patient across several Dutch healthcare facilities in different cities, over 18 months [42]. Eleven patients ultimately acquired the outbreak strain from a hospitalized index patient, with several generations of transmission complicated by patient movement between facilities. Sequence analysis and recognition of clonality informed the epidemiological investigation, and, later, use of a clone-specific PCR enabled rapid screening and management of additional suspected cases [42].

The rapid regional spread of $bla_{KPC}+$ *Enterobacteriacaeae* in the New York City metropolitan area in the mid-2000s led to endemicity of these organisms in many healthcare facilities in the region, followed closely by a national healthcare-associated epidemic in Israel [43, 44]. Kreiswirth and colleagues sequenced six $bla_{KPC}+$ plasmids from three species of *Enterobacteriacaeae* isolated from hospitals in the New York City region between 2003 and 2010. The team found that the organisms harbored plasmids that were similar to the epidemic bla_{KPC}-carrying plasmid *pKpQIL* and that all likely evolved from a common ancestor. The team developed a *pKpQIL*-specific PCR and implemented it to screen hundreds of healthcare-associated isolates from New York and New Jersey, learning that approximately a third of the isolates carried *pKpQIL*-like plasmids. Their analysis had implications beyond just the mid-Atlantic United States, as one sequenced bla_{KPC}-carrying plasmid from 2003 appeared to be a precursor of the plasmid from the predominant $bla_{KPC}+$ clone in Israeli. This suggests that an isolate containing this plasmid was carried by international travel from the New York region to Israel in the early 2000s, leading to a clonal healthcare-associated epidemic throughout Israel [17].

Retrospective sequencing of isolates across healthcare facilities has enhanced knowledge of the complexity of regional spread and selection of resistant clones, [45] and perhaps of suspected routes of transmission.

Molecular Clocks and the Dynamics of Sampling

The "molecular clock" of an organism refers to the rate of development of gene mutations and is a useful tool for estimating the timing of a transmission. If the molecular clock of a bacterial genome is faster than the rate of transmission in an outbreak, SNP analysis may have sufficient discriminatory power to map transmission among patients in an outbreak. The $bla_{KPC}+$ *K. pneumoniae* outbreak reported by Snitkin was characterized by a molecular clock that enabled investigators to recreate the route of transmission despite the rapid pace of the outbreak [14]. For tuberculosis, the molecular clock is quite slow, estimated at 0.5 SNP per genome per year, making it difficult to formulate a granular map of transmission over short time periods [46, 47].

In the analysis of *C. auris* strains, serial isolates from one patient who had recurrent fungemia while receiving antifungal therapy developed six SNPs over just three weeks, comparable with the degree of genomic similarity among isolates recovered from different patients hospitalized at the same facilities (<10 SNPs) [28].

Whole Genome Sequencing to Elucidate Mycobacterial Transmission

Gardy and colleagues studied a large Canadian TB outbreak in which isolates appeared clonal by the standard typing method, Mycobacterial Interspersed Repetitive Unit-Variable Number of Tandem Repeat (MIRU-VNTR) [48]. Whole genome sequencing and SNP analysis was combined with social network analysis to investigate with greater granularity the dynamics of the outbreak. Genomic analysis alone revealed a chaotic map with many possible connections among patients; addition of the epidemiological data elucidated the transmission dynamics. What had appeared to be a unitary outbreak was in fact two separate outbreaks with distinct lineages, and cases disseminated by superspreaders outnumbered those due to secondary transmission [48].

Whole genome sequencing informed by social network analysis has been used to study other TB outbreaks. In a Norwegian TB outbreak, 22 isolates from cases distributed over a 4-year period had low genomic variability. Indeed, the isolates differed by a mean of one SNV, and the mutation rate was estimated at 1.1 SNV per genome per year. The authors note that although whole genome sequencing defines relatedness of isolates with a resolution far higher than that of MIRU-VNTR, the slow mutation rate of TB means whole genome sequencing may add limited information for establishing the chain of transmission in outbreak investigations [46].

Whole genome sequencing of *M. abscessus* isolates from persons with cystic fibrosis in the United Kingdom has provided startling insights into the transmission of these multidrug-resistant organisms [49]. SNP analysis in combination with social network analysis demonstrated multiple episodes of transmission of a *M. abscessus* subspecies among a cohort of 31 cystic fibrosis patients, many likely occurring within the center in which they received their care. Because of the granularity of whole genome sequencing, investigators were able to discern person-to-person transmission of strains that had mutations conferring additional resistance to antibiotics. The researchers were also able to show that similar isolates of a different *M. abscessus* subspecies did not represent transmission but rather colonization with a dominant circulating clone. The findings prompted enhancement of infection control precautions and initiation of routine microbial surveillance for cystic fibrosis patients at the authors' healthcare facility [49]. Another group studied *M. abscessus* clinical isolates from its cystic fibrosis patient cohort in a similar fashion and found no evidence of transmission, apart from likely spread between a pair of siblings [50].

Whole genome sequencing has been used to pinpoint the origin of nosocomial outbreaks of serious *M. chimaera* infections that have occurred in multiple countries over the past three years with case fatality rates as high as 50% [51, 52]. The infections were quickly traced to aerosols generated by contaminated heater-cooler units used during open-heart surgery, but one mystery was why the problem occurred simultaneously on distant continents and in devices from more than one manufacturer [51–57]. Investigators noted that a significant proportion of sampled units of different brands were contaminated with *M. chimaera*, even in countries where no infections had occurred [53]. Whole genome sequencing confirmed the clonality of isolates from patients and heater-cooler units [51] and in units from different countries that were made by the same manufacturer [53]. These findings pointed to the production facilities as possible point sources of contamination. A public health investigation in Germany discovered nearly identical strains contaminating newly built units at one manufacturing plant [58]. Investigations are still in progress. In the meanwhile, specialists have already concluded that remediation of existing units is not possible [55, 59] and are focusing instead on ways to prevent patient exposure [59] and on improved design of future units.

Whole Genome Sequencing for Foodborne Outbreaks

Whole genome analysis of foodborne bacterial outbreaks provided real-time, actionable output in addition to eye-opening microbiological findings [15, 60, 61]. In a particularly notable example, a Shiga-toxin-producing *Escherichia coli* 0104:H4 caused an enormous outbreak in Germany in 2011, with more than 3,000 cases of infection complicated by an unusually high rate of hemolytic uremic syndrome at 22% [62, 63]. The strain could not be cultured with the methods typically used for the more common Shiga-toxic-producing *E. coli* 0157:H7.

Whole genome sequencing demonstrated that, rather than the expected enterohemorrhagic pathotype of *E. coli*, the German outbreak strain was actually a Shiga-toxin-producing enteroaggregative *E. coli*, a previously rarely encountered strain with characteristics of both *E. coli* pathotypes. During the outbreak, after investigators released the sequence of one patient's isolate into the public domain, open-source whole genome analysis resulted in assembly of the genome within 24 h and the release of strain-specific primers within five days [63]. The strain-specific primers could be used for rapid identification of the outbreak strain, [19] enabling public health authorities to direct clinical and epidemiological resources in a highly targeted manner.

In the United States, a national public health initiative involving real-time whole genome sequencing was deployed in 2013 as an investigative tool and to monitor for *Listeria* outbreaks. In the first two years of use, GenomeTrakr, the collaborative, multiagency project, identified and solved five and nine outbreaks of listeriosis, respectively, compared with two in the year preceding the sequencing initiative [64]. This network is a model for use of real-time sequencing to make urgent public health interventions.

How Can Whole Genome Sequencing Generate Actionable Data?

The channeling of resources into implementing whole genome sequencing for public health and hospital infection control investigations is paying dividends in scientific understanding of the spread of resistance and the enormous consequences that can arise from a single introduction of a pathogen to a new environment [14, 17, 24]. A remaining challenge is to identify concrete steps that can be taken in response to real-time sequencing data and that could change the course of an outbreak. One example of such a response is the aforementioned use of GenomeTrakr to detect and rapidly halt transmission of *Listeria* [64].

In the 2011 *K. pneumoniae* outbreak at the NIH Clinical Center, real-time genome sequencing and analysis of the early isolates directed the investigation away from a point source or multiple independent introductions of the organism and toward a more complex web of person-to-person transmission. The information prompted several rounds of whole-hospital patient screening for carriage of the outbreak strain. This large-scale screening identified the last few colonized patients and was associated with interruption of transmission [14]. Although the sequencing output did lead to useful action, the action was application of a blanket measure (screening all inpatients). The granularity of sequencing data merits development of targeted epidemiological strategies that take advantage of the precise, high-resolution data.

Mellmann et al. attempted to do just that in a prospective study conducted in a large German teaching hospital. The investigators aimed to determine whether actionable data could be gleaned from real-time sequencing of endemic multidrug-resistant organisms, and whether acquiring such data would be cost-effective [65]. MRSA, vancomycin-resistant enterococci, multidrug-resistant *E. coli*, and multidrug-resistant *Pseudomonas aeruginosa* isolates were sequenced and analyzed using core genome MLST over a six-month period. When isolates were found to be nearly identical, epidemiological data were used to confirm or refute the likelihood of transmission. Small clusters of MRSA transmission were identified. Following this baseline analytical period, in which low rates of nosocomial transmission were observed, the investigators discontinued isolation of multidrug-resistant (but carbapenem-susceptible) *E. coli* on all but the highest-risk wards. In a follow-up period under the new isolation conditions, multidrug-resistant organism sequencing demonstrated no increase in documented transmission on those wards, and cost-effectiveness analysis suggested a €317,180 savings driven by the reduction in isolation [65].

Bioinformatics Expertise

Although the cost of sequencing continue to decline, and sequencers and automated assembly and analysis programs become more accessible, there remains a human factor that poses a challenge for incorporating the technique into routine infection control and outbreak investigation. Bioinformatics specialists must have the expertise to handle the large, often fragmented data output associated with sequencing, to select and use the appropriate programs, which may vary by organism and platform, to develop computational pipelines and generate interpretations that are accurate and reproducible. In addition, there is pressure to return sequence analyses in real time, especially when they are central to an outbreak investigation. The cost of bioinformatics expertise can be a substantial barrier and is growing as a proportion of the total cost of sequencing [66].

Conclusion

As computational and bioinformatics experts confront the challenges posed by massive output of sequencing data, the infection control and public health communities must devise ways to translate real-time sequence data into real-time action that can change the course of an outbreak. Whole genome sequencing combined with epidemiologic data has provided a degree of resolution and certainty in elucidating outbreaks that were unimaginable 15 years ago. Now the epidemiology community must find more innovative ways to use this outbreak investigative tool for outbreak control.

Acknowledgment This work was supported by the Intramural Research Program of the NIH Clinical Center.

References

1. International Human Genome Sequencing C. Finishing the euchromatic sequence of the human genome. Nature. 2004;431(7011):931–45.
2. Liu L, Li Y, Li S, et al. Comparison of next-generation sequencing systems. J Biomed Biotechnol. 2012;2012:251364.
3. Metzker ML. Sequencing technologies – the next generation. Nat Rev Genet. 2010;11(1):31–46.
4. Baker M. De novo genome assembly: what every biologist should know. Nat Methods. 2012;9(4):333–7.
5. Roberts RJ, Carneiro MO, Schatz MC. The advantages of SMRT sequencing. Genome Biol. 2013;14(7):405.
6. Conlan S, Thomas PJ, Deming C, et al. Single-molecule sequencing to track plasmid diversity of hospital-associated carbapenemase-producing Enterobacteriaceae. Sci Transl Med. 2014;6(254):254ra126.
7. Tenover FC, Arbeit RD, Goering RV, et al. Interpreting chromosomal DNA restriction patterns produced by pulsed-field gel electrophoresis: criteria for bacterial strain typing. J Clin Microbiol. 1995;33(9):2233–9.
8. van Belkum A. DNA fingerprinting of medically important microorganisms by use of PCR. Clin Microbiol Rev. 1994;7(2):174–84.
9. Larsen AR, Goering R, Stegger M, et al. Two distinct clones of methicillin-resistant *Staphylococcus aureus* (MRSA) with the same USA300 pulsed-field gel electrophoresis profile: a potential pitfall for identification of USA300 community-associated MRSA. J Clin Microbiol. 2009;47(11):3765–8.
10. Larsen MV, Cosentino S, Rasmussen S, et al. Multilocus sequence typing of total-genome-sequenced bacteria. J Clin Microbiol. 2012;50(4):1355–61.
11. National Human Genome Research Institute. Data from the NHGRI Genome Sequencing Program (GSP). Available at: https://www.genome.gov/sequencingcostsdata/. Accessed 2 Feb 2017.
12. Dekker JP, Frank KM. Next-generation epidemiology: using real-time core genome multilocus sequence typing to support infection control policy. J Clin Microbiol. 2016;54(12):2850–3.
13. Kluytmans-van den Bergh MF, Rossen JW, Bruijning-Verhagen PC, et al. Whole-genome multilocus sequence typing of extended-spectrum-beta-lactamase-producing Enterobacteriaceae. J Clin Microbiol. 2016;54(12):2919–27.
14. Snitkin ES, Zelazny AM, Thomas PJ, et al. Tracking a hospital outbreak of carbapenem-resistant *Klebsiella pneumoniae* with whole-genome sequencing. Sci Transl Med. 2012;4:148ra16.
15. Bottichio L, Medus C, Sorenson A, et al. Outbreak of salmonella Oslo infections linked to Persian cucumbers – United States, 2016. MMWR Morb Mortal Wkly Rep. 2016;65(5051):1430–3.
16. Weiss D, Boyd C, Rakeman JL, et al. A large community outbreak of Legionnaires' disease associated with a cooling tower in New York City, 2015. Public Health Rep. 2017;132(2):241–50.
17. Chen L, Chavda KD, Melano RG, et al. Comparative genomic analysis of KPC-encoding pKpQIL-like plasmids and their distribution in New Jersey and New York Hospitals. Antimicrob Agents Chemother. 2014;58(5):2871–7.
18. Mathers AJ, Cox HL, Kitchel B, et al. Molecular dissection of an outbreak of carbapenem-resistant enterobacteriaceae reveals Intergenus KPC carbapenemase transmission through a promiscuous plasmid. MBio. 2011;2(6):e00204–11.
19. Qin J, Cui Y, Zhao X, et al. Identification of the Shiga toxin-producing *Escherichia coli* O104:H4 strain responsible for a food poisoning outbreak in Germany by PCR. J Clin Microbiol. 2011;49(9):3439–40.
20. Yang JY, Brooks S, Meyer JA, et al. Pan-PCR, a computational method for designing bacterium-typing assays based on whole-genome sequence data. J Clin Microbiol. 2013;51(3):752–8.
21. Jenson D, Szabo V, Duke FHIHHLSRT. Cholera in Haiti and other Caribbean regions, 19th century. Emerg Infect Dis. 2011;17(11):2130–5.
22. Mutreja A, Kim DW, Thomson NR, et al. Evidence for several waves of global transmission in the seventh cholera pandemic. Nature. 2011;477(7365):462–5.

23. Chin CS, Sorenson J, Harris JB, et al. The origin of the Haitian cholera outbreak strain. N Engl J Med. 2011;364(1):33–42.

24. Eppinger M, Pearson T, Koenig SS, et al. Genomic epidemiology of the Haitian cholera outbreak: a single introduction followed by rapid, extensive, and continued spread characterized the onset of the epidemic. MBio. 2014;5(6):e01721.

25. Katz JM. The U.N.'s cholera admission and what comes next. New York Times Magazine. 2016 August 19. 2016.

26. Satoh K, Makimura K, Hasumi Y, Nishiyama Y, Uchida K, Yamaguchi H. Candida auris sp. nov., a novel ascomycetous yeast isolated from the external ear canal of an inpatient in a Japanese hospital. Microbiol Immunol. 2009;53(1):41–4.

27. Lockhart SR, Etienne KA, Vallabhaneni S, et al. Simultaneous emergence of multidrug-resistant Candida auris on 3 continents confirmed by whole-genome sequencing and epidemiological analyses. Clin Infect Dis. 2017;64(2):134–40.

28. Vallabhaneni S, Kallen A, Tsay S, et al. Investigation of the first seven reported cases of Candida auris, a globally emerging invasive, multidrug-resistant fungus – United States, May 2013-August 2016. MMWR Morb Mortal Wkly Rep. 2016;65(44):1234–7.

29. Centers for Disease Control and Prevention. Candida auris. Available at: https://www.cdc.gov/fungal/diseases/candidiasis/candida-auris.html. Accessed 20 Mar 2017.

30. Koser CU, Holden MT, Ellington MJ, et al. Rapid whole-genome sequencing for investigation of a neonatal MRSA outbreak. N Engl J Med. 2012;366(24):2267–75.

31. Schlebusch S, Price GR, Gallagher RL, et al. MALDI-TOF MS meets WGS in a VRE outbreak investigation. Eur J Clin Microbiol Infect Dis. 2017;36(3):495–9.

32. Jimenez A, Castro JG, Munoz-Price LS, et al. Outbreak of Klebsiella pneumoniae carbapenemase-producing Citrobacter freundii at a tertiary acute care facility in Miami. Fla Infect Control Hosp Epidemiol. 2017;38(3):320–6.

33. Jauneikaite E, Khan-Orakzai Z, Kapatai G, et al. Nosocomial outbreak of drug-resistant Streptococcus pneumoniae serotype 9V in an adult respiratory medicine ward. J Clin Microbiol. 2017;55(3):776–82.

34. Hagiya H, Aoki K, Akeda Y, et al. Nosocomial transmission of carbapenem-resistant Klebsiella pneumoniae elucidated by single-nucleotide variation analysis: a case investigation. Infection. 2017;45:221–5.

35. Sabat AJ, Hermelijn SM, Akkerboom V, et al. Complete-genome sequencing elucidates outbreak dynamics of CA-MRSA USA300 (ST8-spa t008) in an academic hospital of Paramaribo, Republic of Suriname. Sci Rep. 2017;7:41050.

36. Weterings V, Zhou K, Rossen JW, et al. An outbreak of colistin-resistant Klebsiella pneumoniae carbapenemase-producing Klebsiella pneumoniae in the Netherlands (July to December 2013), with inter-institutional spread. Eur J Clin Microbiol Infect Dis. 2015;34(8):1647–55.

37. Marsh JW, Krauland MG, Nelson JS, et al. Genomic epidemiology of an endoscope-associated outbreak of Klebsiella pneumoniae Carbapenemase (KPC)-producing K. pneumoniae. PLoS One. 2015;10(12):e0144310.

38. Skalova A, Chudejova K, Rotova V, et al. Molecular characterization of OXA-48-like-producing enterobacteriaceae in the Czech Republic and evidence for horizontal transfer of pOXA-48-like plasmids. Antimicrob Agents Chemother. 2017;61(2):e01889–16.

39. Mathers AJ, Stoesser N, Sheppard AE, et al. Klebsiella pneumoniae carbapenemase (KPC)-producing K. pneumoniae at a single institution: insights into endemicity from whole-genome sequencing. Antimicrob Agents Chemother. 2015;59(3):1656–63.

40. Popovich KJ, Snitkin E, Green SJ, et al. Genomic epidemiology of USA300 methicillin-resistant Staphylococcus aureus in an urban community. Clin Infect Dis. 2016;62(1):37–44.

41. Pecora ND, Li N, Allard M, et al. Genomically informed surveillance for carbapenem-resistant Enterobacteriaceae in a health care system. MBio. 2015;6(4):e01030.

42. Zhou K, Lokate M, Deurenberg RH, et al. Use of whole-genome sequencing to trace, control and characterize the regional expansion of extended-spectrum beta-lactamase producing ST15 Klebsiella pneumoniae. Sci Rep. 2016;6:20840.

43. Gupta N, Limbago BM, Patel JB, Kallen AJ. Carbapenem-resistant Enterobacteriaceae: epidemiology and prevention. Clin Infect Dis. 2011;53(1):60–7.

44. Leavitt A, Navon-Venezia S, Chmelnitsky I, Schwaber MJ, Carmeli Y. Emergence of KPC-2 and KPC-3 in carbapenem-resistant Klebsiella pneumoniae strains in an Israeli hospital. Antimicrob Agents Chemother. 2007;51(8):3026–9.

45. Del Franco M, Paone L, Novati R, et al. Molecular epidemiology of carbapenem resistant Enterobacteriaceae in Valle d'Aosta region, Italy, shows the emergence of KPC-2 producing Klebsiella pneumoniae clonal complex 101 (ST101 and ST1789). BMC Microbiol. 2015;15(1):260.

46. Norheim G, Seterelv S, Arnesen TM, et al. Tuberculosis outbreak in an educational institution in Norway. J Clin Microbiol. 2017;55:1327–33.

47. Walker TM, Ip CL, Harrell RH, et al. Whole-genome sequencing to delineate Mycobacterium tuberculosis outbreaks: a retrospective observational study. Lancet Infect Dis. 2013;13(2):137–46.

48. Gardy JL, Johnston JC, Ho Sui SJ, et al. Whole-genome sequencing and social-network analysis of a tuberculosis outbreak. N Engl J Med. 2011;364:730–9.

49. Bryant JM, Grogono DM, Greaves D, et al. Whole-genome sequencing to identify transmission of Mycobacterium abscessus between patients with cystic fibrosis: a retrospective cohort study. Lancet. 2013;381(9877):1551–60.

50. Harris KA, Underwood A, Kenna DT, et al. Whole-genome sequencing and epidemiological analysis do not provide evidence for cross-transmission of mycobacterium abscessus in a cohort of pediatric cystic fibrosis patients. Clin Infect Dis. 2015;60(7):1007–16.

51. Chand M, Lamagni T, Kranzer K, et al. Insidious risk of severe Mycobacterium chimaera infection in cardiac surgery patients. Clin Infect Dis. 2017;64(3):335–42.

52. Kohler P, Kuster SP, Bloemberg G, et al. Healthcare-associated prosthetic heart valve, aortic vascular graft, and disseminated Mycobacterium chimaera infections subsequent to open heart surgery. Eur Heart J. 2015;36(40):2745–53.

53. Svensson E, Jensen ET, Rasmussen EM, Folkvardsen DB, Norman A, Lillebaek T. Mycobacterium chimaera in heater-cooler units in Denmark related to isolates from the United States and United Kingdom. Emerg Infect Dis. 2017;23(3):507–9.

54. Sax H, Bloemberg G, Hasse B, et al. Prolonged outbreak of Mycobacterium chimaera infection after open-chest heart surgery. Clin Infect Dis. 2015;61(1):67–75.

55. Schreiber PW, Kuster SP, Hasse B, et al. Reemergence of Mycobacterium chimaera in heater-cooler units despite intensified cleaning and disinfection protocol. Emerg Infect Dis. 2016;22(10):1830–3.

56. Perkins KM, Lawsin A, Hasan NA, et al. Notes from the field: mycobacterium chimaera contamination of heater-cooler devices used in cardiac surgery – United States. MMWR Morb Mortal Wkly Rep. 2016;65(40):1117–8.

57. Robinson JO, Coombs GW, Speers DJ, et al. Mycobacterium chimaera colonisation of heater-cooler units (HCU) in Western Australia, 2015: investigation of possible iatrogenic infection using whole genome sequencing. Euro Surveill. 2016;21(46):pii=30396.

58. Haller S, Holler C, Jacobshagen A, et al. Contamination during production of heater-cooler units by Mycobacterium chimaera potential cause for invasive cardiovascular infections: results of an

outbreak investigation in Germany, April 2015 to February 2016. Euro Surveill. 2016;21(17):pii=30215.

59. Kanamori H, Weber DJ, Rutala WA. Healthcare-associated Mycobacterium chimaera transmission and infection prevention challenges: role of heater-cooler units as a water source in cardiac surgery. Clin Infect Dis. 2017;64(3):343–6.

60. Chen Y, Luo Y, Curry P, et al. Assessing the genome level diversity of *Listeria monocytogenes* from contaminated ice cream and environmental samples linked to a listeriosis outbreak in the United States. PLoS One. 2017;12(2):e0171389.

61. Jackson KA, Stroika S, Katz LS, et al. Use of whole genome sequencing and patient interviews to link a case of sporadic Listeriosis to consumption of prepackaged lettuce. J Food Prot. 2016;79(5):806–9.

62. Zoufaly A, Cramer JP, Vettorazzi E, et al. Risk factors for development of hemolytic uremic syndrome in a cohort of adult patients with STEC 0104:H4 infection. PLoS One. 2013;8(3):e59209.

63. Rohde H, Qin J, Cui Y, et al. Open-source genomic analysis of shiga-toxin-producing *E. coli* O104:H4. N Engl J Med. 2011;365(8):718–24.

64. Jackson BR, Tarr C, Strain E, et al. Implementation of nationwide real-time whole-genome sequencing to enhance Listeriosis outbreak detection and investigation. Clin Infect Dis. 2016;63(3):380–6.

65. Mellmann A, Bletz S, Boking T, et al. Real-time genome sequencing of resistant bacteria provides precision infection control in an institutional setting. J Clin Microbiol. 2016;54(12):2874–81.

66. Davis-Turak J, Courtney SM, Hazard ES, et al. Genomics pipelines and data integration: challenges and opportunities in the research setting. Expert Rev Mol Diagn. 2017;17(3):225–37.

Viral Hemorrhagic Fever Preparedness

21

Angela Hewlett, Angela M. Vasa, Theodore J. Cieslak,
John J. Lowe, and Shelly Schwedhelm

Introduction

The 2014–2016 outbreak of Ebola virus disease (EVD) in West Africa marked the 25th such occurrence but was noteworthy in its massive scope, causing more human morbidity and mortality than the previous 24 recorded outbreaks combined. As of April 2016, there were 28,652 cases resulting in at least 11,325 deaths, nearly all in the three nations of Guinea, Liberia, and Sierra Leone [1]. Moreover, the 2014–2016 outbreak was the first in which patients, albeit few in number, were afforded sophisticated intensive care in the United States and in Europe. This "high-level containment care" (HLCC) was provided in specially designed purpose-built biocontainment units (BCUs). In this chapter, we explore the history and evolution of biocontainment, discuss its unique engineering and infection control modalities, and offer recommendations for the clinical and operational management of Ebola and other viral hemorrhagic fevers (VHFs).

History of Biocontainment

The modern concept of biocontainment had its birth in 1969 with the convergence of four separate events. In May of that year, Michael Crichton published *The Andromeda Strain*, and, while the work was clearly fictional, it debuted amidst a series of discussions leading up to President Nixon's decision in November of that year to abandon the US offensive biological weapons program. Nixon's decision was a prelude to ratification of the 1972 Biological Weapons Convention and to the US ratification, in 1975, of the Geneva Protocols. At the time, Nixon stated that "the United States has decided to destroy its entire stockpile of biological agents and confine its future biological research program to defensive measures." Implicit in that decision was a shift in the focus of US efforts to defensive and medical countermeasure development that would include an emphasis on the management of patients potentially infected with highly hazardous human pathogens. This medical defense program would fall largely upon the newly created US Army Medical Research Institute of Infectious Diseases (USAMRIID), an entity which would inherit its defensive mission from the old Army Biological Laboratory (ABL).

The year 1969 also witnessed the discovery of Lassa virus by Dr. Jordi Casals-Ariet at Yale University [2]. While attempting to characterize the new virus, Dr. Casals contracted Lassa fever himself and fell critically ill but survived following the administration of convalescent serum from one of his patients. Unfortunately, one of his technicians, Juan Roman, succumbed to the disease while conducting laboratory studies, causing Dr. Casals to move his research to a new maximum-security laboratory at the Communicable Disease Center in Atlanta (now

A. Hewlett (✉)
Division of Infectious Diseases, Internal Medicine, Infectious Diseases, University of Nebraska Medical Center, Omaha, NE 68198, USA

Biocontainment Unit, Nebraska Medicine, Omaha, NE, USA
e-mail: alhewlett@unmc.edu

A.M. Vasa
Biocontainment Unit, Nebraska Medicine, Omaha, NE, USA
e-mail: avasa@nebraskamed.com

T.J. Cieslak
Biocontainment Unit, Nebraska Medicine, Omaha, NE, USA

College of Public Health, Department of Epidemiology, University of Nebraska Medical Center, Omaha, NE, USA
e-mail: ted.cieslak@unmc.edu

J.J. Lowe
Biocontainment Unit, Nebraska Medicine, Omaha, NE, USA

Environmental, Agricultural, and Occupational Health, University of Nebraska Medicine, Omaha, NE, USA
e-mail: jjlowe@unmc.edu

S. Schwedhelm
Biocontainment Unit, Nebraska Medicine, Omaha, NE, USA

Infection Prevention & Emergency Preparedness, Nebraska Medicine, Omaha, NE, USA
e-mail: sschwedh@nebraskamed.com

© Springer International Publishing AG 2018
G. Bearman et al. (eds.), *Infection Prevention*, DOI 10.1007/978-3-319-60980-5_21

the Centers for Disease Control and Prevention) and ushering in a new era of laboratory safety.

Finally, 1969 saw man's first journey to the moon, aboard Apollo 11. In order to guard against the remote possibility that extraterrestrial pathogens might inadvertently accompany the returning astronauts, a new facility, the Lunar Receiving Laboratory (LRL), was constructed, in consultation with ABL experts, at the Johnson Manned Spaceflight Center in Houston. The facility would receive spacecraft, equipment, and lunar samples from Apollo 11 and from future Apollo missions. Moreover, it would serve as a quarantine facility for the returning astronauts from the Apollo 11, 12, and 14 missions.

Included among the assets of the USAMRIID facility was a novel two-bed high-level containment care unit [3]. This unit, often referred to as "the Slammer," presumably owing to the sound produced by the closure of its heavy steel airlock doors, opened in 1971 and included engineering controls analogous to those employed in Biosafety Level 4 (BSL-4) laboratories. The facility was designed to treat infected patients but also to provide confidence and a sense of security to scientists and to the community of Frederick, Maryland, in which it was located.

During the period 1972–1985, 20 individuals were admitted to the Slammer following laboratory or field exposure to a variety of BSL-4 pathogens [4]. A 21st patient (exposed to Ebola in the laboratory) was admitted in 2004 [5]. Of note, none of the 21 patients developed clinical evidence of infection. The Slammer was decommissioned in 2012; a new USAMRIID building, slated to open in 2017, will not house a containment care unit.

The intentional dissemination of anthrax via contaminated mail in October 2001, occurring just weeks after the World Trade Center assault and, ironically, attributed to a troubled USAMRIID scientist, convinced some civilian experts to move in the opposite direction and propose the creation of academic medical center-based HLCC facilities. Outbreaks of severe acute respiratory syndrome (SARS) and monkeypox in the spring of 2003 added impetus to these construction projects, SARS because of its high mortality and apparent transmission via droplet nuclei and monkeypox owing to a resistance among fearful healthcare providers to treat victims of the disease [6].

During 2004–2005, a two-bed facility at Emory University in Atlanta and a ten-bed facility at the University of Nebraska Medical Center in Omaha opened; the facilities employed some (but not all) of the engineering controls contained within the USAMRIID facility. In 2005, leaders from these facilities, as well as USAMRIID and the Centers for Disease Control and Prevention (CDC), published consensus guidelines for the employment of HLCC units [7].

In that same year, the National Institute of Allergy and Infectious Diseases (NIAID) contracted with Saint Patrick Hospital in Missoula MT to construct the first HLCC unit housed outside of a large university-based medical center in order to care for scientists exposed to BSL-3 and BSL-4 pathogens at the NIAID's Rocky Mountain Laboratories in nearby Hamilton [8]. As of this writing, no patients have been cared for in this facility. In 2010, the Special Clinical Studies Unit at the National Institutes of Health adapted its seven-bed clinical research unit in order to provide HLCC. This facility, along with those at Emory and Nebraska, cared for 9 of the 11 victims of the 2014–2016 West African Ebola outbreak managed in the United States. One patient was managed under HLCC conditions at Bellevue Hospital in New York, and one patient was managed at Dallas Presbyterian Hospital.

Germany possesses seven HLCC facilities, four of which cared for EVD victims during the 2014–2016 West African outbreak. Some of these units have experience in treating patients infected with Marburg and Lassa viruses as well. Biocontainment units in Britain, France, Spain, the Netherlands, Norway, Switzerland, and Italy also successfully cared for expatriate patients during the recent EVD outbreak, and European nations have been pioneers in the development of HLCC doctrine [9, 10]. Finally, China, at the height of the SARS outbreak in 2003, constructed a 1000-bed infectious disease treatment facility equipped with engineering controls designed to ameliorate the risk of airborne transmission of the SARS coronavirus [11]. Other nations in the region, such as Singapore and South Korea, are constructing HLCC facilities as well.

Background: Viral Hemorrhagic Fever (VHF)

The viral hemorrhagic fevers (VHFs) are caused by a heterogeneous group of viruses belonging to four taxonomic families and include:

– The filoviruses, Ebola, and Marburg
– The arenaviruses, which can be divided into Old World (Lassa) and New World (Guanarito, Junin, Machupo, Sabia) agents, the latter causing Venezuelan, Argentinian, Bolivian, and Brazilian hemorrhagic fevers, respectively
– The flaviviruses, yellow fever, dengue, Kyasanur Forest, and Omsk
– The bunyaviruses, Crimean-Congo hemorrhagic fever (CCHF), Rift Valley fever (RVF), and a number of hantaviruses which cause hemorrhagic fever with renal syndrome (HFRS; Hantaan, Dobrova, Seoul, and Puumala)

Yellow fever has been known since at least 1647; is distributed throughout tropical Africa, Asia, and South America; and was the first disease shown, by Walter Reed, to be transmitted by mosquitos [12]. The remaining VHFs have, for the most part, been discovered within the last half-century and remain quite limited in their geographic distributions.

Although the VHF viruses share certain microbiologic characteristics (all are lipid-enveloped single-stranded RNA viruses) and derive their name from the fact that some (but not all) patients experience clinically significant hemorrhage, they produce a diverse array of clinical symptoms and vary widely in their virulence. While massive hemorrhage occurs frequently with New World arenaviral infections, as well as RVF, CCHF, certain hantaviruses, and yellow fever, it occurs less frequently with infections due to the filoviruses and rarely in Lassa infections. Renal failure is characteristic of HFRS and yellow fever but otherwise rare. Rash is seen with dengue, Lassa, and filovirus infections, but not with most other VHFs. Icterus is prominent with yellow fever; tremors with the New World arenaviruses; deafness with Lassa. Pulmonary disease is prominent with Kyasanur Forest and Omsk, as well as with certain hantaviruses.

In addition, laboratory findings vary considerably among the VHFs. New World arenaviral infections characteristically cause a profound leukopenia, while HFRS patients often exhibit significant leukocytosis. Thrombocytopenia can be marked in most VHFs but is usually not a prominent feature of Lassa fever. These notable differences in presentation and symptomatology have implications for clinical care and infection control. The prodigious amount of vomiting and diarrhea seen in patients during the 2014–2016 EVD outbreak, coupled with the very low infectious dose and high quantity of viral particles within these bodily fluids, makes meticulous attention to personal protection imperative. Guidelines for the employment of such protection, as well as engineering and other controls, provide the basis for the remainder of this chapter.

It is important to note that the causative agents of most VHFs need be handled under Biosafety Level 4 (BSL-4) conditions in the laboratory [13]. Exceptions include yellow fever, RVF, and the hantaviruses, which require BSL-3 precautions. Patients harboring any of these agents that present the risk of person-to-person transmission ideally should be managed under HLCC conditions. These agents would include the hantaviruses, as well all of the BSL-4 agents except RVF, Kyasanur Forest, and Omsk viruses, which are transmitted to humans only via the bite of infected arthropods.

Facility Design

High-level containment care facilities include enhanced engineering controls with the goal of providing safe and effective care to patients while optimizing infection prevention and control procedures [9]. Two consensus efforts have been conducted to develop recommendations for designing HLCC care units: a US consensus workgroup met in 2005 in order to develop standards for the operation of BCUs and a 2007 European Network for Highly Infectious Diseases

(EuroNHID) project [7, 10]. However, formal standards for HLCC facility design features have not been established.

The design of a HLCC unit should serve to minimize nosocomial transmission of infectious diseases by establishing a contained clinical isolation unit capable of housing all facets of patient care. Hallmark HLCC engineering controls include care units that are physically separated from normal patient care spaces and maintained at negative pressure by independent air handling systems. At least 12 air exchanges per hour in patient rooms are accomplished using dedicated exhaust systems with high efficiency particulate air (HEPA)-filtered effluent air. It is recommended that pressure status of patient care rooms be monitored with audible and visual alarms [14, 15]. Individual patient care rooms should have the equipment necessary to support critically ill patients, self-closing doors, and handwashing sinks [7].

It is important to have established zones for employee donning and doffing, storage of personal protective equipment (PPE), and staff shower-out capability [7]. Additionally, selection of nonporous and seamless construction materials is an ideal design component of HLCCs that both minimizes the risk of environmental contamination and maximizes the ability to clean surfaces when contaminated.

HLCC units should delineate high-risk areas ("Hot" or "Red" zones: patient room, laboratory), intermediate-risk areas ("Warm" or "Yellow" zones: anteroom, decontamination area, waste processing, doffing), and low-risk areas ("Cold" or "Green" zones: nurse station, clean supply room, staff egress changing area). Establishment of these designated zones guides healthcare worker flow as well as implementation of protocols for cleaning, packaging of waste or clinical specimens, and decontamination of medical devices, reducing the potential for contamination as personnel and devices move through the HLCC. Inclusion of laboratory and waste sterilization capabilities within HLCC units are also key features that help minimize the potential of transmission throughout the hospital [16, 17]. A double door pass through autoclave was identified as mandatory for HLCC unit through both consensus efforts [7, 18]. Analogous pass through "dunk tanks" filled with disinfectant solution is useful in moving specimens from the HLCC to the laboratory and is particularly useful in facilities which lack a dedicated "in-unit" laboratory. Implementation of telehealth strategies that enable communication with healthcare workers as well as provide a platform for remote patient assessment is important in reducing the number of healthcare workers with direct patient contact, thus limiting risk.

Administration and Support Services

The intermittent and sporadic utilization of HLCC units necessitates strong leadership. Ideally, a HLCC leadership team should possess a robust set of diverse skills to include expertise in infectious disease and critical care, nursing, emergency management, industrial and environmental hygiene, research, laboratory, hospital administration, and public affairs. This leadership team should meet regularly to strategize and define drill objectives, plan educational efforts, promote research projects, and synchronize collaborative endeavors [19].

A robust activation checklist should be developed and drilled intermittently to assure that departments followed through on tasks assigned and that necessary items can be obtained in a timely fashion. This checklist should address unit stockage and supplies, equipment, medications, facilities activation procedures, and notification of departments and key individuals who will be involved in the activation of the unit and the care of the patient(s).

Numerous communication strategies are adaptable for use by HLCC team members. An electronic alert system with individual key numbers can be used to notify the HLCC team of drills and activation. An email distribution list can be used for less urgent information sharing. In order to organize the response for arriving patients, a modified Hospital Incident Command System (HICS) can be utilized, and the Incident Commander (IC) can support HLCC leaders in completing the activation checklist. Moreover, the IC can facilitate coordination among the multiple agencies often involved in air and ground transport of patients to the patient care unit.

Although each facility may wish to tailor the composition of the HICS team to their own particular needs, and each situation may require adjustment, key team members would typically include logisticians to plan to replenish PPE supply levels and address waste management issues, a public information officer (PIO), medical technical specialists to include infectious disease physicians and nurse leaders to manage the clinical care of the patient and staffing within the patient care unit, a laboratorian to address testing logistics and specimen transport challenges, a clinical research expert to facilitate the use of experimental therapies when necessary, a nurse concierge or other dedicated individual to support family needs, and a behavioral health expert to address staff well-being as well as the psychological and emotional needs of patients and families.

The PIO is charged with responding to media requests, including those from social media sources. Internal messaging within the organization should be done prior to release of any external information. Internal messaging may be directed at administration, employees, and also patients (inpatients and outpatients) and their family members. Press conferences with infectious diseases experts and others involved in patient care should be held to provide timely updates. It is also helpful to establish an information phone line staffed by the state or local health department to answer questions and provide education to the community.

During activation, a concierge nurse or other patient advocate may prove helpful in the support of families of patients. This individual can assist by making advance contact with family members and arranging services such as airport transportation, accommodations, and meals. They can also serve as the liaison with family in the coordination of meetings to discuss the status of the patient, media information, and various other details. Pastoral Care staff should be available upon request during activation.

Staffing: Nursing

The HLCC facilities in the United States that admitted patients infected with Ebola virus disease (EVD) have well developed teams of nurses who are able to provide skilled and effective patient care within their isolation units. Recruiting and retaining qualified nursing staff willing and able to provide care for patients under emotionally and physically demanding HLCC conditions is the cornerstone to building a successful team. The staffing model must take into account the need for specialized nurses to provide quality care. The virulence of the disease in question, its mortality rate, the advanced levels of PPE required, and the propensity for infected patients to require complex interventions all influence the profile of staff selected to care for patients with VHF or other highly hazardous communicable diseases.

The composition of the HLCC nursing team should reflect these needs. The centers in the United States that provided care for EVD patients each required that a percentage of their core nursing staff possess critical care experience, with some institutions relying solely upon critical care nurses to staff their units [20]. In addition to critical care experience, it is essential to have nurses on the core team who have expertise in infectious diseases and have expressed an interest in caring for patients with highly hazardous communicable diseases [21]. The success of the nursing staff starts with a robust selection process. Utilizing a formal interview process to determine qualifications and interest has been proven to be an effective method of selecting staff. Once the interview is complete, the nursing leadership should contact the employee's current manager to discuss their clinical skills, teamwork skills, adaptability, dependability, and critical thinking skills.

When staffing a unit that is only activated intermittently, an important consideration involves creating a process by which staff members can designate their availability on any given day. This can be accomplished in a multitude of ways; however, maintaining a consistent process is key to ensuring staff availability when needed. As the provision of nursing care must occur 24 h a day, 7 days a week, it is important that a schedule be created that accounts for all times. One way to achieve this is to mandate on-call shifts for dedicated staff.

The on-call nurses are required to be at the Unit within 60 min of being notified of activation. Another option is to have each staff member fill out their availability and maintain a balanced schedule several weeks in advance. This allows staff members a level of autonomy to self-schedule.

Considerations for creating a nursing staff matrix include the design of the unit, the waste management strategy, the disease being treated, the acuity of the patient, the level of personal protective equipment (PPE) required, and the time that could be spent in the PPE [20, 22]. An important consideration is the need to minimize the number of staff that enters into the patient care area. The ability to utilize nursing staff in multiple roles can facilitate effective infection control by minimizing the footprint within potentially contaminated areas. In this effort, nursing staff become responsible for tasks that would typically be assigned to ancillary services within the standard hospital system, including routine cleaning and environmental services, phlebotomy, coordinating care needs, and unit clerk roles [20, 23].

Consideration must also be given to the nurse-to-patient ratio necessary to provide safe care to a patient with VHF. The number of staff members required for a standard 12 h nursing shift must take into account the time limitations imposed on each staff member due to the use of advanced PPE. When providing the level of intensive care that these patients can require in addition to wearing PPE, it is necessary to adjust shift times and staffing ratios [24]. The staffing matrix utilized within hospitals that successfully cared for EVD patients differed significantly from standard staffing ratios. Within the Nebraska Biocontainment Unit, six staff members were present on a day shift and five on the night shift (usually three nurses along with respiratory therapists and/or patient care technicians). Healthcare staff was scheduled for 12 h shifts which were broken up into 4 h blocks to allow for the limitation of not wearing PPE for greater than 3–4 h at a time. Designation of roles for each staff member on each shift can clarify expectations and ensure consistency within each role. The use of an autoclave for waste processing may necessitate the inclusion of a dedicated staff member to operate the machine. The Special Communicable Diseases Unit (SCDU) at Emory University utilized two to three nurses to staff the Unit at all times when occupied, and it was recommended that nurses remove ("doff") PPE every 4 h to allow for personal needs and a break. At the highest level of PPE and patient care, three nurses were working in the SCDU at one time, in 12-h shifts. They rotated in 4-h shifts between the patient room, the anteroom, and the nursing desk with each having designated responsibilities [20].

Within each treatment facility, there are unique circumstances which will dictate the most efficient and safe nursing staffing practices. It is important to consider both staff safety and patient safety when determining which guidelines will be used to operate a unit caring for patients with VHF or other highly hazardous communicable infectious disease. Nurses that join these teams must be individuals able to operate outside their normal routine by utilizing critical thinking skills, flexibility, and autonomy. These nurses are required to take responsibility for a wide array of clinical and nonclinical tasks and perform these in demanding clinical situations, which are skills that require practice, exceptional communication, and teamwork.

Staffing: Physicians

Caring for patients with highly hazardous communicable diseases is a true multidisciplinary effort, and choosing and maintaining an effective physician team illustrates this concept well. Each center should tailor their physician team to fit their needs and the culture of the facility. In general, Infectious Diseases specialists have often led physician teams in the biocontainment setting; however this may not be appropriate in every facility. Infectious Diseases specialists monitor and manage infectious complications and coinfections and oversee the administration of antimicrobial agents, including experimental products. Specialists in Critical Care medicine are an important asset in the care of patients with VHF, since some of these patients may have critical illness and require ICU-level care, including mechanical ventilation, vasopressors, and other supportive care measures [25]. Since invasive procedures are often necessary as well, it is critical to ensure that the physician team includes individuals who are experienced and comfortable performing these procedures. This skillset should be assessed by direct consultation with these physicians, since some may not feel comfortable performing invasive procedures in a high-risk isolation environment. Training and drills involving critically ill patients, including performing invasive procedures in PPE, are an integral part of skill assessment and maintenance for the physician team.

It is also important to involve other groups of physicians who may be needed in the care of a patient with VHF. Pediatricians and Pediatric Intensive Care specialists should be identified in the event that a pediatric patient must be cared for under HLCC conditions. Similarly, obstetricians are an important part of the physician team since it is possible that a pregnant and/or laboring patient with suspected or confirmed VHF will need care in the isolation setting. Nephrology specialists have been involved in the care of patients with VHF who developed renal failure, especially those who required dialysis [26]. Relationships with other physician groups, including but not limited to Surgery, Emergency Medicine, General Internal Medicine, and Pathology, should be established as necessary in case consultative needs arise. It is important to note that some physician consultations can occur via telemedicine without the physician entering the patient care room. This serves to limit the number of physicians required to directly evaluate the patient at the bedside in order to decrease the possibility of exposure.

When considering physician staffing models, it is important to note that physicians providing care to patients with EVD or other VHF in the biocontainment setting may be unavailable for prolonged periods of time. This makes the ability to provide clinical care to other patients very difficult. Thus it is important to consider backfilling other clinical responsibilities in order to provide dedicated time to the complex processes of donning and doffing PPE, performing procedures, and other aspects of biocontainment care. The most appropriate way to provide 24-h on-call coverage for patients with VHF must be evaluated, and this will vary depending on the current call structure in the medical facility [27].

The involvement of physicians in training (fellows, residents, etc.) in the care of patients with VHF in the biocontainment setting has been discussed, and generally it is felt that trainees should not be compelled to provide direct care for patients with VHF as a requirement of a clinical rotation due to excessive risk. However, physicians in training have entered the biocontainment setting on a volunteer basis to observe and assist in the management of patients with VHF via the telemedicine system, which provides educational opportunity without excessive risk.

Personal Protective Equipment (PPE)

The use of PPE in clinical care to prevent the transmission of infectious diseases is not a new concept, yet in the context of viral hemorrhagic fever, PPE became the topic of much debate during the 2014–2016 EVD outbreak. Facilities who were tasked with providing care to infected individuals with EVD faced multifaceted challenges related to the selection, procurement, and proper utilization of PPE, along with changing guidelines.

Personal protective equipment is worn to minimize exposure to infectious material and to protect the skin and mucous membranes from exposure to pathogens. PPE reduces, but does not eliminate, the risk of skin and clothing contamination with pathogens among healthcare personnel [28]. Examples of PPE include items such as gowns, gloves, foot and eye protection, respirators, and full body suits. The Occupational Safety and Health Administration (OSHA) requires that employers protect their employees from workplace hazards that might cause injury. Controlling a hazard at its source is the best way to protect employees. Depending on the hazard or workplace conditions, OSHA recommends the use of engineering or work practice controls to manage or eliminate hazards to the greatest extent possible [29]. Installing negative pressure air handlers to place a barrier between the hazard and the employees is an engineering con-

trol; changing the way in which employees perform their work is a work practice control. When engineering, work practice, and administrative controls are not feasible or provide insufficient protection, PPE must be utilized to protect healthcare workers who are providing care to patients with infectious diseases.

There are many variations of PPE available for purchase, and selecting the best version for the environment in which care must be delivered can be daunting. The versions of PPE used in HLCC units differed in the individual pieces used; however, the guiding principles remained the same. For healthcare workers caring for patients with EVD, PPE that fully covers skin and clothing and prevents any exposure of the eyes, nose, and mouth is recommended to reduce the risk of accidental self-contamination of mucous membranes or broken skin [30]. Varying levels of PPE are appropriate for use based upon the acuity of the patient, the volume of infectious bodily fluids (blood, vomitus, diarrheal stool) present, and the potential for aerosolization of these fluids [31]. Providing this level of protection often requires that many pieces of PPE be worn; this can lead to an increased risk of fatigue and overheating.

Centers in the United States that treated patients with EVD in 2014 utilized varying levels of PPE based on this stratified risk assessment [20, 23, 31]. In the Nebraska Biocontainment Unit (NBU), the first level of PPE used completely disposable, and the second level incorporated the use of a powered air-purifying respirator (PAPR). First-level PPE consisted of fluid-impervious Association for the Advancement of Medical Instrumentation (AAMI) level 4 gown, N95 respirator, surgical hood, face shield, knee-high fluid-impervious boots, three pairs of gloves, and the addition of a second splash-resistant apron as needed (Fig. 21.1). The second level of PPE consisted of fluid-impervious coveralls, inner boot liners, outer boot covers, three pairs of gloves, and the PAPR hood with accompanying belt and blower motor. In the Emory University Special Communicable Diseases Unit (SCDU), varying levels of PPE based upon the risk assessment consisted of a completely disposable ensemble as well as a PAPR ensemble. The disposable PPE included a coverall, apron, booties, double gloves, face shield (goggles if face shield is not available), and a surgical mask. The PAPR level of PPE was comprised of a coverall, double gloves, booties, an apron, and the PAPR hood [20] (Fig. 21.2). The equipment available for purchase through each institution may have differed; however, making selections based upon disease transmission and risk factors related to patient care rather than brand-specific products helped to ensure healthcare worker protection.

The donning and doffing procedures require both vigilance and attention to detail. While PPE is effective at decreasing exposure to infected bodily fluids among healthcare workers, these healthcare workers are still at risk if this

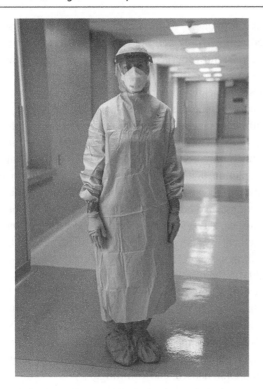

Fig. 21.1 First-level PPE worn in the Nebraska Biocontainment Unit (NBU) while caring for patients with Ebola in 2014

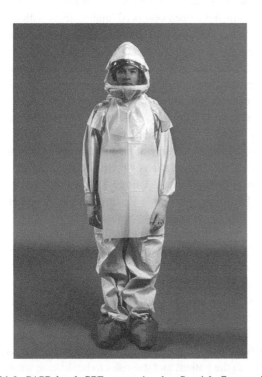

Fig. 21.2 PAPR-level PPE worn in the Special Communicable Diseases Unit (SCDU) while caring for patients with Ebola in 2014

equipment is not removed in a manner that prevents exposure [32]. Detailed guidance with the correct order of donning and doffing equipment should be readily visible on

a chart posted within the patient care area. The process used to don and doff PPE should be followed exactly by all personnel every time it is performed and should be guided by a checklist. All staff members, regardless of title or position, are expected to hold one another accountable for adhering to the policies and procedures, including the appropriate use of PPE [22, 33, 34]. The donning and doffing process should incorporate the use of a donning partner who assists the healthcare worker in appropriate placement of PPE and a doffing partner who assists the healthcare worker in removing their PPE. This doffing partner helps to ensure that all steps in the process are completed in the proper order and technique. The physical exhaustion and emotional fatigue that can accompany the provision of care for patients infected with VHF may further increase the chance of an inadvertent exposure to bodily fluids on the outside of the PPE when performing the doffing process [32]. The CDC also recommends the presence of a trained observer when performing the doffing process [30]. The trained observer is available to provide immediate feedback if there is any inadvertent contamination of the healthcare worker. The doffing process can be complex and is considered to be a vulnerable area in which the healthcare providers may be inadvertently contaminated. Simulation studies conducted using donning and doffing scenarios have shown high rates of self-contamination during the doffing process, especially during the removal of the gown and gloves, emphasizing the need for stringent protocols and supervision during this process [28].

Transportation

The safe transport and prehospital care of patients with EVD or other highly hazardous communicable diseases require enhanced infection control practices, which necessitate sound administrative policies, work practices, and environmental controls implemented through focused education, training, and supervision [35]. HLCC hospitals require partner emergency medical services (EMS) capable of ensuring the safety of the HLCC transport medics and the public through implementation of infection control practices, policies, and procedures [9].

The ambulance environment is defined by confined space with limited air handling, and care is provided with reusable medical devices in acute situations. Emergency vehicles have many compartments, shelves, patient care beds, and other high-touch areas that are difficult to clean. Ambulance cleaning protocols have been established, but environmental contamination with nosocomial organisms continues to be documented [36–38].

A variety of specialized approaches have been established for HLCC transport. These include specialized truck and trailer ambulances (used in Germany), HEPA-filtered ground ambulance positioned aboard a Hercules C130 aircraft (Sweden), road ambulances with stretcher-based isolators (Italy), and road ambulances draped to minimize contamination potential (United States) [39, 40]. HLCC transport medics should receive enhanced education and training on modes of transmission, the availability of vaccines, pre- and postexposure prophylaxis, and treatment modalities. Competency-based training has also been recommended to develop and maintain PPE donning and doffing competency [32, 35, 41]. The transporting HLCC ambulance is commonly supported by an external transport team with extra supplies that facilitates communication with external support agencies (which may include law enforcement, airport operations, public health, and emergency management) and provides guidance for clinical decision-making when required [35, 39]. Transition of the patient from the HLCC transport team to the HLCC unit team should be a highly scripted event, rigorously tested through planning and exercise [35].

Following transition of care, the emergency vehicle should be decontaminated. HLCC facilities have utilized different decontamination methods; however the general principles of surface cleaning performed by personnel in PPE followed by appropriate waste disposal are maintained. Vaporized hydrogen peroxide, chlorine dioxide, and ultraviolet light have all been used or proposed as adjunct decontamination strategies for emergency vehicles [40, 42, 43].

Clinical Care

The clinical care of patients with VHF is largely supportive, and the ability to provide supportive care varies depending on the capabilities of the individual healthcare facility. Generally, healthcare centers caring for patients with VHF should be ready to provide general supportive care and additional aggressive intensive care modalities when necessary and available. Up until recently, little information regarding these care modalities was available given that outbreaks of VHF occurred in resource-limited settings. However during the 2014–2016 EVD outbreak, patients who were managed in resourced settings in the United States and Europe where aggressive supportive care was available had a much lower mortality rate when compared with that noted in previous reports from Africa [44].

The clinical presentation of VHF may vary according to the etiology, the wide range of clinical severity, and multiple patient factors. It is important to note that the clinical presentation of VHF is non-specific; therefore it is important to evaluate patients with possible and confirmed VHF for other causes of symptoms, notably including malaria if the patient has a history of travel to an endemic area.

The delivery of aggressive supportive care requires intravenous access, and the availability of this depends on the resource limitations of the healthcare facility. In resource-limited settings, only peripheral IV placement may be feasible, whereas in resourced settings, central venous catheters (CVCs) are generally utilized. The placement of a CVC also enables healthcare workers to obtain blood samples without repeated venipuncture, reducing the risk of sharps injuries.

Antipyretic agents have been utilized to manage fever in patients with VHF. Oral rehydration solutions and/or intravenous fluids may become necessary given the profound volume depletion that can result from vomiting and diarrhea. Pharmacologic controls such as antiemetic and antidiarrheal medications have been utilized to control nausea, vomiting, and diarrhea. Physical controls such as emesis bags and fecal management systems have been employed as well, since controlling these secretions is an important infection control modality in the healthcare setting.

The monitoring and replacement of electrolytes is also an important aspect of supportive care in patients with VHF, since significant electrolyte disturbances have been observed [45]. Nutritional support is often necessary, and when available, total parenteral nutrition has been utilized in patients with anorexia, nausea, and vomiting.

Patients with respiratory symptoms may require supplemental oxygen. Bleeding complications can be treated with blood products and correction of coagulopathy. Cases of encephalitis have been observed, and patients with agitation may require sedating medications. Patients with VHF may also develop secondary infectious complications including bacterial sepsis, and these infections may be managed with antimicrobial therapy, which is often empiric since the availability of blood cultures is limited [46].

Patients with VHF may present with, or may progress to, critical illness involving multi-organ failure and may require advanced life support including mechanical ventilation and dialysis. These interventions were utilized during the care of patients with EVD in the United States and Europe during the 2014–2016 outbreak [44]. In patients with respiratory failure, airway management was accomplished via intubation by rapid sequence induction and video laryngoscopy [27, 47]. Renal failure was managed with continuous renal replacement therapy (CRRT) in some centers. Vasopressors have been utilized for blood pressure support in patients with VHF. An assessment of the use of other advanced cardiac life support measures like cardioversion and chest compressions should be discussed by healthcare facilities preparing to care for patients with VHF, with consideration of the potential benefits to the patient and the risks to healthcare workers.

There are currently no FDA-approved therapeutic agents available for the treatment of Ebola or Marburg virus disease, although many experimental drugs were used in the treatment of patients with EVD during the 2014–2016 outbreak. Since most of the use of these agents was employed in individuals and very small groups of patients, no definite conclusions can be made regarding efficacy. Nonrandomized single-arm trials were conducted in Africa evaluating certain therapeutics; however one was unable to reach any conclusions on the potential benefit of the viral RNA polymerase inhibitor favipiravir, and another evaluating the small interfering RNAs product TKM-130803 did not demonstrate improvement in survival [48, 49]. A randomized trial involving the triple monoclonal antibody cocktail ZMapp was conducted, but although the estimated effect appeared beneficial, the result did not meet the statistical threshold for efficacy [50]. Similarly, convalescent serum has been used in the management of patients with EVD; however one study did not demonstrate a significant improvement in survival in patients administered convalescent plasma [51]. Ribavarin has been shown to be effective in treatment of Lassa fever [52].

The hospital discharge of patients with VHF is a complicated process and is dependent on many factors, including resolution or significant improvement of symptoms along with correlative virologic laboratory data. Consultation with local and state health authorities and the CDC and/or WHO should occur to determine the recommended disease-specific discharge criteria for patients with VHF.

Laboratory Support

The monitoring of laboratory parameters is a vital part of providing supportive care to patients with VHF, since these patients may have significant laboratory abnormalities on which clinical management is based. This is especially important in patients who are critically ill who require interventions like dialysis where laboratory parameters must be evaluated frequently and closely monitored. The ability to perform laboratory testing in a safe and effective manner requires significant planning prior to implementation.

As a first step, the clinical care team should discuss which laboratory studies are necessary in order to care for the patient with VHF. This potential testing menu should be communicated to laboratory leadership, who should assess each test to determine if the sample can be processed safely. It is essential that the clinical care team have access to a menu of available laboratory tests and detailed information on the collection of specimens, including any special media required or recommended collection times.

Determining the location of the laboratory should take into account the capabilities of the facility. If feasible, laboratory testing should be performed in close proximity to the site of clinical care to eliminate the need for specimen transport, thereby increasing safety and decreasing turnaround time [19, 53]. Point-of-care testing is desirable but is often not comprehensive, and additional testing may need to occur in the core laboratory or a special containment laboratory. It is important

to note that some special containment laboratories may not have the equipment necessary to perform routine laboratory studies such as complete blood counts or metabolic panels, so these tests may need to be performed in the core laboratory if point-of-care testing is not available. A careful risk assessment should occur prior to implementation of any testing in order to minimize risk to the instruments and most importantly the laboratory staff [17].

Viral load monitoring is helpful in patients with VHF, as the degree of viremia may predict the initial severity of disease and provide information on progression of disease during the treatment phase. The viral load is generally a component of discharge criteria as well [54, 55]. The transport of samples to the appropriate reference laboratory for viral load testing is a complicated process, and significant preplanning is necessary in order to facilitate this.

Waste Management

The importance of stringent infection prevention and control, including environmental infection control, is heightened when providing HLCC for patients with VHF due to factors such as low infectious dose and potentially large volume of body fluids containing high concentrations of viral particles. These elements contribute to the significant yet manageable hazards posed by such care. Perspectives and waste management strategies of two HLCC facilities have been reported [16]. Robust packaging and disinfection procedures were employed by these two facilities in order to process EVD-associated solid and liquid patient waste, contaminated patient linens, healthcare worker PPE and linens, contaminated medical devices, and other general medical waste.

Waste, linens, medical equipment, and other items potentially contaminated with pathogens such as Ebola, Lassa, Marburg, and select other VHFs are categorized as Category A Infectious Substances through the United Nations and US Department of Transportation's Hazardous Materials Regulations [56]. Category A Infectious Substances require enhanced packaging and labeling along with security plans in preparation for transport [57]. Materials that are sterilized by autoclaving or incineration are not required to be packaged and shipped as Category A Infectious Substances.

The quantity of waste generated through HLCC is significant with reports of over 1,000 lb of waste generated per patient [58]. Management of such large quantities of infectious waste requires scalable strategies for packaging, storage, and security. Solid waste disposal strategies include autoclaving and incineration. It is important to maintain autoclave validation logs to ensure appropriate function. Several strategies have been employed for the transport of waste from the patient care room, including double bagging of waste and wiping the outside of the bag with bleach prior to transport. Storage in waste-holding containers may be necessary while awaiting transport to the autoclave or incinerator. According to current recommendations, liquid waste can be safely disposed of in the sewer system. However, during the 2014–2016 Ebola outbreak, some facilities utilized pretreatment strategies with a hospital-grade disinfectant prior to disposal of liquid waste [16]. Fluid solidifiers were also used at some facilities in order to dispose of liquid waste into the solid waste stream. Waste should only be handled by trained individuals in full PPE [59].

Environmental cleaning during and after the care of patients with VHF is an important part of protecting healthcare workers, as well as other patients in the facility by maintaining the highest infection control standards. Environmental cleaning for many VHFs, including Ebola, should only be performed by trained individuals, and full PPE should be worn at all times during this process. Daily cleaning of HLCC facilities generally consists of surface cleaning with an EPA-registered disinfectant approved for use against non-enveloped viruses [60]. The terminal cleaning process varies by facility but generally consists of disposal of waste followed by surface cleaning with a hospital-grade disinfectant and disinfection of medical equipment. Some facilities utilize a final decontamination step involving ultraviolet germicidal irradiation or vaporized hydrogen peroxide [16, 61]. This process should be monitored and documented by a trained infection control expert to ensure compliance with all procedures.

Care of the Deceased

The remains of a patient with Ebola virus disease (EVD) are considered highly infectious. It is important to remember that although the patient is deceased, the viral load may remain very high, and body fluids may remain infectious for an extended period of time postmortem [62]. There is significant risk for those who are handling the body if proper procedures and barriers are not employed. Preparing the body for transportation to the mortuary must be done by trained staff in the patient care room as close to the time of death as possible [63].

When providing care for the deceased in the United States, it is most likely that these patients will be in a hospital setting and more stringent controls can be implemented. In addition to federal laws and guidelines that apply to mortuary workers, mortuary practices may also be subject to a variety of state, tribal, territorial, and local regulations. CDC recommends close collaboration with public health officials in the state or local jurisdiction, as well as with the licensed funeral director who has agreed to accept the bagged remains, to safely implement each step of the process [63]. The presence of a memorandum of understanding (MOU) with key ancillary partners can facilitate safe and timely transfer of the remains of deceased patients. It is beneficial for any institution that may provide care for patients with VHF to have an MOU in place with a local mortuary service, crematorium, or cemetery.

The highly infectious nature of the remains of a deceased victim of EVD demands the use of increased protection for the healthcare worker. The recommended PPE for handling such remains includes a powered air-purifying respirator (PAPR), fluid-impervious coveralls, double gloves, and use of an outer apron [64]. Adequate staffing during the care of the deceased is essential for safe execution of the procedures. The patient remains are first prepared and packaged within the patient room (hot zone) and transferred out into the hallway or anteroom (warm zone) and out of the patient care area (cold zone) for transport to final disposition [65]. The body of the deceased should not be washed or embalmed, medical devices should remain in place, and healthcare workers should not attempt to remove them. Autopsies should not be performed unless specifically directed by the state health department and only after consultation with the CDC and state health department officials [63]. Patient remains should be securely contained within the patient care area. The remains should be packaged using established guidance, which currently includes the use of multiple layers [63]. The first layer to form a protective barrier is a standard hospital issued mortuary bag, followed by a heat sealable chlorine-free material, and final securement is achieved by the use of a heavy duty morgue bag. Each protective barrier that is added should be thoroughly disinfected before moving to the next step and again before being transported out of the hot zone. The patient remains should be transferred out of the hot zone with special attention paid to minimizing the cross contamination of zones.

When the remains have been safely processed out of the patient care area, the transport team will assume care of the deceased. The composition of the transport team will vary; however it is important to consider state requirements for chain of custody when developing protocols. Personnel serving on the transport team may include the servicing mortuary staff, state medical examiner, healthcare worker or leadership staff, and law enforcement personnel. Cremation is recommended [63]. Upon completion of cremation, the ashes may be returned to the family of the deceased as the risk of transmission of infection is no longer present [63]. When providing care for the deceased patient, the utmost level of dignity and respect for the deceased patient and his/her family should be maintained.

Evaluation of Persons Under Investigation (PUI)

During the 2014–2016 Ebola outbreak, many healthcare facilities were faced with caring for patients who presented with symptoms compatible with EVD and met certain epidemiologic criteria as defined by the CDC [66, 67]. These patients were termed "persons under investigation."

In order to properly address quick isolation and care of persons under investigation for EVD or other VHF, a travel and symptom triage tool is needed at check in areas within the healthcare environment. The tool can be a paper instrument with simple questions related to travel history and symptoms. Alternatively, a more robust tool can be built within the electronic health record (EHR) to assess travel history, identifying specific countries and providing decision support prompts that then are matched up with presenting symptoms and correlated with CDC case definitions. Alerts then appear within the EHR to notify caregivers of additional precautions required (e.g., give patient mask to wear, notify Infectious Diseases experts, isolate patient in a negative pressure room, etc.). Whatever tool is used, it must be agile and quickly adapted to meet ever-changing emerging pathogen threats.

Once a patient screens positive for travel history and symptoms matching the CDC case definition, a process map can be used to provide step-by-step guidance to healthcare providers using a standardized approach. A protocol should be created for the Emergency Department, as well as for other ambulatory locations (outpatient clinics, radiology, etc.) where patients may present with symptoms. A positive screen result for epidemiologic risk and signs or symptoms consistent with viral hemorrhagic fever should trigger escalating personal protective equipment use and movement to a designated isolation area. The choice of isolation area is determined by each individual facility. A predetermined area within the Emergency Department can be utilized since this is often the point of entry for patients [68]. Notification of appropriate personnel should then occur, including Infection Control professionals, area leadership, a designated Infectious Diseases physician, public health officials, and the laboratory.

Once the patient is isolated, security should be summoned to control the area and to maintain a log of staff entering the isolation zone. Staff in PPE then perform an initial assessment of the patient and obtain additional details and history, including confirmation of epidemiologic history. Specialists may be called in to assess the patient as well, or alternatively this may be accomplished via video technology in an effort to limit the number of individuals who enter the room. Once the exam is completed, a consultation with local public health and CDC should be conducted, and testing requirements should be determined. It is important to ensure that the appropriate collection methods are utilized; these should be clarified with the public health laboratory prior to specimen collection [69].

A PUI may require imaging studies. Bedside studies are preferred from an infection control perspective but are not comprehensive, and additional studies that cannot be per-

formed at the bedside may be necessary. Robust predefined plans for patient transport to cardiac catheterization, CT, MRI, and endoscopy should be developed. In addition, a PUI may require surgical intervention. A predefined plan should be created, which outlines the preoperative timeout briefing, intraoperative care considerations to include type of PPE to be used by the surgical team, instrument handling and care, recovery of patient in the operating room, and subsequent cleaning and disinfection of the space, instruments, and waste management [70]. Although there are no formal guidelines for the management of patients with suspected VHF in the operating room, there is information available from the American College of Surgeons, who recommends against elective surgical procedures but states that emergency operations can be considered [71]. Development of these processes along with defined drills involving the operating room staff will enhance the capability to successfully navigate through care of PUIs in need of surgical care.

Special Populations

Children differ from adults in myriad ways which potentially impact their vulnerability to the viral hemorrhagic fevers and present challenging management issues. Developmentally, children are likely to be frightened by the sight of caregivers in PPE and may flail, tug, and pull at such equipment, creating additional risk for these caregivers. Similarly, young children are unable to cooperate with their management, and the usual pediatric paradigm of family-centered care, which would enlist parents in assisting with such care, may be prohibitively hazardous in the setting of transmissible VHF such as Ebola, Marburg, or Lassa.

From a policy perspective, multiple factors complicate the care of children. Certain medications that might be used in adults are contraindicated in children, are unavailable in liquid preparations, or are unfamiliar to pediatric practitioners. Similarly, the use of investigational drugs may be more problematic in children. Finally, pediatric-specific equipment, doctrine, and HLCC beds are often lacking.

Despite these apparent disadvantages, children have been consistently underrepresented among Ebola victims. In the 1995 Kikwit outbreak, children accounted for 27 of the 315 cases (9%), despite constituting 50% of the Zairean population [72]. Similar findings were obtained during the 2000 outbreak in Gulu, Uganda, where children represented 20 of the 218 cases (9%) [73]. Moreover, these children had a case fatality rate of 40%, not dissimilar to the rate among adults. Finally, in a study performed in Guinea during the 2014–2016 outbreak, 147 of 823 cases (18%) occurred in children, again despite the fact that children constitute 50% of the population of Guinea [74]. While these findings raise the possibility that children may be less susceptible to infection with Ebola (and, perhaps, with other VHFs), it is likely that this diminished susceptibility derives mainly from social factors; young children are less likely to function as primary caregivers to dying family members, are thus less likely to have contact with body fluids, and are less likely to participate in intimate funereal preparations.

Management of the pregnant or laboring patient with VHF is similarly problematic; maternal and infant mortality are extraordinarily high in virtually all of the VHFs, although maternal survival has been reported following fetal loss associated with Ebola infection and uterine evacuation has been shown to improve survival of pregnant women with Lassa fever [75, 76]. Fetal and neonatal loss among women with Lassa fever has been reported to be as high as 87%, and there are no reports of neonates born to Ebola-infected mothers surviving beyond 19 days [76, 77]. Vertical transmission of yellow fever appears to occur very rarely, and few reports of affected pregnant women exist for the remaining VHFs [78]. In light of this paucity of information, it is difficult to make specific recommendations for the management of the pregnant woman with VHF. Nonetheless, meticulous planning must be undertaken by facilities that might be called upon to care for pregnant VHF patients. Such planning should address, among others, questions regarding where and when delivery should occur, what equipment is required, and how complications like bleeding should be managed.

This final question that raises, perhaps, the most vexing issue associated with the care of newborns and children with contagious VHFs is under what circumstances might parents or other nonmedical caregivers be permitted to remain at the beside of an infected child. Parents might assist in reducing the anxious flailing of a toddler, thereby diminishing risk to HCWs. They are also afforded the opportunity to participate in family-centered care, thus emotionally benefitting both parent and child. These considerations must be balanced, however, against the reality that parents then become, in a sense, additional patients, requiring assistance in donning and doffing PPE and running the risk of inadvertent breaks in containment by non-skilled individuals. An expert panel recently met to discuss these considerations, although the subject is likely to remain controversial [79].

Maintenance of Preparedness

Training healthcare workers in the provision of care to patients with VHF presents many challenges. One of the challenges involves maintaining readiness and keeping team members engaged when these specialized patient care areas are not activated. The implementation of a consistent and structured training schedule facilitates staff engagement by incorporating activities of varying intensity. Incorporating complex functional exercises, tabletop exercises, skill-focused drills, competency evaluations, and team-building activities builds a strong foundation from which the patient care team can further develop. Educational sessions on emerging infectious diseases may also be helpful to maintain readiness and interest. Developing an annual training calendar that is available to team members in advance sets the expectation for the team members and also helps to minimize scheduling conflicts for required attendance. Bringing healthcare workers together to train regularly enables the formation of a cohesive functional team rather than a collection of individuals.

When considering the provision of intensive care to patients with EVD, the challenges are heightened. These patients often require invasive interventions which involve the skills of anesthesiologists and critical care physicians, as well as nurses proficient in managing the ongoing care of critically ill patients. The interventions must be implemented while wearing advanced levels of PPE, thus potentially limiting the dexterity of the providers. Training regimens for healthcare workers should allow for the development and refinement of specific policies and procedures, addressing critical issues like donning and doffing PPE, waste processing, the insertion of central venous catheters, endotracheal intubation, the use of continuous renal replacement therapy, Advanced Cardiac Life Support (ACLS) and Pediatric Advanced Life Support (PALS) plans and protocols, and the plan for extraction and provision of care for a provider who has a medical emergency in the patient care area. Providing routine training for key personnel ensures the opportunity for healthcare workers to gain confidence in their ability to perform the procedures, as well as to build a firm foundation of processes for many aspects of care [22]. Developing and exercising detailed policies to guide cares within the unit, as well as maintaining an expert staff, are key components to maintaining preparedness.

Training ensures that healthcare workers are knowledgeable and proficient in donning and doffing PPE before caring for a patient with VHF. Comfort and proficiency when donning and doffing are only achieved by repeatedly practicing correct use of PPE. When providing training and assessing competency in PPE, healthcare workers should perform required duties while wearing PPE. This could include inserting an intravenous device, assisting with perineal care after an incontinent episode, processing waste in the patient care area, or charting an assessment. Training should be customized for the intended audience and effectively relay essential information. Healthcare workers who are unwilling or unable to fulfill these requirements should not be included in the patient care team.

With regard to maintenance of skills, it is imperative that a culture of safety be fostered within the care team, where the focus is on effective teamwork to accomplish the goal of safe, high-quality patient care [80]. All staff must feel empowered to identify and take action to prevent errors from occurring and to improve the patient care environment. This sense of empowerment can be developed during routine training and preparedness exercises in preparation for the reality of patient care.

Conclusions and Future Directions

The provision of care for patients with EVD or other VHF is a complex process necessitating that close attention be paid to multiple infection control modalities. Engineering and facility controls such as negatively pressurized rooms within designated care areas are ideal; however the most important assets needed to provide safe and effective care for patients with VHF or other highly hazardous communicable diseases are a trained team and a collection of well-developed and practiced protocols.

In order to increase preparedness for highly hazardous communicable diseases in the United States following the Ebola outbreak of 2014–2016, the CDC and Department of Health and Human Services (DHHS) developed a three-tiered system to screen and manage patients with suspected or confirmed EVD. Under this system, facilities with high-level containment care capability are designated as "Ebola Treatment Centers" (ETC). As of this writing, approximately 55 such centers have applied for designation and funding; among them are ten designated as regional referral centers by DHHS (one in each of its ten geographic regions) [81]. In addition, other hospitals would be designated as "Ebola Assessment Hospitals" (EAH), able to manage and isolate persons under investigation (PUI) until a diagnosis of Ebola virus disease (EVD) can be confirmed or refuted. Finally, remaining hospitals ("Frontline Facilities") would receive training in order to improve their ability to isolate potential Ebola victims until they could be transferred to an EAH or ETC. Within this network, the provision of patient care can be optimized, protocols practiced and improved, and research on investigational drugs and products streamlined. Although this system represents a vast improvement in hospital preparedness in the United States, isolation bed capacity remains limited [82].

The US Department of Health and Human Services, the Assistant Secretary for Preparedness and Response (ASPR), the Centers for Disease Control and Prevention (CDC), and Emory University, Nebraska Medicine, and Bellevue Hospital Center comprise the National Ebola Training and Education Center (NETEC) [83]. Initiated in 2015, the NETEC program supports the education and training of healthcare facilities in order to enhance preparedness for Ebola and other highly infectious diseases. Although there remains a significant amount of education and work to be done in this area, this collaborative effort, along with the tiered network of hospitals, represents a significant improvement in preparedness.

References

1. Centers for Disease Control and Prevention. http://www.cdc.gov/vhf/ebola/outbreaks/2014-west-africa/index.html. (n.d.). Accessed 2 June 2016.
2. Crawford DH. The invisible enemy: a natural history of viruses. Oxford: Oxford University Press; 2000.
3. Hill EE, McKee KT. Isolation and biocontainment of patients with highly hazardous infectious diseases. J Army Med Dept. 1991;PB8-91-1/2:10–4.
4. Cieslak TJ, Christopher GW, Eitzen EM. The "slammer": isolation and biocontainment of patients exposed to biosafety level 4 pathogens. Clin Infect Dis. 1999;29:1083.
5. Kortepeter MG, Martin JW, Rusnak JM, Cieslak TJ, Warfield KL, Anderson EL, Ranadive MV. Managing potential laboratory exposure to Ebola virus by using a patient biocontainment care unit. Emerg Infect Dis. 2008;14:881–7.
6. Reynolds G. Why were doctors afraid to treat Rebecca McLester? New York Times, April 18, 2004. (n.d.)
7. Smith PW, Anderson AO, Christopher GW, Cieslak TJ, Devreede GJ, et al. Designing a biocontainment unit to care for patients with serious communicable diseases: a consensus statement. Biosecur Bioterror. 2006;4:351–65.
8. Risi GF, Bloom ME, Hoe HP, Arminio T, Carlson P, et al. Preparing a community hospital to manage work-related exposures to infectious agents in biosafety level 3 and 4 laboratories. Emerg Infect Dis. 2010;16:373–8.
9. Bannister B, Puro V, Fusco FM, Heptonstall J, Ippolito G. Framework for the design and operation of high-level isolation units: consensus of the European Network of Infectious Diseases. Lancet Infect Dis. 2009;9:45–56.
10. Brouqui P, Puro V, Fusco FM, et al. Infection control in the management of highly pathogenic infectious diseases: consensus of the European Network of Infectious Diseases. Lancet Infect Dis. 2009;9:301–11.
11. Kahn J. The SARS epidemic: treatment; Beijing hurries to build hospital complex for increasing number of SARS patients. New York Times, 27 April 2003. (n.d.)
12. McNeill JR. Yellow Jack and geopolitics: environment, epidemics, and the struggles for empire in the American tropics, 1650–1825. OAH Mag Hist. 2004;18:9–13.
13. US Department of Health and Human Services. Biosafety in microbiological and biomedical laboratories, 5th ed. 2009.
14. Siegel JD, Rhinehart E, Jackson M, Chiarello L. 2007 guideline for isolation precautions: preventing transmission of infectious agents in health care settings. Am J Infect Control. 2007;35(10):S65–S164.
15. Facility Guidelines Institute. Guidelines for design and construction of hospitals and outpatient facilities. American Hospital Association; 2014.
16. Lowe JJ, Olinger PL, Gibbs SG, et al. Environmental infection control considerations for Ebola. Am J Infect Control. 2015;43(7):747.
17. Iwen PC, Smith PW, Hewlett AL, et al. Safety considerations in the laboratory testing of specimens suspected or known to contain Ebola virus. Am J Clin Pathol. 2015;143(1):4–5.
18. Brouqui P. Facing highly infectious diseases: new trends and current concepts. Clin Microbiol Infect. 2009;15(8):700–5.

19. Smith PW, Boulter KC, Hewlett AL, et al. Planning and response to Ebola virus disease: an integrated approach. Am J Infect Control. 2015;43:441–6.

20. Emory Healthcare. Emory Healthcare Ebola preparedness protocols. http://www.emoryhealthcare.org/ebola-protocol/pdf/ehc-evd-protocols.pdf. (n.d.). Accessed 7 June 2016.

21. Hewlett A, Varkey J, Smith P, Ribner B. Ebola virus disease: preparedness and infection control lessons learned from two biocontainment units. Curr Opin Infect Dis. 2015;28(4):343–8.

22. Vasa A, Schwedhelm M, Johnson D. Critical care for the patient with Ebola virus disease: the Nebraska perspective. J Intensive Crit Care. 2015;1(8):1–5.

23. Nebraska Biocontainment Unit. The Nebraska biocontainment unit policies and procedures. Available from http://netec.org/resources/nbu-policies/. (n.d.). Accessed 10 Mar 2016.

24. Loftus M. Surviving Ebola. Emory medicine. http://emorymedicin-emagazine.emory.edu/issues/2014/fall/features/surviving-ebola/. (n.d.). Accessed 10 Mar 2016.

25. Decker BK, Sevransky JE, Barrett K, Davey RT, Chertow DS. Preparing for critical care services to patients with Ebola. Ann Intern Med. 2014;161:831–2.

26. Connor MJ, Kraft C, Mehta AK, et al. Successful delivery of RRT in Ebola virus disease. J Am Soc Nephrol. 2015;26:31–7.

27. Johnson DW, Sullivan JN, Piquette CA, et al. Lessons learned: critical care management of patients with Ebola in the United States. Crit Care Med. 2015;43:1157–64.

28. Tomas M, Kundrapu S, Thota P, et al. Contamination of health care personnel during removal of personal protective equipment. JAMA Intern Med. 2015;175(12):1904–10.

29. United States Department of Labor-Occupational Safety and Health Administration. OSHA 3151-12R. https://www.osha.gov/Publications/osha3151.html. (n.d.). Accessed 10 Mar 2016.

30. Centers for Disease Control and Prevention. Guidance on Personal Protective Equipment (PPE) to be used by healthcare workers during management of patients with confirmed Ebola or Persons under Investigation (PUIs) for Ebola who are clinically unstable or have bleeding, vomiting, or diarrhea in U.S. hospitals, including procedures for donning and doffing PPE. (2015). http://www.cdc.gov/vhf/ebola/healthcare-us/ppe/guidance.html. Accessed 10 Mar 2016.

31. Beam EL, Schwedhelm S, Boulter KC, et al. Personal protective equipment processes and rationale for the Nebraska biocontainment unit during the 2014 activations for Ebola virus disease. Am J Infect Control. 2016;44:340–2.

32. Fischer W, Hynes N, Perl T. Protecting healthcare workers from Ebola: personal protective equipment is critical but not enough. Ann Intern Med. 2014;161(10):753–4.

33. Beam E, Gibbs SG, Hewlett AL, Iwen PC, Nuss SL, Smith PW. Clinical challenges in isolation care. Am J Nurs. 2015;115(4):44–9.

34. Jelden K, Smith P, Schwedhelm S, et al. Learning from Ebola: interprofessional practice in the Nebraska biocontainment unit. J Interprofessional Educ Pract. 2015;1(3–4):97–9.

35. Isakov A, Miles W, Gibbs S, Lowe J, Jamison A, Swansiger R. Transport and management of patients with confirmed or suspected Ebola virus disease. Ann Emerg Med. 2015;66(3):297–305.

36. Alves DW, Bissell RA. Bacterial pathogens in ambulances: results of unannounced sample collection. Prehospital Emerg Care: Off J Natl Assoc EMS Phys Natl Assoc State EMS Dir. 2008;12(2):218–24.

37. Nigam Y. A preliminary investigation into bacterial contamination of Welsh emergency ambulances. Emerg Med J. 2003. 2003;20(5):479–82.

38. Rettig A. Regulations for disinfection of ambulance services. Osterreichische Schwesternzeitung. 1972;25(10):248–54.

39. Schilling S, Follin P, Jarhall B, et al. European concepts for the domestic transport of highly infectious patients. Clin Microbiol Infect. 2009;15(8):727–33.

40. Lowe JJ, Jelden KC, Schenarts PJ, et al. Considerations for safe EMS transport of patients infected with Ebola virus. Prehosp Emerg Care. 2015;19(2):179–83.

41. Centers for Disease Control and Prevention (CDC). Cluster of severe acute respiratory syndrome cases among protected healthcare workers – Toronto, Canada 2003. MMWR. 2003;52:433–6.

42. Andersen B, Rasch M, Hochlin K, Jensen FH, Wismar P, Fredriksen JE. Decontamination of rooms, medical equipment and ambulances using an aerosol of hydrogen peroxide disinfectant. J Hosp Infect. 2006;62(2):149–55.

43. Lowe JJ, Hewlett AL, Iwen P, Smith PW, Gibbs SG. Evaluation of ambulance decontamination using gaseous chlorine dioxide. Prehosp Emerg Care. 2013;17:401–8.

44. Uyeki TM, Mehta AK, Davey RT, et al. Clinical management of Ebola virus disease in the United States and Europe. N Engl J Med. 2016;374:636–46.

45. Lyon GM, Mehta AK, Varkey JB, et al. Clinical care of two patients with Ebola virus disease in the United States. N Engl J Med. 2014;371:2402–9.

46. Kreuels B, Wichmann D, Emmerich P, et al. A case of severe Ebola virus infection complicated by Gram-negative septicemia. N Engl J Med. 2014;371:2394–401.

47. Wolf T, Kann G, Becker S, et al. Severe Ebola virus disease with vascular leakage and multiorgan failure: treatment of a patient in intensive care. Lancet. 2015;385:1428–35.

48. Sissoko D, Laouenan C, Folkesson E, et al. Experimental treatment with Favipiravir for Ebola virus disease (the JIKI trial): a historically controlled, single-arm proof-of-concept trial in Guinea. PLoS Med. 2016;13(3):e1001967.

49. Dunning J, Sahr F, Rojek A, et al. Experimental treatment of Ebola virus disease with TKM-130803: a single-arm phase 2 clinical trial. PLoS Med. 2016;13(4):e1001997.

50. DOI 10.1056/NEJMoa1604330.

51. van Griensven J, Edwards T, de Lamballerie X, et al. Evaluation of convalescent plasma for Ebola virus disease in Guinea. N Engl J Med. 2016;374:33–42.

52. McCormick JB, King IJ, Webb PA, et al. Lassa fever. N Engl J Med. 1986;314:20–6.

53. Hill CE, Burd EM, Kraft CS, et al. Laboratory test support for Ebola patients within a high-containment facility. Lab Med. 2014;45:e109–11.

54. Bevilacqua N, Nicastri E, Chinello P, et al. Criteria for discharge of patients with Ebola virus diseases in high-income countries. Lancet. 2015;3:e739–40.

55. World Health Organization. Clinical management of patients with viral haemorrhagic fever. A pocket guide for the front-line health worker. http://www.who.int/csr/resources/publications/clinical-management-patients/en/. (n.d.). Accessed 14 June 2016.

56. U.S. Department of Transportation. 49 CFR Parts 171, 172, 173, and 175 Hazardous materials: infectious substances; harmonization with the United Nations recommendations; final rule. https://www.gpo.gov/fdsys/pkg/FR-2006-06-02/pdf/06-4992.pdf. (n.d.). Accessed 5 July 2016.

57. U.S. Department of Transportation. DOT guidance for preparing packages of Ebola contaminated waste for transportation and disposal. http://phmsa.dot.gov/staticfiles/PHMSA/DownloadableFiles/Files/suspected_ebola_patient_packaging_guidance_final.pdf. (n.d.). Accessed 5 July 2016.

58. Lowe JJ, Gibbs SG, Schwedhelm S, et al. Nebraska biocontainment unit perspective on disposal of Ebola medical waste. Am J Infect Control. 2014;30:1–2.

59. Occupational Safety & Health Administration. Safe handling, treatment, transport and disposal of Ebola-contaminated waste. https://

www.osha.gov/Publications/OSHA_FS-3766.pdf. (n.d.). Accessed 5 July 2016.

60. Centers for Disease Control and Prevention. Interim guidance for environmental infection control in hospitals for Ebola virus. http://www.cdc.gov/vhf/ebola/healthcare-us/cleaning/hospitals.html#eight. (n.d.). Accessed 5 July 2016.

61. Jelden KC, Gibbs SG, Smith PW, et al. Nebraska biocontainment unit patient discharge and environmental decontamination following Ebola care. Am J Infect Control. 2015;43:203–5.

62. World Health Organization. New WHO safe and dignified burial protocol – key to reducing Ebola transmission. World Health Organization, Geneva. http://www.who.int/mediacentre/news/notes/2014/ebola-burial-protocol/en. (n.d.). Accessed 3 Mar 2016.

63. Centers for Disease Control and Prevention. Guidance for safe handling of human remains of Ebola patients in U.S. hospitals and mortuaries. http://www.cdc.gov/vhf/ebola/healthcare-us/hospitals/handling-human-remains.html. (n.d.). Accessed 10 Mar 2016.

64. Centers for Disease Control and Prevention. Guidance on Personal Protective Equipment (PPE) to be used by healthcare workers during management of patients with confirmed Ebola or Persons under Investigation (PUIs) for Ebola who are clinically unstable or have bleeding, vomiting, or diarrhea in U.S. hospitals, including procedures for donning and doffing PPE. http://www.cdc.gov/vhf/ebola/healthcare-us/ppe/guidance.html. Accessed 10 Mar 2016. (2015)

65. The Nebraska Biocontainment Unit. The Nebraska biocontainment unit policies and procedures. http://netec.org/resources/nbu-policies/. Accessed 10 Mar 2016.

66. Centers for Disease Control and Prevention. Case definition for Ebola Virus Disease (EVD). http://www.cdc.gov/vhf/ebola/healthcare-us/evaluating-patients/case-definition.html. (n.d.). Accessed 14 June 2016.

67. Fairley JK, Kozarsky PE, Kraft CS, et al. Ebola or not? Evaluating the Ill traveler from Ebola-affected countries in West Africa. Open Forum Infect Dis. 2016;3(1):ofw005. doi:10.1093/ofid/ofw005.

68. Sugalski G, Murano T, Fox A, Rosania A. Development and use of mobile containment units for the evaluation and treatment of potential Ebola virus disease patients in a United States hospital. Acad Emerg Med. 2015;22:616–22.

69. Wadman M, Schwedhelm S, Watson S, et al. Emergency department processes for the evaluation and management of person under investigation for Ebola virus disease. Ann Emerg Med. 2015;66(3):306–14.

70. Schwedhelm MM, Berg K, Emodi M, Shradar M, Hayes K. Ebola surgical protocols enhance safety of patients and personnel. OR Manager. 2015;31(4):7–11.

71. Wren S, Kushner A. Surgical protocol for possible or confirmed Ebola cases. https://www.facs.org/surgeons/ebola/surgical-protocol. (n.d.). Accessed 14 June 2016.

72. Dowell SF. Ebola hemorrhagic fever: why were children spared? Pediatr Infect Dis J. 1996;15:189–91.

73. Mupere E, Kaducu OF, Yoti Z. Ebola hemorrhagic fever among hospitalized children and adolescents in northern Uganda: epidemiologic and clinical observations. Afr Health Sci. 2001;1:60–5.

74. Peacock G, Uyeki TM, Rasmussen SA. Ebola virus disease and children: what pediatric health care professionals need to know. JAMA Pediatr. 2014;168:1087–8.

75. Caluwaerts S, Fautsch T, Lagrou D, et al. Dilemmas in managing pregnant women with Ebola: 2 case reports. Clin Infect Dis. 2016;62:903–5.

76. Price ME, Fisher-Hich SP, Craven RB, McCormick JB. A prospective study of maternal and fetal outcome in acute Lassa fever infection during pregnancy. BMJ. 1988;297:584–7.

77. Nelson JM, Griese SE, Goodman AB, Peacock G. Live neonates born to mothers with Ebola virus disease: a review of the literature. J Perinatol. 2016;36:411–4.

78. Bentlin MR, de Barros Almeida RA, Coelho KI, et al. Perinatal transmission of yellow fever, Brazil, 2009. Emerg Infect Dis. 2011;17:1779–80.

79. Hinton CF, Davies HD, Hocevar SN, et al. Parental presence at the bedside of a child with suspected Ebola: an expert discussion. Clin Pediatr Emerg Med. 2016;17:81–6.

80. Barnsteiner, J. Teaching the culture of safety. Online J Nurs Issues. 2011;(16)5.

81. Centers for Disease Control and Prevention. Hospital preparedness: a tiered approach. http://www.cdc.gov/vhf/ebola/healthcare-us/preparing/current-treatment-centers.html. (n.d.). Accessed 14 June 2016.

82. Herstein JJ, Biddinger PD, Kraft CS, et al. Current capabilities and capacity of Ebola treatment centers in the United States Infect. Control Hosp Epidemiol. 2016;37(3):313–8.

83. National Ebola Training and Education Center. http://netec.org/. (n.d.). Accessed 14 June 2016.

Probiotics and Infection Prevention

Whitney Perry and Shira Doron

Introduction

The World Health Organization accepts a definition of probiotics as "live microorganisms which when administered in adequate amounts confer a health benefit on the host" [1]. Increasing interest in the clinical use of probiotics in the United States is driven both by consumer enthusiasm for products marketed to have potential health benefits and by researchers inspired by the potential to prevent, treat, and mitigate disease. Some commonly studied applications for clinical use of probiotics include antibiotic-associated diarrhea, traveler's diarrhea, and primary and secondary prevention of *Clostridium difficile* colitis. However, a limited number of studies have examined the use of probiotics as a potential tool in the antimicrobial resistance crisis. These studies include trials using probiotics to eliminate vancomycin-resistant Enterococcus colonization and to prevent multidrug-resistant organisms. These topics, along with the safety of probiotics in the healthcare setting, will be discussed in detail in this chapter. Results have been mixed, leading to ongoing controversy regarding the utility of probiotics in these settings.

The conversation is limited by the quality of published studies. Specifically, there is an overall lack of uniformity in nearly all elements of study design which makes generalizability of results difficult for clinicians. One of the challenges is the breadth of organisms included in the probiotic category. Among many others, frequently studied genera include lactobacilli, bifidobacteria, streptococci, and enterococci. Such organisms have been examined individually and in varying combinations, compared with each other and with placebo, and provided in a wide range of doses and formulations. In addition to the variability of intervention, there is also the heterogeneity of populations. An inherent challenge arises in accounting for differing rates of multidrug-resistant organisms and differences in the microbiome by geographic location and by setting (outpatient to inpatient to intensive care unit). Finally, studies to date have been small and short term.

However, despite the challenges to studying and applying data regarding probiotic use, the potential significance is massive and cannot go understated. The unfortunate effects of the increasing trend of healthcare-associated infections include prolonged hospital stay, increased resistance to antimicrobials, high cost to patients as well as the healthcare system, and death. Over 99,000 deaths in the United States were attributed to healthcare-associated infection in 2002 with an estimated economic impact in 2004 of $6.5 billion [2].

In vitro studies have demonstrated various mechanisms by which probiotics are proposed to take effect. Lactobacilli, in particular, have demonstrated production of both antimicrobial substances which inhibit bacterial growth and short-chain fatty acids that are toxic to various bacteria [3, 4]. In addition, they produce hydrogen peroxide which induces an anaerobic environment, thereby indirectly inhibiting bacterial growth [5]. Other probiotics also suppress bacterial growth by competitive colonization, by altering intestinal metabolic activity, by altering mucin production, and by binding toxins [6, 7]. Lastly, studies also have shown lactobacilli to inhibit the adherence of *E. coli*, *Klebsiella*, and *Pseudomonas* in uroepithelial cells [8].

VRE Colonization

Beginning with its first appearance in 1988, and growing rapidly in the 1990s, vancomycin-resistant enterococcus (VRE) has been associated with increased morbidity and

W. Perry (✉)
Division of Internal Medicine, Tufts Medical Center,
800 Washington Street, Boston, MA 02111, USA
e-mail: wperry@tuftsmedicalcenter.org

S. Doron
Division of Geographic Medicine and Infectious Disease,
Tufts Medical Center, Boston, MA, USA
e-mail: sdoron@tuftsmedicalcenter.org

© Springer International Publishing AG 2018
G. Bearman et al. (eds.), *Infection Prevention*, DOI 10.1007/978-3-319-60980-5_22

mortality, particularly in intensive care settings. Risk factors for nosocomial colonization with VRE are prolonged hospital stay, proximity to a patient colonized by VRE, care by a nurse who also cares for patients positive for VRE, longer stay in the ICU, and exposure to a hospital with higher proportion of patients with VRE colonization [9]. Gastrointestinal colonization is most common, though skin colonization is also frequently present. Animal studies have shown that colonization was more easily established following the administration of vancomycin or other antibiotics, and the continuation of antibiotics caused persistence of VRE [9]. The implications of VRE colonization are dramatically stated with data demonstrating that patients with VRE bacteremia have a twofold increase in the relative risk of mortality compared to patients who are bacteremic with vancomycin-susceptible enterococcus [10]. This finding was independent of underlying disease. Given the gravity of the burden of VRE, widespread infection control efforts have been implemented, though permanent elimination from a hospital has not been described. Thus, the role for probiotics is of considerable interest. Promising in vitro studies have led to three prominent in vivo trials.

The first study, published in 2007, looked at 27 VRE-positive patients on the renal ward of a tertiary care hospital who were randomly assigned to receive either yogurt containing Lactobacillus rhamnosus strain GG (LGG) or standard pasteurized yogurt [11]. Stool was obtained weekly three times and again at 8 weeks to assess for VRE clearance. All 11 in the LGG group who completed the study cleared VRE which was striking compared with 1 of the 12 who completed the study in the control arm. In a second phase of the study, these controls were crossed over and given LGG. Eight of the eleven subsequently cleared VRE within 4 weeks.

Of note, this study did not attempt to culture the stool samples for LGG and did not quantify VRE colonization. In addition, by week 8, three of the subjects in the original treatment group again showed VRE positivity. Lastly, there were a disproportionate number of patients receiving concomitant antibiotics in the treatment group (10 of 14) than in the controls (5 of 13) which included linezolid. These factors may have been at least partially responsible for the very strong initial results of this study.

A second study, published in 2011, also had positive results, demonstrating successful clearance of VRE in children given Lactobacillus [12]. The study population was 65 VRE-colonized, inpatient, immunocompetent children (age 0–18), who were randomized to receive 3 billion CFU of LGG or placebo for 21 days. Rectal swabs were obtained for culture at baseline, at weekly intervals for the 3 weeks during intervention, and then at 4 weeks following completion of the intervention. The investigators found a significant difference in the number of children colonized with VRE beginning in week 1. By the third week, 20 of 32 patients in the LGG group were no longer VRE carriers compared with 7 of 29 in the control group ($P = 0.002$). They also observed increased counts of Lactobacillus species (though not LGG specifically) in the stool of children receiving LGG. However, at 4 weeks following completion of the treatment, there was no significant difference in VRE colonization.

In contrast to these two studies, most recently, there has been a third small randomized, double-blind, placebo-controlled clinical trial done to examine the efficacy of LGG for the reduction or elimination of intestinal colonization by VRE [13]. The study included non-critically ill adults who had positive stool culture or rectal swab for VRE within 7 days preceding study enrollment. Strict exclusion criteria applied. Ultimately, 11 adults were randomized to either a group receiving LGG (five subjects) or placebo (six subjects). The intervention group subjects received one capsule of LGG (1×10^{10}) organisms twice daily. Duration was 14 days, and stool samples were collected at days 7, 14, 21, 28, and 56 for quantitative culture of LGG and VRE. No significant differences were observed in VRE colony counts at any time point. LGG was detected by PCR in all samples from subjects in the LGG arm. However, it was only isolated in culture in two of the five subjects in that arm. This was perhaps due to antibiotic administration in this population leaving dead organisms detectable by PCR but not viable by culture. However, the major finding from this study was the lack of effect of LGG on VRE colonization.

The differing outcome of this third study on VRE elimination may be explained by an inadequately powered study, a shorter course of LGG administration (2 weeks rather than 3 or 4), or a sicker population with heavier burden of comorbidities and higher rate of concomitant antibiotic use. In addition, this study used a different formulation for administration of LGG, using a capsule rather than yogurt.

At this point, there remains hope for an important role of Lactobacillus rhamnosus GG in clearing VRE colonization, but questions remain regarding characteristics of the population to be targeted, formulation and length of treatment, and the effect of concomitant antibiotic use.

Prevention of Multidrug-Resistant Organisms

Colonization with multidrug-resistant organisms (MDROs) poses great risk for hospital complications including increased length of stay and increased mortality. Risk factors for acquiring MDROs include placement of central lines, administration of broad-spectrum antibiotics, ventilator use, and nasogastric tubes. Infection is often preceded by colonization. Therefore, there is theoretical benefit in an intervention that will prevent or treat colonization and, in doing so, prevent transmission within high-risk healthcare settings such as the intensive care unit.

In particular, studies with *Lactobacillus rhamnosus* GG (LGG) have demonstrated several behaviors that suggest it may be a promising candidate for clinical application in the intensive care unit. First, its susceptibility profile is key to its success in attaining colonization status of patients in the ICU setting where patients commonly require antimicrobial treatment. While known to be susceptible to penicillin, ampicillin, and erythromycin, studies have demonstrated survival of LGG in the digestive tract of patients treated with such antibiotics [14]. Furthermore, LGG has demonstrated resistance to many other commonly used antibiotics including meropenem, ertapenem, cefoxitin, cefotetan, cefoperazone, ceftrizoxine, bactrim, and metronidazole. In our lab it has, however, displayed susceptibility to piperacillin-tazobactam and imipenem (unpublished data).

In vitro studies show a growth inhibition mechanism involving a filterable low molecular weight fatty acid elaborated by LGG that suppresses the growth of *Staphylococcus*, *Streptococcus*, *Mycobacterium*, *Bacillus*, *Clostridium*, *Listeria*, *Escherichia coli*, and *Salmonella* [4]. Later experiments by our lab demonstrated production by LGG of a substance that inhibits and has bactericidal activity against four different strains of VRE as well as five ESBL-producing *Klebsiella pneumoniae* (as determined by pulsed field gel electrophoresis) (unpublished data).

Putting this data together, LGG provides a promising modality for colonization and survival in the GI tracts of ICU patients, as well as for inhibition of growth and bactericidal activity against multidrug-resistant organisms. This sets the stage for in vivo study of lactobacillus in ICU patients. A recent randomized controlled pilot study by Kwon et al. looked at LGG versus standard of care in preventing gastrointestinal MDRO colonization in the ICU setting. The study took place at a 1250-bed university-affiliated US hospital in 2012–2013 and included patients over the age of 18, in medical or coronary ICUs, with anticipated lengths of stay greater than 48 h. There were extensive exclusion criteria largely based around immunosuppression, invasive devices, and breakdown of the GI tract, among others. A total of 103 patients were randomized to receive either probiotic or placebo. Randomization was not blinded. Probiotic recipients received one capsule of 1×10^{10} cells twice daily for 14 days or until study exit (death or hospital discharge, whichever came first). Stool samples or rectal swabs were obtained for culture at study enrollment, study day 3, and every 3 days until study exit. Included in the outcomes analysis were 70 patients who had at least three specimens available. Primary outcome was the acquisition of gastrointestinal MDRO colonization. Organisms included here were extended-spectrum beta-lactamase-producing and carbapenem-resistant *Enterobacteriaceae*, vancomycin-resistant

enterococci, *Pseudomonas aeruginosa*, and *C. difficile*. Secondary outcomes were safety and loss of MDRO colonization. Results revealed that there was no significant difference in acquisition of MDROs between probiotic (10%) and placebo (15%) groups ($P = 0.72$) [15]. Similarly, there was no difference in loss of colonization. The study was limited by size and duration.

Given a trend of multiple small studies frequently with contradictory conclusions, recent meta-analyses have attempted to synthesize a broader view of the literature. A 2013 meta-analysis published in CHEST by Barraud et al. compared important outcomes in critically ill patients receiving probiotics. Their group assembled data from nine randomized controlled trials from 2002 to 2013. Sample sizes varied from 28 to 259, pooling a total of 1119 patients receiving prebiotics, probiotics, and synbiotics. Primary outcomes were ICU and hospital mortality, and both were found to be uninfluenced by use of probiotics. The quality of the studies was variable. The authors state, however, that their findings with regard to their primary outcomes were robust because heterogeneity was small and findings were consistent among different sensitivity analyses that accounted for the importance of mortality rate and the kind and dose of probiotics used [16].

Interestingly, however, despite a lack of effect on ICU and hospital mortality, Barraud did find that probiotic administration reduced the incidence of ICU-acquired pneumonia (OR, 0.58; 95% CI, 0.42–0.79) and was associated with a shorter ICU course (weighted mean difference, 21.49 days; 95% CI, 22.12–20.87 days). Despite these observations, other secondary outcomes of the meta-analysis yielded negative findings. There was a lack of association between probiotic use and shorter duration of mechanical ventilation (WMD, 20.18 days; 95% CI, 21.72–1.36 days) or shorter hospital stay (WMD, 20.45 days; 95% CI, 21.41–0.52 days) [16].

A 2012 systematic review published in Critical Care Medicine by Petrof et al. drew somewhat more positive conclusions than Barraud based on a larger number of randomized controlled trials. In their analysis, 23 trials met inclusion criteria. They looked at critically ill adults randomized to either probiotic or placebo and assessed outcomes including infections, mortality, and length of stay. Eleven of the included studies documented reduced risk of infectious complications in the probiotic arm of the study (risk ratio 0.82; 95% confidence interval 0.69–0.99; $p = 0.03\%$) [17]. In addition, there were seven trials which examined probiotic effect on ventilator-associated pneumonia. When these were pooled, they concluded that risk of VAP was decreased with probiotic use (risk ratio 0.75; 95% confidence interval 0.59–0.97; $p = 0.03$).

Regarding mortality, though, Petrof's findings were similar but not identical to the Barraud meta-analysis. With probiotics there was a trend toward reduced intensive care unit mortality (risk ratio 0.80; 95% confidence interval 0.59–1.09; $p = 0.16$) but not hospital mortality. Importantly, the authors note that in their analysis, trials of lower methodological quality observed greater treatment effects than those of higher methodological quality. They acknowledge that recommendations are limited based on clinical and statistical heterogeneity.

Overall, the effects of probiotics on multidrug-resistant organisms in clinical settings, specifically in critically ill patients, are uncertain. While the in vitro data aligns, creating anticipation for a major role for probiotics in vivo, the clinical data from existing trials has been less conclusive. Trials to date have been small with nonuniform inclusion and exclusion criteria, variable probiotic intervention, and short-term follow-up. Therefore, even systematic reviews of the topic struggle to draw applicable conclusions. Larger studies looking at effects of single-species preparations are necessary to definitively comment on the utility of probiotics in altering the colonization, and thereby outcomes, of critically ill patients.

Risks of Hospital-Acquired Infection Due to Use of Probiotics

In recent years, amidst ongoing discussion regarding the role of probiotics in the clinical setting, new controversy has developed over the safety of their clinical use. Despite an overall unremarkable record of adverse outcomes over many decades in the world of food and dairy, their evolving applications for more targeted therapeutic use have triggered somewhat of a re-categorization by the US Food and Drug Administration (FDA). A 2010 draft guidance defined probiotics as biotherapeutic products and therefore mandated an Investigational New Drug (IND) application for all clinical research concerning their use. This has prompted reaction from many in the scientific community who have since recognized new barriers to advancing study in this area. Fallout from the new policy has been a decrease in the number of federally funded human interventional studies. This is due, in part, to reticence of probiotic manufacturers in providing required information to the FDA and also to greater challenges for enrollment given the now-extensive exclusion criteria for these studies [18]. In response, the FDA has maintained its stance in a 2013 guidance that as long as a product is being used for purposes beyond nutritive value, taste, or aroma, it should be considered a drug and therefore held to such higher scrutiny [19].

In a similar vein, a 2011 report released by the Agency for Healthcare Research and Quality (AHRQ) stated that while there is no significant evidence to suggest increased risk,

"the current literature is not well equipped to answer questions on the safety of probiotics in intervention studies with confidence" [20]. The report provided a review of the safety of probiotics based on 622 studies and concluded the above based on a general lack of assessment of safety provided by this literature. However, the report has been criticized by some who maintain that this data was not reported because it was not, at the time, required nor considered to be relevant. They contend that the long-standing history of safe use carries a substantial weight that is lost in the report's conclusion and further that data does exist from clinical, animal, and in vitro studies that support this presumption.

One of the landmark trials which has raised concern for the safety of probiotics is the *Probiotic prophylaxis in patients with predicted severe acute pancreatitis* (PROPATRIA) trial which was published in 2008 [21]. In a double-blind, placebo-controlled randomized trial, the study looked at 200 patients in 15 Dutch hospitals with first episode of acute pancreatitis which was predicted at onset to be severe. Subjects were randomized within 72 h to receive either twice-daily multispecies probiotic or placebo via nasojejunal tube for 28 days or until discharge. The primary endpoint was the total number of infectious complications. Secondary endpoints were mortality, necrosectomy, antibiotic resistance, hospital stay, and adverse events. Results were surprisingly striking with no significant difference in infectious complications but mortality rate of 24 of 152 patients (16%) in the treatment arm versus 9 of 144 (6%) in the placebo group with relative risk 2.53 (95% CI 1.22–5.25). Nine patients in the probiotic group and zero in the placebo group developed bowel ischemia, eight of whom had a fatal outcome. The authors concluded that given the lack of effect on infectious complications and an increased risk of mortality, probiotic prophylaxis should not be administered in patients with predicted severe acute pancreatitis.

Results of this study had been unexpected given that it had been inspired by multiple prior studies, and one randomized controlled trial in particular, that had demonstrated positive results with no significant effect on mortality. Olah et al. had looked at an individual probiotic strain, *Lactobacillus plantarum*, in patients with acute pancreatitis and found infected pancreatic necrosis was significantly decreased in the probiotic arm [22]. The PROPATRIA group had hoped to expand on these findings by broadening to a multispecies probiotic intervention and including patients with biliary etiology of pancreatitis.

Given the unforeseen mortality outcome of the PROPATRIA trial, it was followed by a thorough investigation organized by three Dutch National Institutes in 2009 which ultimately concluded that there were no peculiarities about the way the study was performed to explain the high mortality rate in the probiotic arm [23]. In addition, there have been meta-analyses which have systematically reviewed PROPATRIA among related literature and asserted the observed outcome could not have been predicted based on evidence published both before and after the trial [24, 25].

A 2016 perspective article, however, published in Nature Biotechnology uses the existing basic science foundation for the use of probiotics to propose a mechanism for the observed findings of PROPATRIA [26]. It forcefully rebuts the notion that future probiotic use in the acute pancreatitis population is contraindicated. Their proposed explanation for the adverse outcome of the study includes delayed initiation of intervention (within 72 h) and excessive delivery of carbohydrates provided by tube feeds in the inherent presence of digestive pancreatic enzymes. They suggest a complex mechanism for damage that makes the methodology used in the trial design specifically responsible for the outcome. Their conclusion is that we may expect safe use of probiotics in patients with acute pancreatitis if higher doses of probiotic are used, concurrent enteral nutrition is minimized, and early initiation of probiotic therapy (within 24 h) is achieved.

In any case, acute pancreatitis is one of many populations which are potentially at risk with use of probiotics according to the FDA. Others among this list include those who are pregnant, immunosuppressed, have structural heart disease, or have increased potential for translocation of probiotic across the bowel wall. Inpatients are also considered by the FDA to be potentially a high-risk group.

Adverse outcomes of probiotic use have been primarily reported in case reports. There have been over 30 reported cases of fungemia (*Saccharomyces* species), at least 8 cases of bacteremia (lactobacilli species), and among these at least 9 cases of sepsis [18]. Endocarditis and abscess have both been described, and five reports of D-lactic acidosis have been published. Beyond these proven risks, there is theoretical concern regarding excessive immune stimulation provoking autoimmune response as well as lateral gene transfer of resistance traits via plasmid exchange.

Anecdotal reports of *Lactobacillus*-related central line-associated bloodstream infection in our own institution and others in patients receiving probiotics while in the hospital are the basis for our hospital's policy regarding particular attention to hand hygiene. Providers caring for patients with central venous catheters are advised to change gloves after handling probiotic preparations and before manipulating vascular catheters.

Undoubtedly, the climate of safety reporting and investigation is changing as probiotics have become more widely recognized as a therapeutic agent. While this poses increased challenge for researchers, the growing body of data will serve to inform on best uses for probiotics. As research continues, accurate and precise description of adverse events will be critical to their advancement.

Conclusion

While there is increasing interest in the use of probiotics in the treatment and prevention of disease, an abundance of unanswered questions remain. Despite exciting in vitro data, clinical results have been inconsistent. Randomized trials have been small, and subsequent meta-analyses have been limited in their ability to pool data given the variability of study design with respect to organism, dose, and formulation used for intervention, as well as acuity and population of study subjects.

With regard to the specific question of clearance of VRE colonization, there have been only two small clinical trials suggesting the effectiveness of LGG and a third with contrasting results [11–13].

This third study was undoubtedly small with limited power and was performed in a population with a complicated profile of comorbidities and concomitant antibiotic use. It certainly does not rule out the possibility for future LGG use to clear VRE colonization but does prompt careful consideration for future study design to determine whom to target, how to administer intervention, and what outcomes are most important. We are left to wonder – particularly given the positive outcomes of the previous two studies – whether there may be other beneficial effects of the presence of LGG which may not be represented by the primary outcome that was assessed here (growth of LGG in stool culture and quantifying VRE colonization). It would be informative to see the effect of LGG on the full profile of the microbiota and on the intestinal immune and barrier functions.

The topic of probiotic use in the critical care setting to prevent disease from MDROs has been examined with many small, varied trials which systematic reviews have subsequently attempted to pool in order to draw meaningful conclusions. Meta-analyses from 2012 to 2013 with differing inclusion criteria seem to agree on a lack of effect on hospital mortality [16, 17]. They also both comment on a potentially reduced risk of ventilator-associated or ICU-associated pneumonia with probiotic use. However, conclusions regarding other endpoints are variable. Given such a widely heterogeneous group of studies, there is room in this topic for a large, randomized trial which examines a single-species probiotic in order to provide more compelling clinical guidance.

The call for further investigation now comes with the critical requirement for increased vigilance regarding safety data. While in the past there has been inconsistent reporting of safety outcomes, their use has been generally regarded as safe given the overall widespread use without major adverse events. However, the landscape is evolving as the FDA now recognizes probiotic preparations as drug rather than food [19]. Increased scrutiny, perhaps in part inspired by the noteworthy PROPATRIA trial, means that all probiotic studies now require an investigational new drug application to proceed [21]. This has been met with some resistance by critics who argue that the larger body of historical practice and limited body of reported evidence should carry a greater significance than a single trial. Regardless, a new standard has been set as we seek to answer the outstanding questions necessary to guide clinical application of probiotics in the prevention and treatment of disease.

References

1. Guarner F, Schaafsma GJ. Probiotics. Int J Food Microbiol. 1998;39:237–8.
2. World Health Organization. Report on the burden of endemic health care-associated infection worldwide: a systematic review of the literature. *apps.who.int.* [Online] 2011. http://apps.who.int/iris/bitstream/10665/80135/1/9789241501507_eng.pdf
3. Vandenberg PA. Lactic acid bacteria, their metabolic products and interference with microbial growth. FEMS Microbiol Rev. 1993;12:221–38.
4. Silva M, Jacobus NV, Deneke C, Gorbach SL. Antimicrobial substance from a human lactobacillus strain. Antimicrob Agents Chemother. 1987;31:1231–3.
5. Axelsson LT, Chung TC, Dobrogosz WJ, Lindgren SE. Production of a broad spectrum antimicrobial substance by Lactobacillus reuteri. Microb Ecol Health Dis. 1989;2:131–6.
6. Coconnier MH, et al. Inhibition of adhesion on enteroinvasive pathogens to human intestinal Caco-2 cells by lactobacillus acidophilus strain LB decreases bacterial invasion. FEMS Microbiol Lett. 1993;110:299–306.
7. Mack DR, Michail S, Weis, et al. Probiotic inhibit enteropathogenic *E. coli* adherence in vitro by inducing intestinal mucin gene expression. Am J Phys. 1999;276:G–941.
8. Chan RCY, Rei G, Irvin RT, Bruce AW, Costerton JW. Competitive exclusion of uropathogens from uroepithelial cells by Lactobacillus whole cells and cell wall fragments. Infect Immun. 1985;1985:84–9.
9. Murray BE. Vancomycin-resistant enterococcal infections. N Engl J Med. 2000;342:710–21.
10. Vergis EN, et al. Determinants of vancomycin resistance and mortality rates in enterococcal bacteremia. A prospective multicenter study. Ann Intern Med. 2001;135:484–92.
11. Manley KJ, Fraenkel MB, Mayall BC, Power DA. Probiotic treatment of vancomycin-resistant enterococci: a randomised controlled trial. Med J Aust. 2007;186:454–7.
12. Szachta P, Ignys I, Cichy W. An evaluation of the ability of the probiotic strain Lactobacillus rhamnosus GG to eliminate the gastrointestinal carrier state of vancomycin-resistant enterococci in colonized children. J Clin Gastroenterol. 2011;45:872–7.
13. Doron S, Hibberd PL, Goldin B, Thorpe C, McDermott L, Snydman DR. Effect of Lactobacillus rhamnosus GG administration on vancomycin-resistant enterococcus colonization in adults with comorbidities. Antimicrob Agents Chemother. 2015;59:4593–9.
14. Goldin BR, Gorbach SL, Saxelin M, Barakat S, Gualtieri L, Salminen S. Survival of Lactobacillus species (strain GG) in human gastrointestinal tract. Dig Dis Sci. 1992;37:121–8.
15. Kwon JH, Bommarito KM, Reske KA, et al. Randomized controlled trial to determine the impact of probiotic administration on colonization with multidrug-resistant organisms in critically Ill patients. Infect Contr Hosp Epidemiol. 2015;36(12):1451–54.
16. Barraud D, Bolleart PE, Gibot S. Impact of the administration of probiotics on mortality in critically ill patients. Chest. 2013;143:646–55.
17. Petrof E, et al. Probiotics in the critically ill: a systematic review of the randomized trial evidence. Crit Care Med. 2012;40:3290–302.
18. Doron S, Snydman DR. Risk and safety of probiotics. Clin Infect Dis. 2015;60(Suppl 2):S129–34.
19. U.S. Department of Health and Human Services, Food and Drug Administration. Guidance for clinical investigators, sponsors, and IRBs: Investigational New Drug Applications (INDs)—determining whether human research studies can be conducted without an IND. n.d.. www.fda.gov. [Online] September 2013. http://www.fda.gov/downloads/Drugs/Guidances/UCM229175.pdf.
20. Hempel S, Newberry S, Ruelaz A, et al. Safety of probiotics used to reduce risk and prevent or treat disease. Rockville: Agency for Healthcare Resarch and Quality; 2011.
21. Besselink MG, van Santvoort HC, Buskens HC, Boermeester MA, van Goor H, Timmerman HM, Nieuwenhuijs VB, Bollen TL, van Ramshorst B, Witteman BJ, Rosman C, Ploeg RJ, Brink MA, Schaapherder AF, Dejong CH, Wahab PJ, van Laarhoven CJ, van der Harst E, van Eijck CH, Cuesta MA, Akkermans LM, Gooszen HG, Dutch Acute Pancreatitis Study Group. Probiotic prophylaxis in predicted severe acute pancreatitis: a randomised, double blind controlled trial. Lancet. 2008;371:651–9.
22. Olah A, Belagyi T, Issekutz A, Gamal ME, Bengmark S. Randomized clinical trial of specific lactobacillus and fibre supplement to early enteral nutrition in patients with acute pancreatitis. Br J Surg. 2002;89:1103–7.
23. Inspectie voor de Gezondheiszorg, Centrale Commissie Mensgebonden Onderzoek en Voedsel en Waren Autoriteit. Den Haag/Utrect. [Online] 2009. http://www.igz.nl/actueel/nieuws/belangrijketekortkomingenpropatriastudieverbeteringenvoorverantwoordklinischonderzoeknoodzakelijk.aspx
24. Hoojimans CR, De Vries RBM, Rovers MM, Gooszen HG, Ritskes-Hoitinga M. The effects of probiotic supplementation on experimental acute pancreatitis: a systematic review and meta-analysis. PLoS One. 2012;7:e48811.
25. Gou S, Yang Z, Liu T, Wu H, Wang C. Use of probiotics in the treatment of severe acute pancreatitis: a systematic review and meta-analysis of randomized controlled trials. Crit Care. 2014;18:R 57.
26. Bongaerts GPA, Severijnen RVM. A reassessment of the PROPATRIA study and its implications for probiotic therapy. Nat Biotechnol. 2016;34:55–63.

Animals in Healthcare Settings

Rekha K. Murthy, Vivek Pandrangi, and David Jay Weber

Introduction

Animals may be present in healthcare facilities for multiple reasons. Although specific laws regarding the use of service animals in public facilities were established in the United States in 1990, the widespread presence of animals in hospitals, including service animals, animals used to assist in patient therapy, and research animals, has resulted in the increased presence of animals in acute care hospitals and ambulatory medical settings. The role of animals in the transmission of zoonotic pathogens and cross-transmission of human pathogens in these settings remains poorly studied. Until more definitive information is available, healthcare facilities should establish policies and procedures to prioritize patient and healthcare provider safety and to use standard infection prevention and control measures to prevent animal-to-human transmission in healthcare settings. This paper is based on recently published consensus recommendations from a panel of experts, representing the Society of Healthcare Epidemiology of America (SHEA), regarding the management of animals in healthcare (AHC) [1]. However, this paper aims to review the controversies related to animals in healthcare with respect to infection prevention, identify potential steps for mitigation of risks and areas for future study, and provide updated information where available; any opinions noted beyond the consensus SHEA guidance document reflect the opinions of only the authors of this document.

Background

Contact with animals by people is increasing and can occur in a variety of settings including households (pets), occupational exposure (veterinarians, farmers, ranchers, and forestry workers), leisure pursuits (hunting, camping, and fishing), petting zoos, and travel to rural areas in the United States or abroad. Pet ownership is common in the United States. A national poll of pet owners revealed that in 2014, 65% of US households included a pet; dogs and cats represented over 70% of household pets (dogs 40% and cats 32%, respectively) [2]. Patients in healthcare facilities come into contact with animals primarily through the use of animals for animal-assisted activities (animal-assisted activities encompass "pet therapy," "animal-assisted therapy," and pet volunteer programs) and the use of service animals such as guide dogs for the sight impaired. Other reasons for contact with AHC include the use of animals in research or education and personal pet visits to their owners in the hospital (personal pet visitation). Risks to patients from exposure to animals in the healthcare setting may be associated with transmission of pathogens through direct or indirect contact or, less likely, droplet/aerosol transmission (Table 23.1). However, insufficient studies are available to produce generalizable, evidence-based recommendations, and as a result, substantial variations exist in policies and practice across healthcare institutions [1].

Although limited published literature exists on this topic, the SHEA document offers specific guidance on the management of AHC in four categories, animal-assisted activities (AAA), service animals as defined under the Americans with Disabilities Act (ADA), research animals, and personal pet visitation, and recommends that institutions considering

R.K. Murthy (✉)
Department of Medical Affairs and Division of Infectious Diseases, Cedars-Sinai Health System, 8700 Beverly Blvd, Suite 2211, Los Angeles, 90048 CA, USA
e-mail: Rekha.Murthy@cshs.org

V. Pandrangi
Virginia Commonwealth University School of Medicine, Richmond, VA, USA
e-mail: pandrangiv@vcu.edu

D.J. Weber
Division of Infectious Diseases, University of North Carolina at Chapel Hill School of Medicine, Chapel Hill, NC, USA
e-mail: David.Weber@unchealth.unc.edu

G. Bearman et al. (eds.), *Infection Prevention*, DOI 10.1007/978-3-319-60980-5_23

Table 23.1 Selected diseases transmitted by dogs stratified by transmission route

Transmission route	Selected diseases
Direct contact (bites)	Rabies (rabies virus)
	Capnocytophaga canimorsus infection
	Pasteurellosis (*Pasteurella* spp.)
	Staphylococcus aureus, including methicillin-resistant strains
	Streptococcus spp. infection
Direct or indirect contact	Flea bites, mites
	Fungal infection (*Malassezia pachydermatis, Microsporum canis, Trichophyton mentagrophytes*)
	Staphylococcus aureus infection
	Mites (Cheyletiellidae, Sarcoptidae)
Fecal-oral	Campylobacteriosis (*Campylobacter* spp.)
	Paratyphoid (*Salmonella* spp.)
	Giardiasis (*Giardia duodenalis*)
	Salmonellosis (*Salmonella enterica* subsp. *enterica* serotypes)
Droplet	*Chlamydophila psittaci*
Vector-borne	Ticks (dogs passively carry ticks to humans; disease not transmitted directly from dog to human)
	Rocky Mountain spotted fever (*Rickettsia rickettsii*)
	Ehrlichiosis (*Ehrlichia* spp.)
	Fleas
	Dipylidium caninum
	Bartonella henselae

these programs should have policies that include well-organized communication and education directed at healthcare personnel (HCP), patients, and visitors. Table 23.2 represents an overview of the key recommendations from the SHEA expert guidance document.

Risks of Animals in Healthcare

Reasons for concern about AHC stem mainly from general knowledge of zoonotic diseases, case reports, and limited research involving animals in healthcare facilities. Scientific studies addressing the potential risks of animal-to-human transmission of pathogens in the healthcare setting are limited in number, and because animals have generally been excluded from hospitals, the experience gained to date has been mainly from case reports and outbreak investigations [1]. For example, human strains of methicillin-resistant *Staphylococcus aureus* (MRSA) have increasingly been described in cats, dogs, horses, and pigs, with animals potentially acting as sources of MRSA exposure in healthcare

facilities [3]. MRSA is just one of many potential pathogens; a wide range of pathogens exist, including common healthcare-associated pathogens (e.g., *Clostridium difficile*, multidrug-resistant enterococci), emerging infectious diseases (e.g., extended spectrum β-lactamase (ESBL)-producing *Enterobacteriaceae*), common zoonotic pathogens (e.g., *Campylobacter, Salmonella,* and dermatophytes), rare but devastating zoonotic pathogens (e.g., rabies virus), and pathogens associated with bites and scratches (e.g., *Pasteurella* spp., *Capnocytophaga canimorsus,* and *Bartonella* spp.) [3–7].

The SHEA document was developed from an analysis of available data and was intended to provide a set of practical, expert opinion-based recommendations for the management of animals in acute care and ambulatory medical facilities. Except where clear regulatory or legislative mandates exist related to the topic and are noted (e.g., ADA), adoption and implementation of the recommendations is expected to occur at the discretion of individual institutions. In addition, these recommendations have been endorsed by, and incorporated into, animal-assisted therapy training modules by Pet Partners [8].

The following definitions are used in the SHEA document as well as in this paper:

1. Animal-assisted activities (animal-assisted activities): pet therapy, animal-assisted therapy, and other animal-assisted activities. While these practices and their purposes may vary because these animals and their handlers are (or should be) specifically trained, they will be referred to as animal-assisted activities in this document.
2. Service animals: specifically defined in the United States under the Americans with Disabilities Act (ADA).
3. Research animals: animals approved for research by the facility's Institutional Animal Care and Use Committee (IACUC).
4. Personal pet visitation: defined as a personal pet of a patient that is brought into the facility specifically to interact with that individual patient.

In this paper, we address select controversies (Table 23.3) related to AHC with respect to infection prevention, including those identified in the SHEA document as well as others, and suggest potential steps for mitigation of risks as well as potential areas for future study.

Benefits of Animal-Assisted Therapy

Background

Animal-assisted activities (AAA) therapy (also known as "animal-assisted therapy (AAT)" or "pet therapy") is defined as an animal-assisted activities as a personal pet

Table 23.2 Summary of animals in healthcare classification and selected recommendations

	Animal-assisted activities	Service[a]	Research	Personal pet
Program				
Written policy recommended	Yes	Yes	Yes	Yes
Federal legal protection	No	Yes	No	No
Animal visit liaison	Yes	No	IACUC	Yes
Infection prevention and control notification of animal visit/session	Yes	Yes	Yes	Yes
Infection prevention and control consultation for restricted areas	Yes	Yes	Yes	Yes
Visit supervised	Yes	No	Yes	Yes
Visit predetermined	Yes	No	Yes	Yes
Animal and handler/owner				
Performs trained tasks	As indicated for goal-directed interventions or recreational/social purposes	Yes	N/A	No
Specially trained handler	Yes	Yes	Yes	No
Health screening of animals and handlers	Yes	N/A	N/A	No
Documentation of formal training	Yes	No	N/A	No
Animal can be a pet	Yes	No	No	Yes
Animal serves solely for comfort or emotional support	Includes recreational/social purposes	No	N/A	Yes
Identification with ID tag	Yes	Not required	N/A	Yes/no
Animal required to be housebroken	Yes	Yes	N/A	Yes
Permitted animals				
Dogs	Yes	Yes	N/A	Yes
Other animals	Not recommended	Miniature horses	N/A	Not recommended (case-by-case exceptions may apply)

Adapted from 2015 SHEA guidance document [1]

IACUC Institutional Animal Care and Use Committee

[a]Policy to reflect ADA and regulatory compliance. Inquiries limited by ADA to tasks performed for patient

that, with its owner or handler, provides comfort to patients in healthcare facilities [1]. Dogs are almost exclusively utilized in AAA; however, cats, miniature horses, and occasionally other animals have been used for AAA. The use of AAA in hospitals is now well established [1, 9]. In a 2013 survey of the SHEA Research Committee, 337 SHEA members responded and provided information regarding their institutions' policies for AAA. Overall, 89% of US facilities and 67% of non-US facilities provided AAA for their patients [1]. Of the facilities that permitted AAA, all allowed dogs, with 21% of facilities also allowing cats, 5% allowing miniature horses, and 2% allowing primates. This survey also noted that animals were prohibited from visiting in an intensive care unit (73%) and step-down units (39%).

Benefits/Risks

The SHEA guidance documents a review of selected references on AAA (see Table 23.2 in reference 1) [1]. Multiple studies have demonstrated benefits of AAA including enjoyment of canine-assisted ambulation for patients with heart failure (hospital) [10]; decreased loneliness (long-term care) [11]; improved social functioning (psychiatric ward) [12]; decreased fear and anxiety in electroconvulsive therapy (hospital) [13]; reduced anxiety in psychiatric patients (hospital) [14]; improved nutritional uptake in Alzheimer's disease with contact with fish aquariums [15]; improved depressive symptoms in patients with dementia, depression, or psychosis (nursing home) [16]; and decreased perceived pain in children (pediatric hospital) [17]. However, the benefits of AAA in general hospitalized patients have not been adequately assessed in high-quality comparative trials.

Table 23.3 Controversies related to animals in healthcare and potential resolutions

Topic	Argument for	Argument against	Practical resolutions
Benefits of animal-assisted therapy	Improved physical well-being	Risk of physical injury (e.g., bite)	Institutional policy modeled after SHEA guidance document
	Improved emotional well-being	Risk of interference with care (e.g., damage to indwelling device)	Use of specifically trained and evaluated dogs
	Relief of boredom in the healthcare facility	Risk of zoonotic pathogen via director or indirect contact or droplet transmission	Use of specifically trained and evaluated handlers
		Acquisition of healthcare-associated pathogen (e.g., MRSA)	
		Precipitation of allergies	
Role of animals used for emotional support as "service animals"	Possibly improved physical well-being	Not covered by the ADA	Either exclude or require approval by institution designee
	Possibly improved emotional well-being	Unlike ADA, animals are not limited to dogs or miniature horses	Require same conditions as ADA animals (i.e., limit to dogs and miniature horses; housebroken; owner responsible for care, etc.)
		Unlike ADA, specific requirements by owner not delineated (e.g., ADA animals must be housebroken and the owner is responsible for care)	
		Impossible to define specific role for the animal thus potentially allows any person to bring any animal into the facility	Include in institutional policy
Cats	Large segment of pets	Cannot be trained to reliably provide safe interactions with patients	Avoid any direct contact
	Some patients prefer cats	Concerns for increased potential allergenicity	Assure no allergies
		Potential increased risk of bites and scratches	Consider for compassionate use visits only
		Lack of data to demonstrate advantages over dogs	Require transport in a pet container (i.e., not carried)
Pets	Strong bond between the pet and owner	No formal training of owner/designee	Do not allow pets (including healthcare personnel pets)
	Possible positive impact on patient	Inability to reliably restrict to individual patient (potential for pets to encounter health care personnel, visitors, and patients while at facility)	Consider for compassionate use visits only (e.g., terminally ill patients)
	Possible lower risk of adverse events due to patient-pet bond (such as bites and scratches)	Pets not temperament tested	Dogs only
		Do not typically undergo the same degree of health assessment or exclusion practices (e.g., age), as compared to AAT animals	Outline expectations for owner/guardian for hygiene and safety
			Establish facility policy with oversight and restrictions to pet visitation

(continued)

Table 23.3 (continued)

Topic	Argument for	Argument against	Practical resolutions
Research, veterinary, zoo animals	Allows use of equipment/facilities already used for humans	Risk of pathogen transmission to humans (patients or healthcare providers)	Oversight by IACUC
	Mitigates logistics and cost of acquiring separate equipment		Restrictions as appropriate to prevent disease transmission from ill animals
			Environmental disinfection
	Access to new technology for diagnostic and therapeutic use in animals		Ensure surgical instruments and other medical devices not be used on both animals and humans
			Use single-use disposable devices where feasible
			Medical devices that require disinfection or sterilization should be used exclusively for animals
Leeches	Prevention of acute venous congestion	Wound infection with *Aeromonas* species and possible sepsis especially in patients with immunosuppression	Use only FDA-approved leeches (regulated as devices)
	Future potential uses (i.e., osteoarthritis pain reduction)	Multiple side effects including thrombotic microangiopathy, anemia, and allergy	Antibiotic prophylaxis to decrease infection risk
			Avoid use in contraindicated cases
			Disposal as regulated medical waste (i.e., they contain human blood)
Maggots	Exclusively debride necrotic tissue leaving viable tissue intact	Pain	Use only FDA-approved maggots
	Antimicrobial, anti-inflammatory, and promote healing	Infection	Analgesics for pain and physical discomfort
	Low side effect profile	Social stigma	Follow disinfection protocol to decrease infectious risk
			Disposal as regulated medical waste
Aquarium	Visually appealing	Potential reservoir for pathogens that can cause infection during routine cleaning and maintenance	Ensure protocols for appropriate tank hygiene and secure maintenance
			Prohibit from patient care areas
			Keep covered; prevent access by patients
			Ensure professional maintenance
Petting zoo	Enjoyable experience for children	Potential reservoir for pathogens	Prohibit from healthcare facilities
		High level of interaction provides increased infection risk	

The general risks of animals in the hospital have been described above. Additional concerns regarding AAA, especially for immunocompromised patients or patients with host defects, include local infection or seeding of proximal prosthetic joints following licks by a dog [18] and peritonitis in patients with peritoneal dialysis catheters [19].

Mitigation

Recommendations from SHEA and APIC should be followed to reduce the risk of adverse patient outcomes from participating in AAA [1, 9]. The evidence suggests that adherence to these recommendations allows AAA to be safely used in hospitals.

Key recommendations for a safe AAA program include:

1. Facilities should develop a written policy for animal-assisted activities.
2. Only dogs should be used.
3. Animals and handlers should be formally trained and evaluated. Facilities should consider the use of certification by organizations that provide relevant formal training programs (e.g., Pet Partners, Therapy Dogs Incorporated, Therapy Dogs International).
4. Animals and animal handlers should be screened prior to being accepted into a facility animal-assisted activities program.
5. Instruct the animal-assisted activities handler to restrict contact of his or her animal to the patient(s) being visited and to avoid casual contact of their animal with other patients, staff, or the public.
6. Require that every animal-assisted activities handler participate in a formal training program and provide a certificate confirming the training.

Future Research Needs

The great majority of studies claiming benefits of AAA have been low-quality studies and focused on specific patient populations (e.g., psychiatric patients, older patients). Additional high-quality comparative trials, especially in general hospital populations, should be undertaken. Further, most studies did not specifically comment on possible adverse events (e.g., precipitation of allergies, injuries, etc.). It would be useful for additional studies to be specifically designed to collect information on possible adverse events.

Conclusions

AAA is widely used in US hospitals. Many benefits of AAA have been demonstrated in published studies, although many used low-quality designs. However, the weight of evidence suggests properly managed AAA program are both safe for patients and beneficial. Hospitals should adhere to the published recommendations to protect patient safety when implementing an AAA program.

ADA: Role of Animals Used for Emotional Support as "Service Animals"

Background

The Americans with Disabilities Act (ADA) is a US federal law that was passed in 1990 and has been subsequently updated [20]. This law established certain legal rights for persons with disabilities including the need to use service animals and defined the minimum access required by law. Healthcare facilities must comply with the ADA. Under the ADA, "service animals" are defined as "dogs that are individually trained to do work or perform tasks for people with disabilities" [21]. Legal protection extends only to individuals who are disabled; as defined under the ADA, not all patients with medical or psychological conditions are covered. In brief, disability is generally defined by the statute as (1) a physical or mental impairment that substantially limits one or more major life activities, (2) a record of such an impairment, or (3) being regarded as having such an impairment. A guidance provided by the Department of Justice makes clear that service animals under the ADA are "working animals" and not pets, and they are trained to perform specific duties or tasks. "Examples of such work or tasks include guiding people who are blind, alerting people who are deaf, pulling a wheelchair, alerting and protecting a person who is having a seizure, reminding a person with mental illness to take prescribed medications, calming a person with Post Traumatic Stress Disorder (PTSD) during an anxiety attack, or performing other duties.

Service animals are working animals, not pets. The work or task a dog has been trained to provide must be directly related to the person's disability. *Dogs whose sole function is to provide comfort or emotional support do not qualify as service animals under the ADA*" [21]. Thus, healthcare facilities are not legally required to allow animals into the hospital that provide comfort or emotional support to visitors, patients, or healthcare provides.

The Fair Housing Act (1968, revised 1974 and 1988) provides protection against disability discrimination for tenants and renters [22]. The Act also prohibits housing providers from refusing residency to persons with disabilities, or placing conditions on their residency, because they require reasonable accommodations. Included in the Act is the requirement to allow disabled persons to use an assistance animal (i.e., an animal that works, provides assistance, or performs tasks for the benefit of a person with a disability). The Act differs from the ADA in several ways. First, an assistance animal must be accommodated if it "provides emotional support that alleviates one or more identified symptoms or effects of a person's disability." Second, unlike the ADA which only allows dogs or miniature horses, the Fair Housing Act states "while dogs are the most common type of assistance animal, other animals can also be assistance animals." Finally, for purposes of reasonable accommodation requests, "neither the Fair Housing Act nor Section 504 requires an assistance animal to be individually trained or certified." The Fair Housing Act does not extend to hospitals but does include independent living and assisted living facilities. It is unclear whether the Fair Housing Act includes nursing homes.

Although allowing emotional support animals into a hospital is not required by the ADA, hospitals may choose to allow patients and/or visitors to bring such animals into the hospital.

Benefits/Risks

The physical (e.g., lower blood pressure) and social (e.g., improved self-esteem, reduced levels of stress, reduced anxiety) benefits of human-animal interaction have been reported [23]. As most of the studies were uncontrolled and compared pet owners with non-pet owners, substantial bias and/or confounding may have been present in the studies. As noted by Peacock and colleagues, "few controlled studies have been conducted to provide empirical support for positive physical or mental health outcomes gained from interacting with companion animals. Previous research has been largely descriptive and conducted with specific populations of convenience such as the aged" [23].

Despite the limitation of the existing research, there are multiple studies which have reported the benefits of pet ownership. For example, Shoda and colleagues performed a series of studies to assess the positive consequences of pet ownership [24]. They reported the following findings: (1) Study 1 found in a community sample that pet owners fared better on several well-being (e.g., greater self-esteem, more exercise) and individual difference (e.g., greater conscientiousness, less fearful attachment) measures. (2) Study 2 assessed a different community sample and found that owners enjoyed better well-being when their pets fulfilled social needs better, and the support that pets provided complemented rather than competed with human sources. (3) Study 3 brought pet owners into the laboratory and experimentally demonstrated the ability of pets to stave off negativity caused by social rejection.

The risks associated with the use of animals in healthcare facilities to patients, visitors, and HCP have been described above and include physical injuries (e.g., bites and scratches), allergies, and zoonotic infections. Importantly, emotional support animals are unlike service animals in that there are strict criteria that define a service animal (i.e., ability to perform work) that can be observed, while there are no strict observable criteria that define an emotional support animal. Thus, a healthcare facility that allows the use of emotional support animals might find a large number of patients and visitors requesting the use of such animals with an increased risk of physical injuries, zoonotic infections, and/or precipitating allergies. Adoption of the Fair Housing Act standards would also permit the use of a variety of animals (e.g., primates, birds, etc.) which may increase the risk of injuries and zoonotic infections and preclude requirements for training or certification of the animal.

Mitigation

Since there is no legal requirement that hospitals allow the use of emotional support animals in the facility, most hospitals should include a prohibition of such animals in their policy. Hospital wishing to allow the use of emotional support animals should consider applying the same standards as defined in the ADA for service animals. Such standards would include the following: allowing only the use of dogs or miniature horses; requirement that the animal be housebroken; statement that the care of animal is responsibility of the owners or his/her designee (not HCP); statement that the use of such animals be approved by the patient's physician, primary care nurse, and legal and infection preventionist; and that animals that are disruptive or impair patient care are excluded.

Future Research Needs

Two key evidence gaps are the preponderance of anecdotal reports and cross-sectional research designs and failure to control for a host of known influences on human health [25]. Thus, there is a need for well-designed studies to assess the benefits, if any, of companion animals on the physical and emotional well-being of humans. The potential benefits of emotional support animals in specific populations (e.g., persons with anxiety, depression, attention deficit order, etc.) need to be rigorously examined.

There is virtually no research on the benefits, risks, and impact of emotional support animals in healthcare facilities. Hospitals that allow such animals should review and publish the benefits and risks of allowing emotional support animal use. In the longer run, well-designed studies should be undertaken which assess the benefits and risks of emotional support animals in healthcare facilities. These should focus on the use of such animals in psychiatric units, rehabilitation and geriatric units, and hospice units and potentially among long-term patients.

Conclusions

In conclusion, there is no legal requirement that hospitals allow the use of emotional support animals by patients, visitors, or HCP. Allowing such use might lead to substantial increase in the number of animals in the hospital with increased risks of physical injury, allergies, and zoonotic diseases. The evidence supporting the use of emotional support animals is weak, and more rigorously designed studies are required to define the benefits. Hospitals choosing to allow emotional support animals should follow similar requirements as allowed under the ADA.

Cats

Background

As noted above, animals may be present in healthcare facilities for multiple reasons including serving as service animals, animal-assisted therapy (AAT), "pet" visitation, and research. In this section, we will explore whether domestic cats (*Felis catus*) should be allowed in healthcare facilities in one of capacities listed above.

As of 2012, 30.4% of households (*N* = 36,117,000) owned at least one cat [26]. Since, on average, households owning a cat have 2.1 cats, there are ~74,000,000 pet cats in the United States. Although more households own a dog, there are greater than 4,000,000 more pet cats than pet dogs. Importantly, 56.1% of cat owners consider their cats to be family members [27]. Another 41.5% of cat owners consider their cats to be pets or companions. Surveys have reported that the average amount spent on veterinary care per year per cat is either $90 or $1,141 [27].

Benefits/Risks

Over the centuries, cats have provided benefits to humans which include pest control (e.g., reducing numbers of rats and mice) and companionship. Studies have reported that the ownership of cat is useful in maintaining or slightly enhancing activities of daily living in older people [28].

The lifetime risk of at least one emergency room visit due to a cat bite or scratch was 1 in 60 based on a incidence study in North Carolina, 2008–2010 [29]. The overall incidence rate of emergency room visits related to cat bites or scratches was 18.8/100,000 person-years (p-y) [29]. The rate of injuries was more than twofold higher for females than males (26/100,000 p-y vs. 12/100,000 p-y). The incidence rose with increasing age being highest in persons >79 years of age.

Approximately, 5–15% of cat bites or scratches become infected [30]. The most common types of infection are a non-purulent wound with cellulitis, lymphangitis, or both (42%), followed by a purulent wound without abscess formation (39%) and abscesses (19%) [7]. Most cat-related wounds yield a mixture of aerobic and anaerobic organisms. The most common genera isolated from cat bite wounds are *Pasteurella* (75%), followed by *Streptococcus* (46%), *Staphylococcus* (35%), *Neisseria* (35%), *Moraxella* (35%), *Corynebacterium* (28%), *Enterococcus* (12%), and *Bacillus* (11%) [7]. *Pasteurella multocida* is the most common pathogen isolated from cat bite or scratch-related infections, most commonly causes a rapidly evolving cellulitis [31]. As cats have sharp pointed teeth, cat bites may directly inocu-

late pathogens in deeper tissues resulting in tenosynovitis, septic arthritis, osteomyelitis, and meningitis [31]. Several features of cat-related *P. multocida* infection are relevant to the potential use of cats in healthcare facilities [31]. First, immunocompromised patients (e.g., leukemia) are at higher risk of serious infection. Second, cat licks of open wounds or bites/scratches of limbs may result in septic arthritis of more proximal joints if they have been damaged (e.g., rheumatoid arthritis) or the patient has had a joint replacement. Third, cat bites or scratches of tubing used for peritoneal dialysis may result in peritonitis. Finally, transmission by contaminated fomites (e.g., baby's pacifier which was used by a cat as a toy) may lead via indirect transmission to severe infection in patients with host defense abnormalities (e.g., extremes of age, immunocompromised). Cat bites or scratches may also cause an infection by *Bartonella* (cat-scratch disease), *Bacillus anthracis* (anthrax), *Erysipelothrix rhusiopathiae*, *Francisella tularensis* (tularemia), *Yersinia pestis* (plague), and *Sporothrix schenckii* (sporotrichosis) [32]. A number of pathogens may be transmitted to humans from cats including Q fever (direct exposure, inhalation of infected material from parturient or aborted tissue), plague (cat bite/scratch, inhalation), bordetellosis (inhalation), and flea-borne spotted fever and murine typhus (via cat flea) [32]. Fecal-oral transmission from cats may occur with *Campylobacter jejuni* (campylobacteriosis), *Helicobacter* (helicobacteriosis), *Toxoplasma gondii* (toxoplasmosis), *Cryptosporidia* (cryptosporidiosis), *Salmonella* (salmonellosis), *Toxocara cati* (toxocariasis), and *Giardia lamblia* (giardiasis) [32]. Direct contact transmitted diseases include dermatophilosis, scabies, *Cheyletiella* mite infestation, and dermatophytosis [32]. Rabies in domestic animals such as cats is rare in the United States. During 2014, domestic animals accounted for 47.9% of all animals submitted for testing, but only 7.37% (*n* = 445) of all rabies cases reported [33]. Cats accounted for 61.1% (272/445) of the rabid domestic animals reported in 2014, a 10.12% increase compared with the 247 reported in 2013.

Importantly, methicillin-resistant *Staphylococcus aureus* (MRSA) may colonize companion animals including cats which may be transmitted to humans [32]. An outbreak of epidemic MRSA occurred on a rehabilitation geriatric ward [34]. Intensive screening of patients and staff revealed an unusually high carriage rate in the nursing staff (38%), thought to be related to a ward cat which was heavily colonized from the environment. Other healthcare-associated infections or outbreaks due to contact with cats have occasionally been reported. A case of Q fever in a long-term nursing home resident was linked to cat exposure [35]. An outbreak of nosocomial ringworm involving five infants in a neonatal intensive care unit was linked a nurse infected with *Microsporum canis* by her cat [36].

Mitigation

Per the US Department of Justices: "Beginning on March 15, 2011, only dogs are recognized as service animals under titles II and III of the ADA. A service animal is a dog that is individually trained to do work or perform tasks for a person with a disability [37]. In addition to the provisions about service dogs, the Department's revised ADA regulations have a new, separate provision about miniature horses that have been individually trained to do work or perform tasks for people with disabilities (miniature horses generally range in height from 24 to 34 in. measured to the shoulders and generally weigh between 70 and 100 lb) [37]. Thus, healthcare facilities do not need to allow cats into the facility even if a person claims they provide a service function.

Cats, in general, should not serve as an AAT animal [1]. This is because of their temperament (i.e., bite or scratch moving objects); lesser ability to be trained compared to dogs; multitude of potential pathogens that they can transmit via direct contact, bites or scratches, inhalation, fecal-oral exposure, or indirect exposure (i.e., ectoparasites); occasional reports of nosocomial outbreak associated with cats; and lack of protocols for safe use as AAT animals. For similar reasons, cats should, in general, not be allowed in hospitals for "pet" visits. Exceptions for a single "pet" visit may be considered for terminal patients for compassionate reasons (to say goodbye to their pet cat) under strict supervision and with the approval of the patient, the attending physician, and infection prevention.

One potential mitigation strategy would be to allow the use of a declawed cat. However, many people are opposed to declawing because of the pain inflicted on the cat, complications of the procedure, interference with the ability of cat when out of doors to escape predators, and impairment of natural cat behavior. At the present time, there is a bill pending before the New York State legislature that would outlaw declawing of cats [38].

Future Research Needs

A recent review of pet ownership and physical health concluded that "most research on pet therapy/ownership has focused on dogs and to a lesser extent, cats. Essentially all of the laboratory research has been with dogs" [39]. Additional research, including clinical trials, is warranted to determine whether cat ownership is beneficial, especially to older persons. Similarly, almost all the research on the benefits and risks of animal-assisted therapy has focused on dogs. Additional research on the benefits and risks of using cats in AAT is warranted. Healthcare facilities that use cats for AAT should publish their policies and protocols for the safe use of cats and describe whether any adverse events were associated with the use of cats. At the present time, the New York State is considering a law to prohibit declawing of cats.

Conclusions

Domestic cats are the most prevalent pets in the United States. Although less studied than dogs, some studies suggest that cats improve the well-being of older adults. Cats may be the source of many infectious diseases transmitted to humans by bites, scratches, and licks (e.g., *P. multocida*); direct contact (e.g., MRSA); fecal-oral transmission (e.g., toxoplasmosis); inhalation (e.g., Q fever); or ectoparasites. Cats are not recognized under the ADA as approved service animals. Due to their temperament and lesser ability to be trained, in general, cats should not be permitted to serve at AAT animals. Additional research should be undertaken to assess the benefits and risks of using cats as AAT animals.

Research Animals

Background

The advancement of human health through research in basic science as well as clinical and translational science often requires the application of sophisticated equipment and clinical techniques for research animals. Many health science centers may not be able to dedicate some equipment items and facilities solely for animal use due to the logistics and expense associated. Therefore, healthcare institutions may need to consider using equipment and facilities used for humans to also study research animals. In addition, zoos and veterinary facilities may also appeal to human healthcare facilities to diagnose or treat sick or injured animals. In order to accommodate these situations, where applicable, acute care hospitals should establish comprehensive policies and procedures in order to ensure patient and public safety, while enabling safe, effective, and efficient evaluation and treatment of animals.

Benefits/Risks

Animals can serve as a reservoir and vehicle for potentially infectious pathogens; as such, potential pathogens can be transmitted from research animals to humans. Though the focus of this document is on transmission of infectious agents, given the variety of animals that may be used in research settings [40], it should be noted that some animal species may pose additional threats, such as physical injury from large animals or envenomation.

Potential routes of inoculation and the range of pathogens associated with research and veterinary animals are illustrated below:

1. Direct inoculation from percutaneous or mucosal membrane exposure: Blood and body fluids of research and veterinary animals may harbor a variety of pathogens, and reports of transmission to laboratory workers or healthcare providers have been documented. Examples include *Streptobacillus moniliformis* (rat-bite fever) resulting from the bite or scratch of laboratory rodents [41]; herpes B virus encephalitis, transmitted by the bite of certain nonhuman primates [42]; skin and soft tissue infection due to *Pasteurella multocida* from cat bites and scratches and dog bites [43]; and infection due to lymphocytic choriomeningitis virus, associated with exposures to laboratory rodents [44].
2. Inhalation: *Coxiella burnetii* (Q fever) and *Chlamydophila psittaci* (psittacosis) are examples of pathogens that have been spread from laboratory animals to humans [45, 46].
3. Direct contact: Infected mammals may transmit zoophilic dermatophytes (*Microsporum canis*, *Trichophyton mentagrophytes*) to humans through direct contact [47]. Similarly, MRSA has been noted to colonize various domestic animal species and may pose a risk of transmission to humans through contact [3].
4. Fecal-oral: Laboratory animals may carry a large number of pathogens subclinically in the gastrointestinal tracts that can potentially be transmitted via the fecal-oral route. Examples include *Salmonella* sp. (many animal species), *Campylobacter* sp. (mammals, birds, reptiles), and *Cryptosporidium* sp. (mammals, reptiles, primates).
5. Indirect transmission via vectors: Laboratory animals may occasionally harbor ectoparasites (e.g., fleas) that may serve as vectors for transmission of various pathogens to human laboratory personnel or HCP.
6. Indirect contact: Animals may be infected with prions, leading to potential risk for transmission via surgical instruments or medical devices if the same instruments are subsequently used on humans.

Mitigation

In order to minimize the risk of transmission of pathogens to humans, institutions should formulate thorough procedures to safely conduct diagnostic and therapeutic procedures on research animals and animals from veterinary or zoological sources. In doing so, healthcare facilities must ensure human safety takes priority over research project goals. Although accredited healthcare research centers expend significant efforts to ensure research animal well-being and to minimize

the likelihood that research animals harbor human pathogens, the risks cannot be eliminated as many potential pathogens are part of the normal microbiota of animals. At a minimum, the institutions IACUC must have approved all research involving animals, with supervision and monitoring by the institution's Comparative Medicine Department or Infection Control Department to ensure minimal exposure to potentially ill animals, and optimal prevention measures are in place for animal and human interactions, including environmental cleaning protocols for any equipment used in common. Since animals may be infected with prions, surgical instruments and other medical devices should not be used on both animals and humans. Medical devices that require disinfection or sterilization should be used exclusively for animals. Alternatively, single-use disposable devices could be used.

Conclusions and Future Research Needs

As advances in medical research to benefit humans continue to develop, healthcare facilities are increasingly likely to use advanced diagnostic and therapeutic facilities for patients as well as research animals and possibly for zoo and veterinary animals. Healthcare facilities that use research animals should publish their policies and protocols for their safe use and monitor whether any adverse events were associated with their use. Single-use disposable devices are preferred for animal use or instruments or devices that are exclusively dedicated for animals. Future research is needed in this area to assure safe use of facilities at acute care hospitals for research animals.

Pets

Background

For the purposes of this document, "pet" refers to a "personal pet," namely, a domestic animal that is owned by an individual patient that is not a service animal nor an animal used for animal-assisted activities.

It has been estimated that over 60% of American households [48] own at least one pet (dogs 36.5%, cats 304%, birds 3.1%, and horses 1.5%), representing an estimated total of over 157 million companion animals [26]. The benefits associated with pet ownership, brief exposures to pets in various types of clinical and laboratory settings, and as an augmentation to traditional therapy are being increasingly realized and acknowledged [39, 49]. However, the safe management of pet visitation in healthcare facilities has not been systematically studied.

Benefits/Risks

Visitation of patients in healthcare facilities by their own pets potentially offers benefits and challenges. The potential benefits of pet ownership have been discussed in another section [28], and though no studies have specifically addressed the impact of pet visitation when the pet owner is in the healthcare setting, some of the described benefits, such as reduced levels of stress and reduced anxiety, may occur when the pet owner is a patient in the healthcare setting. While pets are less scrutinized and would not necessarily fulfill the requirements for animal-assisted activities visitation programs, the potentially strong human-animal bond and corresponding potential positive impact on the patient lead many facilities to permit this activity. The stronger bond with the pet could accentuate the positive impacts on the patient, and the preestablished relationship between the pet and person could reduce the risk of adverse events such as bites and scratches.

However, pets and their owners typically do not undergo the same (or any) form of training and scrutiny as compared to animal-assisted activities teams. Pets do not typically undergo the same degree of health assessment or exclusion practices (e.g., age) as compared to animals used in animal-assisted activities. Further, while visitation with pets can be restricted, in theory, to only the individual patient, in practice, this may not be the case, as pets could encounter various HCP, visitors, and patients during their time in the facility. Therefore, it cannot necessarily be assumed that the implications of visitation of a personal pet are guaranteed to be restricted to an individual patient. Additionally, pets have typically not been temperament tested, resulting in inconsistency in their behavior in an unfamiliar healthcare environment. Especially concerning would be young animals which may not be housebroken, are generally more excitable, and are more likely to bite or scratch.

Mitigation

Healthcare facilities should have a policy regarding the admittance of pet animals into the facility and an individual that oversees the program. Pets in general should be prohibited from entering healthcare facilities, including pets of HCP, patients, and visitors. Exceptions can be considered when the healthcare team determines that visit with a pet would be of benefit for the patient and can be performed with limited risk to the patient, to other patients, and for the healthcare facility as a whole. Examples of such exceptions may be for compassionate or clinical care purposes (such as terminally ill patient, a patient hospitalized for prolonged period of time, or where the healthcare team determines that a visit with a pet may improve the patient's physical or mental health). Pets of HCP should not be allowed in a healthcare

facility since they may place other HCP at risk (i.e., bites or scratches, allergies).

Risks associated with pet visitation should also be mitigated by limiting pet visitation to dogs, in particular to dogs at least 1 year of age and that are housebroken. Additionally, written information must be provided to the animal's owner/designee outlining the details of the visit, limited duration (1 h), expectations for acceptable and unacceptable practices, and supervisory and hygiene responsibilities of the owner/guardian. Visitation should be restricted for high-risk settings (e.g., patients on isolation precautions or in intensive care or immunocompromised patients).

Future Research Needs

A recent review of pet ownership and physical health concluded that the value of pet ownership as a nonpharmacological treatment modality, augmentation to traditional treatment, and healthy preventive behavior is starting to be realized [39]. However, more investigations, including clinical trials and investigations that more closely examine the underlying mechanism of the pet-health effect, such as oxytocin, are needed. Finally, research is warranted on benefits and risks of pet interactions in the acute care setting.

Conclusions

Pets should in general be excluded from visiting their owners in the healthcare setting. Though pets are prevalent throughout the United States, little data is available to clearly demonstrate that benefits outweigh potential risks associated with pet visitation in the healthcare setting. Unlike animals used in AAT, pets and their owners typically do not undergo the same (or any) form of training and scrutiny as compared to animal-assisted activities teams, nor are they subject to the same degree of health assessment or exclusion practices (e.g., age) as compared to AAT animals. Exceptions may be considered for pet visitation for compassionate reasons on a case-by-case basis at the discretion of the healthcare facility, with close supervision. Additional research should be undertaken to assess the benefits and risks of allowing pets into healthcare facilities.

Medicinal Leeches

Background

Medicinal leeches are used in modern medicine to sustain circulation in the management of acute venous congestion in patients with replantation of digits and ears, and in reconstruction using cutaneous or muscle flaps [1]. Evidence has also demonstrated that leeches might provide therapeutic pain reduction in patients with osteoarthritis [50]. Leech therapy most commonly uses *Hirudo medicinalis* and usually lasts around 2–6 days. Leeches may remove 5–15 mL of blood in this period to prevent congestion, keeping the tissue perfused until venous capillary return is established. Leech saliva released during feeding contains biologically active substances that act as vasodilators, anti-inflammatory mediators, anticoagulants, and analgesics. The most important component of leech saliva is the anticoagulant and bactericidal agent hirudin [51].

Benefits/Risks

Leech therapy (hirudotherapy) is generally considered safe and well tolerated, but contraindications include arterial insufficiency, hematologic disorders, and allergy to leeches. Additionally, infection is a major complication. *Aeromonas hydrophila* is one common pathogen found in the gut of leeches that has been implicated in an incidence of sepsis after leech therapy [52]. Infections from *Vibrio fluvialis* and *Serratia marcescens* have also been reported [53, 54]. In addition to infection, other potential complications that can arise following hirudotherapy include thrombotic microangiopathy, anemia, and continued bleeding [55].

Mitigation

Antimicrobial prophylaxis with trimethoprim-sulfamethoxazole or ciprofloxacin appears to be equally effective for prevention of leech-associated infection of *Aeromonas* spp. [56]. However, antibiotic-resistant *Aeromonas hydrophila* infection following leech therapy has been reported.

Guidelines for using leeches include general storage protocols. Leeches should be stored in a refrigerator or cool, dark place in a glass or plastic container with bottled or distilled, non-chlorinated water as well as a salt additive. Tap water, direct sunlight, and temperatures above 20 °C are contraindicated for leech storage [57]. Unused leeches should be maintained by a pharmacy. Used leeches should never be reused even on the same patient or returned to the pharmacy. They should be disposed of by placement in a labeled, screw capped jar of 20 mL of 8% ethanol for 3 min, have 50 mL of 70% methylated spirit added, and disposed of as regulated (i.e., hazardous) medical waste [1, 58].

Future Research Needs

Further research is needed to understand the role of prophylactic antibiotic therapy to decrease risk of infection. Additionally, it is important to determine conditions in which leech therapy is contraindicated and improve prevention against adverse effects.

Maggot Debridement Therapy

Background

Larval debridement therapy, also known as maggot debridement therapy (MDT), uses sterile larva of the fly *Lucilia sericata* and is implemented around the world to treat wounds that are resistant to conventional therapy. Maggots preferentially digest and remove necrotic tissue, leaving behind healthy tissue. The antimicrobial and anti-inflammatory properties of MDT therapy may also aid in wound healing through disinfection and tissue growth stimulation [59, 60].

Benefits/Risks

MDT has been shown to effectively treat chronic ulcers in diabetics and wounds in patients with malignancies [61, 62]. The most common complaint after MDT in patients is pain due to the hooklike teeth of maggots used for locomotion, but it can be controlled with analgesics [63]. While many clinical uses for MDT have been identified, contraindications include dry wounds, wounds close to large blood vessels, and patients allergic to fly larvae [64].

Mitigation

Before the use of larvae, external disinfection of the fly eggs is necessary to reduce the chance of introducing new bacteria into the wound. One study has yielded a protocol that requires immersing fly eggs for 10 min in 3% Lysol to provide high disinfection efficacy as well as maximum egg survival [65]. Larvae should be bred in a sterile and moist environment. After hatching, larvae should be stored in a refrigerator at 8–10 °C in an insulated box with oxygen and a humid atmosphere or used within 8 h [66]. Used maggots should be disposed of as regulated (i.e., hazardous) medical waste (i.e., placed in a tight-fitting bottle) and incinerated.

Future Research Needs

Large controlled clinical trials assessing benefits, risks, and cost-effectiveness of MDT need to be performed [67]. Further research needs to assess whether single or episodic debridement has better clinical benefits and whether MDT enhances wound healing after debridement is achieved. In order to decrease the social stigma of MDT, further studies should assess if the antimicrobial or anti-inflammatory properties of MDT can be concentrated in a medication or cream.

Aquariums/Fish Tanks

Background

There are many infections that can be acquired in water either by trauma or animal-inflicted injury. Pathogens that can cause these infections include *Aeromonas hydrophila*, *Erysipelothrix rhusiopathiae*, *Mycobacterium marinum*, *Vibrio vulnificus*, *Staphylococcus* species, *Streptococcus* species, and *Sporothrix schenckii* [68].

Benefits/Risks

While aquariums and fish tanks are found by many to be visually appealing, infections pose a serious concern. *M. marinum* infections have been shown to be associated with cleaning fish tanks [69]. One study identified *A. hydrophila* in a patient's goldfish tank as the cause of peritoneal dialysis-related peritonitis [70]. Another study investigated an outbreak of *Salmonella* Paratyphi in which 33 of the 53 patients owned aquariums and purchased tropical fish weeks before exhibiting symptoms. Furthermore, more than half of the pet shop aquariums where the fish were purchased tested positive for *Salmonella* serotypes [71]. Additionally, one public aquarium was found to be the source of an outbreak of Legionnaires' disease [72].

Mitigation

Because fish tanks can be a reservoir for many pathogens, fish tanks should be generally excluded from healthcare facilities, including nonclinical areas; however, aquariums may be permitted if maintained by trained personnel, utilize a closed system, and are implemented with water pumps designed to prevent aerosalization [1]. Patients should never have direct access to the aquarium.

Future Research Needs

Further studies into methods to improve tank hygiene are important to decrease potential for infection.

Petting Zoos

Background

Animal exhibits such as petting zoos provide a popular, managed learning environment that involves interaction with animals such as feeding and other physical contact. Conrad et al. compiled a review of the principal causal organisms of human illness associated with petting zoos and farm environments that includes *Campylobacter*, non-0157 Shiga toxin-producing *Escherichia coli* (STEC), *Yersinia enterocolitica*, *Salmonella*, and *Cryptosporidium* [73]. Transmission risk of enteric infectious diseases and parasites may be higher in children where high-risk behaviors may contribute to pathogen transmission, such as contact with manure and hand-to-mouth behaviors such as thumb-sucking. Controlling transmission is difficult as livestock can shed pathogens such as *E. coli* O157:H7 intermittently; can shed due to stress from confinement, transport, and human interaction; and can carry infectious organisms in their fur, saliva, and hair due to fecal contamination [73]. Additionally, non-typhoidal *Salmonella* species are found in live poultry including baby chicks and ducklings [74]. Lastly, infections spread to humans from pet reptiles have been identified, with 90% of captive reptiles estimated to carry *Salmonella* [73].

Mitigation

As petting zoos and other animal exhibits have been associated with infectious outbreaks, such activities should be prohibited from healthcare facilities [1]. If any exceptions are made for special situations, they should not be conducted as an activity of the healthcare facility to avoid confusion about the healthcare facility's responsibility for legal and regulatory requirements and to protect the patients from possible acquisition of a zoonotic disease.

Future Research Needs

Further research should examine methods of animal vaccination and decontamination. Additionally, facilities should assess allowing children to view animals in an active and enjoyable experience without direct contact.

Conclusions

Recommendations for the safe oversight and management of AHC should comply with legal requirements and minimize the risk of transmission of pathogens from animals to humans when animals are permitted in the healthcare setting. Accordingly, healthcare institutions should ensure appropriate policies, and procedures are implemented regarding the management of AHC and provide education to staff, patients, and visitors as indicated.

As the role of AHC evolves, research is warranted to establish evidence-based guidelines for their management. Carefully designed and conducted studies are needed to better define the benefits and risks of allowing animals in the healthcare setting for specific purposes.

Additionally, there is a need for the systematic evaluation of risks of animals in healthcare based on the category of use (e.g., animal-assisted activities, service animal, research, and personal pet visitation). Prospective tracking of adverse outcomes associated with AHC facilities will help to refine and clarify the approaches to managing the controversies related to AHC. In addition, publication of any outbreaks, clusters, or infections attributable to the presence of AHC facilities should be encouraged. Finally, prospective studies on optimal infection prevention practices for management of animals in healthcare are needed.

References

1. Murthy R, Bearman G, Brown S, Bryant K, Chinn R, Hewlett A, George BG, Goldstein EJ, Holzmann-Pazgal G, Rupp ME, Wiemken T, Weese JS, Weber DJ. Animals in healthcare facilities: recommendations to minimize potential risks. Infect Control Hosp Epidemiol. 2015;36:495–516.
2. Humane Society of the United States. Pets by the numbers. http://www.humanesociety.org/issues/pet_overpopulation/facts/pet_ownership_statistics.html. (n.d.). Accessed 5 Aug 2016.
3. Weese JS, Caldwell F, Willey BM, Kreiswirth BN, McGeer A, Rousseau J, et al. An outbreak of methicillin-resistant *Staphylococcus aureus* skin infections resulting from horse to human transmission in a veterinary hospital. Vet Microbiol. 2006;114:160–4.
4. Lefebvre SL, Reid-Smith RJ, Waltner-Toews D, Weese JS. Incidence of acquisition of methicillin-resistant *Staphylococcus aureus*, Clostridium difficile, and other health-care-associated pathogens by dogs that participate in animal-assisted interventions. J Am Vet Med Assoc. 2009;234:1404–17.
5. Oehler RL, Velez AP, Mizrachi M, Lamarche J, Gompf S. Bite-related and septic syndromes caused by cats and dogs. Lancet Infect Dis. 2009;9:439–47.
6. Heydemann J, Heydemann JS, Antony S. Acute infection of a total knee arthroplasty caused by *Pasteurella multocida*: a case report and a comprehensive review of the literature in the last 10 years. Int J Infect Dis. 2010;14(Suppl 3):e242–5.
7. Abrahamian FM, Goldstein EJ. Microbiology of animal bite wound infections. Clin Microbiol Rev. 2011;24:231–46.
8. Pet partners course on infection prevention and control for AAT https://petpartners.org/learn/online-education/. Accessed 5 Sept 2016.
9. Lefebvre SL, Golab GC, Christensen E, et al. Guidelines for animal-assisted interventions in health care facilities. Am J Infect Control. 2008;36:78–85.
10. Abate SV, Zucconi M, Boxer BA. Impact of canine-assisted ambulation on hospitalized chronic heart failure patients' ambulation outcomes and satisfaction: a pilot study. J Cardiovasc Nurs. 2011;26:224–30.
11. Banks MR, Banks WA. The effects of animal-assisted therapy on loneliness in an elderly population in long-term care facilities. J Gerontol A Biol Sci Med Sci. 2002;57:M428–32.
12. Barak Y, Savorai O, Mavashev S, Beni A. Animal-assisted therapy for elderly schizophrenic patients: a one-year controlled trial. Am J Geriatr Psychiatry. 2001;9:439–42.
13. Barker SB, Pandurangi AK, Best AM. Effects of animal-assisted therapy on patients' anxiety, fear, and depression before ECT. J ECT. 2003;19:38–44.
14. Barker SB, Dawson KS. The effects of animal-assisted therapy on anxiety ratings of hospitalized psychiatric patients. Psychiatr Serv. 1998;49:797–801.
15. Edwards NE, Beck AM. Animal-assisted therapy and nutrition in Alzheimer's disease. West J Nurs Res. 2002;24:697–712.
16. Moretti F, De Ronchi D, Bernabei V, et al. Pet therapy in elderly patients with mental illness. Psychogeriatrics. 2011;11:125–9.
17. Sobo EJ, Seid M, Reyes Gelhard L. Parent-identified barriers to pediatric health care: a process-oriented model. Health Serv Res. 2006;41:148–72.
18. Honnorat E, Seng P, Savini H, Pinelli PO, Simon F, Stein A. Prosthetic joint infection caused by *Pasteurella multocida*: a case series and review of literature. BMC Infect Dis. 2016;16(1):435.
19. Hadley K, Torres AM, Moran J. Schiller B *Bordetella bronchiseptica* peritonitis – beware of the dog! Perit Dial Int. 2009;29(6):670–1.
20. U.S. Department of Labor. American with disabilities act. https://www.dol.gov/general/topic/disability/ada. (n.d.). Accessed 1 Dec 2016.
21. U.S. Department of Justice, Civil Rights Division. ADA requirements: service animals. https://www.ada.gov/service_animals_2010.pdf. (n.d.). Accessed 1 Dec 2016.
22. U,S. Department of Housing and Urban Development. Reasonable accommodations under the fair housing act. http://portal.hud.gov/hudportal/HUD?src=/program_offices/fair_housing_equal_opp/ReasonableAccommodations15. (n.d.). Accessed 1 Dec 2016.
23. Peacock J, Chur-Hansen A, Winefield H. Mental health implications of human attachment to companion animals. J Clin Psychol. 2012;68(3):292–303.
24. McConnell AR, Brown CM, Shoda TM, Stayton LE, Martin CE. Friends with benefits: on the positive consequences of pet ownership. J Pers Soc Psychol. 2011;101(6):1239–5.
25. Chur-Hansen A, Stern C, Winefield H. Gaps in the evidence about companion animals and human health: some suggestions for progress. Int J Evid Based Healthc. 2010;8(3):140–6.
26. AVMA. U.S. pet ownership statistics. https://www.avma.org/KB/Resources/Statistics/Pages/Market-research-statistics-US-pet-ownership.aspx. (n.d.). Accessed 5 Aug 2016.
27. Humane Society of the United States. Pets by the numbers. http://www.humanesociety.org/issues/pet_overpopulation/facts/pet_ownership_statistics.html. (n.d.). Accessed 5 Aug 2016.
28. Raina P, Waltner-Toews D, Bonnett B, Woodward C, Abernathy T. Influence of companion animals on the physical and psychological health of older people: an analysis of a one-year longitudinal study. J Am Geriatr Soc. 1999;47:323–9.
29. Rhea SK, Weber DJ, Poole C, Waller AE, Ising AI, Williams C. Use of statewide emergency department surveillance data to assess inci-

dence of animal bite injuries among humans in North Carolina. J Am Vet Med Assoc. 2014;244:597–603.

30. Weber DJ, Hansen AR. Infections resulting from animal bites. Infect Dis Clin NA. 1991;5:663–80.

31. Weber DJ, Rutala WA, Kaplan SL. *Pasteurella* infections. UpToDate. 2016.

32. Goldstein EJ, Abrahamian FM. Diseases transmitted by cats. Microbiol Spectr. 2015;3(5).

33. Centers for Disease Control and Prevention. Rabies: domestic animals. http://www.cdc.gov/rabies/location/usa/surveillance/domestic_animals.html. (n.d.). Accessed 5 Aug 2016.

34. Scott GM, Thomson R, Malone-Lee J, Ridgway GL. Cross-infection between animals and man: possible feline transmission of Staphylococcus aureus infection in humans? J Hosp Infect. 1988;12:2.

35. Schattner A, Huber R. Zoonosis in the nursing home. J Am Geriatr Soc. 2016;64:685.

36. Drusin LM, Ross BG, Rhodes KH, Krauss AN, Scott RA. Nosocomial ringworm in a neonatal intensive care unit: a nurse and her cat. Infect Control Hosp Epidemiol. 2000;21:605–7.

37. U.S. Department of Justice. ADA requirements, service animals. https://www.ada.gov/service_animals_2010.htm. (n.d.). Accessed 5 Aug 2016.

38. New York State Senate. Senate bill S5084A. Relates to the prohibition of the declawing of cats. https://www.nysenate.gov/legislation/bills/2015/s5084. (n.d.). Accessed 5 Aug 2016.

39. Matchock RL. Pet ownership and physical health. Curr Opin Psychiatry. 2015;28(5):386–92. doi:10.1097/YCO.0000000000000183. Accessed 5 Sept 2016

40. U.S. Department of Agriculture, animal and plant health inspection service, "Annual Report Animal Usage by Fiscal Year," 2 June 2015.

41. Anderson LC, Leary SL, Manning PJ. Rat-bite fever in animal research laboratory personnel. Lab Anim Sci. 1983;33:292–4.

42. Davenport DS, Johnson DR, Holmes GP, Jewett DA, Ross SC, Hilliard JK. Diagnosis and management of human B virus (Herpesvirus simiae) infections in Michigan. Clin Infect Dis. 1994;19:33–41.

43. Wilson BA, Ho M. Pasteurella multocida: from zoonosis to cellular microbiology. Clin Microbiol Rev. 2013;26:631–55.

44. Pedrosa PB, Cardoso TA. Viral infections in workers in hospital and research laboratory settings: a comparative review of infection modes and respective biosafety aspects. Int J Infect Dis. 2011;15:e366–76.

45. Dorsett-Martin WA. Considering Q fever when working with laboratory sheep. Lab Anim (NY). 2010;39:86–9.

46. Saito T, Ohnishi J, Mori Y, Iinuma Y, Ichiyama S, Kohi F. Infection by *Chlamydophilia avium* in an elderly couple working in a pet shop. J Clin Microbiol. 2005;43:3011–3.

47. Aly R. Ecology and epidemiology of dermatophyte infections. J Am Acad Dermatol. 1994;31:S21–5.

48. American pet products association (2015–2016) http://www.humanesociety.org/issues/pet_overpopulation/facts/pet_ownership_statistics.html. Accessed 11 Sept 2016.

49. Cherniack EP, Cherniack AR. The benefit of pets and animal-assisted therapy to the health of older individuals. Curr Gerontol Geriatr Res. 2014;2014:623203.

50. Gunawan F, Wibowo YR, Bunawan NC, Turner JH. Controversy: hirudotherapy (leech therapy) as an alternative treatment for osteoarthritis. Acta Med Indones. 2015;47(2):176–80.

51. Mumcuoglu KY. Recommendations for the use of leeches in reconstructive plastic surgery. Evid Based Complement Alternat Med. 2014;2014:1–7. doi:10.1155/2014/205929.

52. Levine SM, Frangos SG, Hanna B, Colen K, Levine JP. *Aeromonas* septicemia after medicinal leech use following replantation of severed digits. Am J Crit Care. 2010;19:469–71.

53. Varghese MR, Farr RW, Wax MK, Chafin BJ, Owens RM. *Vibrio fluvialis* wound infection associated with medicinal leech therapy. Clin Infect Dis. 1996;22:709–10.

54. Pereira JA, Greig JR, Liddy H, Ion L, Moss ALH. Leech-borne *Serratia marcescens* infection following complex hand injury. Br J Plast Surg. 1998;51(8):640–1.

55. Etemadi J, Ardalan MR, Motavali R, Tubbs RS, Shoja MM. Thrombotic microangiopathy as a complication of medicinal leech therapy. South Med J. 2008;101(8):845–7.

56. Kruer RM, Barton CA, Roberti G, Gilbert B, McMilian WD. Antimicrobial prophylaxis during Hirudo medicinalis therapy: a multicenter study. J Reconstr Microsurg. 2015;31(3):205–9.

57. Bennett-Marsden M, Ng A. Hirudotherapy: a guide to using leeches to drain blood from tissue. Clin Pharm. 2014;6(3):69. doi:10.1211/CP.2014.11136626.

58. Whitaker IS, Izadi D, Oliver DW, Monteath G, Butler PE. *Hirudo Medicinalis* and the plastic surgeon. Br J Plast Surg. 2004;57(4):348–53.

59. Sun X, Jiang K, Chen J, Wu L, Lu H, Wang A, Wang J. A systematic review of maggot debridement therapy for chronically infected wounds and ulcers. Int J Infect Dis. 2014;25:32–7.

60. Klaus K, Steinwedel C. Maggot debridement therapy: advancing to the past in wound care. Medsurg Nurs. 2015;24(6):407–11.

61. Lin Y, Amin A, Donnelly AFW, Amar S. Maggot debridement therapy of a leg wound from Kaposi's sarcoma: a case report. J Glob Oncol. 2015;1(2):92–8.

62. Azad AK, Wan Azizi WS, Adham SA, Yee BL. Maggot debridement therapy for diabetic foot ulcer: experience from maggot treatment centers. Asian J Pharm Pharmacol. 2016;2(1):23–5.

63. Mumcuoglu KY, Davidson E, Avidan A, Gilead L. Pain related to maggot debridement therapy. J Wound Care. 2012;21(8):400–5.

64. Chan DCW, Fong DHF, Leung JYY, Patil NG, Leung GKK. Maggot debridement therapy in chronic wound care. Hong Kong Med J. 2007;13(5):382–6.

65. Brundage AL, Crippen TL, Tomberlin JK. Methods for external disinfection of blow fly (Diptera: Calliphoridae) eggs prior to use in wound debridement therapy. Wound Repair Regen. 2016;24(2):384–93.

66. Richardson M. The benefits of larval therapy in wound care. Nurs Stand. 2004;19(7):70–6.

67. Sherman RA. Mechanisms of maggot-induced wound healing: what do we know, and where do we go from here? Evid Based Complement Alternat Med. 2014;2014:1–13. doi:10.1155/2014/592419.

68. Haddad V, Lupi O, Lonza JP, Tyring SK. Tropical dermatology: marine and aquatic dermatology. J Am Acad Dermatol. 2009;61(5):733–50.

69. Slany M, Jezek P, Bodnarova M. Fish tank granuloma caused by *Mycobacterium marinum* in two aquarists: two case reports. Biomed Res Int. 2013;2013:1–4. doi:10.1155/2013/161329.

70. Hisamachi M, et al. A rare case of peritoneal dialysis-related peritonitis caused by goldfish water tank derived *Aeromonas hydrophila*. Clin Nephrol. 2015;84(7):50–4.

71. Gaulin C, Vincent C, Ismaïl J. Sporadic infections of *Salmonella Paratyphi* B, var. Java associated with fish tanks. Can J Public Health. 2005;96(6):471–4.

72. Greig JE, Carnie JA, Tallis GF, et al. An outbreak of Legionnaires' disease at the Melbourne Aquarium, April 2000: investigation and case-control studies. Med J Aust. 2004;180(11):566–72.

73. Conrad C, Stanford K, Narvaez-Bravo C, Callaway T, Mcallister T. Farm fairs and petting zoos: a review of animal contact as a source of zoonotic enteric disease. Foodborne Pathog Dis. Epub ahead of print December 19, 2016 (doi:10.1089/fpd.2016.2185). (n.d.). Accessed 2 Jan 2017.

74. Centers for Disease Control and Prevention. Three outbreaks of salmonellosis associated with baby poultry from three hatcheries – United States, 2006. MMWR Morb Mortal Wkly Rep. 2007;56(12):273–6.

Decolonization in Infection Control of Gram-Negative Bacilli

24

David Thomas and David Banach

Background

The most common sites of bacterial colonization include the nares, skin, and gastrointestinal tract. Colonization with microorganisms is a normal component of the human microbiome and usually not of significant clinical consequence. Conversely, bacterial colonization with some organisms, including antibiotic-resistant organisms, can lead to subsequent clinical infection caused by the same colonizing organisms. The strategy of decolonization for the prevention of healthcare-associated infections has gained increasing attention over recent decades. The premise is that through localized antibiotic therapy, the burden of organisms at the site of colonization can be diminished, thereby reducing the risk of subsequent infection. Additionally, there may be a potential benefit of decolonization in preventing the spread of microorganisms within the healthcare setting as patients with asymptomatic colonization may serve as reservoirs for infection transmission.

Although much of the published literature focuses on decolonization of Gram-positive organisms, most notably *Staphylococcus aureus*, there is a growing interest in the decolonization strategy for Gram-negative bacilli, particularly multidrug-resistant organisms. Decolonization strategies are often divided into two categories: vertical and horizontal decolonization. Vertical decolonization is a strategy targeted to specific organisms, usually multidrug-resistant organisms. When colonization with a specific organism is identified through clinical culture or active surveillance, decolonization may be considered in an effort to prevent subsequent infection caused by that organism. Horizontal decolonization involves administration of the same decolonization strategy across all patients in a specific unit in an attempt to decrease burden from multiple different organisms. Much of this chapter will focus on horizontal approaches to decolonization, including topical decolonization and the use of selective digestive decontamination for gastrointestinal decolonization (Table 24.1). Some strategies are focused upon patients colonized with specific Gram-negative organisms, such as carbapenem-resistant *Enterobacteriaceae* or multidrug-resistant *Acinetobacter* or *Pseudomonas*.

Skin Decolonization for Gram-Negative Bacilli Infections

Topical decolonization of the skin has become an emerging and increasingly appealing strategy to prevent subsequent bacterial infections by reducing skin microbial burden. Several antiseptic agents have been explored as potential topical decolonizing agents in various clinical settings. Although much of the focus of topical decolonization lies in preventing infections caused by Gram-positive organisms which compose the majority of the skin microbiome, some studies have evaluated the impact of this strategy on the reduction of infections caused by Gram-negative bacteria, including multidrug-resistant organisms. Some topical decolonizing agents that have been explored in the clinical setting, such as hexochlorophane, do not have adequate activity against Gram-negative bacilli. Other agents, such as sodium hypochlorite, have been studied for their utility in reducing methicillin-resistant *Staphylococcus aureus* (MRSA) skin colonization [1]. Triclosan is an antimicrobial agent with Gram-negative activity incorporated into household soaps and skin care products. Its role in decolonization for the control of Gram-negative bacilli is not well established, and its benefit over traditional soap and water in hand hygiene has not been well demonstrated [2].

D. Thomas • D. Banach (✉)
Infectious Diseases, University of Connecticut School of Medicine, 263 Farmington Avenue, Farmington, CT 06030, USA
e-mail: DThomas@uchc.edu; DBanach@uchc.edu

© Springer International Publishing AG 2018
G. Bearman et al. (eds.), *Infection Prevention*, DOI 10.1007/978-3-319-60980-5_24

Table 24.1 Strategies for decolonization of Gram-negative bacilli

Strategy	Examples	Potential advantages	Potential disadvantages
Topical decolonization	Topical chlorhexidine	Well tolerated, has broad activity against both Gram-negative and Gram-positive organisms	Data on clinical utility against preventing infection and transmission of Gram-negative organisms is limited. Potential for emergence of resistant organisms not well understood
Selective oral or digestive decontamination	Aminoglycosides or polymyxin administered orally or the nasogastric tube	Localized antibiotic delivery to the most common site of Gram-negative bacilli colonization, the gastrointestinal tract	Efficacy and optimal regimen not well established in clinical studies. May lead to emergence of resistant organisms. Typically involves antibiotics used as "last resort" for treating organisms with multidrug resistance
Systemic antibiotics	Intravenous antibiotics with broad-spectrum activity	Delivery of high levels of antibiotics to all colonization sites	Significant concern for increased risk of antibiotic-associated adverse effects and the emergence of resistant organisms at colonizing sites

Chlorhexidine Gluconate

The agent with the most experience in topical decolonization is chlorhexidine gluconate (CHG). CHG has a broad spectrum of antimicrobial activity against Gram-positive and Gram-negative organisms and some clinically significant yeast. In clinical practice topical CHG has been used in skin antisepsis prior to surgery or insertion of medical devices, maintenance of intravascular catheters, and hand hygiene. It is available in varying formulations and concentrations, most commonly as a 2–4% concentration solution. Its most common clinical application for decolonization consists of "bathing" patients, usually in the intensive care unit (ICU) setting, using impregnated cloths either daily or at regular intervals.

Several studies, including recently published prospective, randomized clinical trials, have demonstrated a reduction in bloodstream infections [3, 4] and a reduction in the acquisition of MRSA and vancomycin-resistant enterococci (VRE) [3] associated with CHG bathing. Despite its broad activity against many Gram-negative organisms, the data supporting its use in the prevention of both infection and transmission of Gram-negative bacilli is limited. Bundled strategies which have incorporated the use of topical CHG have been effective in controlling outbreaks of *Klebsiella pneumoniae* carbapenemase-producing (KPC) *Klebsiella pneumoniae* [5] and multidrug-resistant *Acinetobacter baumannii* [6]. Data focusing specifically in the specific impact of universal decolonization with topical CHG on reducing Gram-negative bacilli transmission and preventing clinical infection are limited.

A single-center study from Israel evaluated the impact of 4% CHG gluconate washing on *A. baumannii* skin colonization among patients admitted to the medical ICU. In this study, among 320 patients admitted to the ICU, 55 (17%) were colonized with *A. baumannii*. Following CHG washing, subsequent cultures revealed a prevalence of *A. baumannii* colonization among 5.5% of patients at 24 h and (1/55)

1% at 48 h after washing ($p = 0.002$) [7]. In this study, the rate of *A. baumannii bloodstream* infections was reduced as well. Similar findings were seen in a study of trauma patients who underwent daily CHG bathing resulting in lower rates of *A. baumannii* colonization (69% vs. 23%, $p < 0.001$) [8]. CHG bathing coupled with a hand hygiene intervention was associated with decreased rates of *A. baumannii* pneumonia [8]. A subsequent study evaluated the impact of routine CHG bathing on reducing skin burden of *Klebsiella pneumoniae* carbapenemase-producing (KPC) *Klebsiella pneumoniae* among patients at a single long-term acute care hospital. This study found that post-decolonization, rates of skin colonization with *K. pneumoniae* decreased significantly at multiple sites (56% vs. 32%, $p = 0.01$). Additionally, higher skin concentrations of CHG were associated with decreased KPC *K. pneumoniae* colonization [9]. More recently, a single center in France evaluated the impact of 2% CHG washing among ICU patients with a history of a septic event. This study revealed that daily CHG bathing was associated with decreased risk of healthcare-associated infections and decreased incidence of clinical cultures positive with Gram-negative bacilli (relative risk (RR) 0.59, 95% confidence interval (CI) 0.35–0.98) [10].

However, not all studies have demonstrated efficacy of topical CHG in decolonization for Gram-negative bacilli. A recent open-label, controlled trial among ICU patients showed that CHG-impregnated wipes did not prevent colonization with multidrug-resistant Gram-negative organisms, including ESBL-producing *K. pneumoniae* and *E. coli* and MDR *P. aeruginosa* and *A. baumannii* [11]. A large multicenter study in Europe evaluated the use of CHG in combination with intensified hand hygiene through an interrupted time-series model and found that although MRSA acquisition decreased with the intervention, there was no impact on the acquisition of highly resistant *Enterobacteriaceae*, consisting of organisms resistant to third- or fourth-generation cephalosporins [12].

Overall, large studies demonstrated that CHG bathing is well tolerated [3, 4]. The most common adverse effects are skin reactions, usually relatively mild in nature, typically occurring in less than 2% of patients. The impact of topical CHG on the emergence of resistance among Gram-negative bacilli has raised concern. Increasing adoption of universal decolonization with CHG as a horizontal strategy for infection prevention may lead to increasing emergence of isolates resistant to topical antiseptics through selective pressure. Additionally, cross-resistance of CHG with antibiotics that are administered systemically for the treatment of infections has been raised as a separate but related concern. To date, there has been limited effort in evaluating CHG resistance among Gram-negative organisms, and there is no system in place to monitor this on a larger scale. One study suggested a rise in in vitro CHG resistance among *A. baumannii* isolates following introduction of CHG bathing in an ICU [13].

In summary, topical decolonization with CHG may be a useful strategy to reduce the transmission of Gram-negative organisms and in prevention of subsequent infections caused by these bacteria, particularly when used as part of a multifaceted infection prevention program. More data is needed to further evaluate the impact of CHG bathing on preventing infections caused by Gram-negative bacilli in different settings in order to determine the true value of this topical decolonization strategy and the impact on the emergence of CHG resistance associated with widespread use.

Selective Decontamination

Selective digestive decontamination (SDD) is a prophylactic strategy designed to prevent or minimize risk of developing infection, either from endogenous or exogenous sources, as well as utility in reducing mortality in critically ill patient populations [14]. In essence, the goal is eradication or prevention of oropharyngeal and/or intestinal carriage of potentially pathogenic organisms, particularly with attention to aerobic Gram-negative bacteria, including both sensitive and highly resistant strains. In most situations SDD does not include antimicrobial activity against all possible organisms and excludes anaerobes, enterococci, coagulase-negative staphylococci, and the viridans group streptococci.

In recent decades, significant research has been conducted to assess the feasibility and effectiveness of SDD and selective oropharyngeal decontamination (SOD) often combined with systemic, typically intravenous, antimicrobials. As of 2012, there were 66 clinical trials and 11 meta-analyses published since 1983 [14]. It is noteworthy that the majority of these trials were conducted in European countries. Although accumulated data is relatively limited at this time, more trials are being conducted to strengthen the existing body of evidence. Some of the largest individual trials and meta-analyses will be summarized in this section.

From 1999 to 2001, a major trial was undertaken to assess the effectiveness of SDD as well as potential acquisition of resistant bacteria in 934 patients in ICUs in the Netherlands [15]. Patients were randomly assigned to either the treatment group or control group receiving standard treatments over a period of 2 years. The treatment group received a regimen of oral and enteral polymyxin E, tobramycin, and amphotericin B combined with an initial 4-day course of IV cefotaxime. Primary endpoints included mortality in the ICU as well as resistant bacteria acquisition. As a secondary endpoint, patients who survived their stay in the ICU were continued to be followed for the rest of their hospitalization. The SDD group had a lower ICU mortality (15% vs. 23%, $p = 0.002$) and lower overall in-hospital mortality (24% vs. 43%, $p = 0.02$). Additionally, rates of colonization with multidrug organisms were lower in the SDD group compared to the control group. These organisms included resistant Gram-negatives and vancomycin-resistant enterococci. The study concluded that in a setting of low prevalence of resistant organisms, SDD can decrease mortality and decrease colonization with drug-resistant Gram-negative bacterial strains.

Two years later, another trial of SDD versus SOD focused specifically on prevention of respiratory tract colonization and bacteremia with highly resistant organisms [16]. The study was conducted as an open-label clustered group randomized trial in the same 13 ICUs across the Netherlands comparing a regimen of SDD to SOD and standard care. The duration of this study was for 2 years and included 5927 total patients. The overall rate of bacteremia was higher in the standard of care group (13%) compared to SDD (7%) and SOD (9%) groups as were rates of bacteremia caused by highly resistant organisms. It was noted that 128 (15%) patients acquired polymyxin E or cefotaxime-resistant organisms during standard care compared with 74 (8%) patients in the SDD group and 88 (10%) patients in SOD group. Respiratory colonization with highly resistant organisms was also found to occur 38% less in SDD and 32% less frequently in the SOD group. Hence, the authors concluded that widespread use of SDD and SOD in the ICU setting with low levels of endemic antibiotic resistance may be justified.

Another large cluster-randomized trial attempted to compare efficacy of SDD and SOD while stratifying and comparing surgical to nonsurgical ICU patient subpopulations. This included analysis of SDD, SOD, and standard care in these patients [17]. The trial included 5927 patients from the original trial which included 2762 surgical versus 3,165 nonsurgical patients. The primary endpoint was mortality at 28 days. The authors also evaluated other secondary endpoints such as duration of ICU stay, duration of hospitalization, and duration of mechanical ventilation. Using adjusted odds ratios, there was no statistically significant mortality benefit among medical and surgical patients who received SDD. All secondary outcomes were significantly reduced in the surgical patients who received SDD. SOD did not reduce mortality in surgical patients versus standard care (OR 0.97, 95% CI 0.77–1.22); however, the regimen proved more effective in reducing mortality among nonsurgical patients (OR 0.77, 95% CI 0.63–0.94).

As data increased supporting SDD/SOD as a practical measure for reducing morbidity and mortality in the ICU setting, investigators began to focus on highly resistant organisms, recognizing the high mortality rates and limited systemic antibiotic therapies associated with infections caused by these organisms. A recent randomized double-blind, placebo-controlled trial undertaken at the Infectious Diseases Institute at Soroka University in Israel aimed to address this concern in studying the utility of SOD for eradication of known carriers of carbapenem-resistant *Klebsiella pneumoniae* [18]. The trial was conducted at a single tertiary hospital in adult patients with positive rectal swab cultures as well as swabs from the throat, groin, and urine. Patients were selected over a 20-month period with 7-week follow-up. The groups were matched 1:1 and received either the SOD regimen or placebo. The SOD regimen consisted of oral gentamicin and polymyxin E gel with oral solutions of gentamicin and polymyxin E. The placebo arm received a similarly timed regimen but without any active drug component. All subjects were imposed strict contact isolation with samples from 40 patients included in the analysis. There was significant reduction in positive rectal surveillance culture results at 2 weeks post-SOD treatment, with 16.1% reduction in the placebo group versus 61.1% reduction in the SOD arm, respectively (OR 0.13, 95% CI 0.02–0.74). Throat cultures were rendered completely sterile. However, there was no change in colonization rates of the groin and urine cultures associated with SOD, though colonization in these sites increased in the placebo arm. Notably, patients included in this study were the elderly, most with multiple comorbidities. Resistance was monitored in this study, and it was noted there was no appreciable increase in minimum inhibitory concentrations to the antimicrobials included in the SOD regimen.

Another trial aimed at evaluating both efficacy of SDD and SOD and investigating the potential for antibiotic resistance was conducted in the Netherlands as a cluster-randomized crossover trial involving 16 different ICUs averaging 250 patients in each site [19]. The SDD and SOD regimens consisted of oropharyngeal application of a paste containing polymyxin E, tobramycin, and amphotericin B in a 2% concentration every 6 h along with a 10 mL suspension of polymyxin E, tobramycin, and amphotericin B administered by nasogastric tube in the SDD group only. SDD patients also received a 4-day course of intravenous cefotaxime or ceftriaxone. The investigators found there was

significantly lower rate of rectal colonization with highly resistant organisms in the SDD arm versus patients receiving SOD. Specifically, aminoglycoside resistance was 5.6% in SDD and 11.8% in SOD, and among the SDD group, there was a nonsignificant decrease in rectal colonization with ciprofloxacin-resistant organisms and ESBL-producing organisms. There was no difference in mortality or length of stay between the two regimens nor were there notable differences between surgical and nonsurgical cases. The rate of bacteremia caused by aminoglycoside-resistant organisms was lower in the SDD group versus SOD patients (OR 0.54, 95% CI 0.31–0.97).

However, not all findings have supported decontamination, and early arguments included the concern for antibiotic resistance as well as concern that no mortality benefit would be demonstrated. One earlier trial looked at 660 patients on mechanical ventilation in a multidisciplinary ICU over a period of 19 months [20]. The purpose of this study was to evaluate two different drug regimens for use in selective decontamination to determine their impact on mortality as well as the emergence of resistant organisms. The first group received standard of care and served as controls. The second group received a regimen of oral and enteral ofloxacin and amphotericin B. The final group received oral and enteral polymyxin E, tobramycin, and amphotericin B. Results did not support the utilization of decontamination, and mortality was found to be identical in the two groups and was also not significantly related to infection. In addition, increased antimicrobial resistance was noted in both groups. This included a 48% increase in tobramycin-resistant *Enterobacteriaceae* in the third group versus 14% in the first group (p < 0.01) as well as a 50% increase in ofloxacin-resistant *Enterobacteriaceae* in the second group versus 11% in the first group (p < 0.02). The researchers concluded no specific benefit was observed in utilization of decontamination regimens though the emergence of resistance among Gram-negative bacteria was a significant concern.

A prospective trial conducted by de Smet et al. evaluated SDD and SOD in preventing bacteremia using cluster randomization in 13 different ICUs in the Netherlands, becoming the largest trial published on the subject to date [21]. Over the course of 6 months, 5939 total patients were enrolled in the study. These patients, similar to prior studies, were expected to have an ICU stay of at least 72 h and an expected mechanical ventilation time of >48 h. The SDD regimen included 4 days of intravenous cefotaxime and topical application of tobramycin, polymyxin E, and amphotericin B in the oropharynx and stomach. The SOD regimen consisted of the same oropharyngeal paste used for the SDD arm only, with surveillance cultures at admission and biweekly after with no restrictions to these physicians' systemic therapy choices. The primary endpoint of the study was mortality at 28 days. Each ICU applied SDD, SOD, or standard care at random over the course of the study. There was an absolute reduction in mortality SDD and SOD patients, 3.5% and 2.9%, respectively, from standard care. This study was able to show a relatively little difference between effectiveness of SDD and SOD. Moreover, SOD was preferable as the selection for organisms with antibiotic resistance was less in this group. The authors postulated this was due to the SOD regimen not including widespread systemic prophylaxis, hence, minimizing selection of resistant organisms. This was monitored by point-prevalence measurements monthly. For all combinations of therapy matched to pathogens detected, the rate of non-susceptibility was less than 5%. Multidrug resistance was less than 2.5% for two drugs and $\leq 2\%$ for a three-drug regimen. However, it is worth noting that the proportion of patients with *Enterobacteriaceae* in rectal surveillance swabs that were resistant was lower with SDD than with standard care or SOD. Importantly, follow-up data on this study did not demonstrate significant mortality benefit at 1 year with whether SOD or SDD [22].

There have also been several meta-analyses conducted evaluating SOD and SDD. An early example of this was published in 1998 which evaluated trials conducted from as early as 1984 to 1996 assessing various antibiotic regimens for preventing respiratory infections and also looking at total mortality in the ICU setting [23]. Two separate analyses were conducted. The first study included 3361 patients across 16 different trials which assessed systemic versus combined topical and systemic antibiotics for reduction of infection and overall mortality. Another confirmatory analysis which was conducted in 2366 more patients across 17 additional trials that assessed topical versus combination antibiotics for prevention also yielded a clear reduction. Hence, the addition of this analysis revealed an additional mortality benefit to regimens that incorporate a topical agent. Infections were reduced by 65% and mortality by an additional 20% with these regimens.

Another group of investigators subsequently performed a larger meta-analysis evaluating SDD for reducing mortality and bacteremia in 51 RCTs conducted between 1987 and 2005 including over 8000 patients across several ICUs [24]. The analysis included three major outcome measures: overall mortality, bloodstream infections, and infections caused by specific categories of organisms. SDD had a significant effect in reducing rates of mortality (OR 0.80, 95% CI 0.69–0.94), bloodstream infections (OR 0.73, 95% CI 0.59–0.90), and infections caused by Gram-negative organisms (OR 0.39 95% CI 0.24–0.63). There was no significant effect on Gram-positive infections. The authors noted several important limitations to this review. As the trials were never designed to look at bloodstream infections, rather the focus was on respiratory infection, it is possible that bloodstream data was underreported. Additionally, as the analysis sought to establish correlation with overall mortality, this is limited as only studies that included data on bloodstream infections were analyzed.

Given the findings of their prior effort, this group then sought to analyze trials that compared the efficacy of SDD between Gram-positive and Gram-negative organisms in both rates of infection and colonization [25]. Data was analyzed from 54 RCTs this time, including nearly 10,000 patients. SDD was associated with a statistically significant reduction in oropharyngeal and rectal carriage of Gram-negative organisms. It was also found to significantly reduce rates of lower respiratory infections, bacteremia, and also overall infections caused by Gram-negative organisms. As was noted in the prior study, once again, SDD did not significantly reduce either carriage or infection rates in patients with Gram-positive organisms.

These investigators then sought to analyze the overall effectiveness in reducing mortality in all trials using the full SDD protocol, which includes a combination of three different prophylactic maneuvers (i.e., parenteral antimicrobials, enteral antimicrobials, and intensified hand hygiene) combined with surveillance cultures from the rectum and throat to monitor effectiveness and compliance of this multifaceted approach [26]. This is termed the full four-component protocol of selective decontamination of the digestive tract. The authors included all trials comparing enteral SDD/SOD with a parenteral component and usable information by outcome. Twenty-one total RCTs were included with a total of 4902 patients. Overall mortality and late mortality were significantly reduced, whereas early mortality and attributable mortality due to infections were not. The findings were strongly suggestive that the full SDD protocol was effective in reducing mortality in critically ill patients, particularly when full decontamination was obtained given the responsiveness in late mortality rates.

The same year as this study, a Cochrane Review was published evaluating trials studying the effects of SDD on reducing respiratory tract infections as well as overall mortality [27]. The analysis included 36 total trials involving 6914 patients in total. In trials that included both topical and systemic antibiotics in their SDD regimen and in the included trials looking specifically at topical-only regimens, both groups showed statistically significant reduction in the rates of respiratory infections. However, while the combination regimen reduced overall mortality, topical-only regimens did not. Once again, while the authors noted the effectiveness of SDD in preventing morbidity and mortality, they also acknowledged the limited adoption of such protocols due to fears of antibiotic resistance.

Another analysis evaluated SDD use in preventing upper respiratory tracheobronchitis associated with mechanical ventilation [28]. Among 17 different trials with varying interventions for preventing infection, 5 of these RCTs evaluated SDD. This analysis revealed no preventive effect on tracheobronchitis infection rates seen in patients who underwent SDD (OR 0.62, 95% CI 0.31–1.26). In 2010, a large systematic review was conducted evaluating the effectiveness of SDD on multiple organ dysfunction (MOD) which included seven trials with a total of 1270 patients [13]. All included trials compared oropharyngeal and intestinal administration. Of the total patients, 132 out of 637 patients in the SDD group had MOD versus 219 out of 633 in the control group (OR 0.5 95% CI 0.34–0.74). Overall mortality was also measured which demonstrated a nonsignificant reduction (OR 0.82 95% CI 0.51–1.32).

Data on the use of SDD in children is particularly limited. One group of investigators performed a meta-analysis of all trials that compared SDD effectiveness in critically ill children [29]. Four randomized trials were identified with a total of 335 patients included. The investigators chose the diagnosis of pneumonia as the analysis' primary endpoint and also evaluated total number of infections as well as overall mortality. SDD reduced the incidence of pneumonia in children to a statistically significant level. SDD was also found to significantly reduce total number of infections compared to control patients. However, overall mortality was not significantly affected. The authors suggested that larger studies would be required to know the impact of SDD on mortality though suggested that SDD was worthy of consideration in certain at-risk patient populations until more information becomes available.

Another question raised by this research has been in the impact of SDD and SOD on immunocompromised individuals, a group at high risk for infections caused by antibiotic-resistant organisms given their frequent exposure to healthcare settings and systemic antimicrobials. This was the focus of an analysis conducted by investigators at the University of Wisconsin in 2004. The analysis was aimed at analyzing SDD in patients undergoing liver transplantation, particularly with attention to Gram-negative organisms [30]. The majority of included studies found statistically significant benefit in reducing infection from Gram-negative organisms using SDD (RR 0.16 95% CI 0.07–0.37); however, four trials did not demonstrate benefit (RR 0.88 95% CI 0.7–1.1). Additionally, antimicrobial resistance was cited as a major concern by the authors. Overall, they concluded that SDD appears to be beneficial in this type of population though acknowledged that more research is needed.

The emergence of antimicrobial resistance in the setting of selective decontamination remains poorly understood. Several of the large trials previously outlined earlier evaluate this question though data remains conflicting and duration of follow-up was relatively brief. Notably, much of the largest trials on this topic have been performed in the Netherlands, where rates of antibiotic-resistant organisms remain relatively low. A small, retrospective study performed in Germany evaluated the use of SDD using polymyxin E and gentamicin in the management of an outbreak of carbapenem-resistant *Klebsiella pneumoniae* [31]. Although no benefit was realized, rapid emergence of polymyxin E and gentamicin-resistance occurred. This may raise important reservations regarding the use of this strategy in outbreak settings or areas where there are relatively high rates of colonization with multidrug-resistant Gram-negative organisms, particularly given that polymyxins and aminoglycosides remain important potential options in acute infections caused by these organisms.

As mentioned earlier in this section, the amount of research done on this topic has been extensive; however, multiple questions remain. The existing body of literature demonstrates a potential role for selective decontamination in reducing morbidity and mortality from Gram-negative organisms in the ICU. Today results on effectiveness of decontamination have not been consistent, and the regimens studied and study populations included in these studies have varied widely. Additionally, the concern for the emergence of resistance among Gram-negative organisms has not been adequately addressed in the studies performed to date. A major concern stems from the use of some broad-spectrum antibiotics, such as polymyxin E, in decontamination regimens. This antibiotic is considered an option in the treatment of clinical infections caused by highly resistant *Enterobacteriaceae*, *Acinetobacter*, and *Pseudomonas aeruginosa*. More research is needed to demonstrate the efficacy of SOD and SDD and an improved understanding on the impact of these strategies on the emergence of resistance before it can be widely recommended in clinical practice.

Systemic Antibiotics

Based on observational data, there is interest in evaluating the use of systemic, absorbable antibiotics in decolonization of Gram-negative bacilli with or without oral or digestive decontamination. A small, single-center study from Germany described a potential association between duration of shedding of ESBL-producing and Shiga toxin-producing enteroaggregative *E. coli* (STEC) and receipt of azithromycin during an outbreak of STEC [32]. In this setting, azithromycin was given for meningococcal prophylaxis in the setting of administration of eculizumab, used in the treatment of hemolytic uremic syndrome. In retrospective analysis azithromycin was associated with lower frequency of STEC 0104:H4 carriage. A review of five liver transplant recipients in the setting of an outbreak of ESBL-producing *E. coli* included the administration of norfloxacin for 5 days as a component of an outbreak control strategy [33]. In this study a transient reduction of ESBL *E. coli* carriage was identified. Based on the limited data available, the use of systemic antibiotics to reduce colonization with Gram-negative organisms is not recommended.

Investigational Agents for Decolonization

The gastrointestinal microbiome consists of thousands of bacterial species, including Gram-negative bacilli. As knowledge about the microbiome increases, strategies to restore homeostasis within the complex microbiome have been explored. Circumstances in which enteropathogens, including multidrug-resistant Gram-negative bacilli, dominate the microflora may be directly addressed through attempts at restoration of a healthy, diverse microbiome. Two potential strategies that may be incorporated in decolonization for Gram-negative bacilli, specifically the recolonization with a healthy microbiome, include fecal microbiota transplantation and the use of probiotics.

Fecal Microbiota Transplantation

Fecal microbiota transplantation is an attempt to selectively repopulate the intestinal microbiome through infusion of donor microbiota. This strategy has been used in the management of *Clostridium difficile*-associated diarrhea, which is driven by antibiotic use and alterations disrupting the normal gastrointestinal flora [34]. There is a potential interest in FMT in the restoration of the intestinal microbiome in hospitalized patients colonized with multidrug-resistant Gram-negative bacilli. This strategy has been attempted on an individual basis for the eradication of ESBL-producing Gram-negative bacilli [35, 36] with successful short-term decolonization. At this time, more study is needed to evaluate the efficacy and potential adverse consequences of this decolonization strategy before it can be recommended on a wider scale.

Probiotics

Probiotics are live bacteria which confer a health benefit on the consumer. Several different organisms have been identified as potential probiotics, and their use in clinical settings is varied. Clinical trials have evaluated their use in the treatment of acute infectious diarrhea [37], including antibiotic-associated diarrhea [38] and *C. difficile*-associated diarrhea [39]. The activity of *Lactobacillus* species against Gram-negative bacilli has raised interest in their use in decolonization. In vitro activity against *E. coli*, including ESBL-producing strains, has been demonstrated [40]. At this time, the therapeutic role of probiotics in the treatment of infections caused by Gram-negative bacteria has yet to be demonstrated in clinical studies. There may be a potential role of probiotics in the restoration of the intestinal microbiome following an oral decolonization regimen. However, to date, the role of probiotics in the reestablishment of the microbiome in the setting of decolonization is uncertain though remains an important area of future study.

Conclusions

Decolonization may be an effective strategy to reduce infections caused by Gram-negative bacilli and reduce healthcare-associated transmission of these organisms. Topical decolonization and selective digestive and oral decontamination of the gastrointestinal tract have been effective, though data has not been conclusive and no consensus has been reached regarding the optimal decolonization strategy and the most appropriate setting for its use. Additionally, the durability of this strategy and the potential emergence of antibiotic-resistant organisms remain important concerns. Although this strategy may be a useful adjunct to other infection prevention strategies, more data is needed before its use can be recommended on a widespread basis.

References

1. Fritz SA, Camins BC, Eisenstein KA, et al. Effectiveness of measures to eradicate *staphylococcus aureus* carriage in patients with community-associated skin and soft-tissue infections: a randomized trial. Infect Control Hosp Epidemiol. 2011;32(9):872–80. doi:10.1086/661285.
2. Giuliano CA, Rybak MJ. Efficacy of triclosan as an antimicrobial hand soap and its potential impact on antimicrobial resistance: a focused review. Pharmacotherapy. 2015;35(3):328–36. doi:10.1002/phar.1553.
3. Climo MW, Sepkowitz KA, Zuccotti G, et al. The effect of daily bathing with chlorhexidine on the acquisition of methicillin-resistant *staphylococcus aureus*, vancomycin-resistant enterococcus, and healthcare-associated bloodstream infections: results of a quasi-experimental multicenter trial. Crit Care Med. 2009;37(6):1858–65. doi:10.1097/CCM.0b013e31819ffe6d.
4. Huang SS, Septimus E, Kleinman K, et al. Targeted versus universal decolonization to prevent ICU infection. N Engl J Med. 2013;368(24):2255–65. doi:10.1056/NEJMoa1207290.
5. Munoz-Price LS, De La Cuesta C, Adams S, et al. Successful eradication of a monoclonal strain of *Klebsiella pneumoniae* during a *K. pneumoniae* carbapenemase-producing *K. pneumoniae* outbreak in a surgical intensive care unit in Miami, Florida. Infect Control Hosp Epidemiol. 2010;31(10):1074–7. doi:10.1086/656243.
6. Apisarnthanarak A, Pinitchai U, Warachan B, Warren DK, Khawcharoenporn T, Hayden MK. Effectiveness of infection prevention measures featuring advanced source control and environmental cleaning to limit transmission of extremely-drug resistant Acinetobacter baumannii in a Thai intensive care unit: an analysis before and after extensive flooding. Am J Infect Control. 2014;42(2):116–21. doi:10.1016/j.ajic.2013.09.025.
7. Borer A, Gilad J, Porat N, et al. Impact of 4% chlorhexidine whole-body washing on multidrug-resistant Acinetobacter baumannii skin colonisation among patients in a medical intensive care unit. J Hosp Infect. 2007;67(2):149–55. doi: S0195-6701(07)00259-9 [pii]
8. Martinez-Resendez MF, Garza-Gonzalez E, Mendoza-Olazaran S, et al. Impact of daily chlorhexidine baths and hand hygiene compliance on nosocomial infection rates in critically ill patients. Am J Infect Control. 2014;42(7):713–7. doi:10.1016/j.ajic.2014.03.354.
9. Lin MY, Lolans K, Blom DW, et al. The effectiveness of routine daily chlorhexidine gluconate bathing in reducing *Klebsiella pneumoniae* carbapenemase-producing Enterobacteriaceae skin burden among long-term acute care hospital patients. Infect Control Hosp Epidemiol. 2014;35(4):440–2. doi:10.1086/675613.

10. Cassir N, Thomas G, Hraiech S, et al. Chlorhexidine daily bathing: impact on health care-associated infections caused by gram-negative bacteria. Am J Infect Control. 2015;43(6):640–3. doi:10.1016/j.ajic.2015.02.010.

11. Boonyasiri A, Thaisiam P, Permpikul C, et al. Effectiveness of chlorhexidine wipes for the prevention of multidrug-resistant bacterial colonization and hospital-acquired infections in intensive care unit patients: a randomized trial in Thailand. Infect Control Hosp Epidemiol. 2016;37(3):245–53. doi:10.1017/ice.2015.285.

12. Derde LP, Cooper BS, Goossens H, et al. Interventions to reduce colonisation and transmission of antimicrobial-resistant bacteria in intensive care units: an interrupted time series study and cluster randomised trial. Lancet Infect Dis. 2014;14(1):31–9. doi:10.1016/S1473-3099(13)70295-0.

13. Mendoza-Olazaran S, Camacho-Ortiz A, Martinez-Resendez MF, Llaca-Diaz JM, Perez-Rodriguez E, Garza-Gonzalez E. Influence of whole-body washing of critically ill patients with chlorhexidine on Acinetobacter baumannii isolates. Am J Infect Control. 2014;42(8):874–8. doi:10.1016/j.ajic.2014.04.009.

14. Silvestri L, van Saene HK. Selective decontamination of the digestive tract: an update of the evidence. HSR Proc Intensive Care Cardiovasc Anesth. 2012;4(1):21–9.

15. de Jonge E, Schultz MJ, Spanjaard L, et al. Effects of selective decontamination of digestive tract on mortality and acquisition of resistant bacteria in intensive care: a randomised controlled trial. Lancet. 2003;362(9389):1011–6. doi: S0140-6736(03)14409-1 [pii]

16. de Smet AM, Kluytmans JA, Blok HE, et al. Selective digestive tract decontamination and selective oropharyngeal decontamination and antibiotic resistance in patients in intensive-care units: an open-label, clustered group-randomised, crossover study. Lancet Infect Dis. 2011;11(5):372–80. doi:10.1016/S1473-3099(11)70035-4.

17. Melsen WG, de Smet AM, Kluytmans JA, Bonten MJ, Dutch SOD-SDD Trialists' Group. Selective decontamination of the oral and digestive tract in surgical versus non-surgical patients in intensive care in a cluster-randomized trial. Br J Surg. 2012;99(2):232–7. doi:10.1002/bjs.7703.

18. Saidel-Odes L, Polachek H, Peled N, et al. A randomized, double-blind, placebo-controlled trial of selective digestive decontamination using oral gentamicin and oral polymyxin E for eradication of carbapenem-resistant Klebsiella pneumoniae carriage. Infect Control Hosp Epidemiol. 2012;33(1):14–9. doi:10.1086/663206.

19. Oostdijk EA, Kesecioglu J, Schultz MJ, et al. Effects of decontamination of the oropharynx and intestinal tract on antibiotic resistance in ICUs: a randomized clinical trial. JAMA. 2014;312(14):1429–37. doi:10.1001/jama.2014.7247.

20. Verwaest C, Verhaegen J, Ferdinande P, et al. Randomized, controlled trial of selective digestive decontamination in 600 mechanically ventilated patients in a multidisciplinary intensive care unit. Crit Care Med. 1997;25(1):63–71.

21. de Smet AM, Kluytmans JA, Cooper BS, et al. Decontamination of the digestive tract and oropharynx in ICU patients. N Engl J Med. 2009;360(1):20–31. doi:10.1056/NEJMoa0800394.

22. Oostdijk EA, de Smet AM, Bonten MJ, Dutch SOD-SDD trialists group. Effects of decontamination of the digestive tract and oropharynx in intensive care unit patients on 1-year survival. Am J Respir Crit Care Med. 2013;188(1):117–20. doi:10.1164/rccm.201209-1733LE.

23. D'Amico R, Pifferi S, Leonetti C, Torri V, Tinazzi A, Liberati A. Effectiveness of antibiotic prophylaxis in critically ill adult patients: systematic review of randomised controlled trials. BMJ. 1998;316(7140):1275–85.

24. Silvestri L, van Saene HK, Milanese M, Gregori D, Gullo A. Selective decontamination of the digestive tract reduces bacterial bloodstream infection and mortality in critically ill patients. Systematic review of randomized, controlled trials. J Hosp Infect. 2007;65(3):187–203. doi: S0195-6701(06)00484-1 [pii]

25. Silvestri L, van Saene HK, Casarin A, Berlot G, Gullo A. Impact of selective decontamination of the digestive tract on carriage and infection due to gram-negative and gram-positive bacteria: a systematic review of randomised controlled trials. Anaesth Intensive Care. 2008;36(3):324–38.

26. Silvestri L, van Saene HK, Weir I, Gullo A. Survival benefit of the full selective digestive decontamination regimen. J Crit Care. 2009;24(3):474.e7–14. doi:10.1016/j.jcrc.2008.11.005.

27. D'Amico R, Pifferi S, Torri V, Brazzi L, Parmelli E, Liberati A. Antibiotic prophylaxis to reduce respiratory tract infections and mortality in adults receiving intensive care. Cochrane Database of Systematic Reviews 2009, Issue 4. Art. No.: CD000022. doi:10.1002/14651858.CD000022.pub3.

28. Agrafiotis M, Siempos II, Falagas ME. Frequency, prevention, outcome and treatment of ventilator-associated tracheobronchitis: systematic review and meta-analysis. Respir Med. 2010;104(3):325–36. doi: S0954-6111(09)00286-8 [pii]

29. Petros A, Silvestri L, Booth R, Taylor N, van Saene H. Selective decontamination of the digestive tract in critically ill children: systematic review and meta-analysis. Pediatr Crit Care Med. 2013;14(1):89–97. doi:10.1097/PCC.0b013e3182417871.

30. Safdar N, Said A, Lucey MR. The role of selective digestive decontamination for reducing infection in patients undergoing liver transplantation: a systematic review and meta-analysis. Liver Transpl. 2004;10(7):817–27. doi:10.1002/lt.20108.

31. Lubbert C, Faucheux S, Becker-Rux D, et al. Rapid emergence of secondary resistance to gentamicin and colistin following selective digestive decontamination in patients with KPC-2-producing Klebsiella pneumoniae: a single-centre experience. Int J Antimicrob Agents. 2013;42(6):565–70. doi:10.1016/j.ijantimicag.2013.08.008.

32. Nitschke M, Sayk F, Hartel C, et al. Association between azithromycin therapy and duration of bacterial shedding among patients with Shiga toxin-producing enteroaggregative Escherichia coli O104:H4. JAMA. 2012;307(10):1046–52. doi:10.1001/jama.2012.264.

33. Paterson DL, Singh N, Rihs JD, Squier C, Rihs BL, Muder RR. Control of an outbreak of infection due to extended-spectrum beta-lactamase – producing Escherichia coli in a liver transplantation unit. Clin Infect Dis. 2001;33(1):126–8. doi: CID000995 [pii]

34. van Nood E, Vrieze A, Nieuwdorp M, et al. Duodenal infusion of donor feces for recurrent clostridium difficile. N Engl J Med. 2013;368(5):407–15. doi:10.1056/NEJMoa1205037.

35. Lagier JC, Million M, Fournier PE, Brouqui P, Raoult D. Faecal microbiota transplantation for stool decolonization of OXA-48 carbapenemase-producing Klebsiella pneumoniae. J Hosp Infect. 2015;90(2):173–4. doi:10.1016/j.jhin.2015.02.013.

36. Singh R, van Nood E, Nieuwdorp M, et al. Donor feces infusion for eradication of extended spectrum beta-lactamase producing Escherichia coli in a patient with end stage renal disease. Clin Microbiol Infect. 2014;20(11):O977–8. doi:10.1111/1469-0691.12683.

37. Allen SJ, Martinez EG, Gregorio GV, Dans LF. Probiotics for treating acute infectious diarrhoea. Cochrane Database of Systematic Reviews 2010, Issue 11. Art. No.: CD003048. doi:10.1002/14651858.CD003048.pub3.

38. Hempel S, Newberry SJ, Maher AR, et al. Probiotics for the prevention and treatment of antibiotic-associated diarrhea: a systematic review and meta-analysis. JAMA. 2012;307(18):1959–69. doi:10.1001/jama.2012.3507.

39. Pillai A, Nelson RL. Probiotics for treatment of Clostridium difficile-associated colitis in adults. Cochrane Database of Systematic Reviews 2008, Issue 1. Art. No.: CD004611. doi:10.1002/14651858.CD004611.pub2.

40. Shim YH, Lee SJ, Lee JW. Antimicrobial activities of lactobacillus strains against uropathogens. Pediatr Int. 2016; doi:10.1111/ped.12949.

Testing Water for *Legionella* Prevention

Brooke K. Decker and Cornelius J. Clancy

Legionellosis consists of two distinct clinical syndromes, a mild flu-like illness called Pontiac fever [1] and a more severe disease that disproportionately affects immunosuppressed hosts, referred to as *Legionella* pneumonia or Legionnaires' disease [2]. Both are clinical manifestations of infection with the waterborne bacteria *Legionella*, in particular *L. pneumophila*, the species most pathogenic to humans [3]. Infection is acquired after aspiration or inhalation of contaminated water. Aspiration is the primary mode of infection in healthcare-associated cases [4].

Approaches to prevention and control of Legionella infection in Allegheny County (PA) health care facilities, one of the first comprehensive recommendations on *Legionella* control in healthcare, was published in 1997. Early in the document, the authors state "It became apparent that there was no uniformity in the evaluation and monitoring of Legionella in hospital water systems…" [5]. Despite the importance of *Legionella* as a cause of human illness and the widespread publicity given to disease outbreaks in healthcare and community settings, this statement regarding controversies in *Legionella* management remains largely true 20 years later. In this chapter, we will review current practices for testing healthcare water systems for *Legionella* prevention, highlighting areas of controversy and uncertainty. We focus on the management of healthcare water systems because these facilities are likely to be most relevant to the interests and professional practices of readers. Healthcare facilities house persons who are most vulnerable to Legionnaires' disease. Not uncommonly, hospitals and healthcare campuses are large, built over decades, and consist of multiple additions and sites of reconstruction. As a result, buildings typically contain highly complex water systems, for which inventory and mapping may be incomplete or inaccurate. The challenges in *Legionella* control presented by these systems are manifold and made more pressing by a particular responsibility to protect the health and safety of patients, visitors, and employees.

How to Test for *Legionella*

Culturing Methods

Environmental testing for *Legionella* most commonly includes swab testing and water cultures. Less commonly, air sampling is performed to explore the association between positive water sources and the potential for nosocomial infection [6, 7]. Water systems may also be cultured for amoebas that carry *Legionella* intracellularly, but such efforts are more of a research tool than standard infection prevention practice.

Legionella bacteria reside in biofilms coating the interior of pipes and fixtures or as free-floating planktonic cells. Fixtures with complex surfaces or mixing of hot and cold water are more likely to harbor *Legionella* [8], since warm water provides an ideal growing temperature [9]. Aerators [10] and electronic faucets (magic eye faucets) [11, 12], in particular, provide additional interior surfaces on which biofilms can develop. The US Centers for Disease Control (CDC) recommends the use of swabs in the investigation of *Legionella* cases [13], based in part on the theoretical consideration that they improve *Legionella* detection within biofilms and subsequently in water samples. While this hypothesis is intuitively appealing, it has not been borne out in testing [14]. In some studies, swabs have been demonstrated to be less sensitive than water cultures [15]. If swab testing is performed, CDC recommends briefly running the water to wet the interior of the fixture. A Dacron or polypropylene-tipped swab should be inserted as far as possible into the fixture followed by a vigorous attempt to disrupt the resident biofilm [13]. Swabs should be stored in water from the same fixture and transported to the lab as soon as possible. Depending on the fixture sampled, some creativity is needed to determine the best location to swab.

B.K. Decker (✉) • C.J. Clancy
Infectious Diseases Section, VA Pittsburgh Healthcare System, University Drive C, Medicine IIIE-U, Pittsburgh, PA 15240, USA
e-mail: brooke.decker@va.gov; cjc76@pitt.edu

© Springer International Publishing AG 2018
G. Bearman et al. (eds.), *Infection Prevention*, DOI 10.1007/978-3-319-60980-5_25

Aerators, moving parts amenable to biofilm, or areas of turbulent or stagnant flow represent good targets for swab collection. Certain point-of-use fixtures (such as those in behavioral health units or some shower heads) may require partial disassembly to access with a swab. Collaboration with plumbing or facilities staff can significantly improve collection process efficiency.

Water collected for the detection of planktonic *Legionella* may be directly plated or filtered. Direct plating is best reserved for non-potable water with a known or suspected high bacterial count. Filtering is superior to centrifugation for improving yield [14] and is most appropriate for water from areas with lower bacterial counts, such as potable water sources where screening a larger volume of water is needed to detect *Legionella*. CDC recommends the use of a 0.2 micron polycarbonate filter. After filtration, the filter is vortexed in a 50 mL centrifuge tube with 5 mL of sterile water, which is plated [6]. If source water has been treated with chlorine, 0.5 mL of 0.1 N sodium thiosulfate per liter should be added in order to neutralize the potential for inhibition of *Legionella* growth. If samples cannot be plated immediately, prompt refrigeration at 4 °C is recommended [6]. For areas without in-house testing, significant error does not appear to occur when samples are appropriately packaged and promptly shipped [16].

Specific guidance for *Legionella* air sampling has been described [6, 17]. Matching sequence types of *Legionella* have been detected in the air and water of healthcare facilities [7]. However, the sensitivity of air sampling and the validity of negative results are not established. As such, air sampling may serve as a complementary approach to water studies in certain situations, but it is not a standard component of healthcare facility *Legionella* testing.

Legionella Growth Requirements

Legionella bacteria require longer incubation time and special media and conditions for detection compared to routine bacterial cultures. *Legionella* media typically include 0.1% alpha-ketoglutarate, which may be more important in limiting oxygen toxicity than in direct metabolism [18]. Both clinical and environmental cultures can be grown on buffered charcoal yeast extract (BCYE), a "nonselective" *Legionella* growth media. Additional supplementation with bovine albumin (ABCYE – BCYE with 1.0% albumin) may increase detection of certain strains, including *L. micdadei* and *L. bozemanii* [19].

Since bacteria other than *Legionella* grow on BCYE, "selective" *Legionella* media with antimicrobial supplementation are useful for water sources with higher bacterial counts. Polymyxin B, cycloheximide, and vancomycin are components of both PCV (polymyxin, cycloheximide,

vancomycin) and GPCV/GVPC media ("G" denotes the addition of glycine to PCV). These selective media reduce the growth of non-*Legionella* bacteria, as well as non-pneumophila *Legionella* species. They are best used for water from areas with high bacteria contamination such as non-potable sources, air sampling, or plating in parallel with "nonselective" media to ensure both sensitivity and the ability to interpret culture results if heavy growth occurs. Colonies that grow on BCYE or PCV media should be inoculated onto media without L-cysteine (BCYE- or PCV-). Growth on BCYE but not on BCYE- is consistent with *Legionella* spp. and should prompt further identification [6]. Additional *Legionella* media include glycine, vancomycin, polymyxin B, and natamycin (GVPN), which substitutes natamycin or anisomycin for cycloheximide as a fungal inhibitory agent that is less toxic to laboratory personnel. Selective *Legionella* agar containing bromocresol purple and bromothymol blue (BCYE with DVGP (dyes, glycine, vancomycin, and polymyxin B) or MWY (the medium of Wadowsky and Yee [20])) may aid in visual identification of *Legionella*.

In addition to special media, *Legionella* selection in a population of bacteria can be improved by exploiting *Legionella*'s relative resistance to low pH. Acid treatment of the specimen before plating reduces overgrowth by non-*Legionella* bacteria. Procedural guidance can be found on the CDC website [6]. There may be little difference in *Legionella* recovery between selective and nonselective media when acid washing is used [14, 21].

After inoculation, *Legionella* plates should be placed in a humidified, 2.5% CO_2 incubator at 35 °C. CDC recommends incubation for 7 days [6], but growth of *Legionella* can take up to 2 weeks [22]. For hospitals with in-house *Legionella* detection capability, it may be reasonable to hold plates longer than 7 days. Ten-day incubation periods are recommended by the International Standards Organization [23] and frequently cited [21, 24]. Incubation longer than 7 days should be considered in circumstances where detection of non-pneumophila *Legionella* species is sought (such as surveillance in an area of immunosuppression or in the investigation of non-pneumophila cases.)

Elite certification is provided by CDC to laboratories that perform to an adequate standard in culturing *Legionella*. Healthcare facilities with the capacity to support in-house *Legionella* culturing should become Elite-certified. In-house *Legionella* surveillance allows for faster notification of positive results and simplifies the collection of strains for typing or other follow-up analyses. Many commercial enterprises perform *Legionella* testing for facilities without in-house capabilities. Hospitals should contract with an Elite Laboratory; infection prevention leadership should be aware of specific culture methods and the duration of incubation and whether these can be modified if desired.

Legionella Burdens Within Positive Water Cultures

Quantitative cultures for *Legionella* hold intuitive appeal as measures of burden within a water system. However, the value of determining *Legionella* concentrations in assessing risk has not been established. Indeed, nosocomial cases of Legionellosis are commonly encountered when counts within culture-positive samples from healthcare facilities are below thresholds for water system treatment proposed by the Occupational Safety and Health Administration (OSHA) for cooling towers [25, 26]. Moreover, an analysis of ELITE-certified labs revealed that quantitation of *Legionella* by colony count varied extensively [27]. Therefore, utilizing a threshold for *Legionella* growth or comparing colony counts between samples has no established clinical value. CDC recommends against using strict CFU/mL thresholds in designating a healthcare facility water system as safe or in triggering remediation [27].

Amoeba Culture

Legionella frequently exist intracellularly in amoeba, and their coexistence within amoeba has been linked to persistence in the setting of adequate biocide levels [28]. Amoebic culture is a sensitive detection method but effort intensive [15]. The correlation between increased sensitivity of *Legionella* detection with amoeba culture and increased patient risk in the setting of this detection has not been established.

Additional Detection Methods

Alternative water testing methods have been suggested, including qPCR and immunomagnetic separation [29]. These strategies aim to better detect *Legionella* in the water, including what has been called viable but nonculturable (VBNC) [30] *Legionella*. It is less clear what risk, if any, *Legionella* that is detectable, but not cultivable, poses to patients.

Which Water to Test

Legionella prefers relatively high temperatures with an optimal range between 32 and 42 °C [9], and strains are more commonly isolated in hot water systems that do not maintain recirculating temperatures greater than 122 °F (50 °C) [9]. Accordingly, most attention in healthcare facilities has focused on sampling hot water systems. CDC recommends testing only hot water [13]. In contrast, the UK Health and Safety Executive Guidance [31] and US Veterans Health Administration [32] require routine sampling of both hot and cold water in healthcare facilities. Areas of increased risk to patients, such as wards that house immunosuppressed hosts or locations that have undergone recent additions of new plumbing into an established system, are reasonable targets for testing. Maintenance or construction involving a water system can result in the disruption of biofilm and the release of planktonic *Legionella*. Construction is a risk factor for *Legionella* outbreaks [25, 33].

A less obvious source of potential water exposure in the hospital setting is the non-potable water systems involved in heating and cooling. Outbreaks occurring in the absence of potable water system positivity should prompt investigation of cooling towers as a potential source [34]. Open cooling towers have been associated with *Legionella* cases [35]. Closed loop cooling systems can also harbor *Legionella*, but patient exposure is less likely outside of a breach of the cooling system (such as in a cold winter if an incompletely drained system freezes). In facilities with open cooling towers, the orientation of the air intake for air handling systems should point away from the cooling tower and be as separated in distance as possible to reduce the potential for inflow of possibly contaminated aerosols.

When to Test

Environmental *Legionella* testing should be performed routinely after detection of a possible or definite hospital-associated case. Such "case-based" testing is recommended by the CDC and allows for the identification of facility sources of *Legionella* risk requiring remediation. Surveillance *Legionella* testing and water system remediation in response to positive cultures have been advocated in the absence of hospital-associated cases, as a means of reducing the risk of nosocomial infections, but remain controversial [36]. Surveillance testing can be further divided into two categories, defined by O'Neill et al. as primary and secondary prevention [37]. Primary prevention is defined as environmental sampling and remediation at institutions without a previous history of nosocomial cases. Secondary prevention occurs in facilities that have had previous cases of *Legionella*, when testing and remediation are performed outside of an immediate investigation into patient cases.

Case Investigation

One or more healthcare-associated cases of *Legionella* warrant investigation of hospital waterworks. Investigations must be multidisciplinary to be complete, including an evaluation of the consistency of engineering controls (pH, biocide levels, temperature), as well as *Legionella* culturing from potential sources of water exposure. Sites of exposure, such as relevant patient care unit(s), restrooms, or showers that might have been used, and any other additional water sources encountered (baths, therapy pools, fountains, etc.) during the incubation period are appropriate targets for sampling [3, 38].

Specific guidance on water system sampling varies greatly by agency, and a recent summary by Parr et al. highlights the differences in primary prevention recommendations [39]. A summary of selected guidance is presented in Table 25.1. For water samples, the first draw of the initial flow of water from the fixture is referred to as "before-flush." The before-flush sample reflects what the patient might experience were they to access the sink. A sample in which the water is allowed to flow for a period of time (e.g., to achieve the maximum temperature) is referred to as "after-flush."

In the absence of consensus on how to obtain samples for testing, it is most reasonable to proceed in a manner consistent with the reasons for sampling. First-draw samples are the logical choice when investigating a patient case. First draw best represents the patient's exposure and includes the fixture as a potential source of *Legionella* colonization. In a study of samples obtained at 0, 5, 10, and 15 min of flushing, the first-draw sample demonstrated the highest yield of *Legionella* [21]. Post-flush samples make sense when the water system is suspected in situations of inadequate engineering control or to validate a remediation of the water system. Institutions investigating an outbreak should consider both "first-draw" and "post-flush" samples in order to ensure that the risks associated with a potentially colonized fixture and the central potable water system are both evaluated.

Surveillance

Routine environmental surveillance for *Legionella* in the absence of definite or possible healthcare-associated cases is controversial. As of this writing, surveillance testing for *Legionella* (in the absence of clinical cases) is not universally required. As mentioned, CDC recommends case-investigation environmental testing in lieu of surveillance strategies. Rather than recommending routine surveillance, the most recent American Society of Heating, Refrigerating, and Air-Conditioning Engineers (ASHRAE, 188-2015) document advocates thoughtful evaluation of water system risk and the generation of a facility-specific water safety plan [40]. Routine surveillance, rather than a case-based approach to environmental detection, has been recommended due to the potential severity of infection, the susceptibility of hospitalized populations, and the advantage of prevention if *Legionella* is detected [5, 41, 42].

Appropriate consideration of patient risk, waterworks complexity, and facility history is necessary before deciding to perform surveillance cultures for *Legionella*. Healthcare facilities contemplating surveillance water testing should first consider if patients at greatest risk for *Legionella* infection are housed at the facility. According to the CDC Healthcare Infection Control Practices Advisory Committee (HICPAC) guidance, patients at greatest risk include transplant patients and those requiring protective environments [38]. CDC/HICPAC guidelines from 2003 state that "water samples from the potable water in the solid-organ transplant and/or PE (protective environment) unit can be performed as part of an overall strategy to prevent Legionnaires disease in PE units." The guidelines suggest that healthcare facilities use periodic potable water culturing as a basis to

Table 25.1 Summary of selected guidance on environmental testing for *Legionella*, requirement and approach

Guideline	Primary surveillance required	Water culture minimum	Swab cultures	First draw	Post-flush	Hot water	Cold water	Hot water tanks/recirculating loops
OSHA 2003 [26]	No	250 mL	Yes	Yes	Yes	Yes	Yes	Yes
WHO 2007 [9]	No	1 L	Yes	Yes	Yes	Yes	Yes	Yes
EWGLI 2011 [56]	No	1 L	Yes	Yes	Yes	Yes	Yes	Yes
UK HSE 2013 [31]	Yes	200 mL	No	Yes	Yes	Yes	Yes	Yes
VHA 1061 2014 [32]	Yes	250 mL	No	Yes	No	Yes	Yes	No
ACHD 2014 [55]	No	1 L	Yes	Yes	Yes	Yes	Yes	Yes
CDC June 2015 [6]	No	1 L	Yes	No	Yes	Yes	No	Yes

Occupational Safety and Health Administration *OSHA*, World Health Organization *WHO*, European Working Group for Legionella Infections *EWGLI*, Veterans Health Administration *VHA*, Allegheny County Health Department *ACHD*, Centers for Disease Control and Prevention *CDC* recommend diagnostic testing to clinicians if positive water cultures are found.

Per the most recent ASHRAE, appropriate high-risk groups include patients with burns, those receiving chemotherapy for cancers or medications that impair immune functioning, solid organ and bone marrow transplantation recipients, and persons with renal disease, diabetes, or chronic lung disease [40]. ASHRAE stops short of recommending *Legionella* testing of water from locations where patients with these conditions are housed. Rather, the guidelines state that the decision of whether to test for *Legionella* should consider the presence of immunosuppressed patients, success in maintaining control limits (biocide, temperature, etc.), and prior history of facility nosocomial legionellosis [40].

A threshold for environmental site positivity was first proposed in a 1983 study, in which the authors suggested that the risk for nosocomial legionellosis within a hospital increased significantly when >30% of sampled sites were culture positive for *Legionella pneumophila* [43]. Based on these data, 30% positivity had been used at many centers as an action threshold for remediation [38]. This practice, however, is controversial. A review of data from peer-reviewed studies reported that the sensitivity and specificity of a 30% threshold relationship for nosocomial legionellosis were only 59% and 74%, respectively. During an outbreak of *Legionella* pneumonia at a Pittsburgh hospital, cases were diagnosed when positivity rates were as low as 4%. The perception that *Legionella* was under control because of positivity rates below the threshold was concluded to have contributed to the duration of the outbreak.

In summary, surveillance testing for *Legionella* is most reasonable in settings with high-risk patients, inadequate environmental controls, and a history of nosocomial legionellosis. In the absence of these factors, decisions on the need for surveillance testing should consider if adequate clinical *Legionella* testing is performed and the risks, benefits, and feasibility of initiating a water sampling program. There is no threshold level of water positivity that signifies a facility is safe from nosocomial acquisition of *Legionella*.

Some jurisdictions and healthcare systems mandate *Legionella* testing. In 2005, New York State required quarterly testing of areas serving patients with transplants or receiving chemotherapy [44]. After a 2015 outbreak of legionellosis in the Bronx, New York City enacted legislation mandating cooling tower registration, testing and treatment, as well as hospital water surveillance and action based on positive results [45]. After a 2011–2012 outbreak at a VA hospital [25], the Department of Veterans Affairs Veterans Health Association released comprehensive requirements for maintaining the safety of hospital water systems. These requirements include quarterly surveillance of both hot and cold water in all buildings in which patients stay overnight

[32]. As of this writing, similar legislation is being discussed in Michigan, in response to a significant increase in legionellosis cases in Genesee County [46].

The tragedy of acquiring a severe, preventable infection like Legionnaire's disease in a healthcare facility is undeniable. Though *Legionella* outbreaks often inspire legislation designed to protect vulnerable citizens seeking medical care, the likelihood of acquiring *Legionella* from a hospital visit is far less than that of acquiring a more mundane (but no less potentially severe) infection related to a catheter or surgery. As resources are always limited, the most rational approach is to develop water system management guidelines based on a hospital's risk and history.

What to Do with Surveillance Results

If *Legionella* surveillance is performed, appropriate responses to positive and negative results are essential. Responses are best defined before testing is undertaken. A decision on how to respond, or change in the planned response, after *Legionella* has been detected has the potential to be perceived as motivated by cost rather than patient safety. Some hospitals have adopted a zero-tolerance policy, remediating water in response to any culture positivity. Such hypervigilant approaches are not feasible at all facilities nor are they likely to be necessary. Infection prevention programs should strive to maintain burdens of *Legionella* as low as possible at all times. However, *Legionella* is a ubiquitous waterborne organism, and long-term sterilization of potable water in endemic areas is not feasible. Where acceptable water-positivity thresholds fall will differ at individual centers, as dictated by factors discussed in the previous section. The need to perform potentially costly remediation is frequently cited as a reason to avoid testing in the absence of documented or suspected cases, provided adequate clinical testing is performed.

Typical immediate strategies to remediate positive *Legionella* cultures include biocide treatment of the water, thermal treatment (heating the water to 160 °F), and flushing each fixture for 5–30 min. These treatments may be followed by a maintenance strategy such as continuous or intermittent prophylactic biocide treatment. Whatever strategy is considered, validation of the effectiveness should follow. In its most basic form, validation includes retesting the fixture after remediation, allowing at least 48–72 h of use to ensure residual biocide does not remain.

L. pneumophila causes approximately 90% of disease [47], but other types of *Legionella* can infect immunosuppressed patients and have been associated with nosocomial cases [48]. Therefore, it is important to consider how non-pneumophila species will be addressed if detected prior to sampling. In locations with immunosuppressed patients, a policy of remediation regardless of *Legionella* species is most conservative. At this time, it is not known if the factors allowing for growth of non-pneumophila species portend future detection of *L. pneumophila* or if they fill a distinct biological niche.

Typing of isolates, if available, is epidemiologically useful and typically performed as part of an outbreak investigation. Sequence-based typing [49–51] has been the gold standard in *Legionella* identification, and more than 2,000 sequence types have been described thus far [52]. Finding identical strains in both a facility location and in the patient's clinical sample implies an association. However, similar *Legionella* sequence types can be found in both the community and a healthcare facility supplied by the same water distribution system. Whole genome sequencing (WGS) has been used in the characterization of outbreak and environmental *Legionella* strains [53]. WGS will likely provide increased granularity for *Legionella* typing compared to SBT, but adequate clinical association between cases and environmental strains will still be needed to differentiate a shared community reservoir vs. facility acquisition in patients spending only part of the incubation period in the positive facility.

For all indications of testing, finding no positive cultures is the ideal and most reassuring finding. Even with negative testing results, however, infection preventionists must maintain vigilance and take care to ensure that water remains safe. *Legionella* is most frequently found from water systems with imperfect engineering control, such as cold water that is too warm, hot water circulating loops that are too cold, infrequently used (stagnant) fixtures, and plumbing dead legs and run-outs. Sampling sites should target areas with engineering risk factors. *Legionella* is a highly seasonal organism, which is more frequently detected in the summer and fall [54]. Case-based sampling should be performed as proximate as possible to the time of exposure, but primary and secondary surveillance is best performed throughout the year. Many sources have recommended quarterly sampling protocols [32, 55]. Additional considerations in the setting of negative surveillance testing might include ensuring that first-draw samples were obtained, obtaining 5-min flush samples in addition to first draw [26], and sampling both hot and cold water sources.

Controversies

The workup of healthcare-associated *Legionella* is rife with controversies; major controversies are listed in Table 25.2. Debate is not limited to just simple concepts such as when, where, and how to perform water sampling. *Legionella* is almost universally found in water systems (manmade or natural), but no level of detectable *Legionella* is considered safe, incentivizing those without nosocomial cases to avoid testing.

Table 25.2 Major controversies in *Legionella* environmental testing

Major controversies	
Surveillance testing for primary prevention	Surveillance testing is not universally recommended, and the detection of *Legionella*, especially non-pneumophila species, in the absence of cases is of unclear significance, and remediation is costly
30% cut off	The percentage of total cultures found to be positive has been suggested as a threshold for concern, but significant outbreaks of Legionnaire's disease have occurred where less than 30% of cultures were positive
Quantitative cultures	Action thresholds using CFU exist but are of uncertain validity in the setting of poor reproducibility and unclear significance

The location where water sampling must occur, central waterworks or point-of-use fixtures, is a subject of debate. It is not generally agreed upon if first draughts of water from the tap should be tested or if the water should be allowed to "equilibrate" prior to collection. Further high-quality data is sorely needed to resolve these controversies on water testing for *Legionella* in the healthcare setting.

Conclusions and Perspectives

All appropriate regulations and requirements should be followed, but in the absence of mandate, the decision to perform primary or secondary *Legionella* surveillance testing should be related to the risk and history of each healthcare facility. A summary of take-home points is listed in Table 25.3. The development of a water safety plan based on a considered facility risk assessment is the recommended first step to approaching hospital water systems [40]. In the absence of standardized guidance, consideration of the reason for testing and system being tested should guide the type, location, and frequency of testing performed and interpretation of the results.

There is a critical need for evidence, free of industry bias and scientifically rigorous, to protect the safety of hospitalized patients and promote the rational development of guidelines. *Legionella* literature is relatively sparse and plagued with limitations, most significantly the retrospective nature of most reports occurring after an outbreak of a seasonal organism. Reports describing June–September outbreak followed by interventions and retesting of a system in January–March should not surprisingly imply that the intervention was highly successful. Unbiased evaluations of *Legionella* prevention systems and treatments across a full year are needed, ideally evaluating *Legionella* control outside of large, highly politicized outbreaks. The rapid initiation of untested requirements and the potential for misappropriating limited resources, in response to political or public relations pressures rather than scientific reasoning, must be avoided.

Table 25.3 Take-home points

Take-home points
Facilities should develop a considered water safety plan based on a facility risk assessment
The decision to perform primary or secondary surveillance should be justified based on above
Even a single possible or definite nosocomial case associated with a facility should prompt environmental testing

References

1. Glick THGM, Berman B, Mallison G, Rhodes WW Jr, Kassanoff I. Pontiac fever. An epidemic of unknown etiology in a health department: I. Clinical and epidemiologic aspects. Am J Epidemiol. 1978;107(2):149–60.
2. Tsai TFFD, Plikaytis BD, McCauley W, Martin SM, Fraser DW. Legionnaires' disease: clinical features of the epidemic in Philadelphia. Ann Intern Med. 1979;90(4):509–17.
3. Legionella (Legionnaires' Disease and Pontiac Fever) [http://www.cdc.gov/legionella/about/index.html].
4. Blatt SPPM, Pace E, Hoffman P, Dolan D, Lauderdale P, Zajac RA, Melcher GP. Nosocomial Legionnaires' disease: aspiration as a primary mode of disease acquisition. Am J Med. 1993;95(1):16–22.
5. Department ACH. Approaches to prevention and control of legionella infection in Allegheny County health care facilities. Allegheny: Allegheny County Health Department; 1997.
6. Legionella (Legionnaires' Disease and Pontiac Fever) [http://www.cdc.gov/legionella/health-depts/inv-tools-cluster/lab-inv-tools/procedures-manual.html].
7. Montagna MTCM, Giglio OD, Spagnolo AM, Napoli C, Cannova L, Deriu MG, Delia SA, Giuliano A, Guida M, Laganà P, Liguori G, Mura I, Pennino F, Rossini A, Tardivo S, Torre I, Torregrossa MV, Villafrate MR, Albertini R, Pasquarella C. Serological and molecular identification of Legionella spp. isolated from water and surrounding air samples in Italian healthcare facilities. Environ Res. 2016;146:47–50.
8. Rhoads WJPA, Edwards MA. Convective mixing in distal pipes exacerbates Legionella pneumophila growth in hot water plumbing. Pathogens. 2016;5(1):E29.
9. Bartram JCY, Lee JV, Pond K, Surman-Lee S. Legionella and the prevention of Legionellosis. Geneva: World Health Organization (WHO); 2007.
10. Cross DFBA, Dimond EG. The faucet aerator – a source of pseudomonas infection. N Engl J Med. 1966;274(25):1430–1.
11. Sydnor ERBG, Gimburg A, Cosgrove SE, Perl TM, Maragakis LL. Electronic-eye faucets: Legionella species contamination in healthcare settings. Infect Control Hosp Epidemiol. 2012;33(3):235–40.
12. Mäkinen R, Miettinen I, Pitkänen T, Kusnetsov J, Pursiainen A, Kovanen S, Riihinen K, Keinänen-Toivola MM. Manual faucets induce more biofilms than electronic faucets. Can J Microbiol. 2013;59(6):407–12.
13. Sampling Procedure and Potential Sampling Sites [http://www.cdc.gov/legionella/downloads/cdc-sampling-procedure.pdf].
14. Ta AC, Stout J, Yu VL, Wagener MM. Comparison of culture methods for monitoring Legionella species in hospital potable water systems and recommendations for standardization of such methods. J Clin Microbiol. 1995;33(8):2118–23.
15. Koziol-Montewka MMA, Stojek N, Palusinska-Szysz M, Danielak M, Wojtowicz M, Niewiedziol J, Koncewicz R, Niedzwiadek J, Paluch-Oles J, Trzeciak H, Drozanski W, Dutkiewicz J. Monitoring legionella species in hospital water systems. Link with disease and evaluation of different detection methods. Ann Agric Environ Med. 2008;15(1):143–7.
16. Flanders WDKK, Shelton BG. Effects of holding time and measurement error on culturing Legionella in environmental water samples. Water Res. 2014;62:293–301.
17. Chang CW, Chou F. Methodologies for quantifying culturable, viable, and total Legionella pneumophila in indoor air. Indoor Air. 2011;21(4):291–9.
18. Weiss E, Westfall H. Substrate utilization by Legionella cells after cryopreservation in phosphate buffer. Appl Environ Microbiol. 1984;48(2):380–5.
19. Morrill WE, Barbaree J, Fields BS, Sanden GN, Martin WT. Increased recovery of Legionella micdadei and Legionella bozemanii on buffered charcoal yeast extract agar supplemented with albumin. J Clin Microbiol. 1990;28(3):616–8.
20. Wadowsky RM, Yee R. Glycine-containing selective medium for isolation of Legionellaceae from environmental specimens. Appl Environ Microbiol. 1981;42(5):768–72.
21. Reinthaler FF, Sattler J, Schaffler-Dullnig K, Weinmayr B, Marth E. Comparative study of procedures for isolation and cultivation of Legionella pneumophila from tap water in hospitals. J Clin Microbiol. 1993;31(5):1213–6.
22. BD: BBL™ BCYE Agar QUALITY CONTROL PROCEDURES. In. Sparks, Maryland: Becton, Dickinson and Company; 2015.
23. (ISO) ISO: ISO 11731-2 Water quality – Detection and enumeration of Legionella. International Organization for Standardization Geneva 2004.
24. Bartie CVS, Nel LH. Identification methods for Legionella from environmental samples. Water Res. 2003;37(6):1362–70.
25. Demirjian A, Lucas C, Garrison LE, Kozak-Muiznieks NA, States S, Brown EW, Wortham JM, Beaudoin A, Casey ML, Marriott C, Ludwig AM, Sonel AF, Muder RR, Hicks LA. The importance of clinical surveillance in detecting Legionnaires' disease outbreaks: a large outbreak in a hospital with a Legionella disinfection system-Pennsylvania, 2011–2012. Clin Infect Dis. 2015;60(11):1596–602.
26. Appendix III: 7-3. Water sampling guidelines [https://www.osha.gov/dts/osta/otm/otm_iii/otm_iii_7.html].
27. Lucas CE, Taylor T Jr, Fields BS. Accuracy and precision of Legionella isolation by US laboratories in the ELITE program pilot study. Water Res. 2011;45(15):4428–36.
28. King CH, Shotts E Jr, Wooley RE, Porter KG. Survival of coliforms and bacterial pathogens within protozoa during chlorination. Appl Environ Microbiol. 1988;54(12):3023–33.
29. Díaz-Flores Á, Montero J, Castro FJ, Alejandres EM, Bayón C, Solís I, Fernández-Lafuente R, Rodríguez G. Comparing methods of determining Legionella spp in complex water matrices. BMC Microbiol. 2015;15:91.
30. Alleron L, Merlet N, Lacombe C, Frère J. Long-term survival of Legionella pneumophila in the viable but nonculturable state after monochloramine treatment. Curr Microbiol. 2008;57(5):497–502.
31. Legionnaires' disease part 2: the control of legionella bacteria in hot and cold water systems. Norwich: Health and Safety Executive; 2014.
32. Affairs DoV: prevention of healthcare-associated legionella disease and scald injury from potable water distribution systems. VHA Directive 1061 2014.
33. Mermel LA, Josephson S, Giorgio CH, Dempsey J, Parenteau S. Association of Legionnaires' disease with construction: contamination of potable water? Infect Control Hosp Epidemiol. 1995;16(2):76–81.
34. Timbury MC, Donaldson J, McCartney AC, Fallon RJ, Sleigh JD, Lyon D, Orange GV, Baird DR, Winter J, Wilson TS. Outbreak of Legionnaires' disease in Glasgow Royal Infirmary: microbiological aspects. J Hyg (Lond). 1986;97(3):393–403.

35. Phares CR, Russell E, Thigpen MC, Service W, Crist MB, Salyers M, Engel J, Benson RF, Fields B, Moore MR. Legionnaires' disease among residents of a long-term care facility: the sentinel event in a community outbreak. Am J Infect Control. 2007;35(5):319–23.

36. Yu VL, Beam T Jr, Lumish RM, Vickers RM, Fleming J, McDermott C, Romano J. Routine culturing for Legionella in the hospital environment may be a good idea: a three-hospital prospective study. Am J Med Sci. 1987;294(2):97–9.

37. O'Neill E, Humphreys H. Surveillance of hospital water and primary prevention of nosocomial legionellosis: what is the evidence? J Hosp Infect. 2005;59(4):273–9.

38. CDC CfDCaP: guidelines for environmental infection control in health-care facilities. Recommendations of CDC and the Healthcare Infection Control Practices Advisory Committee (HICPAC) 2003.

39. Parr A, Whitney E, Berkelman RL. Legionellosis on the rise: a review of guidelines for prevention in the United States. J Public Health Manag Pract. 2015;21(5):E17–26.

40. Legionellosis: risk management for building water systems. ASHRAE 2015, Standard 188–2015.

41. Yu V. Resolving the controversy on environmental cultures for Legionella: a modest proposal. Infect Control Hosp Epidemiol. 1998;19(12):893–7.

42. Patterson WJ, Hay J, McLuckie JC. Colonization of transplant unit water supplies with Legionella and protozoa: precautions required to reduce the risk of legionellosis. J Hosp Infect. 1997;37(1):7–17.

43. Best M, Yu V, Stout J, Goetz A, Muder RR, Taylor F. Legionellaceae in the hospital water-supply. Epidemiological link with disease and evaluation of a method for control of nosocomial legionnaires' disease and Pittsburgh pneumonia. Lancet. 1983;2(8345):307–10.

44. Prevention and control of Legionnaires' disease [http://www.health.ny.gov/press/releases/2005/2005-08-26_legionnaires/hospital_guidelines_legionella.pdf].

45. Protection against Legionella [https://www.health.ny.gov/regulations/emergency/docs/protection_against_legionella.pdf].

46. Services MDoHH: summary of Legionellosis outbreak – Genesee County, June 2014–March 2015.

47. Yu VL, Plouffe J, Pastoris MC, Stout JE, Schousboe M, Widmer A, Summersgill J, File T, Heath CM, Paterson DL, Chereshsky A. Distribution of Legionella species and serogroups isolated by culture in patients with sporadic community-acquired legionellosis: an international collaborative survey. J Infect Dis. 2002;186(1):127–8.

48. Muder RR, Yu V. Infection due to Legionella species other than L. pneumophila. Clin Infect Dis. 2002;35(8):990–8.

49. Gaia V, Fry N, Harrison TG, Peduzzi R. Sequence-based typing of Legionella pneumophila serogroup 1 offers the potential for true portability in legionellosis outbreak investigation. J Clin Microbiol. 2003;41(7):2932–9.

50. Gaia V, Fry N, Afshar B, Lück PC, Meugnier H, Etienne J, Peduzzi R, Harrison TG. Consensus sequence-based scheme for epidemiological typing of clinical and environmental isolates of Legionella pneumophila. J Clin Microbiol. 2005;43(5):2047–52.

51. Ratzow S, Gaia V, Helbig JH, Fry NK, Lück PC. Addition of neuA, the gene encoding N-acylneuraminate cytidylyl transferase, increases the discriminatory ability of the consensus sequence-based scheme for typing Legionella pneumophila serogroup 1 strains. J Clin Microbiol. 2007;45(6):1965–8.

52. EWGLI Sequence-Based Typing (SBT) database for Legionella pneumophila [http://www.hpa-bioinformatics.org.uk/legionella/legionella_sbt/php/sbt_homepage.php].

53. Lévesque S, Plante P, Mendis N, Cantin P, Marchand G, Charest H, Raymond F, Huot C, Goupil-Sormany I, Desbiens F, Faucher SP, Corbeil J, Tremblay C. Genomic characterization of a large outbreak of Legionella pneumophila serogroup 1 strains in Quebec City, 2012. PLoS One. 2014;9(8):e103852.

54. Tobiansky L, Drath A, Dubery B, Koornhof HJ. Seasonality of Legionella isolates from environmental sources. Isr J Med Sci. 1986;22(9):640–3.

55. Initiative ACHDPRH: Updated guidelines for the control of legionella in western Pennsylvania. 2014.

56. (EWGLI) EWGfLI: EWGLI technical guidelines for the investigation, control and prevention of travel associated Legionnaires' Disease. 2011, 1.1.

The Importance of *C. difficile* Colonization in Infection Prevention

Natalia Blanco and Surbhi Leekha

Clostridium difficile infection (CDI) has become the most common healthcare-associated infection in the United States [1]. Initially identified in 1980 as the etiologic agent of antibiotic-associated diarrhea among hospitalized patients, interest in its epidemiology surged in the early 2000s with the emergence of an epidemic strain variably referred to as BI by restriction enzyme analysis, North American PFGE type 1 (NAP1) by PFGE, or PCR ribotype 027 [2]. The strong association of CDI with hospital exposure led to investigation and recognition of transmission in the hospital setting [3, 4] and recommendations for infection control strategies to limit transmission [4]. However, in the United States, rates of CDI continued to increase between 2005 and 2010 and decreased by only 8% from 2011 to 2014 [5]. A 2015 CDC study found that *C. difficile* caused almost half a million infections in the United States in 1 year and was associated with an estimated 15,000 deaths, leading the CDC to name CDI an urgent "drug-resistant threat to the United States" [6, 7].

Current CDI prevention strategies largely focus on *C. difficile* transmission from symptomatic patients. Similar to other epidemiologically significant organisms in the hospital setting such as MRSA, VRE, and multidrug-resistant gram-negative bacteria, asymptomatic colonization with *C. difficile* has been described in several studies as described below. However, unlike other organisms, active surveillance for such asymptomatic colonization is not routinely recommended, is in fact discouraged by many experts [4], and remains an actively debated topic. In this chapter, we will discuss various aspects of *C. difficile* colonization to help readers understand the basis for this controversy.

Prevalence of and Risk Factors for Asymptomatic Colonization with *C. difficile*

Although there is no formal definition, at least one author suggests that asymptomatic colonization with *C. difficile* occurs when the bacteria are present in stool of an individual without CDI symptoms over a period of 7 days [8]. The presence of these bacteria in the absence of symptoms has been associated with the presence of a protective immune response against *C. difficile*. Kyne et al. described a significantly greater detection of IgG serum antibodies against toxin A in asymptomatic carriers than CDI symptomatic patients [9]. Similarly, Loo et al. also associated the presence of serum antibodies against toxin B with healthcare-associated *C. difficile* colonization compared with symptomatic CDI [10].

Several studies have described the frequency of asymptomatic colonization in acute care settings, ranging between 4 and 29% [9–21]. While some of this variability relates to true variation driven by geographic- and patient-related factors, some differences in estimates may be related to the time elapsed from admission to the time when the prevalence study was performed, testing method (whether culture-based, molecular testing, or toxin assay was used to identify colonization), and the inclusion of toxigenic vs. non-toxigenic strains in studies using culture-based detection [11].

C. difficile asymptomatic carriage has been associated with recent hospitalization, chemotherapy, and acid-suppressive medication [10]. In contrast to CDI, several studies have been unable to associate antibiotic use with *C. difficile* carriage [10, 22]. In addition, the *C. difficile* strain or ribotype may play a role in determining if the patient remains asymptomatic after colonization. Loo et al. found 63% of CDI patients in Canadian hospitals carried ribotype 027 compared to 36% of asymptomatic carriers [10]. Similarly, Alasmari et al. reported similar findings among hospitalized patients in St. Louis, Missouri (25% CDI patients vs. 3% asymptomatic carriers had ribotype 027) [22].

N. Blanco • S. Leekha (✉)
Epidemiology and Public Health, University of Maryland School of Medicine, 110 S. Paca Street, 6th Floor, Suite 100, Baltimore, MD 21201, USA
e-mail: nblanco@som.umaryland.edu;
sleekha@som.umaryland.edu

Detection of *C. difficile* Carriers and Its Impact on CDI Rates

The Society for Healthcare Epidemiology of America and the Infectious Diseases Society of America (SHEA/IDSA), the American College of Gastroenterology, and the American Medical Association recommend a multistep laboratory algorithm starting with the detection of glutamate dehydrogenase (GDH), followed by either a confirmatory test for the detection of toxin using an enzyme immunoassay (EIA) or a cell cytotoxicity assay (CCTA) or detection of the toxigenic bacteria through cytotoxigenic culture or nucleic acid amplification testing (NAAT), e.g., PCR [4, 23, 24]. Culture is cumbersome and generally not performed outside of research studies. Although NAAT or PCR is considered to have a higher sensitivity and specificity than EIA [23], as well as a shorter turnaround time than culture or CCTA, NAAT detects the toxin-encoding gene rather than the toxin itself, essentially picking up the presence of toxigenic *C. difficile*, but does not distinguish between CDI symptomatic and asymptomatic individuals [25, 26].

In 2014, 44% of acute care hospitals participating in the National Healthcare Safety Network reported using PCR alone or in combination with other tests for the diagnosis of CDI [27]. The implementation of this more sensitive test has led to 50–100% increases in CDI-reported rates [27]. Considering that colonization with *C. difficile* is five to ten times more common than CDI and that *C. difficile* is responsible for only ~20% of all nosocomial diarrheas, it is likely that some patients diagnosed as CDI positive using a PCR test have diarrhea of a different etiologic origin [27, 28]. Therefore, appropriate identification of only symptomatic patients for CDI testing is essential to avoid "false-positive results" from *C. difficile* carriers.

Association of *C. difficile* Colonization with Subsequent Symptomatic CDI

There is evidence suggesting that asymptomatic *C. difficile* colonization has a protective effect and is associated with a reduced risk of CDI [29]. Shim et al. reviewed four longitudinal studies describing that asymptomatic carriers develop CDI between 0 and 3.9% of the time, while non-colonizers were more likely to develop CDI (1.7–8.0%) [30]. More recently, Zacharioudakis et al. reported the contrary after completing a systematic review and meta-analysis on the topic. Patients colonized with *C. difficile* upon hospital admission had six times higher risk of developing CDI than non-colonizers [31]. This difference might be related to the unknown incubation period for CDI. It is possible that those individuals that go on to develop long-term carriage are protected, while other asymptomatic carriers with more recent

acquisition might still remain susceptible to development of symptomatic CDI. Although further research is needed to better understand this association, this study highlights the need for developing preventive measures toward *C. difficile*-colonized patients.

Contribution of Asymptomatically Colonized Patients to In-Hospital CDI Transmission

While several studies have evaluated prevalence of asymptomatic colonization, fewer studies have investigated hospital-based transmission from these colonized patients and particularly whether such transmissions contribute to active CDI. In one of the earliest studies looking at the role of asymptomatic patients in *C. difficile* transmission in the pre-hypervirulent strain era, Clabots et al. (1992) cultured 634 stool samples and used restriction endonuclease analysis to distinguish between strains. They found that hospital acquisition of a *C. difficile* strain was preceded by introduction of that strain to the ward by an asymptomatic admission in 84% of cases [14]. In contrast, when Walters et al. (1982) conducted a study during an outbreak of pseudomembranous colitis in an ICU, investigators traced the outbreak to a single symptomatic patient and associated environmental contamination [32]. No asymptomatic carriers were found among patients or staff during that outbreak [32].

More recently, studies have been able to take advantage of more sophisticated techniques such as MLVA (multiple locus variable number tandem repeat analysis) or whole genome sequencing to evaluate the relatedness of strains and improve the understanding of transmission. Curry et al. used MLVA to determine the genetic relationship between isolates of asymptomatic carriers and CDI cases after screening 3006 patients at the University of Pittsburgh Medical Center Presbyterian in 2009. Of 59 incident nosocomial CDI cases identified, 30% were associated with previous CDI cases and 29% with asymptomatic carriers [33]. Eyre et al. applied whole genome sequencing to 1223 strains from 1250 cases with symptomatic CDI in either healthcare or community settings in Oxfordshire, UK, between September 2007 and March 2011. In their analysis, 45% of cases were genetically distinct from all other cases preceding that case. The authors concluded that the presence of a reservoir of asymptomatically colonized patients was a potential explanation for this finding [34, 35]. However, the study was limited by inclusion of only toxin-positive CDI cases detected by EIA. Given that EIA has low sensitivity in CDI diagnosis, it is possible that a significant proportion of CDI cases were not considered as sources of subsequent cases. In follow-up to the above, the investigators conducted a small prospective study to assess the potential for transmission from asymptomatically colonized patients in the hospital setting. Stool cultures were performed at admission and sequentially every 3 days between February and June 2012 at two hospitals in the UK. They were able to enroll 132 of 227 patients hospitalized during the study period. They found an initial, at-admission colonization prevalence of 14/132 (11%), and an additional four patients developed colonization over the course of the study [36]. Using whole genome sequencing, only two patients on the same ward were found to be asymptomatically colonized with similar isolates. The authors concluded that this could either be due to transmission from one asymptomatic patient to another or transmission to both patients from a third common source that had not been cultured [36]. The relatively small sample size, short follow-up time, and lack of culturing of nearly half the patients were important limitations of this study.

Similarly, Durham et al. estimated the effect of hospital- and community-based transmission of *C. difficile* using a mathematical CDI transmission model [37]. The investigators reported that hospitalized patients with CDI transmit *C. difficile* at a rate 15 times that of asymptomatic patients. However, as the authors pointed out, despite the lower transmission rate from asymptomatic patients, these transmissions have a substantial effect on CDI because of the relatively larger reservoir of hospitalized *C. difficile* carriers [37]. Likewise, Lanzas et al. (2011) developed a compartmental mathematical model of CDI transmission using data from six medical wards and published literature. Their results suggested that transmission within the ward solely from patients with symptomatic CDI could not sustain the new *C. difficile* colonizations [38].

HCW and Environmental Contamination Related to Asymptomatically Colonized Patients

Evaluation of HCW and environmental contamination related to asymptomatically colonized patients is also important to better delineate the potential role played by asymptomatic carriers in CDI transmission. Several studies have been conducted in this regard. Faden et al. conducted a study in a neonatal intensive care unit (NICU); investigators identified asymptomatic colonization among 9/35 (26%) neonates. A total of 150 cultures of various environmental surfaces were obtained in the NICU and in infant, adolescent, and hematology/ oncology units; none of the included units had any identified cases of CDI during the study period, and units other than the NICU were not assessed for asymptomatic colonization among patients [39]. None of 91 surfaces sampled in non-NICU locations were positive. Seven (12%) of 59 surfaces in the NICU were positive for *C. difficile* (five diaper scales, one infant scale, and a refrigerator). The authors concluded that overall environmental contamination was low in the pediatric setting [39].

At a Veteran Affairs Medical Center, Guerrero et al. (2013) performed rectal swab, skin, and environmental cultures among 149 of 160 patients in eight wards as part of a point prevalence survey in order to identify asymptomatically colonized patients. The prevalence of skin and/or environmental contamination was significantly lower in asymptomatic carriers (3/18, 17%) compared to patients with CDI (5/6, 83%; $P = 0.007$) [40]. However, 18 of 149 (12%) patients were found to be carriers of toxigenic *C. difficile*, while 6 patients (4%) were identified with active CDI [40]. This suggests again that even with lower rates of environmental contamination, because *C. difficile* carriers outnumber CDI patients, they may have a greater overall potential to influence *C. difficile* transmission [40].

Furthermore, in a similar study conducted among residents of a long-term care facility, 35/68 (51%) asymptomatic patients were found to be asymptomatically colonized with toxigenic *C. difficile*. Skin and environmental contamination was found to occur for 61% and 59% of asymptomatic carriers. Using PFGE, 13/15 (87%) of *C. difficile* isolates recovered from the skin, and 11/19 (58%) of isolates from the environment were found to match the patient's isolate. In addition, *C. difficile* was transferred to hands (donning sterile gloves) after contact with the skin of 8 (57%) of 14 patients who had positive skin culture results [41].

Together these results suggest that there is high potential for *C. difficile* to be transmitted from asymptomatic patients to both HCW skin and the environment, creating the potential for onward transmission and infection in susceptible patients. However, because environmental contamination appears more strongly associated with symptomatic patients, and can persist for long periods, the relative contribution to new cases from asymptomatic carriers via the environment remains unquantified.

Impact of Strain Type on the Role of Asymptomatic Colonization

The major difference between *C. difficile* and other antibiotic-resistant microorganisms is that *C. difficile* produces spores. Since these spores are resistant to antibiotics and most hospital-used disinfectants, they become an additional challenge for CDI control and prevention [42]. Among patients with CDI, hypervirulent strains such as ribotype 027 have been shown to produce greater amount of spore than non-hypervirulent strains [43]. Furthermore, although this topic has not been fully explored, some early evidence suggests that certain strains may be more likely to be associated with symptomatic CDI and greater environmental contamination. Samore et al. (1996) prospectively obtained stool cultures from selected epidemiologically linked contacts, as well as cultures of the environment of index cases with symptomatic CDI over a 6-month period.

C. difficile isolates were analyzed by PFGE or by restriction enzyme analysis if unclear by PFGE. The investigators identified 98 index cases of *C. difficile* toxin-associated diarrhea, including 26 outbreak-related cases. Transmission to personnel or patient contacts of the strain cultured from the corresponding index case was strongly associated with the intensity of environmental contamination [44]. A total of 31 index strains were found; however, a single strain was predominant among isolates associated with heavy environmental contamination, with personnel carriage, and with development of symptomatic illness among prospectively identified contacts suggesting that strain type has an important role in environmental contamination, transmission, and disease [44].

Effect of Targeting Asymptomatically Colonized Patients for Infection Prevention Interventions

Contact Precautions and Active Surveillance

The use of gloves when providing care to CDI patients has been shown to reduce CDI rates. Johnson et al. evaluated the impact of the implementation of an intensive education program regarding glove use during CDI patient care in two hospital wards. A significant decrease in the incidence of CDI was observed from 7.7 cases/1000 patient discharges before the intervention to 1.5/1000 during the 6 months of intervention [45]. Moreover, the point prevalence of asymptomatic *C. difficile* carriage was also reduced significantly on the intervention wards in the post-intervention period (from 27% to 9.3%) [45]. Although there is insufficient evidence showing the effectiveness of gown use to reduce CDI, its use is recommended as part of "contact precautions" [29]. Current guidelines for symptomatic CDI patients suggest contact precautions until diarrhea resolves [4]. However, research has shown prolonged shedding continues beyond resolution of symptoms. Sethi et al. reported recurrent shedding up to a month after CDI treatment. These results provide support to recommend continuation of contact precautions until hospital discharge [46].

To date, only one study has evaluated the use of active surveillance and contact precautions for asymptomatic *C difficile* colonization. Longtin et al. conducted a quasi-experimental study in a Canadian acute care facility between November 19, 2013, and March 7, 2015. Admission screening was conducted by detecting the *tcdB* gene by PCR on rectal swabs. Three hundred sixty-eight out of 7599 (4.8%) screened were identified as carriers and placed under contact precautions [47]. The authors detected a significant effect of the intervention, represented by a gradual progressive decrease in the healthcare-associated CDI (HA CDI) by an overall magnitude of 7.2 HA CDIs per 10,000 patient-days [47].

Although this study is unique in exploring this topic, it still has limitations. The intervention was nonrandomized and was based in a single center, and compliance with isolation precautions was not assessed [47]. In addition, the authors did not report the strain relatedness between carriers and CDI cases or the proportion of *C. difficile* carriers that progressed to CDI. Therefore, as Crobach et al. pointed out, it is hard to distinguish if the observed reduction is due to less progression from colonization to symptomatic disease, less spread from carriers, or less spread from symptomatic CDI cases [48].

Treatment of *C. difficile* Asymptomatic Carriers

Antibiotic therapy is a primary risk factor for CDI, and treating *C. difficile* asymptomatic individuals may lead to CDI development and transmission to others [30]. Lawley et al. described the effect of clindamycin treatment on asymptomatic carriers using a mice model. According to the authors, antibiotic treatment triggers a highly contagious supershedding state, which is described by *C. difficile* overgrowth and spore shedding, parallel to a decrease of the gut microbiota diversity [30]. Similarly, Kundrapu et al. reported that among patients diagnosed with CDI but that did not meet the clinical criteria for testing ($n = 30$), skin and environmental contamination was common only in those who had prior antibiotic exposure in the previous 90 days. None of those who were not previously exposed to antibiotics had skin or environmental spores [49]. These studies highlight the importance of antibiotic stewardship not only on development of disease but also on potentially decreasing shedding from asymptomatic carriers and preventing further transmission.

Antimicrobial therapy has also been shown not to be effective in decolonizing *C. difficile* carriers. Johnson et al. conducted a randomized study where 30 asymptomatic *C. difficile* carriers were assigned to received vancomycin, metronidazole, or placebo as treatment. Although vancomycin treatment was temporarily effective to reduce shedding, it was associated with a higher rate of *C. difficile* carriage after 2 months of treatment in comparison to individuals that received the placebo [50]. Furthermore, metronidazole was not effective in eliminating carriage even immediately after treatment [50].

Additionally, there is very limited research specifically on the intervention of treating *C. difficile* carriers as a measure of preventing and reducing CDI [29]. In one of the oldest studies reported in 1987, Delmée et al. observed that after completely renovating and cleaning a leukemia unit and treating all *C. difficile* carriers with vancomycin, their positive toxin assays went from 9.9% to 1.2% [51]. However, this does not take into account the potential impact of environmental cleaning and less detection of *C. difficile* rather than true reduction of symptomatic CDI. In contrast, Bender et al. (1986) observed no effect of treating *C. difficile* carriers with metronidazole on the incidence of new CDAD cases at a chronic care facility during an outbreak [52]. These results are in agreement with Johnson et al., who also observed no effect of metronidazole treatment of asymptomatic carriers [50]. Therefore, evidence to date recommends against treating asymptomatic *C. difficile* carriers [27].

In summary, asymptomatic colonization with *C. difficile* is prevalent in healthcare facilities. Further research of the role played by *C. difficile* carriers in *C. difficile* nosocomial spread and the most effective management of these individuals to prevent *C. difficile* transmission is essential to inform and improve CDI prevention and control guidelines.

References

1. Magill SS, Edwards JR, Bamberg W, Beldavs ZG, Dumyati G, Kainer MA, et al. Multistate point-prevalence survey of health care-associated infections. N Engl J Med. 2014;370(13):1198–208.
2. McDonald LC, Killgore G, Thompson A, Owens RC Jr, Kazakova SV, Sambol SP, et al. An epidemic, toxin gene-variant strain of Clostridium difficile. N Engl J Med. 2005;353(23):2433–41.
3. Kumar N, Miyajima F, He M, Roberts P, Swale A, Ellison L, et al. Genome-based infection tracking reveals dynamics of Clostridium difficile transmission and disease recurrence. Clin Infect Dis. 2016;62(6):746–52.
4. Cohen SH, Gerding DN, Johnson S, Kelly CP, Loo VG, McDonald LC, et al. Clinical practice guidelines for Clostridium difficile infection in adults: 2010 update by the society for healthcare epidemiology of America (SHEA) and the infectious diseases society of America (IDSA). Infect Control Hosp Epidemiol. 2010;31(5):431–55.
5. National and State Healthcare Associated Infections Progress Report-2013: Centers for Disease Control and Prevention. (2015).
6. Lessa FC, Mu Y, Bamberg WM, Beldavs ZG, Dumyati GK, Dunn JR, et al. Burden of Clostridium difficile infection in the United States. N Engl J Med. 2015;372(9):825–34.
7. CDC. Biggest threats. In; (2016).
8. Galdys A, Curry SR, Harrison LH. Asymptomatic Clostridium difficile colonization as a reservoir for Clostridium difficile infection. Expert Rev Anti-Infect Ther. 2014;12(8):967–80.
9. Kyne L, Warny M, Qamar A, Kelly CP. Asymptomatic carriage of Clostridium difficile adn serum levels of IgG antibody against toxin A. NEJM. 2000;342(6):390–7.
10. Loo VG, Poirier L, Lamothe F, Michaud S, Turgeon N, Toye B, et al. Host and pathogen factors for Clostridium difficile infection and colonization. N Engl J Med. 2011;365(18):1693–703.
11. Furuya-Kanamori L, Marquess J, Yakob L, Riley TV, Paterson DL, Foster NF, et al. Asymptomatic Clostridium difficile colonization: epidemiology and clinical implications. BMC Infect Dis. 2015;15:516.
12. McFarland L, Surawicz CM, Stamm WE. Risk factors for Clostridium difficile carriage and C. difficile-associated diarrhea in a cohort of hospitalized patients. J Infect dis. 1990;162(3):678–84.
13. Barbut F, Corthier G, Charpak Y, Cerf M, Monteil H, Fosse T, et al. Prevalence and pathogenicity of Clostridium difficile in hospitalized patients. Arch Intern Med. 1996;156:1449–54.
14. Clabots CR, Johnson S, Olson MM, Peterson LR, Gerding DN. Acquisition of Clostridium difficile by hospitalized patients: evidence for colonized new admissions as a source of infection. J Infect dis. 1992;166:561–7.
15. Gerding DN, Olsen MA, Peterson LR, Teasley DG, Gebhard RL, Schwartz ML. Clostridium difficile- Associated Diarrhea and colitis in adults. Arch Intern Med. 1986;146:95–100.
16. Heard SR, O'Farrell S, Holland D, Crook S, Barnett MJ, Tabaqchali S. The epidemiology of Clostridium difficile with use of a typing scheme: nosocomial acquisition and cross-infection among immunocompromised patients. J Infect Dis. 1986;153(1):159–62.
17. Johnson S, Clabots CR, Linn FV, Olson MM, Peterson LR, Gerding DN. Nosocomial Clostridium difficile colonisation and disease. Lancet. 1990;336:97–100.
18. McFarland L, Mulligan ME, Kwok RYY, Stamm WE. Nosocomial acquisition of Clostridium difficile infection. N Engl J Med. 1989;320:204–10.
19. Samore MH, DeGirolami PC, Tlucko A, Lichtenberg DA, Melvin ZA, Karchmer AW. Clostridium difficile colonization and diarrhea at a tertiary care hospital. CID. 1994;18:181–7.
20. Hung YP, Tsai PJ, Hung KH, Liu HC, Lee CI, Lin HJ, et al. Impact of toxigenic Clostridium difficile colonization and infection among hospitalized adults at a district hospital in southern Taiwan. PLoS One. 2012;7(8):e42415.
21. Leekha S, Aronhalt KC, Sloan LM, Patel R, Orenstein R. Asymptomatic Clostridium difficile colonization in a tertiary care hospital: admission prevalence and risk factors. Am J Infect Control. 2013;41(5):390–3.
22. Alasmari F, Seiler SM, Hink T, Burnham CA, Dubberke ER. Prevalence and risk factors for asymptomatic Clostridium difficile carriage. Clin Infect Dis. 2014;59(2):216–22.
23. Surawicz CM, Brandt LJ, Binion DG, Ananthakrishnan AN, Curry SR, Gilligan PH, et al. Guidelines for diagnosis, treatment, and prevention of Clostridium difficile infections. Am J Gastroenterol. 2013;108(4):478–98. quiz 499
24. Bagdasarian N, Rao K, Malani PN. Diagnosis and treatment of Clostridium difficile in adults: a systematic review. JAMA. 2015;313(4):398–408.
25. Burnham CA, Carroll KC. Diagnosis of Clostridium difficile infection: an ongoing conundrum for clinicians and for clinical laboratories. Clin Microbiol Rev. 2013;26(3):604–30.
26. Gilligan PH. Contemporary approaches for the laboratory diagnosis of Clostridium difficile infections. Semin Colon Rectal Surg. 2014;25(3):137–42.
27. Polage CR, Gyorke CE, Kennedy MA, Leslie JL, Chin DL, Wang S, et al. Overdiagnosis of Clostridium difficile infection in the molecular test era. JAMA Intern Med. 2015;175(11):1792–801.
28. Polage CR, Solnick JV, Cohen SH. Nosocomial diarrhea: evaluation and treatment of causes other than Clostridium difficile. Clin Infect Dis. 2012;55(7):982–9.
29. Gerding DN, Muto CA, Owens RC Jr. Measures to control and prevent Clostridium difficile infection. CID. 2008;46:S43–9.
30. Shim JK, Johnson S, Samore MH, Bliss DZ, Gerding DN. Primary symptomless colonisation by Clostridium difficile and decreased risk of subsequent diarrhoea. Lancet. 1998;351(9103):633–6.
31. Zacharioudakis IM, Zervou FN, Pliakos EE, Ziakas PD, Mylonakis E. Colonization with toxinogenic C. difficile upon hospital admission, and risk of infection: a systematic review and meta-analysis. Am J Gastroenterol. 2015;110(3):381–90. quiz 391
32. Walters BAJ, Stafford R, Roberts RK. Contamination and Crossi nf ect ion with Clostridium difficile in an intensive care unit*. Aust NZ J Med. 1982;12:255–8.
33. Curry SR, Muto CA, Schlackman JL, Pasculle AW, Shutt KA, Marsh JW, et al. Use of multilocus variable number of tandem repeats analysis genotyping to determine the role of asymptomatic

carriers in Clostridium difficile transmission. Clin Infect Dis. 2013;57(8):1094–102.

34. Eyre DW, Cule ML, Wilson DJ, Griffiths D, Vaughan A, O'Connor L, et al. Diverse sources of C. difficile infection identified on whole-genome sequencing. N Engl J Med. 2013;369(13):1195–205.

35. Walker AS, Eyre DW, Wyllie DH, Dingle KE, Harding RM, O'Connor L, et al. Characterisation of Clostridium difficile hospital ward-based transmission using extensive epidemiological data and molecular typing. PLoS Med. 2012;9(2):e1001172.

36. Chang Y-F, Eyre DW, Griffiths D, Vaughan A, Golubchik T, Acharya M, et al. Asymptomatic Clostridium difficile colonisation and onward transmission. PLoS ONE. 2013;8(11):e78445.

37. Durham DP, Olsen MA, Dubberke ER, Galvani AP, Townsend JP. Quantifying transmission of Clostridium difficile within and outside healthcare settings. Emerg Infect Dis. 2016;22(4):608–16.

38. Lanzas C, Dubberke ER, Lu Z, Reske KA, Grohn YT. Epidemiological model for Clostridium difficile transmission in healthcare settings. Infect Control Hosp Epidemiol. 2011;32(6):553–61.

39. Faden HS, Dryja D. Importance of asymptomatic shedding of Clostridium difficile in environmental contamination of a neonatal intensive care unit. Am J Infect Control. 2015;43(8):887–8.

40. Guerrero DM, Becker JC, Eckstein EC, Kundrapu S, Deshpande A, Sethi AK, et al. Asymptomatic carriage of toxigenic Clostridium difficile by hospitalized patients. J Hosp Infect. 2013;85(2):155–8.

41. Riggs MM, Sethi AK, Zabarsky TF, Eckstein EC, Jump RL, Donskey CJ. Asymptomatic carriers are a potential source for transmission of epidemic and nonepidemic Clostridium difficile strains among long-term care facility residents. Clin Infect Dis. 2007;45(8):992–8.

42. Dubberke ER, Carling P, Carrico R, Donskey CJ, Loo VG, McDonald LC, et al. Strategies to prevent Clostridium difficile infections in acute care hospitals: 2014 update. Infect Control Hosp Epidemiol. 2014;35(6):628–45.

43. Merrigan M, Venugopal A, Mallozzi M, Roxas B, Viswanathan VK, Johnson S, et al. Human hypervirulent Clostridium difficile strains exhibit increased sporulation as well as robust toxin production. J Bacteriol. 2010;192(19):4904–11.

44. Samore MH, Venkataraman L, DeGirolami PC, Arbeit RD, Karchmer AW. Clinical and molecular epidemiology of sporadic and clustered cases of nosocomial Clostridium difficile diarrhea. Am J Med. 1996;100:32–40.

45. Johnson S, Gerding DN, Olson MM, Weiler MD, Hughes RA, Clabots CR, et al. Prospective, controlled study of vinyl glove use to interrupt Clostridium difficile nosocomial transmission. Am J Med. 1990;88(2):137–40.

46. Sethi AK, Al-Nassir WN, Nerandzic MM, Bobulsky GS, Donskey CJ. Persistence of skin contamination and environmental shedding of Clostridium difficile during and after treatment of C. difficile infection. Infect Control Hosp Epidemiol. 2010;31(1):21–7.

47. Longtin Y, Paquet-Bolduc B, Gilca R, Garenc C, Fortin E, Longtin J, et al. Effect of detecting and isolating Clostridium difficile carriers at hospital admission on the incidence of C difficile infections: a quasi-experimental controlled study. JAMA Intern Med. 2016;176(6):796–804.

48. Crobach MJT, Terveer EM, Kuijper EJ. Letter to editor: effect of detecting and isolating asymptomatic Clostridium difficile carriers. JAMA Intern Med. 2016;176(10):1572–3.

49. Kundrapu S, Sunkesula V, Tomas M, Donskey CJ. Skin and environmental contamination in patients diagnosed with Clostridium difficile infection but not meeting clinical criteria for testing. Infect Control Hosp Epidemiol. 2015;36(11):1348–50.

50. Johnson S, Homann SR, Bettin KM, Quick JN, Clabots CR, Peterson LR, et al. Treatment of asymptomatic Clostridium difficile carriers (fecal excretors) with vancomycin or metronidazole. Ann Int Med. 1992;117:297–302.

51. Delmée M, Vandercam VA, Michaux JL. Epidemiology and prevention of Clostridium difficile infections in a leukemia unit. Eur J Clin Microbiol. 1987;6(6):623–7.

52. Bender BS, Laughon BE, Gaydos C, Forman MS, Bennet R, Greenough WB III, et al. Is Clostridium difficile endemic in chronic- care facilities? Lancet. 1986;328(8497):11–3.

Mandatory Influenza Vaccination of Healthcare Personnel

27

Bryan D. Harris and Thomas R. Talbot

Introduction

Healthcare-associated transmission of influenza has been documented in many different patient populations and clinical settings [1] including neonatal intensive care units [2–7], pediatric wards [8–11], adult and pediatric transplant units [12–15], infectious disease units [16, 17], general medical wards [18–20], geriatric wards and long-term care facilities [21–25], oncology units [26, 27], pulmonary rehabilitation centers [28], and emergency departments [29]. In many of these outbreaks, infections occurred in unvaccinated healthcare personnel (HCP), and HCP were linked epidemiologically to further transmission of influenza. Such outbreaks may result in increased patient morbidity, mortality, length of hospitalization, and costs and may disrupt the essential services of a healthcare facility during a season when the patient census and HCP absenteeism are high [18].

Recognizing that there is no perfectly effective measure to prevent the nosocomial transmission of influenza, a multi-faceted approach is needed. Such practices should include appropriate isolation of infected patients, high patient vaccination rates, and dedication to basic infection prevention measures such as handwashing, restriction of ill visitors and HCP, and respiratory hygiene and cough etiquette. While these practices seem to be well supported, other strategies, such as mandatory vaccination of HCPs as a condition of employment, have been more controversial. This review will discuss some of the controversial aspects of mandating influenza vaccines for HCP by addressing frequently cited reasons for rejection of such policies. The legal framework for mandatory vaccination is outside the scope of this chapter, but some excellent reviews on this topic are recommended [30, 31].

B.D. Harris • T.R. Talbot (✉)
Department of Medicine, Vanderbilt University Medical Center, 1161 21st Avenue South, A2200 Medical Center North, Nashville, TN 37232, USA
e-mail: bryan.d.harris@vanderbilt.edu; tom.talbot@vanderbilt.edu

History of Mandatory Influenza Vaccination for HCP

At the start of this century, despite efforts to promote HCP influenza vaccination by government agencies, regulatory groups, professional societies, and visible vaccine champions, influenza vaccination rates among US HCP remained low. Prior to the 2009–2010 influenza season, despite increased awareness of the importance of HCP influenza vaccination and large-scale, resource-intensive voluntary vaccination campaigns at most healthcare facilities, vaccination rates remained around 45%. A combination of several factors have led to an increased focus on HCP influenza immunization and the use of various strategies (including mandatory vaccination +/− masking of unvaccinated HCP) in order to improve vaccination rates. Namely, the perception of HCP immunization, and specifically HCP influenza immunization, has evolved from that of an employee health benefit to an important measure of a healthcare facility's quality and patient safety program. In addition, the emergence of novel influenza (e.g., the 2009 H1N1 influenza pandemic) and the importance of preventing healthcare-associated transmission of such pathogens helped alter the approach to and perceptions of the importance of HCP influenza vaccination.

Since 2005, an increasing number of facilities have considered HCP immunization as a mandatory condition of employment. The move to mandate HCP influenza immunization gained traction in 2005, when Virginia Mason Medical Center (VMMC) revised its institutional policy to require influenza immunization as a condition of employment [32]. This innovative program was implemented despite vaccination rates well above the national rate. The Washington State Nurses Association (WSNA) filed a grievance against VMMC arguing that the decision to alter a policy that resulted in termination of employment violated the collective bargaining agreement. An arbitrator found in favor of the WSNA, but VMMC's subsequent implementation of mandatory masking for unvaccinated employees was upheld after

© Springer International Publishing AG 2018
G. Bearman et al. (eds.), *Infection Prevention*, DOI 10.1007/978-3-319-60980-5_27

WSNA challenge. With the mandate, influenza immunization rates of VMMC employees rose to 98.9%, and, notably, the rates in the unionized nurses, who were exempt from the vaccination mandate, rose to 95.8%.

Subsequently, more institutions and healthcare systems have implemented similar programs. Every facility/system that has implemented a mandatory HCP influenza immunization program and has reported their experiences has noted rates above 85% (and above 90% in most instances) following the mandate [33–38]. Of note, not all "mandatory" programs are the same. Variation exists regarding requirements for unvaccinated HCP to wear a mask during the influenza season, varying exemption allowances and review (e.g., only medical vs. allowances for personal belief exemption), and the consequences for non-compliance. Some facilities have also moved to use of the less-punitive term "universal" to describe their still-mandatory program in which HCPs are required to either receive an annual influenza immunization or meet specified exemptions (which may include medical, religious, and/or personal belief exemptions).

The use of policies where influenza immunization is a condition of employment is increasing in the USA, based on an annual survey of HCP conducted by the CDC. The percent of respondents who reported working at an institution where there was an employer vaccination requirement (with no specific mention about masking policies) increased from 20.9% during the 2011–2012 influenza season to 40.1% during the 2014–2015 season [39]. In addition, during the 2014–2015 influenza season, the HCP vaccination rate was 44% in clinical settings where influenza vaccines were not required, promoted, or offered on site, while the HCP vaccination rate was 96% in clinical settings where vaccination was required [39]. While some HCPs have had their employment terminated due to vaccine refusal, the actual reported number of HCP dismissed has been very small compared with the thousands of HCP encompassed by these policies.

With the growing interest in HCP influenza immunization, the use of state regulation and legislation surrounding the topic has also increased. As of June 2011, 20 states had enacted laws that address influenza vaccination of certain categories of the HCP workforce [40]. In most cases, the laws require healthcare facilities to develop and implement influenza programs, but more specific requirements for HCP to be immunized are rare. More than half of the laws require employers to "provide," "arrange for," "ensure," or "offer" influenza immunizations to HCP, while half of the state laws regulate only HCP in long-term care facilities [40].

California was one of the first states to require influenza vaccination of acute care HCP in 2006, but the regulation does not specify the means through which the hospitals should enforce requirements. A Colorado regulation required incremental levels of HCP vaccination coverage over the course of several years (reaching 90% by December 31,

2014), and if a facility is unable to achieve these levels, immunization must be mandated (allowing for medical exemption) with mask use required for unvaccinated HCP [41]. Rhode Island also has a regulation that covers all vaccines recommended for HCP, including influenza [42], and requires unvaccinated persons to wear masks during patient care [43, 44]. In 2013, after a failed attempt during the 2009 H1N1 influenza pandemic, the state of New York tried a different tactic, passing a regulation requiring "all unvaccinated personnel in health care and residential facilities and agencies to wear surgical or procedure masks in areas where patients or residents may be present" during the time when the Commissioner of Health determines that influenza is prevalent [45, 46].

The concept of requiring influenza immunization as a condition of HCP employment has now been endorsed by a growing list of professional societies and quality organizations, including every major US infectious diseases and infection prevention organization (Table 27.1) [38]. Those that explicitly endorse masking for unvaccinated HCP are noted in the table with an asterisk. Notably, in 2015, the American Nurses Association (ANA), a group that initially had not supported influenza immunization as a condition of employment, reversed their position and endorsed such a policy for the safety of HCP and their patients [47–49]. They also noted that "[i]ndividuals who are exempted from vaccination may be required to adopt measures or practices in the workplace to reduce the chance of disease transmission" which may include masking.

Finally, HCP immunization data are now used as part of formal assessments of healthcare facility quality (i.e., the US

Table 27.1 Selected national organizations recommending HCP influenza immunization as a condition of employment

American Academy of Family Physicians (AAFP)*
American Academy of Pediatrics (AAP)
American College of Physicians (ACP)*
American Hospital Association (AHA)*
American Medical Directors Association (AMDA)
American Nurses Association (ANA)
American Pharmacists Association
American Public Health Association (APHA)
Association for Professionals in Infection Control and Epidemiology (APIC)*
Infectious Diseases Society of America (IDSA)*
National Association of County & City Health Officials (NACCHO)
National Business Group on Health*
National Foundation for Infectious Diseases (NFID)
National Patient Safety Foundation (NPSF)*
Society for Healthcare Epidemiology of America (SHEA)
United States Department of Defense

*Specifically endorses masking of unvaccinated HCP

News & World Report assessment of the Best Children's Hospitals in America which utilizes HCP influenza immunization rates in its analysis [50]) and in accreditation standards. The Joint Commission, for example, revised its influenza immunization standard to include an expectation that facilities "[s]et incremental influenza vaccination goals, consistent with achieving the 90% rate established in the national influenza initiatives for 2020" [51]. While not explicitly endorsing mandatory immunization, these programs have emphasized the importance of HCP immunization as a core safety intervention.

The use of such programs, while increasing across the USA, is not without some controversy. In the following sections, we will address some of the espoused concerns regarding mandatory HCP influenza immunization.

"Healthcare-Associated Influenza Is Not a Problem"

The need for mandatory HCP influenza vaccination presupposes that healthcare-associated influenza, both in HCP and patients, has a considerable incidence. Unfortunately, comprehensive estimations of the burden of healthcare-associated influenza have been hindered by the lack of a standardized definition for this outcome, varying methods of surveillance, and lack of recognition of influenza as a cause of nosocomial respiratory failure by clinicians which leads to a lack of testing for the pathogen [1]. There have been, however, a few recent studies that better define the burden of healthcare-associated influenza. A prospective laboratory-based surveillance program in Canada examined laboratory-confirmed influenza among hospitalized adults and found that 17.3% of all influenza cases were healthcare-associated [52]. Many outbreaks of healthcare-associated influenza are likely not reported in the literature, but several have been and are well reviewed by Voirin et al. through 2009 [1].

Healthcare-associated influenza is also not an included target of most infection prevention surveillance programs, so data on disease incidence in key populations are not generally captured in a systematic manner outside of controlled studies. Additionally, even when tests are sent for influenza in patients who have been hospitalized, influenza antigen testing from nasal swabs is often used. These tests have notoriously low sensitivity compared to tests such as polymerase chain reaction (PCR) [53]. So at the present time, the burden of nosocomial influenza has indeed not been well assessed; however, one should not conclude that these cases do not occur nor that these events do not result in substantial patient harm, as evidenced by the reports of nosocomial outbreaks of influenza cited earlier in this chapter which describe numerous cases of patients who contracted influenza in the healthcare setting.

Data do indicate that exposure to ill HCP and ill patients infected with influenza increases a hospitalized patient's risk of developing healthcare-associated influenza. Using the clinical endpoint of influenza-like illness (ILI, which will capture non-influenza infections as well), Vanhems et al. noted that the relative risk of developing healthcare-associated ILI (HA-ILI) was significantly increased based on exposure to HCP and patients with identified ILI. Specifically, for patients exposed to at least one contagious HCP compared with those with no documented exposure in the hospital, the relative risk (RR) of HA-ILI was 5.48 (95% confidence interval [CI], 2.09–14.37); for patients exposed to at least one contagious patient, the RR was 17.96 (95% CI, 10.07–32.03); and for patients exposed to at least one contagious patient and one contagious HCP, the RR was 34.75 (95% CI, 17.70–68.25) [54].

"Influenza Is Not a Major Problem Among HCP"

Data regarding the incidence of influenza specifically among HCP is also sparse. While one would expect the incidence to be at least as high as the general population during a given influenza season, there is reason to believe the rate could be higher due to the nature of the occupational exposure. There are several reasons why capturing this rate accurately is very challenging. Issues surrounding sick day policies and the ability for employers to actively assess reasons for taking time off are significant. Specifically, due to restrictions on an employer's ability to request detailed specifications of illness (related to privacy and other appropriate employee protections), surveillance for employee influenza infections is often only based on passive reporting by the employee. In addition, many time off policies bundle days off due to illness with days off for other reasons (e.g., an aggregate "paid time off" system where employees are given an allotted number of days to take off work for any reason, including vacation or illness), making tracking of HCP influenza and days missed due to infection extremely challenging.

There have been some attempts to quantify the burden of HCP influenza infection. Often ILI is used as the surrogate for influenza infection with the recognition that other respiratory viruses can cause this syndrome and that actual laboratory-confirmed influenza infection may not present with the classic signs and symptoms on ILI. Henkle et al., however, utilized laboratory testing to confirm infections as part of a prospective surveillance study of 1834 HCP and noted that 15.7% developed an acute respiratory infection during that season with 3.1% due to influenza [55]. Other ecological studies have linked influenza vaccination with lower rates of absenteeism [56]. One study examined the risk factors for influenza acquisition among 133 nurses during flu season, and notably failure to receive the flu vaccine increased the risk of symptomatic influenza acquisition with an odds ratio of 4.82 (p = 0.007) [57].

"Mandatory Programs Have Never Been Shown to Impact Healthcare-Associated Influenza"

The impact of mandatory influenza immunization programs has repeatedly been shown to lead to high immunization rates [32–37, 58–60], and implementation of a mandatory program (in the setting of a multifaceted influenza infection control program and often with the use of masking for unvaccinated HCP) is arguably the most effective strategy to increase immunization rates above desired targets. Data on the impact of mandatory influenza vaccination and HCP absenteeism/sick days are also starting to emerge. Researchers at the Denver Health Medical Center reported a decrease in employee absences during the influenza season following implementation of their mandatory program when compared to prior seasons of similar influenza activity [61]. In an analysis of the province-wide vaccination with masking policy in British Columbia, researchers noted a significantly reduced rate of HCP absenteeism due to all-cause illness in vaccinated vs. unvaccinated HCP during the first season of the policy [56]. This study is limited due to its observational nature and analysis of only a single year of the program, but the initial difference in absenteeism with the new policy is informative.

Despite these important findings, some have advocated that the optimal evidence to support mandatory vaccination policies would demonstrate that vaccination of HCP leads to improved patient outcomes. Indeed, vaccination of HCP practicing in long-term care settings has been significantly associated with reductions in patient mortality in multiple large-scale clinical trials. Three cluster randomized trials demonstrated that HCP vaccination was associated with a statistically significant decrease in mortality among nursing home patients [62–64]. One study, performed in 44 facilities and involving over 1700 HCP and 2600 residents, reported a significant decrease in patient mortality, influenza-like illness (ILI), ILI consultations with general practitioners, and ILI hospitalizations during a moderate influenza season among residents of homes in the HCP vaccination arm compared with those residing in control facilities [64]. These reductions were noted even in the setting of high resident vaccination rates (78.2% in the intervention homes vs. 71.4% in the control facilities). A fourth study, conducted in France among 40 facilities that included nearly 3500 residents and 2000 HCP, noted a significant reduction in the risk of all-cause patient mortality between the two study arms even after adjustment for resident age, resident vaccination status,

resident disability score, and Charlson comorbidity index (odds ratio = 0.80) [65].

These investigations do have some limitations, including concerns about outcome assessment in both study arms, vaccination ascertainment in both study arms, infrequent laboratory confirmation of influenza, and lack of a significant impact on laboratory-confirmed influenza. Nonetheless, this striking mortality benefit for patients in long-term care facilities from vaccination of their HCP is remarkably consistent across all four studies. In addition, after formalized assessment and consideration of this evidence base using the Grading of Recommendations Assessment, Development and Evaluation (GRADE) approach, Ahmed et al. noted that pooled risk ratios for all-cause mortality and ILI were 0.71 (95% CI 0.59–0.85) and 0.58 (95% CI, 0.46–0.73) [66] with the use of HCP influenza vaccination.

Some have argued that the studies noted above do not provide evidence that vaccinating HCP against influenza protects patients in the acute care setting, calling for similar studies in each unique patient population. This stance, however, ignores several key points. First, performing a similar trial in the acute care setting would be exceedingly challenging and resource intensive, given the increased number of HCP-patient interactions, the shorter length of stay, and the difficulty attributing influenza acquisition due to healthcare-associated exposure. Second and more importantly, the biological rationale for vaccination of HCP to reduce influenza spread does not vary by practice setting. While in a long-term care facility, the interactions may be more prolonged and frequent in nature; in an acute care setting, the patient has interactions with many more unique HCP, each of whom could be shedding influenza at the time of contact.

Data from randomized controlled trials clearly show the impact of influenza vaccination on the risk of infection in HCP themselves. In a randomized controlled trial, vaccination was 88% effective in preventing laboratory-confirmed influenza in HCP [67]. In addition, studies have examined interventions to reduce healthcare-associated transmission of influenza, which is one of the major aspects of transmission to HCP. In a susceptible-exposed-infected-recovered (SEIR) model, vaccination of HCP was the second most effective strategy in preventing influenza transmission in the hospital by reducing number of cases 6–19% only behind handwashing with an 11–27% case reduction [68].

Thankfully, data are emerging that illustrate an effect on patient outcomes as a result of vaccination of acute care HCP. One of the earliest studies on the effect of HCP influenza vaccination on patient outcomes came out of the University of Virginia. Salgado et al. noted a significant correlation between increasing HCP influenza vaccination rates and reducing healthcare-associated influenza among patients [69]. The study is limited by the ecologic study design but suggests an important impact. More recently, investigators at

MD Anderson Cancer Center examined the impact of increasing HCP influenza immunization over the course of 8 years. Of note, the institution implemented a mandatory vaccine with masking policy during the study period. The proportion of influenza infections that were healthcare associated among patients significantly decreased and was significantly associated with increased HCP vaccination rates [70]. A cluster randomized trial in the Netherlands of HCP at six medical centers, where the intervention arms offered vaccination to HCP vs. no vaccination at control facilities, noted a significantly lower rate of healthcare-associated influenza among internal medicine patients at the facilities with the higher rates of HCP influenza vaccination (3.9% vs. 9.7% of patients) [71].

In a study encompassing seven influenza seasons and over 62,000 hospitalized patients, a significant association was noted between increasing influenza vaccine coverage among HCP and decreasing healthcare-associated ILI among patients at an Italian acute care hospital. Specifically, as vaccination coverage dropped from 13.2% to 3.1%, the frequency of healthcare-associated ILI in patients increased from 1.1 to 5.7% ($p < 0.001$) [72]. Finally, a nested case-control study in France noted a significant association between lower rates of laboratory-confirmed healthcare-associated influenza among patients and higher ($\geq$35%) vaccination rates among HCP [73]. These data suggest that the immunization of HCP reduces mortality and ILI in the patients they care for and, furthermore, reduces influenza in the HCP themselves.

"The Influenza Vaccine Is Not Efficacious Enough to Warrant a Mandate"

The CDC notes that, on average, the influenza vaccine's efficacy is 50–60% [74], and some have argued that a lack of optimal efficacy suggests that such a vaccine should not be mandated. Many studies, particularly those performed prior to the past decade, utilized less specific outcomes (e.g., all-cause pneumonia and influenza based on administrative coding) or diagnostic testing (e.g., rapid antigen testing which has poor sensitivity in some populations such as older adults) as markers for influenza infection. In addition, the selection of the control population is critical due to other unmeasured biases that can affect interpretation of the vaccine impact. For example, using a control population of all older adults that compares the effect of vaccination on medically attended visits for respiratory infection may be biased in that those persons who receive an annual influenza vaccine may be more likely to visit their physician when ill (healthy user bias). Those studies that use highly sensitive laboratory testing for influenza (e.g., PCR) and have a comparable control population (e.g., adults hospitalized for non-influenza

respiratory illnesses) provide a far more accurate assessment of true influenza infection upon which to base effectiveness.

The most detailed summary of the vaccine effectiveness data was provided by Osterholm, where the effectiveness was estimated as 59% for the trivalent inactivated vaccine in adults aged 18–65 years [75]. Therefore, while not as effective as other vaccines such as the measles-mumps-rubella vaccine, the influenza vaccine has moderate benefit that may vary based upon the specific host and their ability to mount an immune response to the vaccine as well as the degree of antigen match of the vaccine to the circulating wild-type strains. This makes it even more imperative that vaccine rates are maximized to contribute to the herd immunity and prevent transmission of the virus, especially in the healthcare setting.

Some have taken this lack of optimal efficacy to also argue that the basics of infection prevention such as hand-washing are substantially more important than vaccination and that mandatory vaccination may not be needed until a more effective vaccine is produced [76, 77]. It is not known whether HCP feel that protection from the vaccine may make them more likely to undervalue basic infection prevention policies [78]. While influenza vaccine may provide some protection against influenza, it would indeed not protect against other respiratory viruses (to which no vaccine exist). Basic infection control practices thus remain important and must not be underemphasized in this debate.

"Influenza Vaccine Safety Is Still a Concern"

Healthcare organizations have both an ethical obligation and a regulatory obligation to ensure a safe workplace. In creating a mandatory vaccination policy, one must consider the safety of the employee, and as part of discussions regarding mandating influenza vaccination for HCP, the risk of harm to the HCP has often been appropriately considered. When compared to the risks of severe outcomes from influenza, the risk of receiving the influenza vaccine each year is far outweighed by the benefits. The vaccine can cause local side effects such as a sore arm or redness, but these symptoms are often very limited and can be easily mitigated with symptom-controlling medications and therapies. Rarely, as with any medication or therapeutic compound, a severe reaction may occur, such as allergy to a vaccine component. Some studies have found a possible small association of injectable influenza vaccine with Guillain-Barré syndrome (GBS). Overall, these studies estimated the risk for GBS after vaccination as fewer than one or two cases of GBS per one million people vaccinated. Other studies have not found any such association [79]. GBS also rarely occurs after influenza infection. Even though GBS adverse outcome is rare, GBS is more common following influenza illness than following vaccination [80].

Concerns such as acquisition of influenza from the vaccine, exposure to toxicities related to compounds reportedly contained in the vaccine (such as formaldehyde or mercury), and confusion about how the vaccine is manufactured (e.g., utilizes aborted fetal cells) are unfounded when examining the scientific evidence. The fear that some individuals have regarding influenza vaccine is amplified by nonscientific and errant claims of adverse effects that are published in nonconventional sources, such as websites and alternative media. This can make implementing a HCP influenza program challenging and requires the program leaders to examine the scientific evidence when assessing claims about vaccine harm while also being respectful when educating HCP with such concerns.

veillance period, but whether those individuals served as sources for additional cases was not known.

While influenza is clearly detectable in the nasopharynx of asymptomatic persons, there is some debate as to how important of a role this plays in transmission (i.e., is there shedding and spread outside of the nasopharynx if no symptoms are present). One nuance with this debate, however, is that even if an asymptomatic person does not result in transmission of virus to others, the development of symptoms, even mild ones, can facilitate spread. For example, the infected HCP initially without symptoms but detectable virus in their upper airway who starts to develop mild rhinorrhea may unknowingly start to spread the virus to others.

"There's No Risk for Influenza Transmission from Asymptomatic HCP"

Even if HCP were perfectly adherent to staying home when ill, studies have shown that influenza virus is detectable in the upper airway and nasopharynx of influenza-infected persons up to several days prior to symptom onset. Much of this data comes from studies of household contacts of an influenza-infected index case with prospective viral surveillance and symptom capture to examine secondary transmission in the household. A study from Hong Kong from 2008 to 2014 followed a cohort of 824 households with an identified 224 cases of secondary influenza infection that developed in the household setting, examining the relationship between symptoms and viral shedding (as detected on nasal and throat swabs) [81]. Of note, only 35% of these cases reported a febrile illness that met the classic definition of an ILI, reinforcing the poor sensitivity of that entity as a surrogate for laboratory-confirmed influenza. Viral shedding without symptoms varied somewhat by influenza strain type. Shedding was detected before onset of respiratory symptoms in influenza A-infected persons but peaked on the first 2 days of clinical illness, while influenza B shedding peaked up to 2 days prior to symptom onset. The authors noted that "[t]he start of viral shedding before symptom onset, albeit at low levels as demonstrated by both PCR and $TCID_{50}$, indicates the potential for influenza virus transmission in the presymptomatic phase of the illness before it becomes clinically apparent."

In addition to the potential spread of virus in the presymptomatic phase, up to 70% of cases may be asymptomatic [82]. A second study in Hong Kong detected viral shedding by PCR testing in the absence of any reported signs or symptoms in 14% of 59 subjects under prospective viral surveillance among household contacts of an index influenza-infected case [83]. A study in New York during the 2009 H1N1 influenza A pandemic noted that serologically confirmed infection occurred in 19% of household contacts [84]. Twenty-eight percent of those infected were asymptomatic during the sur-

"Masking Unvaccinated HCP Is Punitive and Not Evidenced Based"

Influenza is primarily spread through large droplets produced when infected individuals cough, sneeze, and even talk. These droplets can reach others up to approximately 6 ft away [85]. To reduce such transmission of influenza, many mandatory HCP influenza vaccination programs require unvaccinated HCP to wear a mask while in specific areas of the facility during periods when influenza is actively circulating in the community. Masking of HCPs has been shown to halt outbreaks of influenza in healthcare environments [13], and outbreaks of many respiratory diseases that spread similarly via droplets have been shown to abate with the introduction of masking of staff members. Even outside of the healthcare environment, masking has been shown to be effective in reducing influenza transmission among household members in settings with low influenza vaccination rates [86].

Masking of unvaccinated HCP is done for at least two reasons. First, masking may reduce the risk of primary infection of workers caring for patients with influenza. This, however, is not the primary reason for masking as HCP may become infected outside of the healthcare environment as influenza is often a community-acquired disease. The primary reason for masking is to reduce the transmission of influenza from an infected HCP to an uninfected patient (aka "source control"). Some argue that once symptoms develop, the HCP will just stay home or leave work, but in reality that often does not happen. Data consistently show that HCPs, even with classic ILI with fever (a far more severe illness than mild upper respiratory symptoms), still come to work and work while ill for several days [57, 87–89]. To expect that a HCP who starts to have mild respiratory symptoms will suddenly remove themselves from work is unrealistic and not the experience of most occupational and infection prevention programs.

Critics of masking programs have raised concerns that requiring some HCPs to wear a mask could be interpreted as punitive or stigmatizing, especially to those who request personal belief exemptions. In addition, concerns have been raised that requiring a mask reveals details about the HCP's personal health history to others, which would violate their privacy. In contrast, in healthcare settings, there are often numerous reasons for HCP to wear a mask, including in HCP with nonfebrile respiratory illnesses. In addition, the masking does not identify or target specifically why a person is unvaccinated (i.e., due to medical contraindications vs. religious/personal belief exemptions). Clearly, implementation and communication about a masking requirement must be done thoughtfully and fairly. A nice example is the Hospital Corporation of America (HCA) program, which uses stickers to denote visually those who require masking [37, 90]. As part of the program, they provided stickers to both vaccinated and unvaccinated HCP, and both carried the tag line "because I care," emphasizing that either intervention (vaccination or masking) is done with patient safety in mind.

Mandatory vaccination or mask policies should be part of multifaceted programs that include an array of infection prevention interventions such as use of hand hygiene, respiratory hygiene and cough etiquette, early (at initial point of facility contact) identification and isolation of patients suspected of having a contagious respiratory infection, restriction of ill visitors and HCP, and patient vaccination. The goal of the vaccine or mask policy is to use and require strategies that will reduce and minimize viral shedding from infected HCP, including those who may not have symptoms. Both vaccination and masking will impede the shedding of respiratory viruses from the upper airway. The vaccine does this by reducing one's likelihood of becoming infected with the virus in the first place and may also result in less viral shedding in those that do become infected as a result of the less severe illness that occurs. Masking also meets this goal by serving as a physical barrier to shedding from the upper airway. One key difference between the vaccine's effect and the effect of masking and the reason why vaccination is clearly preferred is that the vaccine's impact occurs wherever the HCP may contact influenza (i.e., either in the community or at work). A vaccinated individual has a lower risk of ever becoming infected to begin with. The mask will only serve its purpose when actually worn, so unless a HCP wears the mask all of the time, including when outside of the healthcare facility, influenza acquisition can still occur.

In the development of mandatory HCP influenza policies that use masking for unvaccinated HCP, however, facility leaders should attempt to ameliorate some of the potential issues surrounding such a policy. For example, accommodations for mask wearing in instances where the mask could impede the delivery of care to patients (e.g., in speech pathologists where visualization of the face and mouth is an important facet of therapy) should be made.

Conclusions

Healthcare-associated influenza infection is an understudied but important problem. While the true burden of disease is unknown, it is theoretically significant. Many healthcare professions take an oath to "first do no harm" to their patients. In this light, practices which can keep patients safe should be maximized to the greatest extent that is practical. Vaccination of HCP against influenza is a very low-risk practice which can protect the individual HCP from morbidity and lost work time due to a reduction in HCP infection. Likewise, masking of all symptomatic HCP (regardless of vaccine status) and universal masking for those without the modest benefit of vaccine protection has the potential to protect patients and colleagues from being exposed to infectious droplets, which can halt the chain of transmission. The data that are currently available support the practice of mandatory influenza vaccination for HCP, as best reflected by the decision in 2015 by the National Patient Safety Foundation (NPSF) Board to anoint the inaugural "must do's" for all HCP to ensure patient safety: handwashing and HCP influenza vaccination [91].

References

1. Voirin N, Barret B, Metzger MH, Vanhems P. Hospital-acquired influenza: a synthesis using the outbreak reports and intervention studies of nosocomial infection (ORION) statement. J Hosp Infect. 2009;71(1):1–14.
2. Munoz FM, Campbell JR, Atmar RL, et al. Influenza a virus outbreak in a neonatal intensive care unit. Pediatr Infect Dis J. 1999;18(9):811–5.
3. Meibalane R, Sedmak GV, Sasidharan P, Garg P, Grausz JP. Outbreak of influenza in a neonatal intensive care unit. J Pediatr. 1977;91(6):974–6.
4. Bauer CR, Elie K, Spence L, Stern L. Hong Kong influenza in a neonatal unit. JAMA. 1973;223(11):1233–5.
5. Cunney RJ, Bialachowski A, Thornley D, Smaill FM, Pennie RA. An outbreak of influenza A in a neonatal intensive care unit. Infect Control Hosp Epidemiol. 2000;21(7):449–54.
6. Sagrera X, Ginovart G, Raspall F, et al. Outbreaks of influenza A virus infection in neonatal intensive care units. Pediatr Infect Dis J. 2002;21(3):196–200.
7. Maltezou HC, Drancourt M. Nosocomial influenza in children. J Hosp Infect. 2003;55(2):83–91.
8. Serwint JR, Miller RM, Korsch BM. Influenza type A and B infections in hospitalized pediatric patients. Who should be immunized? Am J Dis Child. 1991;145(6):623–6.
9. Slinger R, Dennis P. Nosocomial influenza at a Canadian pediatric hospital from 1995 to 1999: opportunities for prevention. Infect Control Hosp Epidemiol. 2002;23(10):627–9.
10. Hall CB, Douglas RG Jr. Nosocomial influenza infection as a cause of intercurrent fevers in infants. Pediatrics. 1975;55(5):673–7.
11. Wenzel RP, Deal EC, Hendley JO. Hospital-acquired viral respiratory illness on a pediatric ward. Pediatrics. 1977;60(3):367–71.
12. Mauch TJ, Bratton S, Myers T, Krane E, Gentry SR, Kashtan CE. Influenza B virus infection in pediatric solid organ transplant recipients. Pediatrics. 1994;94(2 Pt 1):225–9.

13. Weinstock DM, Eagan J, Malak SA, et al. Control of influenza A on a bone marrow transplant unit. Infect Control Hosp Epidemiol. 2000;21(11):730–2.

14. Whimbey E, Elting LS, Couch RB, et al. Influenza A virus infections among hospitalized adult bone marrow transplant recipients. Bone Marrow Transplant. 1994;13(4):437–40.

15. Malavaud S, Malavaud B, Sandres K, et al. Nosocomial outbreak of influenza virus a (H3N2) infection in a solid organ transplant department. Transplantation. 2001;72(3):535–7.

16. Horcajada JP, Pumarola T, Martinez JA, et al. A nosocomial outbreak of influenza during a period without influenza epidemic activity. Eur Respir J. 2003;21(2):303–7.

17. Barlow G, Nathwani D. Nosocomial influenza infection. Lancet. 2000;355(9210):1187.

18. Sartor C, Zandotti C, Romain F, et al. Disruption of services in an internal medicine unit due to a nosocomial influenza outbreak. Infect Control Hosp Epidemiol. 2002;23(10):615–9.

19. Van Voris LP, Belshe RB, Shaffer JL. Nosocomial influenza B virus infection in the elderly. Ann Intern Med. 1982;96(2):153–8.

20. Bean B, Rhame FS, Hughes RS, Weiler MD, Peterson LR, Gerding DN. Influenza B: hospital activity during a community epidemic. Diagn Microbiol Infect Dis. 1983;1(3):177–83.

21. Morens DM, Rash VM. Lessons from a nursing home outbreak of influenza A. Infect Control Hosp Epidemiol. 1995;16(5):275–80.

22. Nabeshima A, Ikematsu H, Yamaga S, Hayashi J, Hara H, Kashiwagi S. An outbreak of influenza A (H3N2) among hospitalized geriatric patients. Kansenshogaku Zasshi. 1996;70(8):801–7.

23. Everts RJ, Hanger HC, Jennings LC, Hawkins A, Sainsbury R. Outbreaks of influenza A among elderly hospital inpatients. N Z med J. 1996;109(1026):272–4.

24. Staynor K, Foster G, McArthur M, McGeer A, Petric M, Simor AE. Influenza A outbreak in a nursing home: the value of early diagnosis and the use of amantadine hydrochloride. Can J Infect Control. 1994;9(4):109–11.

25. Drinka PJ, Gravenstein S, Krause P, Nest L, Dissing M, Shult P. Reintroduction of influenza A to a nursing building. Infect Control Hosp Epidemiol. 2000;21(11):732–5.

26. Kempe A, Hall CB, MacDonald NE, et al. Influenza in children with cancer. J Pediatr. 1989;115(1):33–9.

27. Schepetiuk S, Papanaoum K, Qiao M. Spread of influenza A virus infection in hospitalised patients with cancer. Aust NZ J Med. 1998;28(4):475–6.

28. Berg HF, Van Gendt J, Rimmelzwaan GF, Peeters MF, Van Keulen P. Nosocomial influenza infection among post-influenza-vaccinated patients with severe pulmonary diseases. J Inf Secur. 2003;46(2):129–32.

29. Weingarten S, Friedlander M, Rascon D, Ault M, Morgan M, Meyer RD. Influenza surveillance in an acute-care hospital. Arch Intern Med. 1988;148(1):113–6.

30. Ottenberg AL, Wu JT, Poland GA, Jacobson RM, Koenig BA, Tilburt JC. Vaccinating health care workers against influenza: the ethical and legal rationale for a mandate. Am J Public Health. 2011;101(2):212–6.

31. Randall LH, Curran EA, Omer SB. Legal considerations surrounding mandatory influenza vaccination for healthcare workers in the United States. Vaccine. 2013;31(14):1771–6.

32. Rakita RM, Hagar BA, Crome P, Lammert JK. Mandatory influenza vaccination of healthcare workers: a 5-year study. Infect Control Hosp Epidemiol. 2010;31(9):881–8.

33. Babcock HM, Gemeinhart N, Jones M, Dunagan WC, Woeltje KF. Mandatory influenza vaccination of health care workers: translating policy to practice. Clin Infect Dis. 2010;50(4):459–64.

34. Feemster KA, Prasad P, Smith MJ, et al. Employee designation and health care worker support of an influenza vaccine mandate at a large pediatric tertiary care hospital. Vaccine. 2011;29(9):1762–9.

35. Karanfil LV, Bahner J, Hovatter J, Thomas WL. Championing patient safety through mandatory influenza vaccination for all healthcare personnel and affiliated physicians. Infect Control Hosp Epidemiol. 2011;32(4):375–9.

36. Quan K, Tehrani DM, Dickey L, et al. Voluntary to mandatory: evolution of strategies and attitudes toward influenza vaccination of healthcare personnel. Infect Control Hosp Epidemiol. 2012;33(1):63–70.

37. Septimus EJ, Perlin JB, Cormier SB, Moody JA, Hickok JD. A multifaceted mandatory patient safety program and seasonal influenza vaccination of health care workers in community hospitals. JAMA. 2011;305(10):999–1000.

38. Immunization Action Coalition. Honor roll for patient safety mandatory influenza vaccination for healthcare workers. Accessed 11 June 2013 at http://www.immunize.org/honor-roll/

39. Black CL, Yue X, Ball SW, et al. Influenza vaccination coverage among health care personnel – United States, 2014-15 influenza season. MMWR Morb Mortal Wkly Rep. 2015;64(36):993–9.

40. Stewart AM, Cox MA. State law and influenza vaccination of health care personnel. Vaccine. 31(5):827–32.

41. Colorado Department of Public Health and Environment. Standards for Hospitals and Health Facilities, Chapter II General Lincensure Standards, Part 10 Influenza Immunization of Healthcare Workers. Accessed 11 June 2013 at http://www.colorado.gov/cs/Satellite/CDPHE-Main/CBON/1251607568722

42. Rhode Island Department of Public Health. Rules and regulations pertaining to immunization, testing, and health screening for health care workers. Accessed 11 June 2013 at http://sos.ri.gov/documents/archives/regdocs/released/pdf/DOH/7083.pdf

43. Service Employees International Union. Case 1:12-cv-00894-ML-PAS Document 1: SEIU Healthcare Employees Uniion [sic], District 1199 v. Michael Fine, M.D. and Rhode Island Department of Health. Accessed 12 June 2013 at http://www.seiu1199ne.org/files/2013/01/FluLawsuitRI.pdf

44. Lindley MC, Dube D, Kalayil EJ, Kim H, Paiva K, Raymond P. Qualitative evaluation of Rhode Island's healthcare worker influenza vaccination regulations. Vaccine. 2014;32(45):5962–6.

45. Merenstein DJ, Rosenbaum DJ, Woolf SH. Effects of influenza vaccination of health care workers on mortality of elderly people. J Fam Pract. 2000;49(4):300.

46. Crain's New York Business. State requires health workers to wear flu masks. Accessed 7 June 2013 at http://www.crainsnewyork.com/article/20130411/HEALTH_CARE/130419965

47. Poland GA, Tucker S. The nursing profession and patient safety and healthcare provider influenza immunization: the puzzling stance of the American nursing association. Vaccine. 2012;30(10):1753–5.

48. Bennett JA, Block D. Nursing leadership to ensure patient and health worker protection from influenza. Vaccine. 2012;30(10):1756–8.

49. American Nurses Association. American Nurses Association makes new recommendation that all nurses should be immunized against vaccine-preventable diseases (8/20/15). Accessed on 22 June 2016 at http://www.nursingworld.org/MainMenuCategories/Policy-Advocacy/Positions-and-Resolutions/ANAPositionStatements/Position-Statements-Alphabetically/Immunizations.html

50. Sartor C, Tissot-Dupont H, Zandotti C, Martin F, Roques P, Drancourt M. Use of a mobile cart influenza program for vaccination of hospital employees. Infect Control Hosp Epidemiol. 2004;25(11):918–22.

51. The Joint Commission. New flu vaccination requirement. Accessed on 27 Jul 2016 at https://www.jointcommission.org/chat_blog_post_share__lets_talk_ambulatory_with_michael/new_flu_vaccination_requirement_/

52. Taylor G, Mitchell R, McGeer A, et al. Healthcare-associated influenza in Canadian hospitals from 2006 to 2012. Infect Control Hosp Epidemiol. 2014;35(2):169–75.

53. Prevention CfDCa. Guidance for clinicians on the use of rapid influenza diagnostic tests.

54. Vanhems P, Voirin N, Roche S, et al. Risk of influenza-like illness in an acute health care setting during community influenza

epidemics in 2004–2005, 2005–2006, and 2006–2007: a prospective study. Arch Intern Med. 2011;171(2):151–7.

55. Henkle E, Irving SA, Naleway AL, et al. Comparison of laboratory-confirmed influenza and noninfluenza acute respiratory illness in healthcare personnel during the 2010–2011 influenza season. Infect Control Hosp Epidemiol. 2014;35(5):538–46.

56. Van Buynder PG, Konrad S, Kersteins F, et al. Healthcare worker influenza immunization vaccinate or mask policy: strategies for cost effective implementation and subsequent reductions in staff absenteeism due to illness. Vaccine. 2015;33(13):1625–8.

57. Ng TC, Lee N, Hui SC, Lai R, Ip M. Preventing healthcare workers from acquiring influenza. Infect Control Hosp Epidemiol. 2009;30(3):292–5.

58. Doby E, Stockmann C, Petersen S, et al. Mandatory employee vaccination policy with termination for non-compliance increases vaccine coverage in a large, not-for-profit health system (abstract 432). Presented as poster presentation at IDWeek, San Diego, CA, October 18, 2012 (2012). Accessed on 12 June 2013 at https://idsa.confex.com/idsa/2012/webprogram/Paper35063.html

59. Parada J, Chauhan D, Gaughan B, Koller M, Schleffendorf C, Hindle P. Duh, Why didn't we do this sooner?! Three year experience with mandatory seasonal influenza immunization for all personnel in a University Medical Center (abstract 436). Presented as poster presentation at IDWeek, San Diego, CA, October 18, 2012 (2012). Accessed on 12 June 2013 at https://idsa.confex.com/idsa/2012/webprogram/Paper37822.html

60. Kidd F, Wones R, Momper A, Bechtle M, Lewis M. From 51% to 100%: mandatory seasonal influenza vaccination. Am J Infect Control. 2012;40(2):188–90.

61. Knepper B, Young H, Davis Q, et al. Universal Employee Influenza Vaccination Decreases Employee Sick Days (abstract 95). Presented as oral presentation at IDWeek, San Diego, CA, October 18, 2012 (2012). Accessed on 12 June 2013 at https://idsa.confex.com/idsa/2012/webprogram/Paper37051.html

62. Potter J, Stott DJ, Roberts MA, et al. Influenza vaccination of health care workers in long-term-care hospitals reduces the mortality of elderly patients. J Infect Dis. 1997;175(1):1–6.

63. Carman WF, Elder AG, Wallace LA, et al. Effects of influenza vaccination of health-care workers on mortality of elderly people in long-term care: a randomised controlled trial. Lancet. 2000;355(9198):93–7.

64. Hayward AC, Harling R, Wetten S, et al. Effectiveness of an influenza vaccine programme for care home staff to prevent death, morbidity, and health service use among residents: cluster randomised controlled trial. BMJ. 2006;333(7581):1241.

65. Lemaitre M, Meret T, Rothan-Tondeur M, et al. Effect of influenza vaccination of nursing home staff on mortality of residents: a cluster-randomized trial. J Am Geriatr Soc. 2009;57(9):1580–6.

66. Ahmed F, Lindley MC, Allred N, Weinbaum CM, Grohskopf L. Effect of influenza vaccination of healthcare personnel on morbidity and mortality among patients: systematic review and grading of evidence. Clin Infect Dis. 2014;58(1):50–7.

67. Wilde JA, McMillan JA, Serwint J, Butta J, O'Riordan MA, Steinhoff MC. Effectiveness of influenza vaccine in health care professionals: a randomized trial. JAMA. 1999;281(10):908–13.

68. Blanco N, Eisenberg MC, Stillwell T, Foxman B. What transmission precautions best control influenza spread in a hospital? Am J Epidemiol. 2016.

69. Salgado CD, Giannetta ET, Hayden FG, Farr BM. Preventing nosocomial influenza by improving the vaccine acceptance rate of clinicians. Infect Control Hosp Epidemiol. 2004;25(11):923–8.

70. Frenzel E, Chemaly RF, Ariza-Heredia E, et al. Association of increased influenza vaccination in health care workers with a reduction in nosocomial influenza infections in cancer patients. Am J Infect Control. 2016;

71. Riphagen-Dalhuisen J, Burgerhof JG, Frijstein G, et al. Hospital-based cluster randomised controlled trial to assess effects of a multi-faceted programme on influenza vaccine coverage among hospital healthcare workers and nosocomial influenza in the Netherlands, 2009 to 2011. Euro Surveill. 2013;18(26):20512.

72. Amodio E, Restivo V, Firenze A, Mammina C, Tramuto F, Vitale F. Can influenza vaccination coverage among healthcare workers influence the risk of nosocomial influenza-like illness in hospitalized patients? J Hosp Infect. 2014;86(3):182–7.

73. Benet T, Regis C, Voirin N, et al. Influenza vaccination of healthcare workers in acute-care hospitals: a case-control study of its effect on hospital-acquired influenza among patients. BMC Infect Dis. 2012;12:30.

74. Centers for Disease Control and Prevention. Vaccine effectiveness – how well does the flu vaccine work?. Available at http://www.cdc.gov/flu/about/qa/vaccineeffect.htm. Accessed on 23 June 2016. .

75. Osterholm MT, Kelley NS, Sommer A, Belongia EA. Efficacy and effectiveness of influenza vaccines: a systematic review and meta-analysis. Lancet Infect Dis. 2012;12(1):36–44.

76. Buchta WG. Research doesn't support mandatory influenza vaccination. WMJ. 2012;111(3):96.

77. Gardam M, Lemieux C. Mandatory influenza vaccination? First we need a better vaccine. CMAJ. 2013;185(8):639–40.

78. Converso AR. Point counterpoint: mandatory flu vaccination for health care workers. Am J Nurs. 2010;110(1):27.

79. Ghaderi S, Gunnes N, Bakken IJ, Magnus P, Trogstad L, Haberg SE. Risk of Guillain-Barre syndrome after exposure to pandemic influenza A (H1N1)pdm09 vaccination or infection: a Norwegian population-based cohort study. Eur J Epidemiol. 2016;31(1):67–72.

80. Centers for Disease Control and Prevention. Flu vaccine safety information. Available at http://www.cdc.gov/flu/protect/vaccine/general.htm. Accessed on 23 June 2016.

81. Ip DK, Lau LL, Chan KH, et al. The dynamic relationship between clinical symptomatology and viral shedding in naturally acquired seasonal and pandemic influenza virus infections. Clin Infect Dis. 2016;62(4):431–7.

82. Hayward AC, Fragaszy EB, Bermingham A, et al. Comparative community burden and severity of seasonal and pandemic influenza: results of the flu watch cohort study. Lancet Respir Med. 2014;2(6):445–54.

83. Lau LL, Cowling BJ, Fang VJ, et al. Viral shedding and clinical illness in naturally acquired influenza virus infections. J Infect dis. 2010;201(10):1509–16.

84. Jackson ML, France AM, Hancock K, et al. Serologically confirmed household transmission of 2009 pandemic influenza A (H1N1) virus during the first pandemic wave – New York City, April–May 2009. Clin Infect Dis. 2011;53(5):455–62.

85. Centers for Disease Control and Prevention. How flu spreads. Available at http://www.cdc.gov/flu/about/disease/spread.htm. Accessed on 7 Nov 2016.

86. Cowling BJ, Chan KH, Fang VJ, et al. Facemasks and hand hygiene to prevent influenza transmission in households: a cluster randomized trial. Ann Intern Med. 2009;151(7):437–46.

87. Jena AB, Meltzer DO, Press VG, Arora VM. Why physicians work when sick. Arch Intern Med. 2012;172(14):1107–8.

88. Widera E, Chang A, Chen HL. Presenteeism: a public health hazard. J Gen Intern Med. 2010;25(11):1244–7.

89. Jena AB, Baldwin DC Jr, Daugherty SR, Meltzer DO, Arora VM. Presenteeism among resident physicians. JAMA. 2010;304(11):1166–8.

90. Talbot TR, Babcock H, Caplan AL, et al. Revised SHEA position paper: influenza vaccination of healthcare personnel. Infect Control Hosp Epidemiol. 2010;31(10):987–95.

91. Health Affairs Blog. The 'Must Do' List: certain patient safety rules should not be elective. August 20, 2015. Available at http://healthaffairs.org/blog/2015/08/20/the-must-do-list-certain-patient-safety-rules-should-not-be-elective/. Accessed on 30 May 2016.

Controversies in Healthcare-Associated Infection Surveillance

Geetika Sood and Surbhi Leekha

Good surveillance of healthcare-associated infections (HAIs) is the foundation for driving improvement in HAI rates. Participation in surveillance networks and feedback of infection rates have been shown to reduce healthcare-associated infections [1–5]. In the United States, the CDC's National Healthcare Safety Network (NHSN) serves as the national resource for definitions to be used in HAI surveillance. Over the last 10 years with the broad implementation of mandatory surveillance, HAI rates in the United States have decreased [6].

In traditional surveillance, trained infection control practitioners use standard definitions and manually review medical records of patients at risk for healthcare infections. While it is generally accepted that surveillance using standardized definitions and criteria is essential to describing the HAI burden and guiding action, there are several limitations of current surveillance methods. We describe some of these limitations below (and summarized in Table 28.1), with examples of specific HAI types where applicable. We then describe various strategies that have been considered or are being studied to improve the quality of HAI surveillance (summarized in Table 28.2).

Variability and Subjectivity in HAI Surveillance

Variability in defining and finding HAIs results from several issues and can produce different HAI rates in the same population. A well-recognized contributor to this problem is that surveillance definitions include several subjective criteria leading to inherent variability in the application of these definitions between observers. Several studies have quantified this difference by using standardized case vignettes and found significant interobserver variability in applying these definitions [7–10]. Further, case finding is also dependent on the effort of the practitioner and other surveillance processes such as availability of post-discharge data or use of algorithms that restrict surveillance to patients with positive microbiologic reports [11, 12]. While some variation and subjectivity in these definitions is expected and should be understood by hospital infection prevention programs, an entirely new dimension has been added since the wide use of HAI data in public reporting, inter-hospital comparison, and financial reimbursement.

The best example of the impact of subjectivity comes from central line-associated bloodstream infection (CLABSI) surveillance which involves identifying patients who have a central line with bacteremia. Infection preventionists then determine if the bacteremia is due to the central line or from a secondary site of infection. The considerable variability in this process has been demonstrated in several studies. In one study, investigators took the same cases, presented them to different infection preventionists for adjudication, and found significant interobserver variability (kappa = 0.42) [9]. There have been multiple state audits of CLABSI surveillance, and most have found a lower sensitivity of CLABSI detection by hospital reporting compared to external audits but high specificity [9, 12–16]. Further, hospitals with lower rates of infections had greater discordance with auditors' findings [17]. These results create some concern that some of the reduction seen in CLABSIs may be due to misclassification of central line-associated bacteremias as secondary bacteremias from other sites rather than a true improvement in the care of patients with central lines. Encouragingly, two large studies found a reduction in total bacteremia rates along with a reduction in CLABSIs [18, 19].

G. Sood
Department of Medicine, Division of Infectious Diseases, Johns Hopkins University, Baltimore, MD, USA
e-mail: gsood1@jhmi.edu

S. Leekha (✉)
Epidemiology and Public Health, University of Maryland School of Medicine, 110 S. Paca Street, 6th Floor, Suite 100, Baltimore, MD 21201, USA
e-mail: sleekha@epi.umaryland.edu

© Springer International Publishing AG 2018
G. Bearman et al. (eds.), *Infection Prevention*, DOI 10.1007/978-3-319-60980-5_28

Table 28.1 Summary of challenges and controversies in HAI surveillance and potential strategies to improve HAI surveillance

Issue/controversy	Potential strategies to improve HAI surveillance
Surveillance affected by interobserver variability and subjectivity	Use of administrative data
	Algorithmic approach
	Use of objective laboratory test metric
Surveillance is resource intensive	Use of administrative data
	Algorithmic approach
	Use of objective laboratory test metric
Surveillance data are not clinically meaningful	Use well-studied process measures
	Measure related outcome measures
Choice of denominator affects validity of surveillance	Risk adjustment for number of devices should be considered
	Consider multiple denominators for internal use
Lack of appropriate risk adjustment	Improve risk adjustment based on patient-specific factors

Ventilator-associated pneumonia (VAP) is one of the most difficult HAIs to define both clinically and through surveillance definitions. This makes it very difficult to develop a diagnostic gold standard for comparison. In one study reviewing patients who had received antibiotics for VAP, a multidisciplinary review panel found that only 50% of them had VAP by their consensus diagnosis [20]. The NHSN surveillance definition prior to 2012 utilized clinical data for the diagnosis of VAP and was highly subjective. Many of the signs and symptoms of VAP are relatively non-specific and subject to interpretation [21]. For example, it is difficult to define what constitutes consolidation on chest radiography or purulent sputum or even a change in cough. As expected, in this scenario, there is considerable interobserver variability in VAP surveillance [10]. Similar to CLABSI, interpreting clinical findings more strictly or including subjective clinical data to define VAP may result in reduced rates without actual improvement in care [22]. Host factors and underlying clinical illnesses commonly seen in intensive care unit patients such as atelectasis, pulmonary edema, and acute respiratory distress syndrome also have the potential to confound the interpretation of these clinical variables. In one study, modeling different patient populations with these comorbid conditions but similar acute presentations altered the apparent prevalence of VAP from 6 to 31.6% [21]. Case finding approaches vary between institutions and introduce another layer or variability in surveillance. Some institutions use different screening algorithms, such as identifying patients with positive sputum cultures or

bronchoalveolar lavage for VAP surveillance, which reduces case finding by limiting the scope of cases reviewed and would change the apparent prevalence of these HAIs compared to institutions with broader screening criteria [22].

Catheter-associated urinary tract infections (CAUTIs) may be expected to perform better since there is less subjective data interpretation in the NHSN definition; however this is not always the case. The description of urinary symptoms is often poorly documented in the medical record [23]. Additionally, while there is less data interpretation required, the non-specific nature of fevers can cause an overdiagnosis of CAUTI in patients who are more likely to have fevers such as in the burn population or in certain immunosuppressed patient populations. Al-Qas Hanna et al. found a strong association of systemic inflammatory response syndrome and NHSN-defined CAUTI and also showed that a hypothetical increase in the prevalence of fever or culturing practices from other causes would increase the number of NHSN-defined CAUTIs suggesting that frequency of culturing causes a significant change in CAUTI rates [24]. Leekha et al. also found a strong association between NHSN-defined CAUTI and concurrent alternate sources of fever and low agreement between NHSN-defined and clinical CAUTI, suggesting poor specificity of the NHSN CAUTI definition which can be thus heavily influenced by variable culturing practices at different institutions [25].

Surgical site infection (SSI) surveillance is less likely to be biased by surveillance definitions as the criteria for SSI through NHSN definitions are fairly straightforward. However, one of the greatest variabilities in SSI surveillance is the robustness of post-discharge surveillance. Most SSIs are diagnosed after discharge [26–28]. For prosthetic joint infections, only 4% were identified during the index admission; 50% of SSIs were identified through post-discharge surveillance, and 40% were readmitted [29]. Limiting HAI surveillance to the operative hospital alone would miss 17% of SSIs after joint arthroplasty [30].

If hospitals do not have access to outpatient visits or readmissions to their own or other hospitals, case finding may be severely compromised, and SSI rates may be underreported. Different hospitals use different methods to find cases [31, 32]. Some hospitals use surveys with surgeons or patients, and only 40% of hospitals surveyed use postoperative clinic where many surgical site infections are identified [31, 32].

In summary, there are many differences in surveillance methods which can have a significant impact on reported HAI infection rates. These differing approaches to surveillance can create opportunities for intentional and unintentional "gaming" that can impact hospital ranking and influence hospital reimbursement in the era of pay-for-performance [32].

Table 28.2 Summary of pros and cons of strategies to improve HAI surveillance

Strategy to improve HAI surveillance	Pro	Con
Use of administrative data	No requirement for additional chart review, therefore fewer resources needed	Poor specificity compared to traditional surveillance
	Readily available almost all hospitals	
	Moderate to high sensitivity for HAI detection compared to traditional surveillance	
Algorithmic approach	Increases objectivity and efficiency of data collection	Relies on accurate documentation and electronic capture of clinical data
Objective laboratory test-based metric	Does not rely on subjective adjudication	Metric based on positive tests can be affected by variability in culturing practices
	Improves efficiency of data collection	
		May be affected by community prevalence of disease
		Requires risk adjustment
		May not always represent clinical outcome of true infection (e.g., *C. difficile* colonization vs. disease)
Process measures	Clinically more meaningful than some infection outcomes	Requires agreement and data on which process measures are most closely related to outcome of interest; process improvement has historically not always been associated with improvement in outcome (e.g., SSI and SCIP)
	Usually easier to measure	
	Minimal subjective adjudication	
Related outcome measures	Clinically more meaningful than some infection outcomes (e.g., VAE vs. VAP)	May not always correlate well with infection outcome
Better risk adjustment	Levels the playing field for publicly reported and pay-for-performance HAI metrics	Requires large datasets with accurate information on patient characteristics ("case mix") and risk factors for infection

HAI Surveillance Is Resource Intensive

A second issue with traditional HAI surveillance is that diligent application of standard definitions and criteria is time-consuming and cumbersome [33]. Traditionally, infection prevention programs have been heavily surveillance focused, allowing little time for infection preventionists to engage in process improvement. This has become even more important with carefully scrutinized publicly reported HAI rates including independent audits of hospital HAI surveillance by state and other regulatory bodies. This creates a larger need for efficient surveillance methodology that help can free up valuable IP time for guiding implementation of evidence-based practice at the bedside.

HAI Surveillance Is Not Clinically Meaningful

Feedback of HAI rates to bedside clinicians is an important component of surveillance programs. For surveillance data to be meaningful to clinicians, the measured metrics should be related to true patient outcomes and be able to accurately discern improvement. This is not always the case.

While this may occur for several reasons including the subjectivity of definitions highlighted in the previous section, another important contributor to change in the measured or observed HAI rates is the change in clinical or laboratory testing practices. This has been seen in certain

institutions where screening urinalysis on admission has reduced the catheter-associated urinary tract infection rates that were considered "hospital acquired" but may have caused more harm through inappropriate antibiotic use [24, 34].

Reducing unnecessary culturing can also "lower" the measured infection rates, e.g., reduction in measured CAUTI rates in response to less urine culturing [35]. While this may have a positive impact on antimicrobial stewardship, it does not reflect a true change in CAUTI incidence and makes interpretation of concurrent infection prevention interventions difficult.

Similarly, the type of laboratory test used for *C. difficile* testing can greatly impact the observed CDI rates: specifically, institutions that use a highly sensitive nucleic acid amplification test (NAAT) will have higher rates than those that use a less sensitive assay for *C. difficile* toxin detection. In 2014, 44% of acute care hospitals reporting to NHSN were using PCR alone or in combination with other tests for CDI diagnosis; the use of NAAT-based testing has been associated with 50–100% increases in reported CDI rates [36–38]. This can potentially provide a negative incentive to hospitals by leading them toward the use of a less sensitive test. Therefore, these "false" measures have the ability to influence clinical practice with respect to testing rather than promoting a patient-centric model of improving the clinical quality of care. As these metrics diverge from clinical definitions, it becomes more difficult to effectively engage the frontline staff in process improvement efforts.

Other Threats to Validity of HAI Surveillance Metrics: Choice of Denominator and Risk Adjustment

The choice of denominators can also have an impact on the measurement of HAI rates and may mask a true impact of quality improvement efforts. By reducing device days, you reduce the denominator and thus appear to have an increased rate when the actual numbers of infections may be decreased [39]. This may cause clinicians and patients to falsely conclude that there has been no benefit to patient outcomes, when in fact there has been considerable benefit. This could be partially mitigated by using patient days rather than device days [40, 41]. One comparative study looking AHRQ random sample chart review with numbers of chart reviewed as a denominator showed a significant decrease in CAUTIs as compared to NHSN rates which had not decreased over the same time period [42].

Another issue with the device-day denominator for CLABSI is that the denominator uses the total monthly device days. Therefore, this denominator will be the same regardless of whether 100 patients have catheters for 1 day each or 5 patients have catheters for 20 days each. These scenarios represent very different risks and performance improvement outcomes as the duration of catheter use is the strongest risk factor for CLABSI, but this important patient-level risk difference is not captured by the composite denominator. Another device-denominator issue specific to CLABSI relates to the number of central lines per patient. The risk of CLABSI in an individual patient also increases with a larger number of central lines in place [43]; however, the current denominator only accounts for one central line per day. Further, the difference in duration and number of indwelling central lines may also be a function of patient groups with a variety of different host factors, not all which may be preventable. For example, patients with short gut syndrome who are chronically TPN dependent or burn patients who are central line dependent and subject to transient bacteremias are a much higher-risk group for "CLABSIs" than patients in a cardiac intensive care unit who have temporary central lines for a few days. Thus far, risk adjustment in device-associated infections has been based on patient unit location and not on individual host factors. Recent data suggests that patient comorbid conditions from billing codes could be explored for risk adjustment for CLABSI [44].

Similarly, patients with more comorbidities are more likely to develop HAI and surgical site infections [45, 46]. Hospitals that perform surgeries on higher-risk patients are therefore more likely to have higher rates of infection. In one study where investigators used the percent of high-risk procedures as a surrogate marker for complexity of patients, risk adjusting for volume of high-risk procedures (as defined by the volume of procedures with an expected infection rate greater than 3%), surgeon volume, and distance from a referral center reduced the observed rate of infection in the larger hospitals [47]. Older NHSN SSI risk adjustment ("NNIS" risk index) used risk stratification based on American Society of Anesthesiology score, wound class, and duration of surgery. While higher NNIS risk scores were associated with higher SSI rates in general, their ability to discriminate within categories of similar procedures was limited [46]. Although NHSN has revised SSI risk models to be procedure specific, these models are still deficient in patient-specific risk factors [48]. Clinical variables that are not available through NHSN may better predict infection for patients [48, 49]. In a study comparing different models of risk adjustment including patient comorbidities, incorporation of these comorbidities improved the ability of the model to predict surgical site infections but still had [50] relatively low discriminatory power [49]. Nevertheless, these risk adjustment models can make a difference to hospital rankings [51, 52]. As we understand and incorporate patient risk factors into models to determine the expected number of infections in a particular patient population, the change of rates and rankings from crude to adjusted may be even greater.

The importance of risk adjustment should not be minimized as this can change the comparative rankings of hospitals [53]. As an example, the recent consumer report rankings of hospitals found that no academic institution was ranked among the best in class. This may be due to intrinsic differences in the quality of care delivered but may also be due to different populations in primary hospitals vs tertiary or quaternary care hospitals. Therefore, valid HAI risk adjustment models that appropriately account for large variabilities in intrinsic patient-related HAI risk across hospitals are urgently needed [54].

To overcome some of the limitations of current HAI surveillance described above, several approaches have been developed and tested. Here we describe some of these approaches along with their advantages and limitations using examples where applicable.

Use of Administrative Data Approaches

One strategy to overcome the subjectivity and resource-intensive nature of surveillance has been to leverage already available administrative coding and billing data for surveillance for HAI surveillance [55]. This approach is appealing as all US hospitals are already collecting these data in a standardized format. These data could also be potentially used to capture events across multiple healthcare sites. These models can be risk adjusted and propensity score adjusted providing more robust predictive models.

This approach has been used by US News & World Report in their hospital rankings.

Administrative data has been used to stratify hospitals for surgical site infection rates after cardiac artery bypass surgery (CABG) by looking at combinations of diagnosis and prescribing codes [56]. When comparing claims data with traditional surveillance for SSI post CABG, the claims-based surveillance increased the sensitivity by 50% [57]. Seventy-six percent of all cases were identified after discharge, and traditional surveillance only identified 42% of these post-discharge cases thus demonstrating the increased sensitivity of claims-based data [57]. The sensitivity and specificity of administrative data compared to traditional surveillance depends on the screening algorithm used for traditional surveillance. Hospitals often use positive cultures to select for further review for surgical site infections. In such cases, claims data may significantly improve case finding. The use of claims data can also identify infections that are diagnosed in outpatient settings like post-cesarean section infections or post-breast surgery infection [58]. For coronary artery bypass graft surgery, using administrative data to identify surgical site infections found significantly more cases compared to traditional surveillance using culture data to screen cases. However, the administrative data filter still missed 3 out of 22 cases identified by traditional surveillance [59]. The sensitivity and specificity of using claims data can also be refined by the use of more sophisticated diagnostic codes. When more sophisticated combinations of administrative data codes were used to evaluate hospital rankings for surgical site infections after primary arthroplasty, the claims-based ranking for the highest and lowest decile hospitals was found to be correlated to the difference in manual review-confirmed SSIs between the high-performing and low-performing hospitals [60]. However, upon chart review, even when using better diagnostic codes, only 40% of patients identified with an SSI based on claims data had an SSI after chart review [60]. This increase in sensitivity at the cost of specificity is consistent with results from a comparison of surgical site infections and surgical complications identified from Medicare claims data compared to chart review through National Surgical Quality Improvement Program (NSQIP). Claims data resulted in 48–84% false positives. Interestingly, the sensitivity of detecting complications was also variable using administrative data [61]. The Pennsylvania experience highlights the inaccuracies in using administrative data to assess the prevalence of healthcare-associated infections [62]. In 2004, 12,000 HAIs were identified through traditional surveillance and 115,000 HAIs through coding data [63]. The initial assumption was that hospitals were underreporting infection. After further review, it was determined that trained professionals identified all HAIs, as did administrative data, but only 10% of the HAIs identified through

administrative review were true hospital-acquired infections [62]. Generally, administrative data is more likely to be useful in ruling out surgical site infections and ventilator-associated pneumonia [64].

Specific codes may be used to improve the specificity of this approach [65]. Codes for orders for cultures, radiologic studies, and administration of antibiotics are strongly correlated with the presence of an NHSN surgical site infection [66]. Antibiotic administration alone improves the specificity of claims-based models for detecting surgical site infections [67, 68].

For central line-associated bloodstream infections and MRSA infections, administrative data performs poorly and did not increase case finding [69–74]. While these approaches overestimate the absolute number of infections, they have less interobserver variability compared to traditional surveillance [75–77]. This may be an acceptable trade off in the era of public reporting.

For *Clostridium difficile* infection, several studies found poor positive predictive values for cases found through administrative data compared with clinical surveillance [78, 79]. Findings of individual studies are consistent with two meta-analyses comparing the use of administrative data with traditional surveillance for various HAIs that found moderate sensitivity and low positive predictive values, with device-associated infections performed particularly poorly [80, 81].

Algorithmic Approach to HAI Surveillance

Another approach to simplify surveillance is to use the electronic medical record to aid or replace traditional surveillance methods. Rule-based computer algorithms that use clinical data such as microbiology reports, admission-transfer-discharge data or vital signs, or even administrative billing data can identify patients at high risk for having an HAI which can then be refined with traditional surveillance [82]. The benefit of this approach is that the number of cases that need to be reviewed is reduced, and thus this approach allows for infection prevention resources to be used for process improvement initiatives rather than surveillance.

This approach has been used with good efficiency with a high sensitivity for surgical site infections [68, 83]. For prosthetic joint infections, using diagnosis codes for infection combined with antibiotic administration data refined by manual surveillance, the number of infections found was double compared to traditional surveillance alone [55, 65].

In some algorithms, the entire surveillance process can be fully automated. This approach has the advantage of eliminating subjective interpretation from surveillance but may impact sensitivity and specificity of case finding. An automated system to detect CAUTIs and CLABSIs resulted in good negative predictive value but poor positive predictive value [84–86]. In a multicenter evaluation of computer surveillance vs traditional surveillance for central line-associated bloodstream infections, there was better interobserver variability with computer surveillance but poor correlation between computer surveillance and traditional surveillance [17, 87]. However, for many types of HAI, several data elements for HAI definitions rely on clinical documentation such as wound description or pain which can be very variable and difficult to find and may not be documented systemically in a way that can be queried [83]. While fully automated surveillance for most HAIs is not imminent, more sophisticated probabilistic models are being developed and studied for surveillance [77, 88, 89].

Objective Lab ID Approaches

Lab ID has been used as an objective metric for hospital-acquired MRSA bacteremia and *Clostridium difficile* infection in the current NHSN surveillance system. The advantage of this approach is that it does not rely on any subjective criteria. Such metrics are most useful when a positive test result is both sensitive and specific in measuring true infection. Theoretically, MRSA bacteremia represents a good measurement of a clinically valid test result that indicates severe and invasive MRSA infection. However, similar to other HAI metrics, its drawbacks include lack of appropriate risk adjustment and variability in clinical testing strategies.

C. difficile rates are associated with greater severity of illness assessed through case mix index [90]. This association remains even after adjustment for medical school affiliation, hospital size, type of test used, and community prevalence [90]. Risk adjustment for MRSA bacteremia can also change hospital rankings; in one study, adjusting for comorbidities, low education zip codes, and discharge to other healthcare facilities resulted in significant changes in rates and rankings of hospitals [91].

Testing strategies also significantly impact rates. Although positive *C. difficile* tests in an ideal clinical setting would also reflect true *C. difficile* disease, that metric is heavily influenced by the sensitivity of the type of test used and testing frequency. Importantly, a positive *C. difficile* laboratory test does not distinguish colonization from infection and is therefore particularly problematic when used in the absence of an appropriate clinical indication as up to 25% of hospitalized patients are colonized with *C. difficile* [92]. As described above, molecular testing for *C. difficile* is significantly more sensitive in detecting colonization and infection, and hospitals that have switched from toxin tests to PCR tests have seen an increase in their *C. difficile* rates [36, 38].

Additionally the community prevalence of *C. difficile* and especially MRSA heavily influence the rates of hospital-acquired infections [93, 94]. Conversely many cases of MRSA infection and *Clostridium difficile* occur after hospital discharge [95–97]. For MRSA bacteremia, including patients who had been discharged from the facility within the last 30 days tripled the rate of hospital-acquired bacteremia and altered hospital ranking [98]. Including post-discharge CDI doubled the rates of hospital-onset *C. difficile* infection [96].

Hospital-onset bacteremia, a more global measure encompassing all positive blood cultures (as opposed to limiting to those caused by certain pathogens or associated with central lines), also seems to show promise as an objective, lab-based, and clinically relevant HAI metric [99].

Clinically Meaningful Measures for HAI Surveillance

An evolving approach is to use related outcome measures as proxy markers that do not measure the infection outcome but are meaningful and considered important elements of high-quality care. This approach has been used for ventilator-associated events [100]. In 2013, the CDC moved from surveillance for ventilator-associated pneumonia to a more inclusive ventilator-associated event (VAE) surveillance that was predicated on worsening oxygenation as indicated by changes in positive end expiratory pressure (PEEP) or supplemental oxygen requirement [101, 102]. This definition had greater interobserver agreement and took significantly less time [102]. When compared to traditional surveillance for VAP, this case definition was similarly associated with an increased length of stay in the ICU and the hospital, but VAE cases were associated with increased mortality, whereas the VAP cases were not [100]. However, although a seemingly promising clinical endpoint, fully electronic surveillance for VAE was subject to small differences in electronic records [103]. Additionally the newer definition does not correlate well with clinical VAP particularly in certain types of ICUs making it more difficult to provide clinically useful feedback to bedside staff [104].

To overcome limitations of measuring HAI outcomes, measures of processes that are known to lead to or prevent HAIs can sometimes be clinically meaningful and less subject to biases that affect outcome determination. For example, a large trial of spontaneous breathing trials found a significant association between compliance with this metric and clinically meaningful outcomes such as days of assisted ventilation, days in the ICU, and mortality, suggesting that this measure could be a useful adjunct for VAP surveillance [105].

Similarly, device utilization ratio, defined as the number of catheter days over the number of patient days, may be an important adjunct to surveillance of catheter-associated

HAI. Device utilization has the advantages of being objective and of being able to measure device-related harm beyond the infection outcome and directly reflect the impact of efforts at reducing unnecessary devices [41]. However, the accuracy and validity of this measure would still rely on accurate documentation of device presence, as well as appropriate risk adjustment for patient severity of illness.

Finally, the methodology for selection of process measures needs to be dynamic. As an example, key process measures thought to be important for SSI prevention received considerable attention under the Surgical Care Improvement Project (SCIP) in the early 2000s and became part of required reporting for all hospitals. However, in several studies, despite high compliance with SCIP measures, minimal impact on SSIs was noted [106–109], demonstrating that periodic reevaluation of key processes is critical, particularly when those processes are tied to regulatory reporting.

Conclusion

Surveillance and feedback of infection rates are an important component of any effective infection prevention program. The added financial and reputational risks for these publicly reported rates have made it even more important to understand the variability in the way that surveillance is conducted and to develop a robust and fair surveillance strategy that allows infection prevention programs to focus on prevention.

References

1. Maruthappu M, Trehan A, Barnett-Vanes A, McCulloch P, Carty MJ. The impact of feedback of surgical outcome data on surgical performance: a systematic review. World J Surg. 2015;39(4):879–89.
2. Schroder C, Schwab F, Behnke M, et al. Epidemiology of healthcare associated infections in Germany: nearly 20 years of surveillance. Int J Med Microbiol. 2015;305(7):799–806.
3. Haley RW, Culver DH, White JW, et al. The efficacy of infection surveillance and control programs in preventing nosocomial infections in US hospitals. Am J Epidemiol. 1985;121(2):182–205.
4. Gaynes R, Richards C, Edwards J, et al. Feeding back surveillance data to prevent hospital-acquired infections. Emerg Infect Dis. 2001;7(2):295–8.
5. Brandt C, Sohr D, Behnke M, Daschner F, Ruden H, Gastmeier P. Reduction of surgical site infection rates associated with active surveillance. Infect Control Hosp Epidemiol. 2006;27(12):1347–51.
6. Kanamori H, Weber DJ, DiBiase LM, et al. Longitudinal trends in all healthcare-associated infections through comprehensive hospital-wide surveillance and infection control measures over the past 12 years: substantial burden of healthcare-associated infections outside of intensive care units and "other" types of infection. Infect Control Hosp Epidemiol. 2015;36(10):1139–47.
7. Schroder C, Behnke M, Gastmeier P, Schwab F, Geffers C. Case vignettes to evaluate the accuracy of identifying healthcare-

8. Russo PL, Barnett AG, Cheng AC, Richards M, Graves N, Hall L. Differences in identifying healthcare associated infections using clinical vignettes and the influence of respondent characteristics: a cross-sectional survey of Australian infection prevention staff. Antimicrob Resist Infect Control. 2015;4:29.
9. Mayer J, Greene T, Howell J, et al. Agreement in classifying bloodstream infections among multiple reviewers conducting surveillance. Clin Infect Dis. 2012;55(3):364–70.
10. Klompas M. Interobserver variability in ventilator-associated pneumonia surveillance. Am J Infect Control. 2010;38(3):237–9.
11. Gastmeier P, Brauer H, Hauer T, Schumacher M, Daschner F, Ruden H. How many nosocomial infections are missed if identification is restricted to patients with either microbiology reports or antibiotic administration? Infect Control Hosp Epidemiol. 1999;20(2):124–7.
12. Niedner MF, National Association of Children's H, Related Institutions Pediatric Intensive Care Unit Patient Care FG. The harder you look, the more you find: catheter-associated bloodstream infection surveillance variability. Am J Infect Control. 2010;38(8):585–95.
13. Thompson DL, Makvandi M, Baumbach J. Validation of central line-associated bloodstream infection data in a voluntary reporting state: New Mexico. Am J Infect Control. 2013;41(2):122–5.
14. Backman LA, Melchreit R, Rodriguez R. Validation of the surveillance and reporting of central line-associated bloodstream infection data to a state health department. Am J Infect Control. 2010;38(10):832–8.
15. Rich KL, Reese SM, Bol KA, Gilmartin HM, Janosz T. Assessment of the quality of publicly reported central line-associated bloodstream infection data in Colorado, 2010. Am J Infect Control. 2013;41(10):874–9.
16. Oh JY, Cunningham MC, Beldavs ZG, et al. Statewide validation of hospital-reported central line-associated bloodstream infections: Oregon, 2009. Infect Control Hosp Epidemiol. 2012;33(5):439–45.
17. Lin MY, Woeltje KF, Khan YM, et al. Multicenter evaluation of computer automated versus traditional surveillance of hospital-acquired bloodstream infections. Infect Control Hosp Epidemiol. 2014;35(12):1483–90.
18. Thompson ND, Yeh LL, Magill SS, Ostroff SM, Fridkin SK. Investigating systematic misclassification of central line-associated bloodstream infection (CLABSI) to secondary bloodstream infection during health care-associated infection reporting. Am J Med Qual. 2013;28(1):56–9.
19. Leekha S, Li S, Thom KA, et al. Comparison of total hospital-acquired bloodstream infections to central line-associated bloodstream infections and implications for outcome measures in infection control. Infect Control Hosp Epidemiol. 2013;34(9):984–6.
20. Nussenblatt V, Avdic E, Berenholtz S, et al. Ventilator-associated pneumonia: overdiagnosis and treatment are common in medical and surgical intensive care units. Infect Control Hosp Epidemiol. 2014;35(3):278–84.
21. Klompas M, Kulldorff M, Platt R. Risk of misleading ventilator-associated pneumonia rates with use of standard clinical and microbiological criteria. Clin Infect Dis. 2008;46(9):1443–6.
22. Klompas M. Eight initiatives that misleadingly lower ventilator-associated pneumonia rates. Am J Infect Control. 2012;40(5):408–10.
23. Mithoowani S, Celetti SJ, Irfan N, Brooks A, Mertz D. Inadequate documentation of urinary tract infection symptoms in the medical chart. Am J Infect Control. 2015;43(11):1252–4.
24. Al-Qas Hanna F, Sambirska O, Iyer S, Szpunar S, Fakih MG. Clinician practice and the National Healthcare Safety

Network definition for the diagnosis of catheter-associated urinary tract infection. Am J Infect Control. 2013;41(12):1173–7.

25. Leekha S, Preas MA, Hebden J. Association of National Healthcare Safety Network – defined catheter-associated urinary tract infections with alternate sources of fever. Infect Control Hosp Epidemiol. 2015;36(10):1236–8.

26. Sands K, Vineyard G, Platt R. Surgical site infections occurring after hospital discharge. J Infect Dis. 1996;173(4):963–70.

27. Daneman N, Lu H, Redelmeier DA. Discharge after discharge: predicting surgical site infections after patients leave hospital. J Hosp Infect. 2010;75(3):188–94.

28. Tanner J, Khan D, Aplin C, Ball J, Thomas M, Bankart J. Post-discharge surveillance to identify colorectal surgical site infection rates and related costs. J Hosp Infect. 2009;72(3):243–50.

29. Barnes S, Salemi C, Fithian D, et al. An enhanced benchmark for prosthetic joint replacement infection rates. Am J Infect Control. 2006;34(10):669–72.

30. Yokoe DS, Avery TR, Platt R, Huang SS. Reporting surgical site infections following total hip and knee arthroplasty: impact of limiting surveillance to the operative hospital. Clin Infect Dis. 2013;57(9):1282–8.

31. Zarate R, Birnbaum D. Postdischarge surgical site infection surveillance practices in Washington acute care hospitals. Infect Control Hosp Epidemiol. 2012;33(1):87–9.

32. Reese SM, Knepper BC, Price CS, Young HL. An evaluation of surgical site infection surveillance methods for colon surgery and hysterectomy in Colorado hospitals. Infect Control Hosp Epidemiol. 2015;36(3):353–5.

33. Parrillo SL. The burden of National Healthcare Safety Network (NHSN) reporting on the infection Preventionist: a community hospital perspective. Am J Infect Control. 2015;43(6, Supplement):S17.

34. Adherence to the Centers for Disease Control and Prevention's (CDC's) Infection definitions and criteria is needed to ensure accuracy, completeness, and comparability of infection information. http://www.cdc.gov/nhsn/cms/cms-reporting.html. 2016. Accessed Nov 2016.

35. Epstein L, Edwards JR, Halpin AL, et al. Evaluation of a novel intervention to reduce unnecessary urine cultures in intensive care units at a tertiary Care Hospital in Maryland, 2011–2014. Infect Control Hosp Epidemiol. 2016;37(5):606–9.

36. Longtin Y, Trottier S, Brochu G, et al. Impact of the type of diagnostic assay on Clostridium difficile infection and complication rates in a mandatory reporting program. Clin Infect Dis. 2013;56(1):67–73.

37. Fong KS, Fatica C, Hall G, et al. Impact of PCR testing for Clostridium difficile on incident rates and potential on public reporting: is the playing field level? Infect Control Hosp Epidemiol. 2011;32(9):932–3.

38. Moehring RW, Lofgren ET, Anderson DJ. Impact of change to molecular testing for Clostridium difficile infection on healthcare facility-associated incidence rates. Infect Control Hosp Epidemiol. 2013;34(10):1055–61.

39. Wright MO, Kharasch M, Beaumont JL, Peterson LR, Robicsek A. Reporting catheter-associated urinary tract infections: denominator matters. Infect Control Hosp Epidemiol. 2011;32(7):635–40.

40. Horstman MJ, Li YF, Almenoff PL, Freyberg RW, Trautner BW. Denominator doesn't matter: standardizing healthcare-associated infection rates by bed days or device days. Infect Control Hosp Epidemiol. 2015;36(6):710–6.

41. Fakih MG, Gould CV, Trautner BW, et al. Beyond infection: device utilization ratio as a performance measure for urinary catheter harm. Infect Control Hosp Epidemiol. 2016;37(3):327–33.

42. Calderon LE, Kavanagh KT, Rice MK. Questionable validity of the catheter-associated urinary tract infection metric used for value-based purchasing. Am J Infect Control. 2015;43(10):1050–2.

43. Scheithauer S, Hafner H, Schroder J, et al. Simultaneous placement of multiple central lines increases central line-associated bloodstream infection rates. Am J Infect Control. 2013;41(2):113–7.

44. Pepin CS, Thom KA, Sorkin JD, et al. Risk factors for central-line-associated bloodstream infections: a focus on comorbid conditions. Infect Control Hosp Epidemiol. 2015;36(4):479–81.

45. Kanerva M, Ollgren J, Lyytikainen O, Finnish Prevalence Survey Study G. Interhospital differences and case-mix in a nationwide prevalence survey. J Hosp Infect. 2010;76(2):135–8.

46. Anderson DJ, Chen LF, Sexton DJ, Kaye KS. Complex surgical site infections and the devilish details of risk adjustment: important implications for public reporting. Infect Control Hosp Epidemiol. 2008;29(10):941–6.

47. Anderson DJ, Hartwig MG, Pappas T, et al. Surgical volume and the risk of surgical site infection in community hospitals: size matters. Ann Surg. 2008;247(2):343–9.

48. Mu Y, Edwards JR, Horan TC, Berrios-Torres SI, Fridkin SK. Improving risk-adjusted measures of surgical site infection for the national healthcare safety network. Infect Control Hosp Epidemiol. 2011;32(10):970–86.

49. Moehring RW, Anderson DJ. "But my patients are different!": risk adjustment in 2012 and beyond. Infect Control Hosp Epidemiol. 2011;32(10):987–9.

50. Jackson SS, Leekha S, Pineles L, et al. Improving risk adjustment above current centers for disease control and prevention methodology using electronically available comorbid conditions. Infect Control Hosp Epidemiol. 2016;37(10):1173–8.

51. Daneman N, Simor AE, Redelmeier DA. Validation of a modified version of the national nosocomial infections surveillance system risk index for health services research. Infect Control Hosp Epidemiol. 2009;30(6):563–9.

52. Morgan DM, Swenson CW, Streifel KM, et al. Surgical site infection following hysterectomy: adjusted rankings in a regional collaborative. Am J Obstet Gynecol. 2016;214(2):259 e1–8.

53. Kritsotakis EI, Dimitriadis I, Roumbelaki M, et al. Case-mix adjustment approach to benchmarking prevalence rates of nosocomial infection in hospitals in Cyprus and Greece. Infect Control Hosp Epidemiol. 2008;29(8):685–92.

54. Steinberg SM, Popa MR, Michalek JA, Bethel MJ, Ellison EC. Comparison of risk adjustment methodologies in surgical quality improvement. Surgery. 2008;144(4):662–7. discussion -7

55. Calderwood MS, Ma A, Khan YM, et al. Use of Medicare diagnosis and procedure codes to improve detection of surgical site infections following hip arthroplasty, knee arthroplasty, and vascular surgery. Infect Control Hosp Epidemiol. 2012;33(1):40–9.

56. Huang SS, Livingston JM, Rawson NS, Schmaltz S, Platt R. Developing algorithms for healthcare insurers to systematically monitor surgical site infection rates. BMC Med Res Methodol. 2007;7:20.

57. Sands KE, Yokoe DS, Hooper DC, et al. Detection of postoperative surgical-site infections: comparison of health plan-based surveillance with hospital-based programs. Infect Control Hosp Epidemiol. 2003;24(10):741–3.

58. Miner AL, Sands KE, Yokoe DS, et al. Enhanced identification of postoperative infections among outpatients. Emerg Infect Dis. 2004;10(11):1931–7.

59. Apte M, Landers T, Furuya Y, Hyman S, Larson E. Comparison of two computer algorithms to identify surgical site infections. Surg Infect. 2011;12(6):459–64.

60. Calderwood MS, Kleinman K, Bratzler DW, et al. Use of Medicare claims to identify US hospitals with a high rate of surgical site infection after hip arthroplasty. Infect Control Hosp Epidemiol. 2013;34(1):31–9.

61. Lawson EH, Louie R, Zingmond DS, et al. A comparison of clinical registry versus administrative claims data for reporting of 30-day surgical complications. Ann Surg. 2012;256(6):973–81.

62. Sherman ER, Heydon KH, St John KH, et al. Administrative data fail to accurately identify cases of healthcare-associated infection. Infect Control Hosp Epidemiol. 2006;27(4):332–7.

63. Brennan PJ. In the beginning there was...heat. Infect Control Hosp Epidemiol. 2006;27(4):329–31.

64. Stevenson KB, Khan Y, Dickman J, et al. Administrative coding data, compared with CDC/NHSN criteria, are poor indicators of health care-associated infections. Am J Infect Control. 2008;36(3):155–64.

65. Bolon MK, Hooper D, Stevenson KB, et al. Improved surveillance for surgical site infections after orthopedic implantation procedures: extending applications for automated data. Clin Infect Dis. 2009;48(9):1223–9.

66. Branch-Elliman W, Strymish J, Itani KM, Gupta K. Using clinical variables to guide surgical site infection detection: a novel surveillance strategy. Am J Infect Control. 2014;42(12):1291–5.

67. Yokoe DS, Shapiro M, Simchen E, Platt R. Use of antibiotic exposure to detect postoperative infections. Infect Control Hosp Epidemiol. 1998;19(5):317–22.

68. Sands K, Vineyard G, Livingston J, Christiansen C, Platt R. Efficient identification of postdischarge surgical site infections: use of automated pharmacy dispensing information, administrative data, and medical record information. J Infect dis. 1999;179(2):434–41.

69. Tehrani DM, Russell D, Brown J, et al. Discord among performance measures for central line-associated bloodstream infection. Infect Control Hosp Epidemiol. 2013;34(2):176–83.

70. Moehring RW, Staheli R, Miller BA, Chen LF, Sexton DJ, Anderson DJ. Central line-associated infections as defined by the Centers for Medicare and Medicaid Services' Hospital-acquired condition versus standard infection control surveillance: why hospital compare seems conflicted. Infect Control Hosp Epidemiol. 2013;34(3):238–44.

71. Schweizer ML, Eber MR, Laxminarayan R, et al. Validity of ICD-9-CM coding for identifying incident methicillin-resistant Staphylococcus aureus (MRSA) infections: is MRSA infection coded as a chronic disease? Infect Control Hosp Epidemiol. 2011;32(2):148–54.

72. Schaefer MK, Ellingson K, Conover C, et al. Evaluation of international classification of diseases, ninth revision, clinical modification codes for reporting methicillin-resistant Staphylococcus aureus infections at a hospital in Illinois. Infect Control Hosp Epidemiol. 2010;31(5):463–8.

73. Wright SB, Huskins WC, Dokholyan RS, Goldmann DA, Platt R. Administrative databases provide inaccurate data for surveillance of long-term central venous catheter-associated infections. Infect Control Hosp Epidemiol. 2003;24(12):946–9.

74. Cevasco M, Borzecki AM, O'Brien WJ, et al. Validity of the AHRQ patient safety indicator "central venous catheter-related bloodstream infections". J Am Coll Surg. 2011;212(6):984–90.

75. Woeltje KF, McMullen KM, Butler AM, Goris AJ, Doherty JA. Electronic surveillance for healthcare-associated central line-associated bloodstream infections outside the intensive care unit. Infect Control Hosp Epidemiol. 2011;32(11):1086–90.

76. Leal J, Gregson DB, Ross T, Flemons WW, Church DL, Laupland KB. Development of a novel electronic surveillance system for monitoring of bloodstream infections. Infect Control Hosp Epidemiol. 2010;31(7):740–7.

77. Hota B, Malpiedi P, Fridkin SK, Martin J, Trick W. Probabilistic measurement of central line-associated bloodstream infections. Infect Control Hosp Epidemiol. 2016;37(2):149–55.

78. Schmiedeskamp M, Harpe S, Polk R, Oinonen M, Pakyz A. Use of international classification of diseases, ninth revision, clinical modification codes and medication use data to identify nosocomial Clostridium difficile infection. Infect Control Hosp Epidemiol. 2009;30(11):1070–6.

79. Dubberke ER, Reske KA, McDonald LC, Fraser VJ. ICD-9 codes and surveillance for Clostridium difficile-associated disease. Emerg Infect Dis. 2006;12(10):1576–9.

80. Goto M, Ohl ME, Schweizer ML, Perencevich EN. Accuracy of administrative code data for the surveillance of healthcare-associated infections: a systematic review and meta-analysis. Clin Infect Dis. 2014;58(5):688–96.

81. van Mourik MS, van Duijn PJ, Moons KG, Bonten MJ, Lee GM. Accuracy of administrative data for surveillance of healthcare-associated infections: a systematic review. BMJ Open. 2015;5(8):e008424.

82. Freeman R, Moore LS, Garcia Alvarez L, Charlett A, Holmes A. Advances in electronic surveillance for healthcare-associated infections in the 21st century: a systematic review. J Hosp Infect. 2013;84(2):106–19.

83. van Mourik MS, Troelstra A, van Solinge WW, Moons KG, Bonten MJ. Automated surveillance for healthcare-associated infections: opportunities for improvement. Clin Infect Dis. 2013;57(1):85–93.

84. Wald HL, Bandle B, Richard A, Min S. Accuracy of electronic surveillance of catheter-associated urinary tract infection at an academic medical center. Infect Control Hosp Epidemiol. 2014;35(6):685–91.

85. Choudhuri JA, Pergamit RF, Chan JD, et al. An electronic catheter-associated urinary tract infection surveillance tool. Infect Control Hosp Epidemiol. 2011;32(8):757–62.

86. Snyders RE, Goris AJ, Gase KA, Leone CL, Doherty JA, Woeltje KF. Increasing the reliability of fully automated surveillance for central line-associated bloodstream infections. Infect Control Hosp Epidemiol. 2015;36(12):1396–400.

87. Lin MY, Hota B, Khan YM, et al. Quality of traditional surveillance for public reporting of nosocomial bloodstream infection rates. JAMA. 2010;304(18):2035–41.

88. Platt R, Yokoe DS, Sands KE. Automated methods for surveillance of surgical site infections. Emerg Infect Dis. 2001;7(2):212–6.

89. Rochefort CM, Buckeridge DL, Forster AJ. Accuracy of using automated methods for detecting adverse events from electronic health record data: a research protocol. Implement Sci. 2015;10:5.

90. Thompson ND, Edwards JR, Dudeck MA, Fridkin SK, Magill SS. Evaluating the use of the case mix index for risk adjustment of healthcare-associated infection data: an illustration using Clostridium difficile infection data from the National Healthcare Safety Network. Infect Control Hosp Epidemiol. 2016;37(1):19–25.

91. Tehrani DM, Phelan MJ, Cao C, et al. Substantial shifts in ranking of California hospitals by hospital-associated methicillin-resistant Staphylococcus aureus infection following adjustment for hospital characteristics and case mix. Infect Control Hosp Epidemiol. 2014;35(10):1263–70.

92. Carroll KC, Bartlett JG. Biology of Clostridium Difficile: implications for epidemiology and diagnosis. Annu Rev Microbiol. 2011;65:501–21.

93. Murphy CR, Hudson LO, Spratt BG, et al. Predictors of hospitals with endemic community-associated methicillin-resistant Staphylococcus aureus. Infect Control Hosp Epidemiol. 2013;34(6):581–7.

94. Zilberberg MD, Tabak YP, Sievert DM, et al. Using electronic health information to risk-stratify rates of Clostridium difficile infection in US hospitals. Infect Control Hosp Epidemiol. 2011;32(7):649–55.

95. Epstein L, Mu Y, Belflower R, et al. Risk factors for invasive methicillin-resistant Staphylococcus aureus infection after recent discharge from an acute-care hospitalization, 2011–2013. Clin Infect Dis. 2016;62(1):45–52.

96. Murphy CR, Avery TR, Dubberke ER, Huang SS. Frequent hospital readmissions for Clostridium difficile infection and the impact on estimates of hospital-associated C. difficile burden. Infect Control Hosp Epidemiol. 2012;33(1):20–8.

97. Huang SS, Hinrichsen VL, Datta R, et al. Methicillin-resistant Staphylococcus aureus infection and hospitalization in high-risk patients in the year following detection. PLoS One. 2011;6(9):e24340.

98. Avery TR, Kleinman KP, Klompas M, Aschengrau A, Huang SS. Inclusion of 30-day postdischarge detection triples the incidence of hospital-onset methicillin-resistant Staphylococcus aureus. Infect Control Hosp Epidemiol. 2012;33(2):114–21.

99. Rock C, Thom KA, Harris AD, et al. A multicenter longitudinal study of hospital-onset bacteremia: time for a new quality outcome measure? Infect Control Hosp Epidemiol. 2016;37(2):143–8.

100. Klompas M, Khan Y, Kleinman K, et al. Multicenter evaluation of a novel surveillance paradigm for complications of mechanical ventilation. PLoS One. 2011;6(3):e18062.

101. Klompas M. Complications of mechanical ventilation – the CDC's new surveillance paradigm. N Engl J Med. 2013;368(16):1472–5.

102. Klompas M, Kleinman K, Khan Y, et al. Rapid and reproducible surveillance for ventilator-associated pneumonia. Clin Infect Dis. 2012;54(3):370–7.

103. Klein Klouwenberg PM, van Mourik MS, Ong DS, et al. Electronic implementation of a novel surveillance paradigm for ventilator-associated events. Feasibility and validation. Am J Respir Crit Care Med. 2014;189(8):947–55.

104. Stoeppel CM, Eriksson EA, Hawkins K, et al. Applicability of the National Healthcare Safety Network's surveillance definition of ventilator-associated events in the surgical intensive care unit: a 1-year review. J Trauma Acute Care Surg. 2014;77(6):934–7.

105. Girard TD, Kress JP, Fuchs BD, et al. Efficacy and safety of a paired sedation and ventilator weaning protocol for mechanically ventilated patients in intensive care (awakening and breathing controlled trial): a randomised controlled trial. Lancet. 2008;371(9607):126–34.

106. Hawn MT, Vick CC, Richman J, et al. Surgical site infection prevention: time to move beyond the surgical care improvement program. Ann Surg. 2011;254(3):494–9. discussion 9–501

107. Dua A, Desai SS, Seabrook GR, et al. The effect of surgical care improvement project measures on national trends on surgical site infections in open vascular procedures. J Vasc Surg. 2014;60(6):1635–9.

108. Munday GS, Deveaux P, Roberts H, Fry DE, Polk HC. Impact of implementation of the surgical care improvement project and future strategies for improving quality in surgery. Am J Surg. 2014;208(5):835–40.

109. Cataife G, Weinberg DA, Wong HH, Kahn KL. The effect of surgical care improvement project (SCIP) compliance on surgical site infections (SSI). Med Care. 2014;52(2 Suppl 1):S66–73.

Chlorhexidine Gluconate Bathing Outside the Intensive Care Unit

Megan Buller and Kyle J. Popovich

Introduction

Chlorhexidine gluconate is a biguanide antiseptic with both bacteriostatic and bactericidal activities against gram-positive and gram-negative bacteria (both aerobes and anaerobes), fungi, and some enveloped viruses, but is not sporicidal [1]. One of the benefits is that it maintains residual activity for hours after it is applied [2, 3]. It has been employed with increased frequency in healthcare settings for infection control and prevention. Over the last decade, several studies have documented the success of daily chlorhexidine (CHG) bathing as a means of source control in intensive care unit (ICU) settings. Daily CHG bathing in the medical ICU has been associated with a reduction in patient colonization with potential pathogens as well as a decrease in contamination of healthcare worker hands, thus likely reducing transmission of these potential pathogens to other patients (i.e., "source control") [4]. In addition, daily CHG bathing in various types of ICUs (medical, surgical, trauma) has led to reductions in healthcare-associated infections, including those due to multidrug-resistant organisms such as vancomycin-resistant *Enterococci* (VRE) and methicillin-resistant *Staphylococcus aureus* (MRSA) [5]. As a result of the several studies demonstrating the effectiveness of CHG bathing in ICUs, several hospitals across the United States now use CHG for patient bathing in the ICU. This has prompted extension of the use of CHG from the ICU to hospital wards

and ambulatory, institutional, and community populations. There may be a significant value of CHG bathing outside the ICU for both infection control and infection prevention. However, it is also essential to recognize the potential challenges of CHG bathing in more mobile and healthy patient populations.

Hospitalized Patients

Hospital Wards

Individuals admitted to acute care hospitals in non-ICU settings still remain at risk for healthcare-associated infections [6]. Since bathing with CHG in the ICUs has been shown to be beneficial in reducing line-related bacteremia [7] as well as colonization with potential pathogens such as MRSA and VRE [5, 8], it begs the question as to whether daily CHG bathing would be effective in patients on general hospital wards. Patients on hospital wards may still have central lines in place (e.g., short-term femoral/internal jugular/subclavian Central venous catheter (CVC), Peripherally inserted central catheter (PICC) lines, and dialysis access) which put them at continued risk for line-associated bloodstream infections. Hospitalized non-ICU patients may undergo invasive procedures such as cardiac catheterizations, paracenteses, and thoracenteses as well as surgery, and therefore "source control" (i.e., reducing potential pathogens on patient skin and thus limiting the opportunity for contamination of healthcare worker hands and the surrounding environment) may be of value. Finally, as healthcare workers' compliance with hand hygiene remains overall poor, enhanced infection control interventions such as CHG bathing may be needed [9].

In a study by Climo et al., the impact of daily CHG bathing on acquisition of multidrug-resistant organisms (MDROs, in this case VRE and MRSA) was examined along with incidence of hospital-acquired bloodstream infections in various ICUs (medical, coronary care, surgical, cardiac surgery) and bone marrow transplant units [5]. Daily CHG

M. Buller
OhioHealth Physician Group-Infectious Diseases,
Columbus, OH, USA
e-mail: Megan.Buller@OhioHealth.com

K.J. Popovich (✉)
Internal Medicine, Infectious Disease, Rush University Medical Center and Stroger Hospital of Cook County,
600 South Paulina Suite 143, Chicago, IL 60612, USA
e-mail: kyle_popovich@rush.edu

© Springer International Publishing AG 2018
G. Bearman et al. (eds.), *Infection Prevention*, DOI 10.1007/978-3-319-60980-5_29

bathing was associated with a significant decline in the acquisition of MDROs and in hospital-acquired bloodstream infections. This finding was most notable for individuals with prolonged lengths of stay in the unit. Frequently non-ICU level patients are hospitalized for extended periods of time as well, providing them more opportunity to develop nosocomial infections. In patients with prolonged hospitalizations, CHG bathing offers an attractive consideration for reducing healthcare-associated infections on hospital wards.

In a study by Kassakian et al. looking at general medicine wards, daily use of CHG bathing resulted in a reduction in the composite outcome of MRSA and VRE healthcare-associated infections in comparison to daily bathing with soap and water; no decrease in *Clostridium difficile* infections was observed [6]. In this before-after study, bathing for both study arms was performed by certified nursing assistants, and there were no direct bathing compliance observations but rather an estimation of compliance by purchasing records. Nonetheless, the results suggest a possible role for CHG bathing on units.

A before-after study by Bass et al. examined daily bathing with 2% CHG-impregnated cloths for patients on a hematology/oncology ward [10]. In this study, patients were given instructions on proper usage of the cloths and then were responsible for self-application. The authors noted a reduction in VRE colonization, but the association did not attain statistical significance. Compliance with cloths was not monitored in this study, making it unclear why a more significant decline in colonization was not observed. Further evaluation of CHG bathing on hospital wards that includes an assessment of patient compliance as well as reasons for noncompliance is needed.

A study by Wendt et al. enrolled MRSA carriers at the University Hospital of Heidelberg (inpatients as well as outpatients) and from surrounding nursing homes and randomized them to receive either 5 days of whole-body washing with 4% CHG solution or placebo (both study arms received nasal mupirocin and oral CHG) [11]. They observed only a reduction in inguinal MRSA colonization; colonization at multiple body sites was associated with eradication failure. Of note, bathing could be performed by a healthcare worker or by the patient (with instructions from study staff), and thus compliance could be a factor in the apparent reduced effectiveness of CHG in this study. However, this study highlights potential patient populations (those with prolonged colonization with MRSA at multiple body sites) where optimal compliance with CHG may be essential for efficacy.

Long-Term Care Facilities

Long-term acute care hospitals (LTACHs) were created in the 1990s to transition stable but ill patients from acute care hospitals to a facility where high-level care and rehabilitation could continue to be provided [12]. More so than nursing homes, LTACHs frequently have ICU-equivalent patients (e.g., patients on ventilators, patients receiving tube feeds, hemodialysis, medications through central lines, specialized wound care), many of them with prolonged lengths of stay. These factors can lead to colonization and infection with MDROs including carbapenem-resistant *Enterobacteriaceae* (CRE) which can be a significant problem in this patient population [9]. LTACHs have been found to be critical components of regional outbreaks and spread of MDROs [13], hence optimization of infection control and prevention in this population is essential.

A study by Munoz-Price et al. used a quasi-experimental design to examine daily 2% CHG bathing in LTACH patients using a pre-intervention, intervention, and post-intervention phase. They observed a significant reduction in CVC-associated bloodstream infections during the intervention period and an increase in infections in the post-intervention period, supporting the efficacy of CHG in this population [12]. Another study by Hayden et al. utilized 2% CHG cloths for bathing of LTACH patients as a component of an infection prevention bundle (including admission and every other week screening for *Klebsiella pneumoniae* carbapenemase [KPC] rectal colonization, cohorting of colonized patients into specific geographic regions, and institution of a hand hygiene improvement campaign) [9]. This bundle was associated with a significant decline in the rate of KPC colonization at multiple body sites (inguinal region, upper back, antecubital fossa, axilla, neck), KPC bacteremia, all-cause bacteremia, and blood culture contamination [9, 14]. However, as this was a study utilizing an infection control bundle, we do not know the individual benefit of CHG bathing for the outcomes measured.

Preoperative Use

Surgical site infections have been identified as one of the most common causes of nosocomial infection, one of the most significant post-operative complications, and reason for increased morbidity and cost to the patient [15]. CHG is not inactivated by blood or serum proteins and has persistent activity following application, making it an ideal agent to reduce bacterial burden preoperatively [3]. Although multiple studies have been done looking at the actual risk reduction in surgical site infection and have failed to demonstrate a statistically significant decrease in the rates of SSI, bathing with CHG is still often used preoperatively [16]. Current CDC recommendations are based on the 1999 *Guideline for Prevention of Surgical Site Infection* which endorses use of preoperative antiseptic shower or bath with chlorhexidine-containing solution (category 1B) given data that CHG significantly reduces skin microbial counts and therefore would theoretically decrease surgical site infections [17].

Outpatients

While MRSA was once typically seen solely in healthcare facilities, over the past 15 years, colonization and infection with MRSA have been observed in community populations, many without prior healthcare exposures (so-called community-associated MRSA or CA-MRSA) [18]. By pulsed-field gel electrophoresis, USA300 has been identified as the most common strain of CA-MRSA [19]. With the emergence of CA-MRSA, several studies have examined the role of CHG outside the healthcare settings. Most infections due to CA-MRSA are skin and skin structure infections (SSTIs) although more serious infections (e.g., bacteremia, necrotizing pneumonia, necrotizing fasciitis) have been reported. Outbreaks of CA-MRSA have been reported in distinct community populations (military recruits, inmates in correctional facilities, amateur and professional athletes) with the common feature of these patient groups being close person-to-person contact, crowded living conditions, suboptimal hygiene, and increased opportunities for skin breakdown [20].

In the inpatient setting, colonization with MRSA has been associated with an increased risk of MRSA infection (up to fourfold over colonization with MSSA in one meta-analysis [21]), and there have been reports of a strong correlation between *S. aureus* strains identified as colonizing the nares later being isolated from the bloodstream of those same patients, supporting endogenous flora as the source of infection [22]. Several outpatient studies have included decolonization as a component of an outpatient infection prevention strategy, particularly in cases where individuals have recurrent SSTIs. Miller et al. recently published data that in a subset of patients with *S. aureus* skin infection at the time of enrollment, not only did >60% have prior skin infection in the year prior to their enrollment, but 51% had reported recurrent, relapsed, or new skin infection at the 6-month follow-up visit [23].

The following sections will take a closer look at studies examining the use of CHG in nonhospital settings and highlight the potential complexities of CHG use in outpatients. However, as outlined in the Infectious Diseases Society of America (IDSA) MRSA treatment guidelines [24], reinforcement of infection control strategies (i.e., early identification of infection, good hand hygiene, adequate wound care, avoidance of shared personal items, washing clothes and towels at appropriate temperature, and avoiding contact sports until healed [20]) is a critical component of control and prevention, and decolonization can be considered when the standard strategies are unsuccessful.

Outpatient Clinics

Chlorhexidine gluconate has been used among outpatients as part of a decolonization regimen for individuals with CA-MRSA infection, particularly recurrent SSTIs. Providers have also used intranasal mupirocin with or without CHG for decolonization, as a way to target nasal colonization with MRSA. There has been increasing evidence, though, that extra-nasal colonization with MRSA may be important, and

therefore inclusion of topical antiseptics that can target relevant extra-nasal sites may be needed. The IDSA clinical practice guidelines for the management of MRSA infections recommend considering a decolonization regimen only after standard infection control practices have been optimized and infection or ongoing transmission is still occurring. In this situation, the guidelines suggest decolonization utilizing intranasal mupirocin with or without topical body decolonization (chlorhexidine, bleach baths) [24]. Decolonization, though, can be transient, and some of these individuals live or work in an environment where they may be at high risk of recolonization. In a study by Doebbeling et al., recurrence of nasal *S. aureus* colonization following 5 days of intranasal mupirocin occurred in 48% of individuals at 6 months and 53% at a year, with 36% of individuals being recolonized with a new strain and 34% with the same strain [25]. In addition, there is concern for the development of mupirocin resistance with widespread use [26, 27].

Military

In the military setting, chlorhexidine bathing may be a useful component of infection control as military personnel (especially recruits in the training phase of their careers) are required to live in close quarters and have higher potential for skin breakdown given rigorous training activities and outdoor exposure and the potential for reduced access to optimal hygiene [2, 28]. All of these factors increase the risk for SSTIs including those due to *S. aureus*. At one military training facility, it was estimated that one in ten recruits would develop a SSTI sometime during their training, with MRSA being the most common organism cultured [29]. In a study of soldiers, Ellis et al. observed that colonization with CA-MRSA significantly increased the chance of subsequent MRSA infection in comparison to methicillin-susceptible *Staphylococcus aureus* (MSSA) infection risk with prior MSSA colonization [30]. The goal of infection control should be focused not only on decreasing individual risk of development of SSTIs in this population, which depending on severity can contribute to significant loss of days and delay in training, but also reducing the person-to-person transmission that can potentially hamper the efficacy of the larger unit [28, 31]. Several studies have examined different strategies incorporating use of CHG-containing wipes or body washes into the military routine, mostly in conjunction with other interventions (e.g., instruction on hygiene, provision of personal soap and first aid kits, and ensuring adequate time for bathing) [2, 28, 29, 31, 32].

Morisson et al. conducted a retrospective observational study to assess the rates of overall SSTIs and MRSA-SSTIs pre- and post-implementation of a facility-wide infection prevention intervention that included the use of 4% chlorhexidine gluconate body wash (upon arrival to the training site and then an additional six times over the 13 weeks of training) in addition to instruction on hand hygiene, provision of soap and first aid kits, and allotment of adequate time for showering [28]. Even though the study is limited by the lack of a control group, they did observe a significant decrease in the incidence of SSTIs and culture-proven MRSA-SSTIs with the intervention.

Whitman et al. conducted a cluster-randomized, double-blind, controlled trial of CHG bathing in military recruits to determine its effects on MRSA colonization and infection [2, 33]. Recruits were randomized into thrice weekly usage of 2% CHG-impregnated cloths vs thrice weekly control cloths. There was no significant difference in rates of SSTI between the two groups, and the overall rates of nasal carriage of *S. aureus* increased from study initiation, although to a lesser extent in the CHG group. Incidence of colonization with MRSA in the CHG group was half that of the non-CHG group (2.6% vs. 6%, $P = 0.03$) [2]. Within the subset of those recruits who acquired MRSA, there was significantly less acquisition of USA300 strains in the CHG group in comparison to the control group, suggesting that CHG may have led to reduced USA300 MRSA transmission during the study [33]. One of the major limitations of this study was the relatively poor self-reported adherence with CHG cloths. Poor adherence, in addition to factors such as inability to ensure proper application technique and impact of sweating and frequent showering on duration of antimicrobial effect of CHG wipes (even with optimal use) make it difficult to assess the efficacy of the wipes themselves as well as ideal interval of use. Nevertheless, this study highlights a potential role for CHG in this population but demonstrates the many challenges with CHG bathing among outpatients [2, 32].

In a separate analysis, Ellis et al. examined rates of SSTI and MRSA-SSTI in US Army trainees randomized to standard hygiene education arm, enhanced standard hygiene education plus first aid kit arm, and once weekly CHG 4% body wash plus enhanced standard education arm [29]. The authors were unable to show a significant decrease in the rate of SSTI or culture-confirmed MRSA-SSTI between the study groups; however, CHG was used only weekly in this study which may account for the observed lack of benefit.

It remains unclear what the optimal frequency of bathing with CHG is for the military population, although as the studies highlight there are potentially logistical issues with daily CHG use. These studies also demonstrate that adherence with CHG bathing may be more challenging with a larger, healthier, and more mobile population.

Correctional Facilities

Detainees in correctional facilities are also at risk for CA-MRSA due to overcrowding, increased opportunity for skin abrasions, and reduced opportunity for optimal hygiene and infection control practices [34]. Several outbreaks in both jails (characterized by shorter-term stays and high turnover) and prisons (long-term stay) have been reported. Three of the largest documented outbreaks occurred in correctional facilities in Georgia (state detention center, prison, and county jail), California (county jail system), and Texas (Texas Department of Criminal Justice) [34]. During investigations of these outbreaks [34], lapses in basic infection prevention measures were identified including limited access to soap for handwashing and bathing, inappropriate laundry machine temperatures, and inadequate wound care. Included in the intervention during the outbreak at the Georgia detention center were daily CHG baths (body wash; percent CHG was not defined) for all inmates in conjunction with increased access to hand soap, education on skin and hand hygiene, provision of wound care supplies, and instruction on proper wound care [35]. Antibiotic treatment and 5 days of intranasal mupirocin were provided to inmates who had active infection (abscess or "MRSA skin infection"). No further MRSA infections were diagnosed in the subsequent post-intervention period (a time frame of 11.5 weeks).

A randomized controlled trial by David et al. evaluated the impact of bathing with 2% CHG cloths on the rates of *S. aureus* carriage in the nares and hands of inmates in a jail in Dallas, Texas [36]. There were three study arms: (1) thrice weekly bathing with 2% CHG cloths, (2) thrice weekly bathing with water-containing cloths, and (3) no skin treatment. While the authors did observe a significant decrease in overall *S. aureus* carriage, there was no significant difference in MRSA colonization when compared to the use of water-soaked, non-CHG wipes. Although this study reported relatively high adherence to the recommended intervention, there was no direct observation on how well the participants applied the wipes, and it remains unclear if thrice weekly bathing in this study setting is enough. This study also highlights the significant challenges in studies done outside of the healthcare settings; some inmates changed locations during the study which then assigned them to different study arms, and merging of certain jail units affected exposures. Nevertheless, given the overcrowding of correctional facilities and the reported association of incarceration exposure and MRSA, interventions such as the ones performed in this study warrant further investigation.

Athletes: Amateur and Professional

In 2003, an outbreak of MRSA-SSTI was reported in the St. Louis Rams professional football team [37]. The subsequent investigation revealed USA300 as the predominant strain in the outbreak. High-contact sports such as football, rugby, wrestling, and fencing are identified as activities with increased risk for MRSA outbreaks among participants [38] and thus potential targets for enhanced infection control and prevention strategies. Sports such as these are associated with increased opportunity for skin breakdown as well as close person-to-person contact. Team sports can be associated with injuries (due to falls and equipment), as well as sharing of sporting equipment, towels, and whirlpools, which may also increase the risk for MRSA infection [39].

American football is the most studied of all of these sports, with outbreaks at the high school through the professional level reported. In one study of high school football players, incision and drainage were performed on 18 of 21 lesions, and 4 of 13 players required hospitalization for IV antibiotics [40]. Outbreaks of MRSA at the collegiate level also demonstrated high numbers of affected athletes requiring incision and drainage and even hospital admission for further management [41, 42]. In these outbreaks, often the most common cause of SSTI has been USA300 MRSA [38, 40–42].

In several of the outbreak investigations of athletic teams, MRSA was rarely isolated from nasal colonization surveillance swabs of individuals with infection [41, 42], making it unclear if extra-nasal MRSA colonization played a role in infection or if infections were due to a "hit and run" by virulent MRSA strains [43]. From outbreak investigations of football players, the following risk factors were associated with increased relative risk for infection: turf abrasions, body shaving, and playing certain positions (lineman or linebacker in the Rams outbreak, cornerback or wide receiver in the outbreak at a Connecticut university) [37, 41, 42]. During the outbreak investigation for the St. Louis Rams, they also found that members of opposing teams had developed abscesses with the same strain of MRSA (USA300 MRSA), suggesting person-to-person transmission during their matchup [37]. As seen with the other outbreaks mentioned in this chapter, lapses in team hygiene were noted; trainers lacked access to regular hand hygiene products, towels were shared among team members, there was lack of showering prior to whirlpool use, and infrequent cleansing of weight room and therapy equipment was also documented. Implementation of various hygiene processes (i.e., provided soap dispensers for routine handwashing, appropriate wound care, active surveillance for infection, requiring players to shower before whirlpool use, and restricting case patients with active infection from play until wounds were healed) occurred in response to several of the reported outbreaks [37, 42]. It is unknown if CHG bathing could be utilized in high-risk sports settings for infection prevention.

Challenges

As evidenced by the studies discussed, there are many challenges to both studying and even implementing use of chlorhexidine in various non-ICU setting. Many reference adherence as one of the main limitations to their studies,

while ability to perform the recommended procedures, access to necessary supplies, and concern for use of incompatible products are other identified areas where real-life implementation may be difficult.

Adherence and Technique

Studies have suggested that to gain maximal effect from CHG body-cleansing products (i.e., skin concentrations high enough to kill significant pathogens), washing with the right amount of force for the right duration of time is likely required [44]. The LTACH study by Lin et al. demonstrated the small subset of patients who were bathed with proper technique had much higher CHG skin concentrations and better elimination of KPC from difficult-to-treat body sites [14].

Some pre-operative providers use instructional forms on how to use the product and allow patients to affix stickers documenting use [16]. Studies have also looked at the use of electronic alerts to remind patients to perform their preoperative bathing and found higher composite levels of CHG on the skin in patients who received alerts, which was suggestive of increased compliance in that group [45].

Avoidance of Incompatible Products

Many commercially available lotions and skincare products can cause reduced activity of chlorhexidine gluconate [46], and concomitant use of these products is discouraged. On hospital wards, staff can be encouraged to monitor patients for use of these products and provide appropriate replacements. In nonhospital settings practitioners would need to educate patients on limiting the use of products that reduce CHG activity although compliance with this would be more challenging to measure.

Concerns with CHG Resistance

With increased use of CHG in ICUs, there has been concern about development of resistance. There is no defined CLSI breakpoint for CHG, making determination of resistance difficult. The $qacA$ and $qacB$ genes (encode for efflux pumps) found in $S.$ $aureus$ have been seen associated with higher CHG MICs (minimum inhibitory concentration) and MBCs (minimum bactericidal concentration) and have been proposed as a cause of decolonization failure although this has not been widely demonstrated [47]. Of greater concern is potential for decreased susceptibility to CHG in gram-negative organisms as they have inherently higher MICs to CHG than gram positives [48]. CHG skin concentrations that have been measured on patients following appropriate application of CHG-containing products still greatly surpass the MICs for both gram-positive as well as gram-negative organisms, so the true significance of high MICs is not well defined [1, 47, 48]. In the REDUCE MRSA trial where isolates from several ICUs across multiple hospitals were analyzed, resistance to CHG as detected by qacA/qacB carriage and MIC was infrequent [49]. So far, it appears that resistance to CHG is relatively rare, but as usage continues to increase, it is essential that we continue to monitor for emergence of resistant organisms.

Conclusion

Several studies have documented the effectiveness of CHG in ICU populations. However, there may be at-risk groups of patients outside of the ICU—both in the hospital and in community settings—that may benefit from CHG bathing. There are increased challenges in implementing CHG bathing in non-ICU populations, and it is unclear what the optimal frequency of use is when CHG is utilized in congregate living populations (i.e., individuals in correctional facilities or those in the military). As drug-resistant pathogens continue to be of increased significance not only in the hospital but also in community settings, enhanced infection control strategies such as CHG bathing may be of value. Resistance to CHG has so far been infrequent, and CHG itself is largely well tolerated, making it an attractive option for infection prevention and control. Future studies need to understand why compliance with CHG is often challenging in certain outpatient populations and why some prior investigations failed to see the same beneficial effects with CHG used that has been seen in the ICU. While we conduct these studies, though, simple infection control measures such as hand hygiene, proper wound care, and antibiotic stewardship need to be reinforced in both community and hospital settings.

References

1. Milstone AM, Passaretti CL, Perl TM. Chlorhexidine: expanding the armamentarium for infection control and prevention. Clin Infect Dis. 2008;46(2):274–81.
2. Whitman TJ, Herlihy RK, Schlett CD, et al. Chlorhexidine-impregnated cloths to prevent skin and soft-tissue infection in marine recruits: a cluster-randomized, double-blind, controlled effectiveness trial. Infect Control Hosp Epidemiol. 2010;31(12):1207–15.
3. Edmiston CE Jr, Krepel CJ, Seabrook GR, Lewis BD, Brown KR, Towne JB. Preoperative shower revisited: can high topical antiseptic levels be achieved on the skin surface before surgical admission? J Am Coll Surg. 2008;207(2):233–9.
4. Vernon MO, Hayden MK, Trick WE, et al. Chlorhexidine gluconate to cleanse patients in a medical intensive care unit: the effectiveness of source control to reduce the bioburden of vancomycin-resistant enterococci. Arch Intern Med. 2006;166(3):306–12.
5. Climo MW, Yokoe DS, Warren DK, et al. Effect of daily chlorhexidine bathing on hospital-acquired infection. N Engl J Med. 2013;368(6):533–42.
6. Kassakian SZ, Mermel LA, Jefferson JA, Parenteau SL, Machan JT. Impact of chlorhexidine bathing on hospital-acquired infections among general medical patients. Infect Control Hosp Epidemiol. 2011;32(3):238–43.
7. Popovich KJ, Hota B, Hayes R, Weinstein RA, Hayden MK. Effectiveness of routine patient cleansing with chlorhexidine gluconate for infection prevention in the medical intensive care unit. Infect Control Hosp Epidemiol. 2009;30(10):959–63.
8. Rupp ME, Cavalieri RJ, Lyden E, et al. Effect of hospital-wide chlorhexidine patient bathing on healthcare-associated infections. Infect Control Hosp Epidemiol. 2012;33(11):1094–100.
9. Hayden MK, Lin MY, Lolans K, et al. Prevention of colonization and infection by klebsiella pneumoniae carbapenemase-producing enterobacteriaceae in long-term acute-care hospitals. Clin Infect Dis. 2015;60(8):1153–61.
10. Bass P, Karki S, Rhodes D, et al. Impact of chlorhexidine-impregnated washcloths on reducing incidence of vancomycin-resistant enterococci colonization in hematology-oncology patients. Am J Infect Control. 2013;41(4):345–8.
11. Wendt C, Schinke S, Wurttemberger M, Oberdorfer K, Bock-Hensley O, von Baum H. Value of whole-body washing with chlorhexidine for the eradication of methicillin-resistant staphylococcus aureus: a randomized, placebo-controlled, double-blind clinical trial. Infect Control Hosp Epidemiol. 2007;28(9):1036–43.
12. Munoz-Price LS, Hota B, Stemer A, Weinstein RA. Prevention of bloodstream infections by use of daily chlorhexidine baths for patients at a long-term acute care hospital. Infect Control Hosp Epidemiol. 2009;30(11):1031–5.
13. Won SY, Munoz-Price LS, Lolans K, et al. Emergence and rapid regional spread of klebsiella pneumoniae Carbapenemase–producing enterobacteriaceae. Clin Infect Dis. 2011;53(6):532–40.
14. Lin MY, Lolans K, Blom DW, et al. The effectiveness of routine daily chlorhexidine gluconate bathing in reducing klebsiella pneumoniae carbapenemase-producing enterobacteriaceae skin burden among long-term acute care hospital patients. Infect Control Hosp Epidemiol. 2014;35(4):440–2.
15. Webster J, Osborne S. Preoperative bathing or showering with skin antiseptics to prevent surgical site infection. Cochrane Database Syst Rev. 2015;2:CD004985.
16. Edmiston CE Jr, Bruden B, Rucinski MC, Henen C, Graham MB, Lewis BL. Reducing the risk of surgical site infections: does chlorhexidine gluconate provide a risk reduction benefit? Am J Infect Control. 2013;41(5 Suppl):S49–55.
17. Mangram AJ, Horan TC, Pearson ML, Silver LC, Jarvis WR. Guideline for prevention of surgical site infection, 1999. Hospital infection control practices advisory committee. Infect Control Hosp Epidemiol. 1999;20(4):250–78. quiz 279–80
18. Fridkin SK, Hageman JC, Morrison M, et al. Methicillin-resistant staphylococcus aureus disease in three communities. N Engl J Med. 2005;352(14):1436–44.
19. McDougal LK, Steward CD, Killgore GE, Chaitram JM, McAllister SK, Tenover FC. Pulsed-field gel electrophoresis typing of oxacillin-resistant staphylococcus aureus isolates from the united states: establishing a national database. J Clin Microbiol. 2003;41(11):5113–20.
20. Popovich KJ, Hota B, Weinstein RA. Treatment of community-associated methicillin-resistant staphylococcus aureus. Curr Infect Dis Rep. 2008;10(5):411–20.
21. Safdar N, Bradley EA. The risk of infection after nasal colonization with staphylococcus aureus. Am J Med. 2008;121(4):310–5.
22. von Eiff C, Becker K, Machka K, Stammer H, Peters G. Nasal carriage as a source of staphylococcus aureus bacteremia. Study group. N Engl J Med. 2001;344(1):11–6.

23. Miller LG, Eells SJ, David MZ, et al. Staphylococcus aureus skin infection recurrences among household members: an examination of host, behavioral, and pathogen-level predictors. Clin Infect Dis. 2015;60(5):753–63.

24. Liu C, Bayer A, Cosgrove SE, et al. Clinical practice guidelines by the infectious diseases society of america for the treatment of methicillin-resistant staphylococcus aureus infections in adults and children. Clin Infect Dis. 2011;52(3):e18–55.

25. Doebbeling BN, Reagan DR, Pfaller MA, Houston AK, Hollis RJ, Wenzel RP. Long-term efficacy of intranasal mupirocin ointment. A prospective cohort study of staphylococcus aureus carriage. Arch Intern Med. 1994;154(13):1505–8.

26. Fritz SA, Hogan PG, Camins BC, et al. Mupirocin and chlorhexidine resistance in staphylococcus aureus in patients with community-onset skin and soft tissue infections. Antimicrob Agents Chemother. 2013;57(1):559–68.

27. Septimus EJ, Schweizer ML. Decolonization in prevention of health care-associated infections. Clin Microbiol Rev. 2016;29(2):201–22.

28. Morrison SM, Blaesing CR, Millar EV, et al. Evaluation of methicillin-resistant staphylococcus aureus skin and soft-tissue infection prevention strategies at a military training center. Infect Control Hosp Epidemiol. 2013;34(8):841–3.

29. Ellis MW, Schlett CD, Millar EV, et al. Hygiene strategies to prevent methicillin-resistant staphylococcus aureus skin and soft tissue infections: a cluster-randomized controlled trial among high-risk military trainees. Clin Infect Dis. 2014;58(11):1540–8.

30. Ellis MW, Hospenthal DR, Dooley DP, Gray PJ, Murray CK. Natural history of community-acquired methicillin-resistant staphylococcus aureus colonization and infection in soldiers. Clin Infect Dis. 2004;39(7):971–9.

31. Millar EV, Chen WJ, Schlett CD, et al. Frequent use of chlorhexidine-based body wash associated with a reduction in methicillin-resistant staphylococcus aureus nasal colonization among military trainees. Antimicrob Agents Chemother. 2015;59(2):943–9.

32. Popovich KJ. Lessons from a community-based infection prevention study. Infect Control Hosp Epidemiol. 2010;31(12):1216–8.

33. Whitman TJ, Schlett CD, Grandits GA, et al. Chlorhexidine gluconate reduces transmission of methicillin-resistant staphylococcus aureus USA300 among marine recruits. Infect Control Hosp Epidemiol. 2012;33(8):809–16.

34. Centers for Disease Control and Prevention (CDC). Methicillin-resistant staphylococcus aureus infections in correctional facilities – georgia, california, and texas, 2001–2003. MMWR Morb Mortal Wkly Rep. 2003;52(41):992–6.

35. Wootton SH, Arnold K, Hill HA, et al. Intervention to reduce the incidence of methicillin-resistant staphylococcus aureus skin infections in a correctional facility in georgia. Infect Control Hosp Epidemiol. 2004;25(5):402–7.

36. David MZ, Siegel JD, Henderson J, et al. A randomized, controlled trial of chlorhexidine-soaked cloths to reduce methicillin-resistant and methicillin-susceptible staphylococcus aureus carriage prevalence in an urban jail. Infect Control Hosp Epidemiol. 2014;35(12):1466–73.

37. Kazakova SV, Hageman JC, Matava M, et al. A clone of methicillin-resistant staphylococcus aureus among professional football players. N Engl J Med. 2005;352(5):468–75.

38. Centers for Disease Control and Prevention (CDC). Methicillin-resistant staphylococcus aureus infections among competitive sports participants – colorado, indiana, pennsylvania, and los angeles county, 2000–2003. MMWR Morb Mortal Wkly Rep. 2003;52(33):793–5.

39. Weber JT. Community-associated methicillin-resistant staphylococcus aureus. Clin Infect Dis. 2005;41(Suppl 4):S269–72.

40. Rihn JA, Posfay-Barbe K, Harner CD, et al. Community-acquired methicillin-resistant staphylococcus aureus outbreak in a local high school football team unsuccessful interventions. Pediatr Infect Dis J. 2005;24(9):841–3.

41. Bowers AL, Huffman GR, Sennett BJ. Methicillin-resistant staphylococcus aureus infections in collegiate football players. Med Sci Sports Exerc. 2008;40(8):1362–7.

42. Begier EM, Frenette K, Barrett NL, et al. A high-morbidity outbreak of methicillin-resistant staphylococcus aureus among players on a college football team, facilitated by cosmetic body shaving and turf burns. Clin Infect Dis. 2004;39(10):1446–53.

43. Hota B, Ellenbogen C, Hayden MK, Aroutcheva A, Rice TW, Weinstein RA. Community-associated methicillin-resistant staphylococcus aureus skin and soft tissue infections at a public hospital: do public housing and incarceration amplify transmission? Arch Intern Med. 2007;167(10):1026–33.

44. Popovich KJ, Lyles R, Hayes R, et al. Relationship between chlorhexidine gluconate skin concentration and microbial density on the skin of critically ill patients bathed daily with chlorhexidine gluconate. Infect Control Hosp Epidemiol. 2012;33(9):889–96.

45. Edmiston CE Jr, Krepel CJ, Edmiston SE, et al. Empowering the surgical patient: a randomized, prospective analysis of an innovative strategy for improving patient compliance with preadmission showering protocol. J Am Coll Surg. 2014;219(2):256–64.

46. What the Experts Say: Chlorhexidine Gluconate (CHG) skin preps: Benefits and Compatibility. Sage Products website. http://www.sageproducts.com/education/pdf/20785.pdf. Accessed 2 Apr 2016.

47. McDanel JS, Murphy CR, Diekema DJ, et al. Chlorhexidine and mupirocin susceptibilities of methicillin-resistant staphylococcus aureus from colonized nursing home residents. Antimicrob Agents Chemother. 2013;57(1):552–8.

48. Naparstek L, Carmeli Y, Chmelnitsky I, Banin E, Navon-Venezia S. Reduced susceptibility to chlorhexidine among extremely-drug-resistant strains of klebsiella pneumoniae. J Hosp Infect. 2012;81(1):15–9.

49. Lolans K, Haffenreffer K, Avery T, et al. 636Chlorhexidine (CHG) and mupirocin susceptibility of methicillin-resistant staphylococcus aureus (MRSA) isolates in the REDUCE-MRSA trial. Open Forum Infect Dis. 2014;1(Suppl 1):S30–S31.0l.

Pranavi V. Sreeramoju and Jose Cadena

Standard precautions including hand hygiene and proper use of personal protective equipment, as well as isolation precautions, are foundational strategies to prevent transmission of pathogens in hospitals and other healthcare settings. The common types of isolation precautions, based on known or suspected modes of transmission, are contact, droplet, and airborne isolation. Airborne isolation, in contrast to droplet isolation, is intended to break the chain of transmission of pathogens carried in aerosol particles less than 5 μ in size [1]. The term respiratory isolation is confusing as it may be used to mean droplet or airborne isolation, and we recommend against the use of this term. The pathogens transmitted via airborne route are tuberculosis (TB), varicella, measles, severe acute respiratory syndrome coronavirus (SARS-CoV), Middle East respiratory syndrome coronavirus (MERS-CoV), hemorrhagic fever viruses such as Ebola, and highly pathogenic avian influenza viruses such as H5N1 and H7N9 [2]. Airborne isolation is also employed for novel and emerging pathogens whose transmission is unknown. In contrast, droplet isolation is used for pathogens/diseases such as diphtheria, epiglottitis, or meningitis for the first 24 h of treatment, and pertussis and influenza [1].

P.V. Sreeramoju (✉)
Internal Medicine-Infectious Diseases, UT Southwestern Medical Center, 5323 Harry Hines Blvd, Dallas, TX 75390, USA
e-mail: Pranavi.Sreeramoju@UTSouthwestern.edu

J. Cadena
Medicine/Infectious Diseases, University of Texas Health Science at San Antonio and South Texas Veterans Healthcare System, San Antonio, TX, USA
e-mail: CADENAZULUAG@uthscsa.edu

Airborne Isolation Precautions and Personal Protective Equipment

Airborne transmission can be classified into obligate (under natural conditions, transmission occurs only through the airborne route, e.g., *Mycobacterium tuberculosis*), preferential (multiple transmission routes are possible, but small particle inhalation is the most common route, e.g., influenza, MERS-CoV, SARS-CoV), and opportunistic (infection usually occurs through other routes but may occur through small particles under special circumstances, e.g., *Legionella*) [1].

The three major components of airborne isolation precautions as a strategy for reducing transmission of aerosol transmissible diseases are (1) physical space and engineering controls, (2) healthcare personnel respiratory protection and personal protective equipment, and (3) clinical protocols, policies, procedures, and regulatory considerations.

Physical Space and Engineering Controls

Because aerosol particles remain suspended in air, pathogens transmitted via airborne route can spread across hospital floors and across long distances. Therefore, physical space and engineering controls such as proper ventilation; air handling including air exchanges and air flow management, i.e., negative pressure air flow; and high-efficiency particulate filtration are the cornerstone for preventing airborne transmission. Measures such as ultraviolet lights are also effective when used as an adjunct. Portable HEPA filters can also be used in certain situations. When combined with appropriate use of respiratory protection, airborne transmission can be prevented effectively. Physical space controls gained particular importance in recent years as research into transmission of emerging pathogens such as coronaviruses (MERS and SARS) and influenza viruses (e.g., highly pathogenic

© Springer International Publishing AG 2018
G. Bearman et al. (eds.), *Infection Prevention*, DOI 10.1007/978-3-319-60980-5_30

avian influenza) identified potential for airborne transmission. A complete discussion of physical space and engineering controls is beyond the scope of this chapter.

Personal Protective Equipment and Healthcare Personnel Respiratory Protection

Respiratory protection against infectious airborne and droplet particles is an important part of the occupational safety of workers in healthcare settings. Some infections can be transmitted through the airborne route, where an infectious patient produces small particles, <5 μm, which are neutrally buoyant and can remain suspended in the air for prolonged periods of time, traveling relatively long distances, and are inhaled by a susceptible individual, reaching the alveolar tissue, and potentially leading to the transmission. This has been observed in Canada during the SARS epidemic (42% of cases were in HCW and resulted from transmission from patients), in New York during the surge of HIV-related TB transmission, and MERS-CoV in the Arabian Peninsula, all of which led to a significant infection rate of healthcare workers [2, 3].

The most important piece of personal protective equipment to prevent infection from airborne pathogens is a respirator. In addition to prevention of airborne transmission of pathogens, these respirators are also used for protection against chemical, radiological, and nuclear materials [4]. The discussion in this chapter will be limited to respiratory protection against infectious pathogens.

It is important to understand the different levels of protection offered by different types of equipment. Face masks are not considered respiratory protection as they are usually designed to protect from large particles and not smaller aerosol particles [4].

Respirators are classified based on specific factors as follows [5, 6]:

1. By air supply: Air-purifying respirators which remove contaminants and pathogens from the air one breathes and air-supplying respirators which provide clean air from an uncontaminated surface.
2. By whether they require a tight seal between respirator and the wearer's face and/or neck: Tight fitting and loose fitting. The tight-fitting respirators need a tight seal between the face and the respirator. Employers who require tight-fitting respirators to be worn in the workplace are required to have respirator fit testing programs in place.
3. By power requirement: Non-powered or powered. All air-supplying respirators are powered, while air-purifying respirators may be powered or non-powered.
4. By type of facepiece: Half mask facepiece respirator that covers the nose and mouth or a full facepiece respirator that covers the nose, mouth, and eyes.

5. By reusability: Disposable or reusable (elastomeric – they have replaceable filters or cartridges, and the surface can be cleaned).
6. By splash protection: Surgical respirators which have surgical mask material on the outside to protect the wearer from splashes (e.g., surgical N95 respirators) vs. medical respirators.
7. By pressure type: Negative pressure (commonest type) which is tight fitting and generates negative pressure inside the facepiece relative to ambient air or positive pressure respirator which is used in an airplane to supply oxygen.

The commonly used N95 respirator (Figs. 30.1 and 30.2.) is a negative pressure, non-powered, air-purifying, particulate, tight-fitting, disposable respirator which may be a medical or surgical (have surgical mask material on the outside to protect the wearer from splashes) respirator. It is also called the N95 mask or dust mask. It is useful to know that particulate respirators are classified as not resistant to oil, N; resistant to oil, R; or oil proof, P. Depending on percent filter efficiency of the air particles they filter, they are designated as 95, 99, or 100, thus resulting in nine classes of non-powered air-purifying particulate filters. An air-purifying respirator can have an air-purifying filter, cartridge, or canister, and it can have a quarter mask facepiece, half mask facepiece, or a full mask facepiece. Powered air-purifying respirators (PAPRs) use a blower to force ambient air through air-purifying elements and then

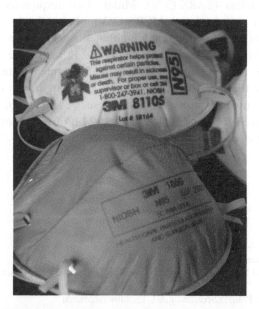

Fig. 30.1 Picture of N95 respirator masks or respirators. This image depicts a still life composed of two N95-type face masks, or respirators, at left, one turquoise (foreground), the other white. The N95 respirator works as an air-purifying respirator (APR), also known as a filtering facepiece respirator, and is certified by the National Institute for Occupational Safety and Health (NIOSH). Content providers(s): CDC/Debora Cartagena; this image is in the public domain and thus free of any copyright restrictions (Image accessed on 3/17/2017 at URL https://phil.cdc.gov/phil/home.asp)

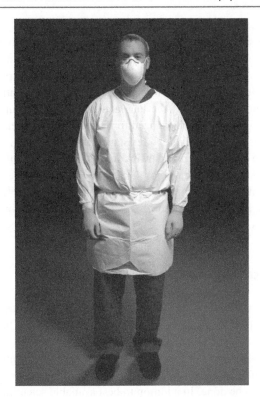

Fig. 30.2 Powered air-purifying respirator. This image depicts a right lateral view of a laboratory technician wearing garments usually worn by field techs, including a disposable white coverall, a disposable plastic apron, head covering, latex gloves, and foot coverings, and is equipped with what is known as a 3 M™ Breathe Easy™ Powered Air Purifying Respirator, PAPR. Content providers(s): CDC/Dr. Todd Parker; this image is in the public domain and thus free of any copyright restrictions (Image accessed on 3/17/2017 at URL https://phil.cdc.gov/phil/home.asp)

through tubing into a hood or helmet. Parts of a PAPR are a half or full facepiece, hood, or helmet, a breathing tube, a canister or cartridge with filter, and a blower. They may be able to provide additional protection compared to the usual N95 respirators if P100 filters are used, because they filter 99.7% of particles 0.3 μm in diameter and provide full face and neck protection including eyes and ears. Others such as supplied air respirators (as in airlines) or the self-contained breathing apparatus (SCBA) such as those used by divers are rarely necessary for a hospital respiratory protection program or pandemic preparedness. The reader is encouraged to look up resources from CDC, NIOSH, and OSHA [4–6] for a more detailed description of the different types of respirators. The respirator classes are given an assigned protection factor value which is applicable when the respirators are properly selected and used in compliance with the OSHA Respiratory Protection standard (29 CFR 1910.134), with properly selected filters or canisters, as needed. A higher APF value is expected to provide greater respiratory protection to employees. For example, a common N95 respirator has an APF of 5, a full facepiece PAPR has an APF of 1,000, and a full facepiece SCBA has an APF of 10,000 [6].

The minimum respiratory protection required is an N95 respirator for routine patient care and aerosol-generating procedures in patients with diseases requiring airborne precautions, viral hemorrhagic fever, and possibly for emerging novel pathogens and pandemic influenza. This minimum respiratory protection is also required for aerosol-generating procedures in patients with seasonal influenza and droplet precautions. PAPRs used by first receivers need to be the most protective type of PAPR equipped with a filter and chemical cartridge. Surgical respirators (without exhalation valves) should be selected for use in environments where a sterile field is needed. The CDC isolation guidelines recommend the use of N95 masks (able to filter 95% or more of the particles <5 μm in size, as well as larger particles) or powered air-purifying respirator (PAPR) [1]. The World Health Organization has similar guidelines for protection of healthcare workers facing acute respiratory illnesses of concern such as SARS [7].

PAPRs are used not only in healthcare but in many other industries.

Pros and Cons of PAPRs

PAPRs do not require fit testing and are not affected by facial hair. They have a higher assigned protection factor and therefore useful in high-hazard situations. Patients can see the wearer's face, and they are easier for communication than an N95 respirator. Reusable respiratory protection equipment has advantages when dealing with pandemic events of potential airborne transmission (such as pandemic influenza or spread of coronavirus such as MERS). In the setting of a pandemic, it is likely that a very large volume of disposable N95 masks would be required to provide protection to every healthcare worker (including not only physicians and nurses but also any other individual, paid or not, who may share air space with individuals with potentially infections transmitted through the airborne route). In these situations, reusable equipment may be more advantageous. They have the disadvantages of being heavy to wear, interfering with stethoscope use, being noisy and sometimes making communication difficult, needing batteries or electricity, and potential for contamination with infectious material, thereby requiring decontamination and reprocessing between uses [8]. There are also theoretical concerns about how PAPRs may affect the wearer's performance. Some of this data comes from nonmedical use of respirators. Visual acuity may decrease, up to 75% in some reports, and visual range may be diminished. More concerning is the potential impact on steadiness and even cognitive impairment (although most studies have failed to prove this) during use due to thermal burden (when temperature rises over 85 °F, there is decreased reaction time, and this correlates with unsafe work behaviors) especially in hot environments [9–12]. A study performed by AlGhamri et al. [13] found no cognitive impairment in individuals using N95 or PAPRs while performing predetermined tasks but found a negative effect in cognitive function when using negative pressure, full-face respirators. This study was limited by a small sample size and the lack of experience with respirator use by many of the studied subjects. A previous study showed that the use of a PAPR was associated with a potential decline in speech intelligibility, but this did not reach statistical significance when compared to other respiratory protection equipment or no respiratory protection at all. Even though full-face PAPRs do not require fit testing, they need to be properly size fitted. PAPRs are not exempt from limitations in their capacity to protect individuals when they are not properly size fitted. Gao et al. evaluated the level of protection provided by a PAPR in manikins, using different sizes of full-face masks. They found decreased protection when the manikins were not fitted with a properly sized full-face mask [12].

Baracco et al. developed a model to evaluate the cost of three options for respiratory protection requiring airborne isolation in the setting of a severe airborne pandemic event [14]. They compared the cost of stockpiling N95 masks, PAPRs, and reusable elastomeric half-face respirator. They took into account the storage space required, the half-life of the equipment, and the maintenance required, in the setting of a massive event requiring about six million contacts per one million population during the pandemic event. They based their model on assumptions derived from the 1918 influenza pandemic event. They found that the cost of stockpiling PAPRs is likely to be higher than the stockpiling of N95 masks, given the need not only of storage but also maintenance and battery care. Most batteries lose charging capacity over time and need to be replaced. Disposable batteries usually have a longer half-life, but only 10 h of battery life, and are more expensive. These batteries are usually made for the equipment, and regular batteries are not usually utilized. PAPRs need a larger storing area, need to be cleaned between uses, and the batteries expire, requiring battery recharging stations within reasonable access from the patient care areas. They are also more expensive, with each PAPR causing upwards of $1000.

Pros and Cons of N95 Respirators

N95 masks work for most people and have the advantage of being disposable. The disadvantages are that they need respiratory fit testing annually in addition to the costs of storing. They are also not suitable for those with beards and those who have undergone facial surgery. The cost of mask fit testing is $18–20 per person using qualitative method. The cost of each mask is $0.73. For an organization that needs to fit test 5000 persons per year, the direct costs would be close to $100,000 per year. According to Susan Johnson, "The sheer number of staff who must be fitted (>8000 annually) is a challenge" [15].

Advantages of the N95 mask include that they allow the use of stethoscopes, are easily available, are inexpensive, and allow for better communication. Disadvantages of N95 include the need for periodic fitting, risk of decreased protection with inappropriate fitting or facial hair, accumulation of moisture, exposure of the face and neck, need to purchase masks on different sizes, need for frequent replacement, and decreased tolerance due to resistance when breathing.

The cost of N95 masks was composed in 25–40% of long-term warehouse storage costs. In addition, many studies omit the costs of N95 issuing and training on their use. Table 30.1 highlights the key differences between N95 respirators and PAPRs.

Clinical Protocols, Policies, and Procedures

Robust clinical protocols, policies, and procedures are necessary to manage airborne infectious diseases in any healthcare facility. Clinical protocols need to be based on best available scientific evidence. While policies offer guiding principles, procedures offer step by step direction on what needs to be done. In addition to best available scientific evidence, regulatory considerations need to be factored in during the development of policies and procedures. The facility plan for managing highly communicable emerging infectious diseases needs to include an incident command structure, policies, screening and signage, triage and plan for inpatient care, staff training, availability supplies, storage, and maintenance. The plan must detail methods for controlling exposure to aerosol transmissible pathogens are airborne isolation to minimize the number of employees exposed, minimize the amount of infectious aerosol in the air through placement of mask on a patient and use of closed suctioning systems to minimize dispersion of aerosol, and protecting employees who must be exposed through vaccination if available, and use of personal protective equipment.

Regulatory Standards

Regulatory standards for respiratory protection are mostly set by the Occupational Safety and Health Administration (OSHA) [6, 16]. The OSHA standard 29 CFR 1910.134 requires that employers establish and maintain a respiratory protection program for workplaces in which workers may be exposed to respiratory hazards, and respiratory protection is used as an exposure control method. The OSHA recommends a hierarchy of controls – prevention or substitution, engineering controls, administrative controls and work practices, and, lastly, respiratory protection/personal protective equipment. One of the OSHA requirements is that the employer makes available respiratory protection gear in any

Table 30.1 Considerations and controversies regarding the use of N95 respirators vs. PAPRS for respiratory protection in healthcare settings

	N95 respirator	PAPR
Cost and preparedness	*Advantages:*	*Advantages:*
	• Disposable	• Does not need fit testing program
	• Lower cost of stockpiling	
	Disadvantages:	*Disadvantages:*
	• Needs fit testing program	• Needs power supply/battery chargers
	• Need to purchase different sizes – cost of fitting	• Units can be expensive (>$1000 per piece)
	• Large volumes of disposable N95 masks may be required during pandemic	• Needs maintenance, which can be expensive
	• Cost of storage given volume	• Need to be properly size fitted, although no formal fitting program is required
		• Need disinfection and cleaning between uses
Training	Requires training	Needs special training
		Disadvantage:
		• May increase body temperature
Contraindications for use	*Disadvantages:*	*Advantage:*
	• Decreased protection with facial hair	• Can be used with facial hair
	• Decreased protection with increased moisture	
	• Not suitable for people with some facial surgeries	
Issues during use	*Advantages:*	*Advantages:*
	• Does not interfere with stethoscope use	• Faces are visible
	• Not heavy	• Reusable
	Disadvantages:	*Disadvantages:*
	• Face may not be visible	• Interferes with stethoscope use
	• Can impair communication	• Heavy to wear
	• Appropriateness of fitting may change with weight changes and facial hair	• Can impair communications
	• Exposure of the face and neck, with limited protection of mucous membranes	• Can affect performance of the wearer, decreasing visual acuity
	• Need for frequent replacement	• Additional protection, including coverage of mucous membranes available
	• Decrease endurance of the wearer due to resistance when breathing	• Can be noisy

workplace where respiratory protection may be required. This includes the presence of a program to select the type of respirators, ensure its proper maintenance, employee fitting if tight-fitting respirators are used, use during potential emergencies, cleaning/storage/maintenance of the respiratory protection equipment, training of employees on respirator use, risks of exposures, and evaluation of effectiveness of the program. It is required that respirators are fitted. The standard requires employees to be fit tested prior to the initial use of a respirator, annually, and whenever a different respirator facepiece (size, style, model, or make) is used. Furthermore, personal protective equipment must be provided at no cost to the employee.

Professionals in infection control and occupational health, as well as hospital administrators, need to be knowledgeable about and comply with regulations governing respiratory protection programs in their respective hospitals. While OSHA stipulates federal standards that are followed by the Centers for Medicare and Medicaid Services and most organizations, the Joint Commission requires that each healthcare facility clearly outlines elements of their respiratory protection program in their policies and procedures and demonstrates compliance [15]. Furthermore, there is considerable variation among states and organizations, especially those which are public, county-owned, or state-owned teaching institutions. The Centers for Disease Control and Prevention recommends that healthcare facilities follow their respective federal, state, or local regulations as it is not a regulatory agency [17]. It is important to know these nuances. Studies show that hospitals are experiencing challenges with the implementation of their respiratory protection programs. Twenty-four states have state-approved OSHA plans. These state-level plans incorporate regulations that are at least as strict as those set forth by OSHA at the federal level.

In August 2009, during the peak of H1N1 pandemic, California enacted the nation's first occupational standard for aerosol transmissible diseases [18]. The standard requires, among other things, that hospitals care for patients with pandemic influenza using respiratory protection that includes an N95 respirator at a minimum. In addition to variation in state-level plans, recent studies in Minnesota, Illinois, and New York have demonstrated a wide variation in interpretation and implementation at the hospital level [19, 20].

PAPR-Only Approach?

The most common approach in healthcare settings for respiratory protection is the use of N95 respirator masks along with employee fit-testing program which could be expensive. An alternative approach used in some settings is the use of PAPRs only, which eliminate the need for employee fit testing, if the PAPRs selected do not have a tight-fitting face piece.

Use of respirator masks vs. PAPRs depends on the following variables in any given facility:

1. Ease of use
2. Training and competencies, e.g., respirator fit testing annually
3. Cleaning between uses for PAPRs
4. Volume of patients and anticipated frequency of use
5. Storage/maintenance/repair and disposal
6. Annual costs
7. Regulatory standards
8. Level of protection needed
9. Intensity of contact and nature of healthcare personnel-patient interaction, including performance of any surgical procedures or aerosol-generating procedures (e.g., intubation, resuscitation, bronchoscopy, autopsy, aspiration of the respiratory tract)
10. Availability of engineering controls

Implementation Approaches in Different Hospitals and Health Systems

PAPRs are generally specified for high-hazard procedures because they reduce risk more than the N95 respirators. The APF for loose-fitting PAPRs is 25 and for full facepiece tight-fitting PAPRs is 1000, which is more than the APF for a typical N95 respirator mask which is 10. In a workshop conducted by the Institute of Medicine in 2015 [8], the participating experts noted that PAPR use is increasing in facilities across the nation. In a study (REACH II Public Health Practice Study – Respirator Evaluation in Acute Care Hospitals 2010–2012) that evaluated hospitals' respiratory

protection programs and respirator usage in six states across the USA, CA, MI, MN, IL, NY, NC, more than 85% of the participating hospital managers and unit managers said their facilities had PAPRs available for use, while 30% of the healthcare personnel themselves were not aware of how to access a PAPR in their facility [8]. More than 40% of the healthcare personnel did not know what would happen if someone failed a fit test. A major finding of the study was that healthcare personnel were largely unaware of appropriate use of respiratory PPE and that the employer focus was on fit testing rather than training on proper use. PAPRs do not require fit testing, allow the patients to see their full face, and they accommodate facial hair. The disadvantage is they do not allow the use of a stethoscope. That being said, each PAPR costs about $1800, and there are costs associated with cleaning and disinfection between use and annual maintenance. Many experts are not convinced that there is a scientific basis for respirator fit testing annually as OSHA stipulates.

Before we decide on taking a PAPR-only approach in any health system, we need to recognize the unanswered questions in the area of healthcare worker respiratory protection. The key unanswered questions are:

PPE Choice and Safety

What PPE is required for aerosol-generating procedures?

What donning and doffing procedures are the safest and in what order? What is the clinical evidence on the safety of repeated donning and doffing of respiratory protection? Research is needed to strengthen the evidence of the effectiveness of PAPRs and of specific donning and doffing protocols.

What is the clinical evidence on the safety of different levels of wear compliance for respiratory protection?

How do we verify that improved filtration efficiency translates into enhanced healthcare worker safety?

What's the best way to use PAPRs in a sterile field?

How does an appropriate protection factor translate into adequate protection in actual clinical practice?

How does the respiratory physiology of a healthcare worker change during PAPR use?

Maintenance of PAPR

What are the appropriate procedures for the disinfection of PAPR components? Which components need to be disposable?

Indications for Use

What is the relative contribution of potential modes of transmission? Droplet, opportunistic airborne, or airborne transmission?

How strong is the evidence that respiratory worker safety translates to safer and healthier workers and patients?

Cost-Effectiveness for Routine Clinical Care and Pandemic Preparedness

What is the epidemiologic threshold at which the cost of N95 + annual fit testing outweighs use of PAPRs?

What should be the adequate size and composition of respiratory protective device stockpile?

PAPR Design

How can PAPRs be better designed so they are more useful to healthcare?

How do we decrease noise, simplify cleaning and storage requirements, and improve battery life?

How do we improve products such as stethoscopes so that they are compatible with PAPRs?

When Would PAPR-Only Approach Work?

For ongoing respiratory protection to prevent transmission of TB and other airborne infections in the hospital, the expenses associated with annual respirator fit testing program may justify a PAPR-only approach. This is particularly true in healthcare facilities with a very low incidence of TB, and many such facilities are currently moving toward a PAPR-only approach for ongoing respiratory protection. This PAPR-only approach may not work in facilities with a high incidence of TB and a high volume of patients unless a seamless process for availability of PAPRs, cleaning and disinfection between uses, a maintenance plan, operational ownership plan, and training plan are fully established. In these facilities, a combination approach with N95 masks and PAPRs may be appropriate.

Pandemic situations present different challenges compared to ongoing prevention of infections potentially transmissible by the airborne route in facilities. Experts note that "given the high cost per unit, PAPR availability will always be a problem in the event of a major outbreak or act of bioterrorism. Health care facilities need to have dual systems for N95 respirators and PAPRs, and they need to train health care workers to use both" [8]. Studies have found that stockpiling PAPRs was the most expensive strategy for a pandemic scenario. Furthermore, respirators do not eliminate the need for negatively pressured rooms or ultraviolet lights or the costs associated with triage and screening in pandemic situations. Therefore, for pandemic situations, a combination approach is probably better, and the proportion of N95 vs. PAPR needs to be customized per the local needs of the hospital.

References

1. Siegel JD, Rhinehart E, Jackson M, Chiarello L, The Healthcare InfectionControl Practices Advisory Committee. 2007. Guideline for isolation precautions: preventing transmission of infectious agents in healthcare settings http://www.cdc.gov/ncidod/dhqp/pdf/isolation2007.pdf

2. Weber DJ, Rutala WA, Fischer WA, Kanamori H, Sickbert-Bennett EE. Emerging infectious diseases: focus on infection control issues for novel coronaviruses (severe acute respiratory syndrome-CoV and Middle East respiratory syndrome-CoV), hemorrhagic fever viruses (Lassa and Ebola), and highly pathogenic avian influenza viruses, A(H5N1) and A(H7N9). Am J Infect Control. 2016;44(5Suppl):e91–e100.

3. Wear compliance and donning/doffing of respiratory protection for Bioaerosols or infectious agents: a review of the effectiveness, safety, and guidelines [Internet]. Ottawa (ON): Canadian Agency for Drugs and Technologies in Health; 2014 Aug 19. Available from http://www.ncbi.nlm.nih.gov/books/NBK253733/PubMed

4. CDC and NIOSH hospital respiratory protection program toolkit. Available at: http://www.cdc.gov/niosh/docs/2015-117/pdfs/2015-117.pdf. Accessed 27 Jan 2017.

5. United States Department of Labor, OSHA. Respirator types. Available at: https://www.osha.gov/video/respiratory_protection/resptypes_transcript.html Accessed 27 Jan 2017.

6. OSHA. Assigned protection factors for the revised respiratory protection standard. Available at: https://www.osha.gov/Publications/3352-APF-respirators.html. Accessed 27 Jan 2017.

7. World Health Organization. Infection prevention and control of epidemic- and pandemic-prone acute respiratory infections in healthcare. WHO, Geneva (2014) http://apps.who.int.libproxy.uthscsa.edu/iris/bitstream/10665/112656/1/9789241507134_eng.pdf?ua=1

8. Board on Health Sciences Policy, Institute of Medicine. The use and effectiveness of powered air purifying respirators in health care: workshop summary. Washington, DC: National Academies Press (US); 2015. PubMed

9. Cuta K. Powered air purifying respirators: versatility beyond respiratory protection. Occup Health Saf. 2014;83(11):20. 22

10. Roberts V. To PAPR or not to PAPR? Can J Respir Ther. 2014 Fall;50(3):87–90.

11. Radonovich LJ Jr, Yanke R, Cheng J, Bender B. Diminished speech intelligibility associated with certain types of respirators worn by healthcare workers. J Occup Environ Hyg. 2010 Jan;7(1):63–70.

12. Gao S, McKay RT, Yermakov M, Kim J, Reponen T, He X, Kimura K, Grinshpun SA. Performance of an improperly sized and stretched-out loose-fitting powered air-purifying respirator: manikin-based study. J Occup Environ Hyg. 2016;13(3):169–76.

13. AlGhamri AA, Murray SL, Samaranayake VA. The effects of wearing respirators on human fine motor, visual, and cognitive performance. Ergonomics. 2013;56(5):791–802.

14. Baracco G, Eisert S, Eagan A, Radonovich L. Comparative cost of stockpiling various types of respiratory protective devices to protect the health care workforce during an influenza pandemic. Disaster Med Public Health Prep. 2015 Jun;9(3):313–8.

15. The Joint Commission. Implementing hospital respiratory protection programs: strategies from the field. Oakbrook Terrace: The Joint Commission; 2014. http://www.jointcommission.org. Accessed 17 Mar 2017

16. OSHA. Personal protective equipment, general requirements. Available at: https://www.osha.gov/pls/oshaweb/owadisp.show_document?p_table=STANDARDS&p_id=9777

17. Centers for Disease Control and Prevention. Tuberculosis factsheets. Available at: https://www.cdc.gov/tb/publications/factsheets/prevention/rphcs.htm. Accessed 17 Mar 2017.

18. California Code of Regulations, Title 8, Section 5199. Aerosol Transmissible Diseases. Available at https://www.dir.ca.gov/Title8/5199.html. Accessed 17 Mar 2017.

19. Brosseau LM, Conroy LM, Sietsema M, Cline K, Durski K. Evaluation of Minnesota and Illinois hospital respiratory protection programs and health care worker respirator use. J Occup Environ Hyg. 2015;12(1):1–15.

20. Hines L, Rees E, Pavelchak N. Respiratory protection policies and practices among the health care workforce exposed to influenza in New York State: evaluating emergency preparedness for the next pandemic. Am J Infect Control. 2014;42(3):240–5.

Donning and Doffing of Personal Protective Equipment (PPE): Is Training Necessary?

31

Michelle Doll, Michael P. Stevens, and Gonzalo Bearman

Introduction

The use of personal protective equipment (PPE) to provide care to patients on "contact" isolation precautions is a standard infection prevention practice. This is despite the fact that limited data exists to show such practices are effective in preventing transmission of organisms from patient to patient [1–3]. Yet contamination of healthcare providers after interaction with the patient care environment has been well documented in the ICU setting, where multidrug-resistant organisms similar to those colonizing patients can be found on the gloves and gowns of healthcare workers after providing care [4, 5]. Several human factors presumably limit effectiveness of contact precautions as they are currently practiced including poor adherence [6]. More recently, technique in PPE donning and doffing has become recognized as a widespread opportunity for improvement among healthcare providers [7].

Self-Contamination

Self-contamination risk when doffing PPE was highlighted during the Ebola virus outbreak of 2014 [8]. Yet well before this crisis, Casanova et al. observed high rates of self-contamination using gowns, gloves, goggles, and masks in PPE donning and doffing simulations [9]. They contaminated PPE with both a nonpathogenic RNA virus and a fluorescing tracer and found the virus was transferred to the volunteers' skin or clothing 100 % of the time while using the current standard method [10] for donning and doffing PPE advised by the Centers for Disease Control (Fig. 31.1). Transfer of the synthetic tracer occurred less frequently, but exact concentrations and technique of application are not discussed in detail in this report [9]. While the CDC method for doffing PPE is clearly not 100% effective in preventing potential pathogen transfer, it has been shown to be better than most provider-driven doffing procedures [11, 12]. Healthcare providers doffing PPE contaminated with a liquid fluorescent marker performed a series of PPE doffing simulations using various gown materials and either their own doffing method or the CDC recommended method. The CDC method was found to be superior in preventing small stains to the front of underlying clothing, while it was ineffective in preventing larger area stains to the back [11]. The CDC method was further evaluated in a study by Tomas et al. in a series of 435 doffing observations in which the contamination rates, as defined as transfer of fluorescent lotion to skin or clothing, occurred over twice as frequently in those using a doffing procedure other than the CDC recommended method (70% vs. 30% self-contamination rates) [12].

Self-contamination when doffing PPE has implications for patient and provider safety. Interventions to improve PPE removal technique are widely employed in the context of care for hemorrhagic fevers such as extensive provider training, paired and observed donning and doffing procedures, and ongoing practice to ensure skills are maintained [13]. However, training for PPE use in general inpatient health-

M. Doll (✉) • M.P. Stevens
Department of Internal Medicine-Division of Infectious Diseases, VCU Medical Center, 1300 East Marshall Street, North Hospital, 2nd Floor, Room 2-100, P.O. Box 980019, Richmond, VA 23298, USA

Infectious Diseases/Epidemiology, Virginia Commonwealth University Health System, Richmond, VA, USA
e-mail: michelle.doll@vcuhealth.org; michael.stevens@vcuhealth.org

G. Bearman
VCUHS Epidemiology and Infection Control, North Hospital, 2nd Floor, Room 2-073, 1300 East Marshall Street, Richmond, VA 23298-0019, USA
e-mail: gonzalo.bearman@vcuhealth.org

© Springer International Publishing AG 2018
G. Bearman et al. (eds.), *Infection Prevention*, DOI 10.1007/978-3-319-60980-5_31

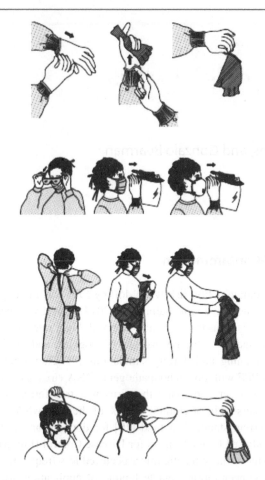

Fig. 31.1 Centers for disease control diagram illustrating the sequencing for removing, or doffing, personal protective equipment (Reprinted from Siegel et al. [10], Copyright 2007, with permission from Elsevier)

Types of Training and PPE

Training to improve the use of PPE has taken a variety of forms. The simplest examples are educational campaigns, similar to those traditionally used to promote adherence. Training can also take the form of hands-on practice of the procedures involved in donning and doffing PPE. Finally, enhanced training with the use of technology and/or feedback has been employed to strengthen experiential learning. Results are mixed and likely highly dependent on the type of intervention and the quality of the implementation. The Cochrane Group conducted a systematic review of training interventions for respiratory PPE use in the workplace that included occupational health and industry literature as well as healthcare settings. They found very low quality evidence that training in the form of either education, or physical practice, was able to improve correct use of respiratory PPE [14]. However, as the complexity of PPE increases, so do the potential benefits of training interventions. For practical reasons, centers involved in the care of patients with known or suspected Ebola developed intensive, protocolized training procedures for donning and doffing complex PPE. A recent study designed to validate CDC recommendations [13] for PPE use in the care of patients with Ebola hemorrhagic fever concluded that the strategies including detailed step-by-step instructions, trained observers, doffing assistants, and frequent hand hygiene were effective in preventing self-contamination with bacteriophage MS2 [15]. However, some virus was found on gloves, hands, and scrubs of several participants after doffing [15]. Similar to PPE for Ebola, Hazmat-type PPE for first responders is complex and requires step-by-step instruction for appropriate use. Paramedic students were recently found to have a 0% error rate after completing training for Level C PPE when assessed by direct observation by trained evaluators [16]. On the other hand, doffing of Ebola-type PPE after a 40 min training session among otherwise untrained medical staff was shown to result in high rates of infection control breaches [17].

care settings is expected to be met with more skepticism. Contact precautions requiring gowns and gloves for the provision of patient care are controversial in their own right; to require training for these procedures pushes the debate even further. The central question relates to the effectiveness of contact precautions for preventing acquisitions of healthcare-acquired infectious agents; these questions have not been definitely answered in the scientific literature. Thus any benefit from a training program will be difficult to assess in terms of hard outcomes. There may be decreased self-contamination, but proving that this reduced bioburden is clinically meaningful will be more difficult. Nevertheless, high rates of self-contamination while using PPE arguably defeat the purpose of the intervention and may be implicated in the difficulty in showing benefit to PPE use in general, in terms of decreasing disease transmission. Finally, self-contamination is a problem that is distinct from general adherence issues, since providers who are faithfully following infection prevention policies could be inadvertently be putting themselves and patients at risk, rather than intentionally neglecting recommendations.

Training for Reduction of Self-Contamination in the Acute Care Hospital

In contrast to PPE for the care of patients within public health emergency settings, PPE for use on isolation precautions in acute care hospitals is relatively simple at first glance. Many providers may not even be aware that specific procedures exist for donning and doffing [18]. However, observations of PPE use on medical units suggest that there is a need for increased education and training regarding choice of PPE [19] and avoidance of contact with the outer surface of PPE during patient care or doffing [18, 20]. Additional observations of simulated isolation care using PPE have identified improper PPE technique even when volunteers were well aware that they were being observed [21]. In defense of healthcare providers, there appears to be a lack of emphasis on proper PPE use; many providers have never had PPE training of any kind [8, 22], and those who have had training report a focus on choice of PPE for various clinical situations over technique in using PPE [22].

Training that emphasizes recommended PPE procedures has been effective in improving PPE technique and/or decreasing contamination rates in several studies [8, 23–25]. Hung et al. developed and trialed a computer simulation program in which participants led an animated figure through donning and doffing five-part PPE for a respiratory isolation scenario [23]. The simulation program also asked the participants knowledge questions throughout the drag-and-click simulation. Participants using the computer simulation training were compared against a control group without access to the simulation; both groups attended a standard demonstration of donning/doffing procedures. Participants' donning and doffing techniques were evaluated before and after all training interventions. The study found that adding computer simulation training to conventional demonstration significantly improved PPE evaluation scores, albeit in a small, single-center study [23]. Unfortunately, it is not entirely clear how the participants were scored in their evaluations [23]. Some training studies focus on an outcome of proper PPE selection for the clinical situation and proper order of application [26]. While these are important considerations, they do not address the issue of technique for avoidance of self-contamination.

A series of quasi experimental studies that use hands-on experiential learning have shown promising effects on participants [8, 24]. An educational program consisting of a 10 min instructional video, followed by a practice session, in which participants donned and doffed PPE that was contaminated with fluorescent lotion, was evaluated with pre- and post-intervention doffing evaluations [8]. The investigators found that the training program reduced healthcare worker self-contamination rates by 68%. Furthermore, this result appears to be durable, with sustained rates at 1 and 3 months reported despite no additional provision of training [8]. Using the same training program, another study evaluated self-contamination rates after participants provided simulated patient care to a mannequin that was "contaminated" with fluorescent dye and bacteriophage MS2 [24]. There were equal amounts of spread of the surrogate contamination throughout the room and onto PPE of providers; however, the training program effectively decreased transfer of both

markers to the skin and clothing of providers after doffing [24]. Of note, in both studies, while self-contamination rates using fluorescent lotion fell from 60% to 19% [8] and 30% to 3% [24], respectively, there is clearly some residual transfer. Complete, consistent avoidance of self-contamination when using PPE may not be attainable.

Limitations of the Available Data

A meta-analysis of PPE that included studies on PPE removal, training, and use concluded that the body of literature to date offered very low evidence to support training for PPE. The analysis was only able to include a handful of studies as most reports on the topic were observational, lacking control groups, or lacking details about the interventions or outcomes [25]. Another issue is the use of various surrogate markers for potentially infectious organisms. It is unclear if simulation results would correspond to real self-contamination with infectious agents in the hospital and patient environment. Furthermore, it is unclear if fluorescent dye contamination correlates with contamination with actual organisms. Some studies that have used both dye and bacteriophages found good correlation in transfer rates between the two [8], while others have demonstrated that the virus is transferred much more readily to provider skin/clothing than the fluorescent dye [9]. Some of this discrepancy might be explained by different methods of application of the fluorescing substance, as well different quantities and formulations: spray, gel, lotion, and powder. A summary of the current knowledge and unanswered questions is presented in Table 31.1.

Conclusion

As our world becomes increasingly interconnected and the patients in our hospitals become ever more complex, effective infection prevention practices are critical for public and patient safety. When it comes to the use of personal protective equipment, opportunities for improvement exist. Although the proportional impact on hospital cross transmission secondary to poor personal protective equipment use is not known, the risk is not nil and should not be overlooked. There is an urgent need for rigorous assessment of existing PPE with a focus on application and technique. In the meantime, healthcare centers must reexamine existing PPE programs to ensure that they meet the educational needs of healthcare workers to provide care that is safe for themselves and safe for others.

Table 31.1 Existing knowledge and important knowledge gaps that contribute to the controversy regarding the importance of training to optimize use of personal protective equipment

Existing knowledge	Unanswered questions
Healthcare worker PPE choice is often inappropriate to the clinical situation [19, 20, 23, 26]	What is the best training method to ensure appropriate PPE choice?
	Can this method be utilized to train entire organizations?
Healthcare worker donning and doffing techniques are inconsistent with recommended practices [11, 12, 18]	What is the best training method to ensure optimal donning and doffing techniques?
	Can this method be utilized to train entire organizations?
Fluorescent markers and bacteriophages are transferred from PPE to provider skin and clothing during doffing activities [9, 11, 12, 15, 17, 24]	Does self-contamination during provider doffing of PPE lead to transmission events within the hospital?
	Does self-contamination lead to increased surface contamination, or bioburden, on hospital units?
Compliance with PPE for contact precautions in the hospital is suboptimal [6]	What benefit of a large-scale training program on PPE effectiveness can be expected in real-world settings?
	Is the potential benefit of training worth the effort of implementing a large-scale program?

PPE personal protective equipment

References

1. Lopez-Alcalde J, Mateos-Mazon M, Guevara M, et al. Gloves, gowns and masks for reducing the transmission of meticillin-resistant Staphylococcus aureus (MRSA) in the hospital setting. Cochrane Database Syst Rev. 2015;(7):CD007087. doi:CD007087
2. Cohen CC, Cohen B, Shang J. Effectiveness of contact precautions against multidrug-resistant organism transmission in acute care: a systematic review of the literature. J Hosp Infect. 2015;90:275–84.
3. De Angelis G, Cataldo MA, De Waure C, et al. Infection control and prevention measures to reduce the spread of vancomycin-resistant enterococci in hospitalized patients: a systematic review and meta-analysis. J Antimicrob Chemother. 2014;69:1185–92.
4. Morgan DJ, Liang SY, Smith CL, et al. Frequent multidrug-resistant Acinetobacter baumannii contamination of gloves, gowns, and hands of healthcare workers. Infect Control Hosp Epidemiol. 2010;31:716–21.
5. Snyder GM, Thom KA, Furuno JP, et al. Detection of methicillin-resistant Staphylococcus aureus and vancomycin-resistant enterococci on the gowns and gloves of healthcare workers. Infect Control Hosp Epidemiol. 2008;29:583–9.
6. Dhar S, Marchaim D, Tansek R, et al. Contact precautions: more is not necessarily better. Infect Control Hosp Epidemiol. 2014;35:213–21.
7. Doll M, Bearman GB. The increasing visibility of the threat of health care worker self-contamination. JAMA Intern Med. 2015;175(12).
8. Edmond MB, Diekema DJ, Perencevich EN. Ebola virus disease and the need for new personal protective equipment. JAMA. 2014;312:2495–6.
9. Casanova L, Alfano-Sobsey E, Rutala WA, Weber DJ, Sobsey M. Virus transfer from personal protective equipment to healthcare employees' skin and clothing. Emerg Infect Dis. 2008;14:1291–3.
10. Siegel JD, Rhinehart E, Jackson M, Chiarello L, Health Care Infection Control Practices Advisory Committee. 2007 guideline for isolation precautions: preventing transmission of infectious agents in health care settings. Am J Infect Control. 2007;35:S65–164.
11. Guo YP, Li Y, Wong PL. Environment and body contamination: a comparison of two different removal methods in three types of personal protective clothing. Am J Infect Control. 2014;42:e39–45.
12. Tomas ME, Kundrapu S, Thota P, et al. Contamination of health care personnel during removal of personal protective equipment. JAMA Intern Med. 2015;175:1904–10.
13. Guidance on personal protective equipment (PPE) to be used by healthcare workers during management of patient with confirmed Ebola or persons under investigation (PUIs) for Ebola, who are clinically unstable or have bleeding, vomiting, or diarrhea in U.S. hospitals, including procedures for donning and doffing PPE. Centers for Disease Control. https://www.cdc.gov/vhf/ebola/healthcare-us/ppe/guidance.html. Published 2015. Accessed 3 Mar 2017.
14. Luong Thanh BY, Laopaiboon M, Koh D, Sakunkoo P, Moe H. Behavioural interventions to promote workers' use of respiratory protective equipment. Cochrane Database Syst Rev. 2016;12:CD010157.
15. Casanova LM, Teal LJ, Sickbert-Bennett EE, et al. Assessment of self-contamination during removal of personal protective equipment for Ebola patient care. Infect Control Hosp Epidemiol. 2016;37:1156–61.
16. Northington WE, Mahoney GM, Hahn ME, Suyama J, Hostler D. Training retention of level C personal protective equipment use by emergency medical services personnel. Acad Emerg Med. 2007;14:846–9.
17. Lim SM, Cha WC, Chae MK, Jo IJ. Contamination during doffing of personal protective equipment by healthcare providers. Clin Exp Emerg Med. 2015;2:162–7.
18. Doll M, Feldman M, Hartigan S, et al. Acceptability and necessity of training for optimal personal protective equipment use. Infect Control Hosp Epidemiol. 2017;38:226–9.
19. Mitchell R, Roth V, Gravel D, et al. Are health care workers protected? An observational study of selection and removal of personal protective equipment in Canadian acute care hospitals. Am J Infect Control. 2013;41:240–4.
20. Zellmer C, Van Hoof S, Safdar N. Variation in health care worker removal of personal protective equipment. Am J Infect Control. 2015;43:750–1.
21. Beam EL, Gibbs SG, Hewlett AL, Iwen PC, Nuss SL, Smith PW. Method for investigating nursing behaviors related to isolation care. Am J Infect Control. 2014;42:1152–6.
22. John A, Tomas ME, Hari A, Wilson BM, Donskey CJ. Do medical students receive training in correct use of personal protective equipment? Med Educ Online. 2017;22:1264125.
23. Hung PP, Choi KS, Chiang VC. Using interactive computer simulation for teaching the proper use of personal protective equipment. Comput Inform Nurs. 2015;33:49–57.
24. Alhmidi H, Koganti S, Tomas ME, Cadnum JL, Jencson A, Donskey CJ. A pilot study to assess use of fluorescent lotion in patient care simulations to illustrate pathogen dissemination and train personnel in correct use of personal protective equipment. Antimicrob Resist Infect Control. 2016;5:40.
25. Verbeek JH, Ijaz S, Mischke C, et al. Personal protective equipment for preventing highly infectious diseases due to exposure to contaminated body fluids in healthcare staff. Cochrane Database Syst Rev. 2016;4:CD011621.
26. Hon CY, Gamage B, Bryce EA, et al. Personal protective equipment in health care: can online infection control courses transfer knowledge and improve proper selection and use? Am J Infect Control. 2008;36:e33–7.

Rapid Diagnostics in Infection Prevention

Sara Revolinski, Angela M. Huang, and Allison Gibble

Introduction

Significant advancements have been realized over the past few years in the expanding field of rapid diagnostics. Compared to traditional laboratory methods where final results are typically obtained within 48–72 h, rapid tests are able to provide identification within hours of organism growth or, in some cases, sample collection [1]. A paradigm shift in organism and susceptibility identification, rapid diagnostics allow for earlier initiation of targeted antimicrobial therapy in infected patients, resulting in decreased mortality, hospital length of stay, broad-spectrum antimicrobial use, and health system costs [1–5].

Rapid diagnostics may also be employed for infection prevention purposes, in addition to treatment of infections. Rapid identification of colonizing pathogens results in prompt implementation of procedures to prevent subsequent development of infection within a colonized patient or transmission of infection to others. Screening can be employed via passive or active strategies [6]. Passive screening is identification of a pathogen when conducting routine microbiologic techniques on clinical samples, while active screening involves obtaining samples for the direct purpose of identifying asymptomatic infection or colonization [7]. Upon isolate identification, infection prevention bundles that may include implementation of isolation procedures, hand hygiene reinforcement, patient cohorting, decolonization regimens, and utilization of proper environmental cleaning may be employed in order to minimize risk of infection or transmission. Utilization of rapid diagnostic tests may be employed during outbreak situations in a similar manner to mitigate further spread and in some cases determine clonality [8].

Carbapenem-resistant *Enterobacteriaceae* (CRE), methicillin-resistant *Staphylococcus aureus* (MRSA), and vancomycin-resistant *Enterococcus* spp. (VRE) are three relevant pathogens in today's healthcare environment. Data describing 2014 hospital-acquired infections in the United States (US) from the Centers for Disease Control and Prevention (CDC) found carbapenem resistance in 3.6 % of *Enterobacteriaceae*, methicillin resistance in 47.9 % of *S. aureus*, and vancomycin resistance in 29.5 % of *Enterococcus* spp. isolates [9]. In European countries, rates of CRE and VRE continue to increase, while MRSA rates have slightly declined [10]. These organisms may colonize patients causing subsequent infection or transmission to others and are associated with considerable morbidity and mortality [7, 11, 12]. Moreover, treatment options for these organisms are limited and can be associated with significant toxicity; avoiding use of these agents by preventing subsequent infection and transmission would be ideal. Employment of rapid diagnostics to swiftly identify patients colonized with these pathogens may have a significant impact on an individual's health as well as the health of the public.

S. Revolinski (✉)
Department of Pharmacy, Froedtert & The Medical College of Wisconsin, 9200 W. Wisconsin Ave., Milwaukee, WI 53226, USA

Clinical Assistant Professor, Medical College of Wisconsin School of Pharmacy, 8701 Watertown Plank Rd., Milwaukee, WI 53226, USA
e-mail: sara.revolinski@froedtert.com

A.M. Huang • A. Gibble
Department of Pharmacy, Froedtert & The Medical College of Wisconsin, 9200 W. Wisconsin Ave., Milwaukee, WI 53226, USA
e-mail: angela.huang@froedtert.com; Allison.gibble@froedtert.com

Carbapenem-Resistant *Enterobacteriaceae*

Enterobacteriaceae commonly colonize the gastrointestinal tract, skin, and naso- and oropharynx [11]. Colonization with CRE is a significant risk factor for subsequent infection as well as transmission [13]. CRE are an emerging global health concern due to rapid interpersonal transmission and the dearth of antimicrobial agents demonstrating activity [11, 14]. First described in the 1980s, CRE have become endemic in certain areas of the world [15]. Infections due to these organisms are associated with a mortality rate between 24 and 70% [11]. CRE has also been associated with increased hospital stays and healthcare costs [11].

The most concerning mechanism of resistance in these organisms is enzymatic degradation (e.g., carbapenemase), as these resistance genes are typically located on mobile elements within the organism allowing for easy transfer to other bacteria [16]. Carbapenemase-producing organisms are responsible for the majority of CRE outbreaks throughout the world [11, 15]. CRE infections pose a major threat to individual and public health and require rapid identification to ensure initiation of strategies to prevent progression of infection within a colonized patient and transmission to uncolonized patients [16].

Detection of CRE poses several challenges for microbiology laboratories. Identification of CRE using traditional phenotypic methods can take up to 4–6 days after culture collection, which can result in delays in initiation of appropriate infection control strategies, subsequently increasing the risk of infection [17, 18]. Rapid diagnostic tests for CRE identify enzyme-mediated resistance only; phenotypic methods are still required to identify resistance due to porin mutations or efflux pumps [18]. Available rapid tests also are unlikely to identify the entire library of carbapenemase enzymes. Several single and multiplex polymerase chain reaction (PCR) tests have been developed to detect enzyme-mediated carbapenem resistance in *Enterobacteriaceae* from clinical specimens or rectal swabs [18]. PCR utilizes DNA primers to amplify targeted DNA. The amplified DNA is then identified via fluorescent probe attached to the primers [1]. PCRs carry the advantages of early identification and increased sensitivity compared to traditional culture methods [18]. Matrix-assisted laser desorption ionization-time of flight (MALDI-TOF) has also been evaluated to detect carbapenemases by measuring the products created via hydrolysis or the presence of a protein found to be associated with certain plasmids that contain the *Klebsiella pneumoniae* carbapenemase (KPC) [18, 19].

Active surveillance utilizing rapid diagnostic tests for CRE have largely been utilized as part of an infection control bundle to prevent or contain outbreaks within institutions [8, 20–23]. Sample collection has been described at varying time points: upon hospital or intensive care unit (ICU) admission, weekly, or on demand based on identification of a colonized or infected patient. Once a patient is identified as a carrier, further infection control measures may be employed.

The CDC has developed a CRE Toolkit that outlines recommended components of a bundle that should be initiated upon identification. Institutions may elect to utilize components of the bundle that apply to their specific setting [16]. Bundle components include active screening of contacts of the index patient, surveillance of high-risk patients, timely notification upon laboratory identification, education of staff about CRE and reinforcing hand hygiene and environmental cleaning practices, initiation of contact precautions, cohorting of patients and staff, utilizing 2% chlorhexidine gluconate (CHG) for patient bathing, minimizing utilization of invasive devices, communication of CRE status upon transfer, and antimicrobial stewardship. Several studies have demonstrated successful outbreak control and significant reduction in CRE incidence with implementation of bundles such as the one described by the CDC [8, 20, 21, 23–25]. Because bundle components are often implemented simultaneously to mitigate outbreaks, it is difficult to determine the individual impact of each intervention [14]. However, several studies implemented infection control practices sequentially, allowing for analysis of targeted interventions. One of those studies implemented active surveillance with various infection prevention practices in a stepwise fashion over 3 years to help control a KPC outbreak in Greece [20]. In the first year, KPC-positive patients were placed in contact isolation, hand hygiene (washing hands before and after patient contact) was reinforced, and patient cohorting occurred for select cases. During the second year, rapid notification of the medical staff occurred after KPC identification, all colonized and infected patients were cohorted to a particular section of the unit, hand hygiene and contact precaution practices were further enforced with healthcare providers and visitors, and patient transfers were limited. In the final year, nursing staff was also cohorted. Overall rates of KPCs continued to decrease each year, reaching a statistically significant reduction in year 3. A second study in Italy evaluated the implementation of a two-phase infection prevention bundle in response to an outbreak [8]. Upon identification of the index patient, the institution thoroughly cleaned the environment of care and provided education about hand hygiene. Further methods for control had to be applied after rates of CRE continued to increase and included patient and caregiver cohorting, contact precautions, and active monitoring of hand hygiene and environmental cleaning. The outbreak was controlled with no further CRE cases identified 1 month after the second phase was implemented. These stepwise studies suggest that early identification via active surveillance and subsequent cohorting of colonized patients are important components of preventing CRE spread [14].

Research has also been conducted on the impact of infection control bundles on CRE incidence and subsequent infection in areas of high CRE endemicity. One such study evaluated the impact of an infection control bundle (active screening upon admission and weekly thereafter, contact isolation, patient cohorting, CHG bathing, and caregiver education and adherence monitoring) at four long-term acute care hospitals [22]. This study found that bundle implementation significantly decreased rates of CRE colonization, CRE infection including bloodstream infection, and blood culture contamination.

Decolonization regimens function to decrease organism transmission and to prevent progression from colonization to active infection. To date, minimal research has been done regarding decolonization in patients with CRE. Chlorhexidine gluconate, a broad-spectrum antibacterial agent, may be an option for skin decolonization but has been minimally studied for decolonization of gram-negative organisms [14, 26]. Additionally, gram-negative organisms may have higher MICs for CHG compared to gram-positive agents due to the presence of an efflux pump in certain organisms, namely, *A. baumannii* and *E. coli* [27]. A recent study conducted in Thailand found that rates of CRE were similar at all evaluable times (baseline and days 3, 5, 7, and 14) in patients receiving daily 2% CHG application and those receiving baths with non-antibacterial soap [27]. CHG was administered appropriately: a nurse utilized five washcloths to coat skin surfaces from the head to the toe. CHG was not washed off, and use of other skin care agents was prohibited. It should be noted that many of the CRE isolates obtained after initiation of CHG were from perianal swabs and could represent gastrointestinal colonization as opposed to skin colonization, making it difficult to draw conclusions regarding CHG efficacy against CRE. Despite these concerns, CHG may be employed as part of a bundle for infection prevention and is recommended as part of the CDC's CRE Toolkit [16]. Utilization of 2% CHG applications is now commonly employed in high-risk patient populations, regardless of CRE colonization status [16, 28].

Oral decolonization regimens are also a potential infection prevention strategy that may be employed. Nonabsorbable oral antibiotics are desirable for this in order to limit systemic exposure, and gentamicin and colistin (polymyxin E) have largely been studied for this indication [29, 30]. Tascini and colleagues targeted a select patient population found to be KPC positive via rectal swab, including those with planned gastrointestinal surgery or immunosuppression [29]. Patients selected for decolonization received gentamicin 80 mg orally four times daily. Duration of treatment varied, with a median duration of 9 days; however, select patients received over 30 days of therapy. The rate of decolonization in patients receiving oral antibiotics was 68%. Outcomes in these patients were evaluated for 6 months following decolonization and compared to KPC-colonized patients not receiving oral decolonization regimens. Decolonization was associated with a significant reduction in active KPC infections: 15% of successfully decolonized patients developed subsequent infection compared to 73% of continually colonized patients. Lubbert evaluated a combination of gentamicin 80 mg orally four times daily and colistin one million units orally four times daily, in addition to gentamicin and colistin gel applied four times daily to the oropharynx [30]. This regimen was continued for 7 days. Decolonization rates were similar in patients receiving the antibiotics (43%) compared to those who did not (30%). However, this study only evaluated 14 patients with CRE and may not have been adequately powered to detect a difference. Of interest, this study did find a 19% increase in resistance to colistin and a 45% increase in resistance to gentamicin after decolonization. Increased resistance to gentamicin was also seen in the study by Tascini, particularly in patients who remained persistently colonized [29]. There was evidence that some patients did become recolonized after successful decolonization.

The overall goal of providing a decolonization regimen would be to prevent dissemination to clinical infection. One study found significantly less clinical infections caused by KPCs in decolonized patients compared to patients who did not receive the decolonization regimen [29]. Despite this, neither study found a difference in mortality between groups [29, 30]. This could be due to the high prevalence of comorbidities that also may contribute to mortality in CRE-colonized patients.

While utilization of gastrointestinal decolonization is appealing to decrease progression from colonization to infection, there is not enough evidence at this time to support routine use. Further research must be conducted to identify the appropriate patient population and optimal regimen including antibiotic choice and duration, to quantify the impact of decolonization on the development of clinical infection, and to analyze the impact decolonization may have on antimicrobial resistance. The impact on antimicrobial resistance is particularly concerning, as gentamicin and colistin are potential therapeutic options within an already limited antimicrobial arsenal for CRE. Additionally, these studies evaluated the use of gastrointestinal decontamination alone and did not evaluate the concurrent impact of skin decontamination, as the skin is another reservoir for CRE colonization.

Methicillin-Resistant *Staphylococcus aureus*

Staphylococcus aureus is the most frequent pathogen associated with healthcare-acquired infections and is also highly prevalent within the community [31, 32]. Antibiotic resistance is common, and infections caused by MRSA place a large burden on health systems. In 2013, the CDC estimated over 11,000 deaths were attributable to MRSA infection [33]. Patients with hospital-acquired MRSA (HA-MRSA) infections are not only at an increased risk of mortality but also a prolonged hospital stay and increased healthcare costs [34].

MRSA colonization has been associated with acquisition of MRSA infections in the acute care setting, with colonized patients demonstrating over a tenfold greater risk of MRSA infection compared to those who are not colonized [35–37]. The highest MRSA colonization and infection rates within a hospital are found in ICU settings, occurring in up to 21.9% of patients within an ICU, compared to 3.4% in hospitalized patients overall [38]. It has been estimated that 218,000 MRSA infections would occur annually within the ICU setting if no infection prevention activities are employed [39]. Therefore, preventing the spread of this infection within patients and healthcare settings is vital.

Multiple rapid diagnostic tests exist that can be utilized to identify MRSA from clinical and surveillance swab specimens, with PCR being the most utilized [1, 40]. PCR test results for swab samples demonstrate a turnaround time of only 1–2 h [41]. MRSA screening can be performed at multiple anatomical sites including the nares, axillae, groin, perineum, and throat. However, the nares are most commonly utilized because they provide an optimal environment to facilitate *S. aureus* survival and have been shown to be the most sensitive site of detection for MRSA colonization [42, 43].

For infection prevention purposes, rapid diagnostics have typically been employed for active surveillance in high-risk patient populations to quickly identify colonized patients and subsequently implement further measures to mitigate transmission. Additional prevention strategies have been defined by the CDC and the Society for Healthcare Epidemiology of America (SHEA) and include conducting an institutional MRSA risk assessment, rapid reporting of MRSA results, assessment of hand hygiene, implementation of contact precautions, adequate environmental disinfection, identification of patients previously colonized with MRSA (passive surveillance), education of healthcare providers, patients, and families, and reporting MRSA data to key stakeholders within the institution [44, 45].

Several studies have evaluated the utilization of active surveillance and its impact on MRSA infection and transmission. While a majority of the published studies demonstrate a positive association with use of active surveillance, there are some studies that question its overall utility [45]. Because most studies utilizing active surveillance also implemented concurrent infection control interventions, it is difficult to draw conclusions about the benefit of active surveillance alone. For these reasons, the employment of active surveillance cultures is not currently recommended as a core strategy for MRSA infection prevention or transmission, although some states do have legislation requiring its use [28, 45].

Active surveillance has mainly been studied in combination with implementation of contact precautions and decolonization regimens. While no longer current, guidelines published by SHEA in 2003 concluded that active surveillance was essential for limiting the spread of MRSA, as it allowed for implementation of contact precautions [46]. The use of contact precautions for prevention of MRSA transmission is supported in the current SHEA/Infectious Diseases Society of America Practice Recommendation regarding strategies to prevent MRSA transmission and infection, as well as by the CDC [44, 45]. A survey conducted by the SHEA Research Network in 2015 found that over 90% of responding hospitals institute contact precautions for MRSA [47]. Despite this, recent literature questions the efficacy and necessity of contact precautions for MRSA [47, 48]. The majority of studies describing a benefit with contact precautions was retrospective, implemented additional simultaneous prevention practices, and did not contain comparator groups. Studies conducted under more rigorous conditions did not find a reduction in MRSA transmission with use of contact precautions, although maintaining similar rigor in everyday practice may be difficult to achieve. The impact of universal gown and glove use for all patient contact in an ICU population has also been evaluated [49]. This study found that universal gown and glove use reduced the risk of MRSA acquisition compared to routine care. Notably, this study also found increased compliance with hand hygiene when universal contact precautions were employed, which may have impacted results. The cost associated with universal gown and glove use must be taken into account if this strategy is employed. Additionally, initiation of contact precautions has been reported to cause delays in care, decreased frequency of healthcare worker visits, and lower patient satisfaction [47, 49–51]. While data is conflicting, utilization of active surveillance combined with contact precautions may be a strategy that can be utilized to minimize infection progression and transmission.

Multiple studies have investigated the impact of various decolonization strategies in patients admitted to the ICU. MRSA decolonization is typically performed utilizing daily 2% CHG applications with or without topical 2% mupirocin applied to the nares [28, 52–54]. Success rates of these agents vary in the literature and are dependent upon dosing and proper administration. Additionally, colonization can reoccur after a documented successful decolonization regimen. One quasi-experimental study conducting active surveillance upon admission to the ICU with targeted decolonization (topical mupirocin applied to nares three times daily in combination with daily application of 4% CHG, each for 5 days) found that the intervention independently decreased in-hospital MRSA infections and 90-day mortality rates [55]. Another study investigated the impact of three different strategies to prevent MRSA infection within an ICU population: active surveillance and isolation, active surveillance with targeted decolonization, and universal decolonization without active surveillance [28]. The decolonization regimen consisted of mupirocin 2% applied twice daily to each nare with 2% CHG applied daily (for 5 days in the targeted decolonization group and until ICU discharge in the universal decolonization group). Universal decolonization was found to significantly reduce the hazard of any MRSA-positive culture compared to targeted decolonization. Significance was not maintained when looking at MRSA bloodstream infections only, although the hazard of bloodstream infections due to any organism was significantly reduced with universal decolonization. Finally, a group of investigators developed a model, based on the wealth of data from previously published studies, to examine the impact of the various surveillance, isolation, and decolonization practices that have been previously investigated on infection prevention and determine the most fiscally optimal approach. This group found that universal decolonization utilizing combination topical mupirocin and CHG had the highest cost savings and was the most effective decolonization strategy for preventing MRSA infection [39].

Although many studies have been performed exploring a variety of decolonization methods, there is no consensus on the most optimal approach. Additionally, when deciding between universal versus targeted decolonization, the impact on antimicrobial resistance should be taken into consideration. Resistance to both CHG and mupirocin has been described in the literature, and continued use of these agents will only result in further increases in resistance [56–63]. For gram-positive organisms, a higher prevalence of CHG resistance has been identified in units performing daily CHG bathing [58, 59]. One study also found that increasing CHG resistance was associated with the development of bloodstream infections and decreased susceptibility to select antibiotics, including methicillin, ciprofloxacin, clindamycin, and vancomycin [58]. Reported rates of mupirocin resistance in MRSA vary between studies, ranging from as low as 1.6% to as high as 13.2% [60–62]. Increased resistance could eventually lead to increased rates of decolonization failures and decreased efficacy of infection prevention practices [63]. While universal decolonization appears to be the most efficacious and cost-effective method described in recent literature, it is important to practice appropriate antimicrobial stewardship with these agents.

It is possible that other infection prevention strategies may obviate the need for active surveillance, such as optimized hand hygiene and environmental cleaning. For these strategies to work, it is imperative that institutions continually monitor hand hygiene and cleaning compliance, providing regular data and feedback to both administrators and clinicians. The employment of universal decolonization may also limit the benefit of active surveillance; however the consideration of increasing resistance must also be weighed. As there is no definitive conclusion that can be made at this time in regard to active surveillance, institutions must determine the strategies that work best for their needs. Strategies should be modified if found to be ineffective. Additionally, active surveillance can be employed in outbreak settings or when MRSA rates are increasing at an institution that already has good infection prevention processes in place [45].

Vancomycin-Resistant *Enterococcus* spp.

Enterococci are considered to be normal flora of the gastrointestinal tract of humans that generally display low levels of virulence but are intrinsically resistant to several antibiotics such as cephalosporins, aztreonam, and aminoglycosides [7]. In hospitalized patients, especially those that are immunosuppressed or critically ill, enterococci can disseminate and proliferate, causing significant infections such as bloodstream infections and infective endocarditis [64]. In particular, infections caused by vancomycin-resistant enterococci (VRE) are a significant cause of morbidity and mortality globally, especially in high-risk patient populations including ICU, hematology/oncology, and solid organ transplant [7]. Treatment options for VRE infections are limited, and several of these antimicrobials are associated with substantial toxicities [65].

PCR tests are available that detect the presence of *vanA* and *vanB* genes within enterococci [7]. It should be noted that the available PCR tests have poor specificity for *vanB*, which is thought to be due to the presence of that gene in several other anaerobic bacterial isolates. Since stool samples and rectal swabs are submitted for VRE surveillance, it is possible that the PCR may detect *vanB* from another organism colonizing the gastrointestinal tract. PCR tests also do not detect other *van* genes responsible for vancomycin resistance, although *vanA* and *vanB* are known to be the most common.

Strategies utilizing rapid diagnostic tests aimed at identifying high-risk patients colonized with VRE may help prevent spread and progression of infection [66–69]. An active surveillance strategy is useful for initiating contact precautions or patient and staff cohorting to contain the spread of VRE to other patients and is commonly used in outbreak settings. Active surveillance can be done at hospital admission combined with subsequent periodic screenings or when certain criteria are met (e.g., onset of neutropenia). Several studies employ weekly screening while inpatient; however the optimal frequency of conducting surveillance is not well defined [66–69]. Based on a mathematical model, utilizing active surveillance in a 10-bed ICU prevents an average of 46 new cases of VRE colonization in a year, whereas passive surveillance prevents only five cases per year [69]. Immediate isolation of all patients admitted to an ICU with removal only if surveillance cultures were negative may prevent up to 77 cases per year; however the feasibility of this strategy is limited.

The clinical impact of active VRE surveillance to prevent VRE bloodstream infection in ICU patients has been studied with variable results in several reviews and studies. Based on one prospective interventional study, it appears that weekly perirectal VRE screening of high-risk patients (in ICU for more than 4 days, co-colonization with methicillin-resistant *Staphylococcus aureus*) with subsequent initiation of contact precautions in colonized patients may reduce the incidence of VRE bloodstream infection as compared to performing no surveillance [68]. Furthermore, this association has been observed in an outbreak setting, resulting in complete control of VRE outbreak bloodstream infections [70]. Active surveillance programs are also associated with more polyclonal VRE populations, potentially indicating less person-to-person transmission. Based on gross estimation, cost attributable to VRE bacteremia exceeds the cost of screening by $508,000, making the strategy appear cost-effective [68]. However, more recently, the benefit of initiating contact precautions for patients colonized with VRE has been called into question. Several studies have not found a link between application of contact precautions and decreased VRE acquisition [49, 71–74]. It should be noted that hospitals who have discontinued contact precautions institute strict horizontal infection control strategies or bundle interventions such as universal hand hygiene, CHG bathing, environmental cleaning, checklists to prevent catheter-related infections, and antimicrobial stewardship programs [47]. There has only been one study evaluating the impact of a bundle program on incidence of VRE [75]. The authors implemented active surveillance and an automated system to identify carriers, followed by implementation of contact precautions of colonized patients. To reduce the environmental burden of VRE, they also performed terminal disinfection with hydrogen peroxide vapor in rooms of colonized patients, changed the bleach cleaning solution, and used fluorescent markers to audit rooms of discharged patients with VRE. Lastly, education on the rates of multidrug-resistant organisms was provided. This multifaceted approach resulted in a significant decrease in cases of VRE. Notably, the bundle strategy does not allow the authors to determine the impact of each infection control measure separately, but it is likely that the combination of interventions contributed to the overall positive effect.

Several studies have reported a link between VRE colonization in immunocompromised patients and the development of VRE infection [76, 77]. Notably, VRE bloodstream infections in this population have also been associated with increased mortality, and thus prevention of transmission and appropriate empiric treatment of these infections is of the utmost importance. Weekly surveillance for VRE colonization and subsequent isolation has been shown to reduce the incidence of VRE bloodstream infections by up to eightfold in oncology patients [66, 69]. In allogeneic hematopoietic stem cell transplant recipients, surveillance for VRE on admission, with the development of diarrhea, and on ICU admission has also been reported to adequately identify VRE colonization prior to bloodstream infection and requires fewer cultures than weekly surveillance [76]. Thus, this strategy may be employed over weekly surveillance, which may decrease overall costs.

Another strategy used to prevent the spread of VRE is active surveillance combined with patient cohorting. This infection control measure may be more useful in outbreak settings, and the impact of cohorting has not been studied specifically for prevention of VRE colonization or infection [78]. Cohorting may be combined with contact precautions or other bundle strategies for the greatest impact.

As previously mentioned, the presence of VRE colonization can also be used to initiate other prevention measures, such as decolonization using CHG. This strategy is more effective at reducing density of VRE on patients compared to soap and water bathing [79]. When used in clinical settings, universal CHG bathing appears to reduce the acquisition of VRE and the incidence of hospital-acquired VRE bloodstream infection by up to threefold, particularly in the ICU setting [26, 80, 81]. The impact or cost-effectiveness of universal CHG bathing on acquisition of VRE infection has not been studied and should be weighed against the feasibility of such strategies. Universal CHG bathing or CHG bathing targeted at VRE-colonized patients appears to decrease overall rates of VRE bloodstream infection in ICU patients.

The optimal method for conducting VRE screening, including the appropriate populations to target and frequency of screening, has not been well defined. Studies have implemented different strategies with variable outcomes, and thus there are no standardized recommendations surrounding VRE surveillance. However, conducting surveillance and subsequent initiation of contact precautions, cohorting, or horizontal infection control measures appear to prevent spread to other patients and thus decrease overall incidence of VRE bloodstream infection. Additionally, patients colonized with VRE may benefit from undergoing CHG-based decontamination, as this has also been associated with decreased rates of VRE bloodstream infections in the ICU setting. It is important to note that the cost-effectiveness of such strategies is based on crude estimates and may vary based on microbiology equipment used, isolation attire, and labor costs. Lastly, the feasibility of implementing such strategies is dependent on institutional resources and funding, and clinical benefit will depend largely on the prevalence of VRE within each institution. Utilization of rapid diagnostic screening tools in high-risk populations and in outbreak settings with subsequent isolation and decontamination of colonized patients may be the most beneficial.

Clostridium difficile

C. difficile infection (CDI) is increasing in prevalence across the world and is associated with significant morbidity, mortality, and excess healthcare costs [82]. While rapid diagnostic testing has been employed more for diagnostic reasons, it still may be of benefit for infection prevention purposes. Active surveillance for *Clostridium difficile* is not routinely performed nor currently recommended, and there is no evidence outlining what infection prevention activities should be implemented upon positive active surveillance result. However, rapid diagnosis of *C. difficile* in an infected patient may reduce further transmission within a unit, as infection control practices such as isolation, hand hygiene with only soap and water, and utilization of sporicidal cleaners are often implemented upon positive test result. While the CDC suggests implementation of isolation procedures immediately upon suspicion of infection, this may not be routinely employed in all settings. PCR tests to detect *C. difficile* result within 1 h, and demonstrate improved sensitivity compared to toxin enzyme immunoassay (EIA) with or without glutamate dehydrogenase screening [83]. With short turnaround time and high sensitivity, it may be possible to delay isolation until result.

Conclusion

The use of rapid diagnostic tests for infection prevention purposes will continue to be an area of research as the burden of antimicrobial resistance continues to expand. Based on current evidence, the impact of utilizing rapid diagnostics for active surveillance of infection is difficult to ascertain, as rapid diagnostics are typically employed in conjunction with other infection prevention strategies. Nonetheless, early identification of relevant pathogens can function to decrease transmission and mitigate outbreak situations.

Most research has evaluated active surveillance in conjunction with implementation of contact precautions and decolonization. Most institutions in the United States currently employ contact precautions for CRE, MRSA, and VRE. Since CRE is associated with high mortality, rapid transmission, and extremely limited antibiotic options, implementing contact precautions upon identification of this organism may be beneficial. Data regarding use of contact precautions for MRSA and VRE is controversial. Studies showing benefit have been conducted in conjunction with other infection prevention measures, making the attributable benefit of contact precautions difficult to ascertain. Recent studies have found that contact precautions may not be necessary for VRE and MRSA. However, these studies also achieved high hand hygiene compliance which may have impacted the overall results. For institutions electing to remove contact precautions for MRSA or VRE, hand hygiene and environmental cleaning must be emphasized and monitored.

The majority of evidence evaluating decolonization regimens has been conducted in gram-positive organisms, particularly MRSA and VRE. Recent literature appears to support universal decolonization over targeted decolonization in high-risk patients; however the concerns for increasing resistance to mupirocin and CHG must be weighed against the benefits realized in these studies. It should also be noted that there is minimal evidence evaluating alternative

agents for this purpose, another reason why antimicrobial stewardship and targeted surveillance must be considered.

The decision to implement active surveillance utilizing rapid diagnostics is one that must be made on an institutional level and should be based on consideration of current outbreaks, pathogen prevalence, and maintenance of other infection prevention strategies (i.e., hand hygiene and environmental cleaning). Early identification of colonizing pathogens via active surveillance may have a significant impact on controlling progression of infection within a colonized patient as well as transmission within the healthcare environment.

References

1. Bauer KA, Perez KK, Forrest GN, Goff DA. Review of rapid diagnostic tests used by antimicrobial stewardship programs. Clin Infect Dis. 2014;59:S134–45.
2. Huang AM, Newton D, Kunapuli A, et al. Impact of rapid organism identification via matrix-assisted laser desorption/ionization time-of-flight combined with antimicrobial stewardship team intervention in adult patients with bacteremia and candidemia. Clin Infect Dis. 2013;57:1237–45.
3. Perez KK, Olson RJ, Musick WL, et al. Integrating rapid diagnostics and antimicrobial stewardship improves outcomes in patients with antibiotic-resistant gram-negative bacteremia. J Infect. 2014;69:216–25.
4. Sothoron C, Ferreira J, Guzman N, Aldridge P, McCarter YS, Jankowski CA. A stewardship approach to optimize antimicrobial therapy through use of a rapid microarray assay on blood cultures positive for gram-negative bacteria. J Clin Microbiol. 2015;53:3627–9.
5. Suzuki H, Hitomi S, Yaguchi Y, et al. Prospective intervention study with a microarray-based, multiplexed, automated molecular diagnosis instrument (Verigene system) for the rapid diagnosis of bloodstream infections, and its impact on the clinical outcomes. J Infect Chemother. 2015;21:849–56.
6. Perencevich EN, Fisman DN, Lipsitch M, Harris AD, Morris JG Jr, Smith DL. Projected benefits of active surveillance for vancomycin-resistant enterococci in intensive care units. Clin Infect Dis. 2004;38:1108–15.
7. Humphreys H. Controlling the spread of vancomycin-resistant enterococci. Is active screening worthwhile? J Hosp Infect. 2014;88:191–8.
8. Agodi A, Voulgari E, Barchitta M, et al. Containment of an outbreak of KPC-3-producing *Klebsiella pneumoniae* in Italy. J Clin Microbiol. 2011;49:3986–9.
9. Weiner LM, Fridkin SK, Aponte-Torres Z, et al. Vital signs: preventing antibiotic-resistant infections in hospitals – United States, 2014. MMWR Morb Mortal Wkly Rep 2016;65:235–241. http://dx.doi.org/10.15585/mmwr.mm6509e1; http://www.cdc.gov/Other/disclaimer.html.
10. Surveillance report: antimicrobial resistance in Europe, 2014. Available at: http://ecdc.europa.eu/en/publications/Publications/antimicrobial-resistance-europe-2014.pdf. Accessed 31 Mar 2016.
11. Tzouvelekis LS, Markogiannakis A, Psichogiou M, Tassios PT, Daikos GL. Carbapenemases in *Klebsiella pneumonia* and other *Enterobacteriaceae*: an evolving crisis of global dimensions. Clin Microbiol Rev. 2012;25:682–707.
12. U.S. Department of Health and Human Services Centers for Disease Control and Prevention. Antibiotic resistance threats in

the United States, 2013. http://www.cdc.gov/drugresistance/pdf/ar-threats-2013-508.pdf. 23 Apr 2013. Accessed 16 Dec 2015.

13. Tischendorf J, Almeida de Avila R, Safdar N. Risk of infection following colonization with carbapenem-resistant Enterobacteriaceae: a systematic review. Am J Infect Control. 2016; doi:10.1016/j.ajic.2015.12.005.

14. Munoz-Price LS, Quinn JP. Deconstructing the infection control bundles for the containment of carbapenem-resistant *Enterobacteriaceae*. Curr Opin Infect Dis. 2013;26:378–87.

15. Molton JS, Tambyah PA, Ang BS, Ling ML, Fisher DA. The global spread of healthcare-associated multidrug-resistant bacteria: a perspective from Asia. Clin Infect Dis. 2013;56:1310–8.

16. CDC CRE Toolkit. Facility guidance for control of Carbapenem-resistant Enterobacteriaceae. November 2015 update. Available at: http://www.cdc.gov/hai/pdfs/cre/CRE-guidance-508.pdf. Accessed 28 Mar 2016.

17. Humphries RM, McKinnell JA. Continuing challenges for the clinical laboratory for the detection of carbapenem-resistant *Enterobacteriaceae*. J Clin Microbiol. 2015;53:3712–4.

18. Lupo A, Papp-Wallace KM, Sendi P, Bonomo RA, Endimiani A, et al. Non-phenotypic tests to detect and characterize antibiotic resistance mechanisms in Enterobacteriaceae. Diagn Microbiol Infect Dis. 2013;77:179–94.

19. Youn JH, Drake SK, Weingarten RA, Frank KM, Dekker JP, Lau AF. Clinical performance of a matrix-assisted laser desorption ionization-time of flight mass spectrometry method for detection of certain bla_{KPC}-containing plasmids. J Clin Microbiol. 2016;54:35–42.

20. Poulou A, Voulgari E, Vrioni G, et al. Imported *Klebsiella pneumoniae* carbapenemase-producing *K. pneumonia* clones in a greek hospital: impact of infection control measures for restraining their dissemination. J Clin Microbiol. 2012;50:2618–23.

21. Palmore TN, Henderson DK. Managing transmission of carbapenem-resistant Enterobacteriaceae in healthcare settings: a view from the trenches. Clin Infect Dis. 2013;57:1593–9.

22. Hayden MK, Yin MY, Lolans K, et al. Prevention of colonization and infection by *Klebsiella pneumoniae* carbapenemase-producing Enterobacteriaceae in long-term acute-care hospitals. Clin Infect Dis. 2015;60:1153–61.

23. Munoz-Price LS, Hayden MK, Lolans K, et al. Successful control of an outbreak of *Klebsiella pneumoniae* carbapenemase-producing *K. pneumoniae* at a long-term acute care hospital. Infect Control Hosp Epidemiol. 2010;31:341–7.

24. Kochar S, Sheard T, Sharma R, et al. Success of an infection control program to reduce the spread of carbapenem-resistant *Klebsiella pneumoniae*. Infect Control Hosp Epidemiol. 2009;30:447–52.

25. Schwaber MJ, Carmeli Y. An ongoing national intervention to contain the spread of carbapenem-resistant Enterobacteriaceae. Clin Infect Dis. 2014;58:697–703.

26. Climo MW, Yokoe DS, Warren DK, et al. Effect of daily chlorhexidine bathing on hospital-acquired infection. N Engl J Med. 2013;368:533–42.

27. Boonyasiri A, Thaisiam P, Permpikul C, et al. Effectiveness of chlorhexidine wipes for the prevention of multidrug-resistant bacterial colonization and hospital-acquired infections in intensive care unit patients: a randomized trial in Thailand. Infect Control Hosp Epidemiol. 2016;37:245–53.

28. Huang SS, Septimus E, Kleinman K, Moody J, Hickok J, Avery TR, et al. Targeted versus universal decolonization to prevent ICU infection. N Engl J Med. 2013;368:2255–65.

29. Tascini C, Sbrana F, Flammini S, et al. Oral gentamicin gut decontamination for prevention of KPC-producing *Klebsiella pneumonia* infections: relevance of concomitant systemic antibiotic therapy. Antimicrob Agents Chemother. 2014;58:1972–6.

30. Lubbert C, Faucheux S, Becker-Rux D, et al. Rapid emergence of secondary resistance to gentamicin and colistin following selective digestive decontamination in patients with KPC-2-producing

Klebsiella pneumoniae: a single-centre experience. Int J Antimicrob Agents. 2013;42:565–70.

31. Sievert DM, Ricks P, Edwards JR, et al. Antimicrobial-resistant pathogens associated with healthcare-associated infections: summary of data reported to the National Healthcare Safety Network at the Centers for Disease Control and Prevention, 2009–2010. Infect Control Hosp Epidemiol. 2013;34:1–14.

32. Moran GJ, Krishnadasan A, Gorwitz RJ, et al. Methicillin-resistant S. aureus infections among patients in the emergency department. N Engl J Med. 2006;355:666–7.

33. U.S. Department of Health and Human Services Centers for Disease Control and Prevention. Antibiotic resistance threats in the United States, 2013. http://www.cdc.gov/drugresistance/pdf/ar-threats-2013-508.pdf. April 23, 2013. Accessed 16 Dec 2015.

34. Thompson DS, Workman R, Strutt M. Contribution of acquired methicillin-resistant *Staphylococcus aureus* bacteraemia to overall mortality in a general intensive care unit. J Hosp Infect. 2008;70:223–7.

35. von Eiff C, Becker K, Machka K, Stammer H, Peters G. Nasal carriage as a source of *Staphylococcus aureus* bacteremia. N Engl J Med. 2001;344:11–6.

36. Wertheim HFL, Melles DC, Vos MC, Leeuwen WV, Belkum AV, Verbrugh HA, et al. The role of nasal carriage in *Staphylococcus aureus* infections. Lancet Infect Dis. 2005;5:751–62.

37. Gupta K, Martinello RA, Young M, Strymish J, Cho K, Lawler E. MRSA nasal carriage patterns and the subsequent risk of conversion between patterns, infection, and death. PlosOne. 2013;8(1):1–8.

38. Davis KA, Stewart JJ, Crouch HK, Florez CE, Hospenthal DR. Methicillin-resistant *Staphylococcus aureus* (MRSA) nares colonization at hospital admission and its effect on subsequent MRSA infection. Clin Infect Dis. 2004;39:776–82.

39. Gidengil C, Gay C, Huang SS, et al. Cost-effectiveness of strategies to prevent MRSA transmission and infection in an intensive care unit. Infect Control Hosp Epidemiol. 2015;36(1):17–27.

40. French GL. Methods for screening for methicillin-resistant Staphylococcus aureus carriage. Clin Microbiol Infect. 2009;15(7):10–6.

41. Cepheid Xpert MRSA. Available at: http://www.cepheid.com/us/cepheid-solutions/clinical-ivd-tests/healthcare-associated-infections/xpert-mrsa. Accessed 27 Mar 2016.

42. Kluytmans J, van Belkum A, Verbrugh H. Nasal carriage of *Staphylococcus aureus*: epidemiology, underlying mechanisms, and associated risks. Clin Microbiol Rev. 1997;10:505–20.

43. Lautenbach E, Nachamkin I, Hu B, et al. Surveillance cultures for detection of methicillin-resistant Staphylococcus aureus: diagnostic yield of anatomic sites and comparison of provider and patient collected samples. Infect Control Hosp Epidemiol. 2009;30(4):380–2.

44. CDC MRSA Toolkit. Available at: http://www.cdc.gov/hai/pdfs/toolkits/MRSA_toolkit_white_020910_v2.pdf. Accessed 28 Mar 2016.

45. Calfee DP, Salgado CD, Milstone AM, et al. Strategies to prevent methicillin-resistant *Staphylococcus aureus* transmission and infection in acute care hospitals: 2014 update. Infect Control Hosp Epidemiol. 2014;35:772–96.

46. Muto CA, Jernigan JA, Ostrowski BE. SHEA guideline for preventing nosocomial transmission of multidrug-resistant strains of *Staphylococcus aureus* and *Enterococcus*. Infect Control Hosp Epidemiol. 2003;24:362–86.

47. Morgan DJ, Murthy R, Munoz-Price LS, et al. Reconsidering contact precautions for endemic methicillin-resistant *Staphylococcus aureus* and vancomycin-resistant *Enterococcus*. Infect Control Hosp Epidemiol. 2015;36:1163–72.

48. Banach DB, Bearman GM, Morgan DJ, Munoz-Price LS. Infection control precautions for visitors to healthcare facilities. Expert Rev Anti-Infect Ther. 2015;13:1047–50.

49. Harris AD, Pineles L, Belton B, et al. Universal glove and gown use and acquisition of antibiotic-resistant bacteria in the ICU: a randomized trial. JAMA. 2013;310:1571–80.

50. Mclemore A, Bearman G, Edmond M. Effect of contact precautions on wait time from emergency room disposition to inpatient admission. Infect Control Hosp Epidemiol. 2011;32:298–9.

51. Stelfox H, Bates DW, Redelmeier DA. Safety of patients isolated for infection control. JAMA. 2003;290:1899–905.

52. Harbarth S, Liassine N, Dharan S, Herrault P, Auckenthaler R, Pittet D. Risk factors for persistent carriage of methicillin-resistant Staphylococcus aureus. Clin Infect Dis. 2000;31(6):1380–5.

53. Gilpin DF, Small S, Bakkshi S, Kearney MP, Cardwell C, Tunney MM. Efficacy of a standard methicillin-resistant *Staphylococcus aureus* decolonisation protocol in routine clinical practice. J Hosp Infect. 2010;75(2):93–8.

54. Kampf G. The value of using chlorhexidine soap in a controlled trial to eradicate MRSA in colonized patients. J Hosp Infect. 2004;58(1):86–7.

55. Lee YJ, Chen JZ, Lin HC, et al. Impact of active screening for methicillin-resistant Staphylococcus aureus (MRSA) and decolonization on MrSA infections, mortality and medical cost: a quasi-experimental study in surgical intensive care unit. Crit Care. 2015;143(19):1–10.

56. Horner C, Mawer D, Wilcox M. Reduced susceptibility to chlorhexidine in staphylococci: is it increasing and does it matter? J Antimicrob Chemother. 2012;67:2547–59.

57. Wang JT, Sheng WH, Wang JL, et al. Longitudinal analysis of chlorhexidine susceptibilities of nosocomial methicillin-resistant *Staphylococcus aureus* isolates at a teaching hospital in Taiwan. J Antimicrob Chemother. 2008;62:514–7.

58. McNeil JC, Kok EY, Vallejo JG, et al. Clinical and molecular features of decreased chlorhexidine susceptibility among nosocomial *Staphylococcus aureus* isolates at Texas Children's Hospital. Antimicrob Agents Chemother. 2016;60:1121–8.

59. Suwantarat N, Carroll KC, Tekle T, et al. High prevalence of reduced chlorhexidine susceptibility in organisms causing central line-associated bloodstream infections. Infect Control Hosp Epidemiol. 2014;35:1183–6.

60. Jones JC, Rogers TJ, Brookmeyer P, et al. Mupirocin resistance in patients colonized with methicillin-resistant *Staphylococcus aureus* in a surgical intensive care unit. Clin Infect Dis. 2007;45:541–7.

61. Simor AE, Stuart TL, Louie L, et al. Mupirocin-resistant, methicillin-resistant *Staphylococcus aureus* strains in Canadian hospitals. Antimicrob Agents Chemother. 2007;51:3880–6.

62. Miller MA, Dascal A, Portnoy J, Mendelson J. Development of mupirocin resistance among methicillin-resistant *Staphylococcus aureus* after widespread use of nasal mupirocin ointment. Infect Control Hosp Epidemiol. 1996;17:811–3.

63. Lee AS, Macedo-Vinas M, Francois P, et al. Impact of combined low-level mupirocin and genotypic chlorhexidine resistance on persistent methicillin-resistant *Staphylococcus aureus* carriage after decolonization therapy: a case-control study. Clin Infect Dis. 2011;52:1422–30.

64. Arias CA, Murray BE. The rise of enterococcus: beyond vancomycin resistance. Nature. 2012;10:266–78.

65. Arias CA, Contreras GA, Murray BE. Management of multidrug-resistant enterococcal infections. Clin Microbiol Infect. 2010;16:555–62.

66. Huang SS, Rifas-Shiman SL, Pottinger JM, et al. Improving assessment of vancomycin-resistant enterococci by routine screening. J Infect dis. 2007;195:339–46.

67. Shadel BN, Puzniak LA, Gillespeie KN, Lawrence SJ, Kolllef M, Mundy LM. Surveillance for vancomycin-resistant enterococci: type, rates, costs and implications. Infect Control Hosp Epidemiol. 2006;27:1068–75.

68. Muto CA, Giannetta ET, Durbin LJ, Simonton BM, Farr BM. Cost-effectiveness of perirectal surveillance cultures for controlling vancomycin-resistant enterococci. Infect Control Hosp Epidemiol. 2002;23:429–35.

69. Montecalvo MA, Jarvis WR, Uman J, et al. Costs and savings associated with infection control measures that reduced transmission of vancomycin-resistant enterococci in an endemic setting. Infect Control Hosp Epidemiol. 2001;22:437–42.

70. Hachem R, Graviss L, Hanna H, et al. Impact of surveillance for vancomycin-resistant enterococci on controlling a bloodstream outbreak among patients with hematologic malignancy. Infect Control Hosp Epidemiol. 2004;25:391–4.

71. Edmond MB, Masroor N, Stevens MP, Ober J, Bearman G. The impact of discontinuing contact precautions for VRE and MRSA on device-associated infections. The impact of discontinuing contact precautions for VRE and MRSA on device-associated infections. Infect Control Hosp Epidemiol. 2015;36:978–80.

72. Bearman GM, Marra AR, Sessler CN, et al. A controlled trial of universal gloving versus contact precautions for preventing the transmission of multidrug-resistant organisms. Am J Infect Control. 2007;35:650–5.

73. Bearman G, Rosato AE, Duane TM, et al. Trial of universal gloving with emollient-impregnated gloves to promote skin health and prevent the transmission of multidrug-resistant organisms in a surgical intensive care unit. Infect Control Hosp Epidemiol. 2010;31:491–7.

74. De Angelis G, Cataldo MA, De Waure C, et al. Infection control and prevention measures to reduce the spread of vancomycin- resistant enterococci in hospitalized patients: a systematic review and meta-analysis. J Antimicrob Chemother. 2014;69:1185–92.

75. Fisher D, Pang L, Salmon S, et al. A successful vancomycin-resistant enterococci reduction bundle at a Singapore hospital. Infect Control Hosp Epidemiol. 2016;37:107–9.

76. Weinstock DM, Conlon M, Iovino C, et al. Colonization, bloodstream infection, and mortality caused by vancomycin-resistant enterococcus early after allogeneic hematopoietic stem cell transplant. Biol Blood Marrow Transplant. 2007;13:615–21.

77. Zirakzadeh A, Gastineau DA, Mandrekar JM, Burke JP, Johnston PB, Patel R. Vancomycin-resistant enterococcal colonization appears associated with increased mortality among allogeneic hematopoietic stem cell transplant recipients. Bone Marrow Transplant. 2008;41:385–92.

78. Sigel JD, Rhinehart E, Jackson M, Chiarello L, the Healthcare Infection Control Practices Advisory Committee. Management of multidrug-resistant organisms in healthcare settings. Am J Infect Control. 2007;35:S165–93.

79. Vernon MO, Hayden MK, Trick WE, et al. Chlorhexidine gluconate to cleanse patients in a medical intensive care unit: the effectiveness of source control to reduce the bioburden of vancomycin-resistant enterococci. Arch Intern Med. 2006;166:306–12.

80. Climo MW, Sepkowitz KA, Zuccotti G, et al. The effect of daily bathing with chlorhexidine on the acquisition of methicillin-resistant Staphylococcus aureus, vancomycin-resistant enterococcus, and healthcare-associated bloodstream infections: results of a quasi-experimental multicenter trial. Crit Care Med. 2009;37:1858–65.

81. Chen W, Li S, Li L, Wu X, Zhang W. Effects of daily bathing with chlorhexidine and acquired infection of methicillin-resistant *Staphylococcus aureus* and vancomycin-resistant *Enterococcus*: a meta-analysis. J Thorac Dis. 2013;5:518–24.

82. CDC *Clostridium difficile* infections toolkit. Available at: http://www.cdc.gov/hai/pdfs/toolkits/CDItoolkitwhite_clearance_edits.pdf. Accessed 27 Mar 2016.

83. Surawicz CM, Brandt LJ, Binion DG, et al. Guidelines for diagnosis, treatment, and prevention of *Clostridium difficile* infections. Am J Gastroenterol. 2013;108:478–98.

Index

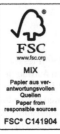

Druck:
Customized Business Services GmbH
im Auftrag der
KNV Zeitfracht GmbH
Ein Unternehmen der Zeitfracht - Gruppe
Ferdinand-Jühlke-Str. 7
99095 Erfurt